THE JOHNS HOPKINS MANUAL
OF GYNECOLOGY AND OBSTETRICS

SECOND EDITION

THE JOHNS HOPKINS MANUAL OF GYNECOLOGY AND OBSTETRICS

SECOND EDITION

Department of Gynecology and Obstetrics
Johns Hopkins University School of Medicine
Baltimore, Maryland

Brandon J. Bankowski, M.D.
Amy E. Hearne, M.D.
Nicholas C. Lambrou, M.D.
Harold E. Fox, M.D., M.Sc.
Edward E. Wallach, M.D.
Editors

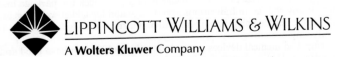

LIPPINCOTT WILLIAMS & WILKINS
A **Wolters Kluwer** Company
Philadelphia · Baltimore · New York · London
Buenos Aires · Hong Kong · Sydney · Tokyo

Acquisitions Editor: Lisa McAllister
Developmental Editor: Brigitte Wilke
Supervising Editor: Mary Ann McLaughlin
Production Editor: Sophia Elaine Battaglia, Silverchair Science + Communications
Marketing Manager: Kate Rubin
Compositor: Silverchair Science + Communications
Printer: Vicks Litho
Cover Illustrator: Patricia Gast

© 2002 by **LIPPINCOTT WILLIAMS & WILKINS**
530 Walnut Street
Philadelphia, PA 19106 USA
LWW.com

Printed in the USA

Library of Congress Cataloging-in-Publication Data

The Johns Hopkins manual of gynecology and obstetrics / edited by Brandon J. Bankowski ... [et al.].-- 2nd ed.
    p. ; cm.
    Includes bibliographical references and index.
    ISBN 0-7817-3595-5
    1. Obstetrics--Handbooks, manuals, etc. 2. Gynecology--Handbooks, manuals, etc. I. Title: Manual of gynecology and obstetrics. II. Bankowski, Brandon J. III. Johns Hopkins University. Dept. of Gynecology and Obstetrics.
    [DNLM: 1. Obstetrics--Handbooks. 2. Genital Diseases, Female--Handbooks. 3. Women's Health--Handbooks. WQ 39 J648 2002]
    RG110 .J64 2002
    618--dc21

                                                                    2001050836

10 9 8 7 6 5 4 3 2 1

DEDICATION

This book is dedicated to the family members—spouses, parents, and children—of the house officers in the Department of Gynecology and Obstetrics at the Johns Hopkins University School of Medicine. The constant support and encouragement of these family members have enabled the development and productivity of these specialists in training.

CONTENTS

SECTION THREE: GYNECOLOGY

SECTION FOUR: REPRODUCTIVE ENDOCRINOLOGY AND INFERTILITY

SECTION FIVE: GYNECOLOGIC ONCOLOGY

SECTION SIX: APPENDIXES

FOREWORD

The inspiration for *The Johns Hopkins Manual of Gynecology and Obstetrics* was the classic *Harriet Lane Handbook* first produced by the residents of the Harriet Lane Pediatric Service at the Johns Hopkins Hospital in 1950 under the leadership of its chief residents, including Dr. Henry Seidel, subsequently Professor of Pediatrics and Dean of Student Affairs. The concept of producing a clinical handbook for busy gynecology and obstetric clinicians was appealing to the gynecology and obstetrics house staff for the following reasons: (1) It supported developing scholarship and academics among the house staff, allowing them to do literature reviews and write chapters that were both scholarly and clinically useful; (2) it encouraged the residents to work together toward a common goal, that of understanding principles of literature review, epidemiology, statistics, and the systematic approach to the evaluation of scientific information; and (3) in an era when support for graduate medical education was increasingly constrained, it provided potential financial resources to be used for furthering resident education (attendance at educational conferences and meetings and seed money for research—all the things that residents need and want to do that take "just a little discretionary money"). Given the long history of contributions from the Department of Gynecology and Obstetrics at Johns Hopkins Hospital, including Williams' *Obstetrics*, TeLinde's *Operative Gynecology*, and similar works by Kelly, Cullen, Novak, Howard and Georgeanna Jones, Woodruff, Rock, and many others, this was a project whose time had come.

Under the supervision of Edward E. Wallach, the first edition was published in 1999. Its success and broad acceptance has led to this second edition and the assurance that *The Johns Hopkins Manual of Gynecology and Obstetrics* has established a place for itself in the pockets of obstetricians and gynecologists throughout their careers. I salute the Gynecology and Obstetrics house staff at the Johns Hopkins Hospital and the current leadership of Dr. Harold E. Fox and Dr. Edward E. Wallach for their continued support of this and other house staff activities. These house staff authors are future leaders of our specialty, who, with their work for this manual, recognize and repay the incredible privilege they have to train and serve "under the Dome."

I am confident that this and future editions of this handbook will continue to serve the Department, our specialty, and the health of women throughout the world.

Timothy R. B. Johnson, M.D.
Bates Professor of the Diseases of Women and Children and Chair,
Department of Obstetrics and Gynecology
Research Scientist, Center for Human Growth and Development
Professor, Women's Studies
University of Michigan
(Fellow 1979–1981; Faculty 1985–1993, Johns Hopkins)

PREFACE

In the century since the founding of its medical school and hospital, Johns Hopkins has devoted itself to the pursuit of excellence in patient care and to the promotion of medical education. During this century, textbooks and journals, authored and edited by leaders in virtually all areas of specialization, have originated from Johns Hopkins. In Obstetrics and Gynecology alone, many of the texts from Johns Hopkins have become classics and stood the test of time, including Williams' *Obstetrics*, now in its twentieth edition; TeLinde's *Operative Gynecology;* Novak's *Textbook of Gynecology;* and Kurman's editorship of Blaustein's *Pathology of the Female Genital Tract.* It has been a given that graduate and postgraduate education go together hand-in-hand with patient care since the doors of Johns Hopkins Hospital were opened in 1889 and its four horsemen—Welch, Osler, Halsted, and Kelly—set the pace for modern medicine. *The Johns Hopkins Manual of Gynecology and Obstetrics* represents a slight variation on this theme. It does not represent the work of a single individual or even a group of leaders in our specialty. Instead, it represents the collaboration of the entire house staff of The Department of Gynecology and Obstetrics, 34 strong, working in conjunction with Johns Hopkins faculty members to provide a contemporary guide to diagnosis and management of clinical problems in obstetrics and gynecology. The planning and construction of this text stems from the curiosity, enthusiasm, and focus of a dedicated resident staff that began with the residents who contributed to the first edition and extends to our current staff of residents. Initially undertaken in 1996, the first volume has been widely circulated not only in the United States, but it has also been distributed in 50 other countries. *The Johns Hopkins Manual of Gynecology and Obstetrics* has even been translated into Portuguese and is currently distributed in Brazil. Now this manual is in its second edition, having proved itself a mainstay for students, house officers, and practitioners. The second edition is updated, expanded, and embellished and includes new chapters on primary care, critical care, obstetric anesthesia, postpartum care, and breast feeding. In addition, the new edition includes sections on frequently used drugs in obstetrics and gynecology, useful Web sites, and OB/GYN Spanish for residents and students. Clearly, the second edition *is* both new and improved. The revisions and expansion serve as a testimony to the dedication of house officers whose timeless activities in the clinics, operating suites, and hospital floors have been supplemented by their preparation of this text, which serves as a valued contribution to medical education and the care of patients.

This manual has a unique legacy in that it has been passed down from the house officers, circa 1998, in the Department of Gynecology and Obstetrics at the Johns Hopkins Hospital and the Johns Hopkins University School of Medicine, to those of the present day. A. Nicholas Morse was instrumental in bringing to completion the first edition of this manual. His commitment to the creation of the manual was remarkable, exceeded only by his painstaking effort to bring the project to fruition. For the outstanding work performed by Dr. Morse, and indeed the hard work of all those who contributed to the first edition, the editors and contributors to this manual are deeply indebted and grateful.

Edward E. Wallach, M.D.
Harold E. Fox, M.D., M.Sc.

Section One. WOMEN'S HEALTH CARE

1. PRIMARY AND PREVENTATIVE CARE

Suzanne Davey Shipman and Harold E. Fox

I. **Role of the obstetrician-gynecologist as primary care provider.** A large percentage of women seeking medical care in the reproductive and postmenopausal age groups look to their obstetrician-gynecologist as their primary care physician.

Past President of ACOG, Dr. Vicki Seltzer stated that "being a woman's primary physician means being able to take care of common problems and placing an emphasis on prevention, wellness, and early detection. I think that more than any other medical specialty, obstetrics and gynecology has emphasized and achieved a great deal in promoting preventive care and general women's wellness" (*Obstet Gynecol,* 91/1, 1998). This chapter provides a quick review of some key components of women's primary care. It is by no means an exhaustive reference.

II. **Role of screening.** Screening plays an important role in prevention, as most deaths among women before the age of 65 are preventable. Screening has two purposes: (1) primary prevention, which is the identification and control of risk factors for disease with the intent of preventing disease before it occurs, and (2) secondary prevention, which is the early diagnosis of disease to prevent or reduce morbidity and mortality once disease has occurred. Criteria for a good screening test include the following: The condition must have a significant effect on the quality and quantity of life, acceptable methods of treatment must be available, the condition must have an asymptomatic period during which detection and treatment significantly reduce the risk for morbidity and mortality, treatment in the asymptomatic phase must yield therapeutic results superior to those obtained by delaying treatment until symptoms develop, tests that are acceptable to patients must be available at a reasonable cost to detect a condition in the asymptomatic period, and the incidence of the condition must be sufficient to justify the cost of the screening.

III. **Leading causes of death and morbidity by age group**

A. **Ages 13–18.** Leading causes of death are motor vehicle accidents, homicide, suicide, and cancer. Leading causes of morbidity are acne; asthma; chlamydia infection; depression; dermatitis; headaches; infective, viral, and parasitic diseases; influenza; injuries; nose, throat, ear, and upper respiratory tract infections; sexual assault; sexually transmitted diseases; and urinary tract infections.

B. **Ages 19–39.** Leading causes of death include accidents and adverse effects, cancer, human immunodeficiency virus infection, and diseases of the heart. Leading causes of morbidity include asthma; back symptoms; breast disease; deformity or orthopedic impairment; depression; diabetes; gynecologic disorders; headache or migraines; hypertension; infective, viral, and parasitic diseases; influenza; injuries; nose, throat, ear, and upper respiratory tract infections; sexual assault and domestic violence; sexually transmitted diseases; skin rash and dermatitis; substance abuse; urinary tract infections; and vaginitis.

C. **Ages 40–64.** Leading causes of death are cancer, diseases of the heart, cerebrovascular diseases, and accidents and their adverse effects. Leading causes of morbidity are arthritis and osteoarthritis; asthma; back symptoms; breast disease; cardiovascular disease; carpal tunnel syndrome; deformity or orthopedic impairment; depression; diabetes; headache; hypertension; infective, viral, and parasitic disease; influenza; injuries; menopause; nose, throat, ear, and upper respiratory tract infections; obesity; skin conditions and dermatitis; substance abuse; urinary tract infections; other

TABLE 1-1. SCREENING (AGES 13–18 YEARS)

History	Physical examination	Laboratory testing
Reason for visit	Height	Periodic
Health status: medical, surgical, family	Weight	Pap testing (yearly when sexually active or by age 18 yrs)
Dietary/nutritional assessment	Blood pressure	
	Secondary sexual characteristics (Tanner staging)	High-risk groups
Physical activity		Hemoglobin level assessment
Use of complementary and alternative medicine	Pelvic examination (yearly when sexually active or by age 18 yrs)	Bacteriuria testing
Tobacco, alcohol, other drug use	Skin	Sexually transmitted disease testing
Abuse/neglect		Human immunodeficiency virus testing
Sexual practices		Genetic testing/counseling
		Rubella titer assessment
		Tuberculosis skin testing
		Lipid profile assessment
		Fasting glucose testing
		Cholesterol testing
		Hepatitis C virus testing

urinary tract conditions (including urinary incontinence); and vision impairment.

D. **Ages 65 and older.** Leading causes of death include diseases of the heart, cancer, cerebrovascular diseases, and chronic obstructive pulmonary diseases. Leading causes of morbidity include arthritis and osteoarthritis; back symptoms; breast cancer; chronic obstructive pulmonary diseases; cardiovascular disease; deformity or orthopedic impairment; degeneration of macula retinae and posterior pole; dementia; depression; diabetes; hearing and vision impairment; hypertension; hypothyroidism and other thyroid diseases; influenza; nose, throat, and upper respiratory tract infections; osteoporosis; skin lesions, dermatoses, and dermatitis; urinary tract infections; other urinary tract conditions (including urinary incontinence); and vertigo.

IV. **Recommendations for preventative examination** (from the American College of Obstetricians and Gynecologists Committee on Primary Care)
   A. Periodic assessment ages 13–18 years (Tables 1-1, 1-2)
   B. Periodic assessment ages 19–39 years (Tables 1-3, 1-4)
   C. Periodic assessment ages 40–64 years (Tables 1-5, 1-6)
   D. Periodic assessment age 65 years and older (Tables 1-7, 1-8)
   E. High-risk groups (Table 1-9)
   F. **Recommended immunizations by age group** (Table 1-10)
V. **Nutrition** (Table 1-11)
VI. **Counseling for prevention.** The office visit or routine health maintenance visit is an ideal time to counsel patients regarding many health-related behaviors. There is evidence in the literature that for some of these behaviors clinical counseling can be an effective way of changing a patient's conduct.
   A. There are many different ways to counsel patients. The following are found in the U.S. Preventive Services Task Force (USPSTF) Guide.

TABLE 1-2. EVALUATION AND COUNSELING (AGES 13–18 YEARS)

Sexuality	Fitness	Psychosocial evaluation	Cardiovascular risk factors	Health/risk behaviors
Development	Hygiene (including dental); fluoride supplementation	Interpersonal/family relationships	Family history	Injury prevention
High-risk behaviors	Dietary/nutritional assessment (including eating disorders)	Sexual identity	Hypertension	Safety belts and helmets
Prevention of unwanted/unintended pregnancy	Exercise: discussion of program	Personal goal development	Dyslipidemia	Recreational hazards
Postponement of sexual involvement	Folic acid supplementation (0.4 mg/day)	Behavioral/learning disorders	Obesity	Firearms
Contraceptive options	Calcium intake	Abuse/neglect	Diabetes mellitus	Hearing
Sexually transmitted diseases		Satisfactory school experience		Skin exposure to ultraviolet rays
Partner selection		Peer relationships		Suicide: depressive symptoms
Barrier protection				Tobacco, alcohol, other drug use

TABLE 1-3. SCREENING (AGES 19–39 YEARS)

History	Physical examination	Laboratory testing
Reason for visit	Height	Periodic
Health status: medical, surgical, family	Weight	Pap testing (at physician and patient discretion after three consecutive normal test results if low risk)
Dietary/nutritional assessment	Blood pressure	
	Neck: adenopathy, thyroid	
Physical activity	Breasts	High-risk groups
Use of complementary and alternative medicine	Abdomen	Hemoglobin level assessment
	Pelvic examination	Bacteriuria testing
Tobacco, alcohol, other drug use	Skin	Mammography
		Fasting glucose testing
Abuse/neglect		Cholesterol testing
Sexual practices		Sexually transmitted disease testing
Urinary and fecal incontinence		Human immunodeficiency virus testing
		Genetic testing/counseling
		Rubella titer assessment
		Tuberculosis skin testing
		Lipid profile assessment
		Thyroid-stimulating hormone testing
		Colonoscopy
		Hepatitis C virus testing

1. Frame the teaching to match the patient's perceptions.
2. Fully inform patients of the purposes and expected effects of interventions and when to expect these effects.
3. Suggest small changes rather than large ones.
4. Be specific.
5. Recognize that it is sometimes easier to add new behaviors than to eliminate established behaviors.
6. Link new behaviors to old behaviors.
7. Use the power of the profession.
8. Get explicit commitments from the patient.
9. Use a combination of strategies.
10. Involve office staff.
11. Refer to sources such as community agencies, national voluntary health organizations (e.g., the American Heart Association and the American Cancer Society), instructional references (e.g., books and videotapes), and, finally, other patients.
12. Monitor progress through follow-up contact.

B. Physician counseling based on the **stages of change**. After the earlier tables are reviewed, many behaviors may be noted that, if changed, could improve a patient's overall health status. The physician must assess whether a patient is ready to make these changes or not. The transtheoreti-

TABLE 1-4. EVALUATION AND COUNSELING (AGES 19–39 YEARS)

Sexuality	Fitness	Psychosocial evaluation	Cardiovascular risk factors	Health/risk behaviors
High-risk behaviors	Hygiene (including dental)	Interpersonal/family relationships	Family history	Injury prevention
Contraceptive options	Dietary/nutritional assessment	Domestic violence	Hypertension	Safety belts and helmets
Genetic counseling	Exercise: discussion of program	Work satisfaction	Dyslipidemia	Occupational hazards
Prevention of unwanted/unintended pregnancy	Folic acid supplementation (0.4 mg/day)	Lifestyle/stress	Obesity	Recreational hazards
Preconception counseling for desired pregnancy	Calcium intake	Sleep disorders	Diabetes mellitus	Firearms
Sexually transmitted diseases			Lifestyle	Hearing
Partner selection				Breast self-examination
Barrier protection				Skin exposure to ultraviolet rays
Sexual functioning				Suicide: depressive symptoms
				Tobacco, alcohol, other drug use

TABLE 1-5. SCREENING (AGES 40–64 YEARS)

History	Physical examination	Laboratory testing
Reason for visit	Height	Periodic
Health status: medical, surgical, family	Weight	Pap testing (at physician and patient discretion after three consecutive normal test results if low risk)
Dietary/nutritional assessment	Blood pressure	
	Oral cavity	
Physical activity	Neck: adenopathy, thyroid	Mammography (every 1–2 yrs until age 50 yrs, yearly beginning at age 50 yrs)
Use of complementary and alternative medicine	Breasts, axillae	
	Abdomen	Cholesterol testing (every 5 yrs beginning at age 45 yrs)
Tobacco, alcohol, other drug use	Pelvic examination	
Abuse/neglect	Rectovaginal examination (beginning at age 50 yrs)	Fecal occult blood testing (beginning at age 50 yrs)
Sexual practices		Sigmoidoscopy (every 3–5 yrs after age 50 yrs)
Urinary and fecal incontinence	Skin	
		Fasting glucose testing (every 3 yrs after age 45 yrs)
		High-risk groups
		Hemoglobin level assessment
		Bacteriuria testing
		Fasting glucose testing
		Sexually transmitted disease testing
		Tuberculosis skin testing
		Lipid profile assessment
		Thyroid-stimulating hormone testing
		Colonoscopy
		Hepatitis C virus testing

cal model of change is based on discrete stages along the continuum of change. These are listed below, with the goals of counseling for each stage.

1. **Precontemplation.** Patients in this stage have no intention of changing their behavior. The goal of counseling in this stage is to introduce ambivalence, so that patients will begin to consider making a change.
2. **Contemplation.** Patients in this stage are considering making a change in their behavior but will often be "riding the fence." For example, the patient may like to smoke but on the other hand may want to quit smoking. The goal of counseling is to explore both sides of the patient's ambivalent attitude and help the patient resolve it (hopefully toward positive change).
3. **Preparation.** Patients in this stage have resolved to make a change and are no longer ambiguous (for example, they may tell you that they are ready to quit smoking). The goal of counseling is to identify successful strategies for change.
4. **Action.** Patients in this stage are actually making a change in their behavior (such as quitting smoking). It may take years of precontempla-

TABLE 1-6. EVALUATION AND COUNSELING (AGES 40–64 YEARS)

Sexuality	Fitness	Psychosocial evaluation	Cardiovascular risk factors	Health/risk behaviors
High-risk behaviors	Hygiene (including dental)	Family relationships	Family history	Hormone replacement therapy
Contraceptive options	Dietary/nutritional assessment	Domestic violence	Hypertension	Injury prevention
Genetic counseling	Exercise: discussion of program	Work satisfaction	Dyslipidemia	Safety belts and helmets
Prevention of unwanted pregnancy	Folic acid supplementation (0.4 mg/day before age 50 yrs)	Retirement planning	Obesity	Occupational hazards
Sexually transmitted diseases	Calcium intake	Lifestyle/stress	Diabetes mellitus	Recreational hazards
Partner selection		Sleep disorders	Lifestyle	Sports involvement
Barrier protection				Firearms
Sexual functioning				Hearing
				Breast self-examination
				Skin exposure to ultraviolet rays
				Suicide: depressive symptoms
				Tobacco, alcohol, other drug use

TABLE 1-7. SCREENING (AGES 65 YEARS AND OLDER)

History	Physical examination	Laboratory testing
Reason for visit	Height	Periodic
Health status: medical, surgical, family	Weight	Pap testing (at physician and patient discretion after three consecutive normal test results if low risk)
Dietary/nutritional assessment	Blood pressure	
Physical activity	Oral cavity	
	Neck: adenopathy, thyroid	Urinalysis
Use of complementary and alternative medicine	Breasts, axillae	Mammography
Tobacco, alcohol, other drug use, and concurrent medication use	Abdomen	Cholesterol testing (every 3–5 yrs before age 75 yrs)
	Pelvic and rectovaginal examination	Fecal occult blood testing
Abuse/neglect	Skin	Sigmoidoscopy (every 3–5 yrs)
Sexual practices		Fasting glucose testing (every 3 yrs)
Urinary and fecal incontinence		High-risk groups
		Hemoglobin level assessment
		Sexually transmitted disease testing
		Human immunodeficiency virus testing
		Tuberculosis skin testing
		Lipid profile assessment
		Thyroid-stimulating hormone testing
		Colonoscopy
		Hepatitis C virus testing

tion and contemplation before the action stage is achieved. The goal of counseling in this stage is to provide solutions to dealing with specific relapse triggers.

    5. **Maintenance.** The goal of counseling in this stage is to solidify the patient's commitment to a continued change (such as maintaining a smoke-free life now that they've successfully quit smoking).

VII. **Screening for asymptomatic coronary artery disease.** There is insufficient evidence to recommend for or against screening of middle-aged and older men and women for asymptomatic coronary artery disease, using resting ECG, ambulatory ECG, or exercise ECG. Emphasizing lifestyle modifications such as diet adjustments, smoking cessation, and BP control is an important part of the routine physical examination.

VIII. **Screening for hypercholesterolemia and other lipid disorders**

    A. According to the updated recommendations for cholesterol management of the National Cholesterol Education Program, serum total cholesterol should be measured in all adults 20 years of age and older at least once every 5 years; high-density lipoprotein (HDL) cholesterol should be measured at the same time if accurate methods are available. These measurements may be made while the patient is nonfasting. In individuals free of

TABLE 1-8. EVALUATION AND COUNSELING (AGES 65 YEARS AND OLDER)

Sexuality	Fitness	Psychosocial evaluation	Cardiovascular risk factors	Health/risk behaviors
Sexual functioning	Hygiene (general and dental)	Neglect/abuse	Hypertension	Hormone replacement therapy
Sexual behaviors	Dietary/nutritional assessment	Lifestyle/stress	Dyslipidemia	Injury prevention
Sexually transmitted diseases	Exercise: discussion of program	Depression/sleep disorders	Obesity	Safety belts and helmets
Partner selection	Calcium intake	Family relationships	Diabetes mellitus	Prevention of falls
Barrier protection		Work/retirement satisfaction	Sedentary lifestyle	Occupational hazards
				Recreational hazards
				Firearms
				Visual acuity/glaucoma
				Hearing
				Breast self-examination
				Skin exposure to ultraviolet rays
				Suicide: depressive symptoms
				Tobacco, alcohol, other drug use

TABLE 1-9. HIGH-RISK GROUPS

High-risk group	Intervention
Persons with diabetes mellitus.	Bacteriuria testing
Individuals with familial lipid disorders, family history of premature coronary heart disease, history of coronary heart disease.	Cholesterol testing
Individuals with history of inflammatory bowel disease or colonic polyps, or family history of familial polyposis, colorectal cancer, or cancer family syndrome.	Colonoscopy
Persons with first-degree relative with diabetes mellitus; individuals with history of gestational diabetes mellitus; those who are obese or hypertensive; members of high-risk ethnic groups (African Americans, Hispanic Americans, Native Americans).	Fasting glucose testing every 3 yrs
Residents in areas with inadequate water fluoridation (<0.7 ppm).	Fluoride supplementation
Persons exposed to teratogens; those considering pregnancy at age 35 or older; persons with history of genetic disorder or birth defect, or partner or family member with such history; persons of African, Acadian, Eastern European Jewish, Mediterranean, or Southeast Asian ancestry.	Genetic testing/counseling
Persons of Caribbean, Latin American, Asian, Mediterranean, or African ancestry; those with history of excessive menstrual flow.	Hemoglobin level assessment
International travelers; illegal drug users; people who work with nonhuman primates; those with chronic liver disease or clotting factor disorders; sexual partners of bisexual men; those not immune to measles, mumps, and rubella; food-service workers; health care workers; day care workers.	Hepatitis A vaccination
Intravenous drug users and their sexual contacts; recipients of clotting factor concentrates; those with occupational exposure to blood or blood products; patients and workers in dialysis units; those with chronic renal or hepatic disease; those with household or sexual contact with hepatitis B virus carriers; persons with history of sexual activity with multiple partners or of sexual contact with sexually active homosexual or bisexual men; international travelers; residents or staff at institutions for the developmentally disabled or correctional institutions.	Hepatitis B vaccination
Persons with history of injecting illegal drugs; recipients of clotting factor concentrates before 1987; persons undergoing long-term hemodialysis; those with persistently abnormal alanine aminotransferase levels; recipients of blood from a donor who later tested positive for HCV infection; recipients of blood or blood-component transfusion or organ transplantation before July 1992; persons with occupational percutaneous or mucosal exposure to HCV-positive blood.	Hepatitis C virus (HCV) testing
Persons seeking treatment for sexually transmitted disease; intravenous drug users; persons with history of prostitution; those with past or present sexual contact with partner who is HIV positive or bisexual or injects drugs; persons born in or long-term residents of an area with high prevalence of HIV infection; recipients of blood transfusion from 1978–1985; individuals with invasive cervical cancer; pregnant women. Women seeking preconception care should be offered testing.	Human immunodeficiency virus (HIV) testing

(continued)

TABLE 1-9. (*continued*)

High-risk group	Intervention
Residents in long-term care facility; persons with chronic cardiopulmonary disorders; those with metabolic diseases (e.g., diabetes mellitus, hemoglobinopathies, immunosuppression, renal dysfunction); health care workers; day care workers; pregnant women who will be in the second or third trimester during the epidemic season. Pregnant women with medical problems should be offered vaccination before the influenza season regardless of stage of pregnancy. Anyone who wishes to reduce the chance of becoming ill with influenza should be offered vaccination.	Influenza vaccination
Individuals with elevated cholesterol level; those with parent or sibling with history of blood cholesterol ≥240 mg/dL; those with sibling, parent, or grandparent with documented premature (<55 yrs) coronary artery disease; those with diabetes mellitus; smokers.	Lipid profile assessment
Those with history of breast cancer; those with first-degree relative (i.e., mother, sister, or daughter) with history of breast cancer or multiple other relatives with history of premenopausal breast or breast and ovarian cancer.	Mammography
Adults born in 1957 or later should be offered vaccination (one dose of MMR) if there is no proof of immunity or documentation of a dose given after first birthday; persons vaccinated in 1963–1967 should be offered revaccination (two doses); health care workers, students entering college, international travelers, and rubella-negative postpartum patients should be offered a second dose.	Measles-mumps-rubella (MMR) vaccination
Persons with chronic illness such as cardiovascular disease, pulmonary disease, diabetes mellitus, alcoholism, chronic liver disease, cerebrospinal fluid leaks, functional or anatomic asplenia; those exposed to an environment in which pneumococcal outbreaks have occurred; immunocompromised patients (e.g., those with HIV infection or hematologic or solid malignancy; those undergoing chemotherapy or steroid therapy); pregnant patients with chronic illness. Revaccination after 5 yrs may be appropriate for certain high-risk groups.	Pneumococcal vaccination
Those of childbearing age with no evidence of immunity.	Rubella titer assessment
Individuals with history of multiple sexual partners or sexual partner with multiple contacts; contacts of person with culture-proven STD; individuals with history of repeated episodes of STD; attendees at clinics for STDs. All sexually active adolescents and other asymptomatic women at high risk for infection should undergo routine screening for chlamydial and gonorrheal infection.	Sexually transmitted disease (STD) testing
Individuals with increased recreational or occupational exposure to sunlight; those with family or personal history of skin cancer; persons with clinical evidence of precursor lesions.	Skin examination
Individuals with strong family history of thyroid disease; those with autoimmune disease (evidence of subclinical hypothyroidism may be related to unfavorable lipid profiles).	Thyroid-stimulating hormone testing

(*continued*)

TABLE 1-9. (*continued*)

High-risk group	Intervention
Individuals with HIV infection; those in close contact with persons known or suspected to have tuberculosis; those with medical risk factors known to increase risk of disease if infected; individuals born in country with high tuberculosis prevalence; medically underserved persons; low-income individuals; alcoholics; intravenous drug users; residents in long-term care facilities (e.g., correctional institution, mental institution, nursing home or facility); health professionals in high-risk health care facilities.	Tuberculosis skin testing
All susceptible adults and adolescents, including health care workers; household contacts of immunocompromised individuals; teachers; day care workers; residents and staff of institutional settings, colleges, prisons, or military installations; international travelers; nonpregnant women of child-bearing age.	Varicella vaccination

Adapted from OB-Gyns revise screening recommendations; expanded testing for diabetes, HIV and Hepatitis C advised [news release]. Washington: American College of Obstetricians and Gynecologists, November 30, 1999, with permission.

TABLE 1-10. RECOMMENDED IMMUNIZATIONS

Ages 13–18 yrs	Ages 19–39 yrs	Ages 40–64 yrs	Ages 65 and older
Periodic	Periodic	Periodic	Periodic
Tetanus-diphtheria booster (once between ages 11 yrs and 16 yrs)	Tetanus-diphtheria booster (once every 10 yrs)	Tetanus-diphtheria booster (every 10 yrs)	Tetanus-diphtheria booster (every 10 yrs)
Hepatitis B vaccine (one series for those not previously immunized)	High-risk groups	High-risk groups	Influenza vaccine (annually)
High-risk groups	Measles-mumps-rubella vaccine	Measles-mumps-rubella vaccine	Pneumococcal vaccine (once)
Influenza vaccine	Hepatitis A vaccine	Hepatitis A vaccine	High-risk groups
Hepatitis A vaccine	Hepatitis B vaccine	Hepatitis B vaccine	Hepatitis A vaccine
Pneumococcal vaccine	Influenza vaccine	Influenza vaccine	Hepatitis B vaccine
Measles-mumps-rubella vaccine	Pneumococcal vaccine	Pneumococcal vaccine	Varicella vaccine
Varicella vaccine	Varicella vaccine	Varicella vaccine	

TABLE 1-11. SELECTED 1989 RECOMMENDED DIETARY ALLOWANCES FOR WOMEN

Nutrient	Nonpregnant 15–18 yrs	Nonpregnant 25–50 yrs	Pregnant	Lactating	Dietary sources
Folic acid (µg)	400	400	400	240	Leafy vegetables, liver
Calcium (mg)	1200	800	1200	1200	Dairy products
Protein (g)	44	50	60	65	Meats, fish, poultry, dairy
Energy (kcal)	2200	2200	2500	2800	Proteins, fats, carbo-hydrates

Adapted from National Research Council. *Recommended dietary allowances*, 10th ed. Washington: National Academy Press, 1989, with permission.

coronary heart disease (CHD), total cholesterol levels below 200 mg/dL are classified as *desirable blood cholesterol*, levels of 200–239 mg/dL as *borderline-high blood cholesterol*, and levels of 240 mg/dL and above as *high blood cholesterol*. The cutpoint that defines high blood cholesterol (240 mg/dL) is a value above which risk for CHD rises more steeply and corresponds approximately to the eightieth percentile of the adult U.S. population (National Health and Nutrition Examination Survey III). An HDL cholesterol level below 35 mg/dL is defined as *low*, and a low HDL cholesterol level constitutes a CHD risk factor. Table 1-12 summarizes these categories.

B. **The National Cholesterol Education Program guidelines** emphasize treating dyslipidemias based on cardiovascular risk factors. One of the first steps in the evaluation of hypercholesterolemia is exclusion of secondary causes of hyperlipidemia.

C. **Assessment of the patient's risk for coronary heart disease** helps determine which treatment should be initiated and how often lipid analysis should be performed. For primary prevention of coronary heart disease, the

TABLE 1-12. RISK CLASSIFICATION OF HYPERCHOLESTEROLEMIA IN PATIENTS WITHOUT CORONARY HEART DISEASE

Classification	Total cholesterol level	LDL cholesterol level	HDL cholesterol level
Desirable	200 mg/dL (5.15 mmol/L)	<130 mg/dL (<3.35 mmol/L)	≥60 mg/dL (≥1.55 mmol/L)
Borderline high risk	200–239 mg/dL (5.15–6.20 mmol/L)	130–159 mg/dL (3.35–4.10 mmol/L)	35–59 mg/dL (0.90–1.55 mmol/L)
High risk	≥240 mg/dL (≥6.20 mmol/L)	≥160 mg/dL (≥4.15 mmol/L)	<35 mg/dL (<0.90 mmol/L)

HDL, high-density lipoprotein; LDL, low-density lipoprotein.
Adapted from National Cholesterol Education Program. Second report of the Expert Panel on Detection, Evaluation, and Treatment of High Blood Cholesterol in Adults (adult treatment panel II). Bethesda, MD: National Cholesterol Education Program, National Institutes of Health, National Heart, Lung, and Blood Institute, 1993:5. DHSS Publication No. (NIH) 93-3095, with permission.

treatment goal is to achieve a low-density lipoprotein (LDL) cholesterol level of less than 160 mg/dL in patients with only one risk factor. The target LDL level in patients with two or more risk factors is 130 mg/dL or less. For patients with documented coronary heart disease, the LDL cholesterol level should be reduced to less than 100 mg/dL. Negative risk factors include the following: age 45 years or older in men, age 55 years or older in women or postmenopausal status without hormone replacement therapy, family history of premature coronary heart disease (definite myocardial infarction or sudden death before age 55 in father or other male first-degree relative or before age 65 in mother or other first-degree female relative), current cigarette smoking, hypertension, HDL cholesterol level below 35 mg/dL, diabetes mellitus. Positive risk factors include HDL cholesterol level above 60 mg/dL.

D. **Treatment.** According to the National Cholesterol Education Program guidelines, dietary modifications, exercise, and weight control are the foundation of the treatment of dyslipidemia. A step II diet, in which the total fat content is less than 30% of total calories and saturated fat is 8–10% of total calories, may help reduce LDL cholesterol levels to the target range in some patients. A high-fiber diet is also therapeutic. The most commonly used options for pharmacologic treatment of dyslipidemia include bile acid–binding resins, HMG-CoA reductase inhibitors, nicotinic acid, and fibric acid derivatives (Table 1-13). In most patients with hypercholesterolemia, β-hydroxy-β-methylglutaryl–coenzyme A reductase inhibitors are the drugs of choice because they reduce LDL cholesterol most effectively. Gemfibrozil or nicotinic acid may be better choices in patients with significant hypertriglyceridemia (Table 1-14). Other possibilities in selected cases are estrogen replacement therapy, plasmapheresis, and even surgery in severe, refractory cases.

IX. **Screening for hypertension**

A. **Hypertension is defined as** a systolic BP of 140 mm Hg or greater, diastolic BP of 90 mm Hg or greater, or requirement for antihypertensive medication. The objective of identifying and treating high BP is to reduce the risk of cardiovascular disease and associated morbidity and mortality. Hypertension is present in an estimated 43 million Americans and is more common in African Americans and older adults. Hypertension is a leading risk factor for coronary heart disease, congestive heart failure, stroke, ruptured aortic aneurysm, renal disease, and retinopathy. These complications of hypertension are among the most common and serious diseases in the United States, and successful efforts to lower BP could thus have substantial impact on population morbidity and mortality. See Table 1-15.

B. **Periodic screening for hypertension** is recommended for all persons 21 years of age or older. The optimal interval for BP screening has not been determined and is left to clinical discretion. Current expert opinion is that adults who are believed to be normotensive should receive BP measurements at least once every 2 years if their last diastolic and systolic BP readings were below 85 and 140 mm Hg, respectively, and annually if the last diastolic BP reading was 85–89 mm Hg. Hypertension should not be diagnosed on the basis of a single measurement. Elevated readings should be confirmed on more than one reading at each of three separate visits. In adults, current BP criteria for the diagnosis of hypertension are an average diastolic pressure of 90 mm Hg or greater or an average systolic pressure of 140 mm Hg or greater, or both. Once hypertension is confirmed, patients should receive appropriate counseling regarding physical activity, weight reduction, dietary sodium intake, and alcohol consumption. Evidence should also be sought for other cardiovascular risk factors, such as elevated serum cholesterol level and smoking, and appropriate intervention should be offered when indicated. The decision to begin drug therapy may include consideration of the level of BP elevation, age, and the presence of other cardiovascular disease risk factors (e.g., tobacco use, hypercholesterolemia), concomitant disease (e.g., diabetes, obesity, peripheral vascular disease), or target-organ damage (e.g., left ven-

TABLE 1-13. CHOLESTEROL-LOWERING AGENTS

Agent	Pregnancy category	Dosage
Bile acid–binding resins		
Cholestyramine (Questran, Questran Lite)	C	Start 4 g qd or bid, max 25 g/dose (divided bid)
Colestipol hydrochloride (Colestid)	?	Start 2 g qd, increase 2 g q1–2 mos
HMG-CoA reductase inhibitors (statins)		
Atorvastatin calcium (Lipitor)	X	Start 10 mg qd, max 80 mg/day
Cerivastatin sodium (Baycol)	X	Start 0.4 mg qpm; 0.2–0.3 mg PO qpm if CrCl <60
Fluvastatin sodium (Lescol)	X	Start 20–40 mg qpm, max 80 mg/day
Lovastatin (Mevacor)	X	Start 20 mg qpm, max 80 mg with evening meal; max 20 mg/day if on niacin, fibrates, or cyclosporine
Pravastatin sodium (Pravachol)	X	10 mg, 20 mg or 40 mg at bedtime, 10 mg/day if liver or renal disease
Simvastatin (Zocor)	X	Start 20 mg qd, max 80 mg/day or 10 mg/day if on niacin, fibrates, or cyclosporine, take with food
Fibric acid analogs		
Clofibrate (Atromid-S)	C	500 mg four times daily
Gemfibrozil (Lopid)	C	600 mg twice daily
Other		
Fenofibrate (Tricor)	C	Start 67 mg qd, double q4–8wks based on response, max 200 mg/day, take with meals
Nicotinic acid	C	Start 50–100 mg bid/tid, increase slowly to max 9 g/day
Niacin (Slo-Niacin)	C	Start 250 mg qd, increase dose q4–7d, max 8 g/day

bid, twice a day; CrCl, creatinine clearance; tid, three times a day; HMG-CoA, β-hydroxy β-methylglutaryl–coenzyme A.

FDA Risk Category C = Either animal studies revealed adverse effects and there are no controlled studies on women, or studies in women and animals are not available.

Category X = Studies in animals or humans have demonstrated fetal abnormalities and the risk of drugs in pregnant women outweighs the benefit.

? = Unknown category.

Note: Lowest maintenance dosages are not necessarily equivalent when switching from one brand to another. Please see Appendix A for discussion of pregnancy categories.

tricular hypertrophy, elevated creatinine level). Antihypertensive drugs should be prescribed in accordance with recent guidelines and with attention to current techniques for improving compliance.

Please refer to a medical text for complete instructions for evaluating and managing hypertension.

X. **Screening for diabetes.** Diabetes mellitus is a heterogeneous group of conditions characterized by hyperglycemia. Diabetes causes complications

TABLE 1-14. SIDE EFFECTS AND CHANGES IN SERUM LIPID VALUES WITH CHOLESTEROL-LOWERING DRUGS

Drug class	Total cholesterol (%)	LDL (%)	HDL (%)	Triglycer-ides	Side effects
HMG-CoA reductase inhibitors	↓ 15–30	↓ 20–60	↑ 5–15	↓ 10–40%	Myositis, myalgia, ↑ transaminase levels
Bile acid–binding resins	↓ 20	↓ 10–20	↑ 3–5	↑ or neutral	Unpalatability, bloating, constipation, heartburn
Nicotinic acid	↓ 25	↓ 10–25	↑ 15–35	↓ 20–50%	Flushing, nausea, glucose intolerance, abnormal liver function test results
Fibric acid analogs	↓ 15	↓ 5–15	↑ 14–20	↓ 20–50%	Nausea, skin rash

↑, increased; ↓, decreased; HDL, high-density lipoprotein; HMG-CoA, β-hydroxy-β-methylglutaryl–coenzyme A; LDL, low-density lipoprotein.

involving the eyes, kidneys, and nerves and is associated with an increased incidence of cardiovascular disease. Diabetes may result from defects in insulin secretion, insulin action, or both.

A. **Diagnostic criteria**

1. Symptoms of diabetes plus casual plasma glucose concentration of 200 mg/dL or more. *Casual* is defined as measured at any time of day with-

TABLE 1-15. CLASSIFICATION OF BLOOD PRESSURE FOR ADULTS AND RECOMMENDATIONS FOR FOLLOW-UP

Category	Systolic (mm Hg)		Diastolic (mm Hg)	Follow-Up Recommended
Optimal	<120	and	<80	Recheck in 2 yrs
Normal	<130	and	<85	Recheck in 2 yrs
High normal	130–139	or	85–89	Recheck in 1 yr
Hypertension				
Stage 1	140–159	or	90–99	Confirm within 2 mos
Stage 2	160–179	or	100–109	Evaluate or refer to source of care within 1 mo
Stage 3	≥180	or	≥110	Evaluate or refer to source of care immediately or within 1 wk depending on clinical situation

Adapted from The Sixth Report of the Joint National Committee on Prevention, Detection, Evaluation, and Treatment of High Blood Pressure. Bethesda, MD: National Institutes of Health, National Heart, Lung, and Blood Institute, National High Blood Pressure Education Program, 1997:11–13. NIH Publication No. 98-4080, with permission.

out regard to time since last meal. The classic symptoms of diabetes include polyuria, polydipsia, and unexplained weight loss; or

2. Fasting plasma glucose level of 126 mg/dL or more. *Fasting* is defined as no caloric intake for at least 8 hours; or

3. Two-hour plasma glucose level of 200 mg/dL or more during an oral glucose tolerance test. The test should be performed as described by the World Health Organization, using a glucose load containing the equivalent of 75 g anhydrous glucose dissolved in water.

4. The term **impaired fasting glucose** has been defined as fasting plasma glucose level of 110 or more and 125 mg/dL or less. Impaired glucose tolerance is defined as a 2-hour plasma glucose value of 140 or more but less than 200 mg/dL during an oral glucose tolerance test.

B. **Criteria for testing for diabetes in asymptomatic, undiagnosed individuals**

1. Testing for diabetes should be considered in all individuals at age 45 years and older; if results are normal, testing should be repeated at 3-year intervals.

2. Testing should be considered at a younger age or should be carried out more frequently in individuals who

   a. are obese (more than 120% of desirable body weight or a body mass index of 27 kg/m^2 or more)

   b. have a first-degree relative with diabetes

   c. are members of a high-risk ethnic population (e.g., African American, Hispanic American, Native American, Asian American, Pacific Islander)

   d. have delivered a baby weighing more than 9 lb or have been diagnosed with gestational diabetes mellitus

   e. are hypertensive (BP of 140/90 or higher)

   f. have an HDL cholesterol level of 35 mg/dL or lower or a triglyceride level of 250 mg/dL or higher or both

   g. on previous testing had impaired glucose tolerance or impaired fasting glucose

3. Please refer to a medical text for guidelines for therapy.

XI. **Screening for breast cancer.** Breast cancer is the most common malignancy among women in the United States; the risk of developing breast cancer increases from 1:25 at age 40 to 1:8 at age 80. In addition to age, other factors that determine a woman's risk for breast cancer include age at menarche, age at first full-term birth, presence of *BRCA1* or *BRCA2* gene, family history of breast cancer, and presence of high-risk benign breast pathology. For those at low risk, the American College of Obstetricians and Gynecologists recommends routine mammography every 1–2 years for women in their 40s and annually thereafter. This is in addition to annual clinical breast examination. The USPSTF recommends routine screening every 1–2 years, with mammography alone or mammography plus annual clinical breast examination for women aged 50–69 years. Mammography interval is still controversial (Table 1-16). For asymptomatic women between the ages of 50 and 69 years, the data support a 30% reduction in breast cancer mortality associated with annual or biennial mammography and clinical breast examination. Controversial data demonstrate a 20% reduction in breast cancer mortality associated with annual mammography among women between the ages of 40 and 49 years. The problem of comorbidity in women older than age 70 complicates data supporting screening recommendations for this cohort of women. Although strong evidence supporting mortality reduction from breast self-examination is lacking, breast self-examination is recommended as a screening modality for breast cancer beginning at age 25.

XII. **Screening for colorectal cancer.** Colorectal cancer is the third most commonly diagnosed cancer and the second leading cause of cancer-related death in the United States. Risk factors for colorectal cancer include a family

TABLE 1-16. BREAST CANCER SCREENING GUIDELINES FOR ASYMPTOMATIC WOMEN 40 YEARS OR OLDER

Screening modality	ACS and ACR	NCI	NCCN	ACP[a]	USPSTF	ACOG
Two-view mammography	Annual	Biennial	Annual	Biennial	Annual or biennial	Annual[b]
Start at age	40 yrs	40 yrs	40 yrs	50 yrs	50 yrs	40 yrs
Upper age	None	69 yrs	None	74 yrs	69 yrs	None
Clinical breast examination	Annual	Encourage	Annual	Encourage	Annual	Annual
Breast self-examination	Monthly	Encourage	Encourage	Encourage	None	Encourage

ACOG, American College of Obstetricians and Gynecologists; ACP, American College of Physicians; ACR, American College of Radiology; ACS, American Cancer Society; NCCN, National Comprehensive Cancer Network; NCI, National Cancer Institute; USPSTF, U.S. Preventive Services Task Force.
[a]*Other recommendations:* American College of Preventive Medicine: same as ACP except no upper age limit to screening.
[b]Mammography every 1–2 years for ages 40–49, yearly beginning at age 50.
Adapted from Overmoyer B. Breast cancer screening. *Med Clin North Am* 1999;83(6):1443–1466, vi–vii, with permission.

history of colorectal cancer, a personal history of colon polyps or cancer, a personal history of inflammatory bowel disease, and the familial polyposis syndromes.
A. According to the USPSTF, screening for colorectal cancer with annual fecal occult blood testing (FOBT) or sigmoidoscopy (periodicity unspecified), or both, is recommended for all persons aged 50 years and older.
B. Other recommendations for screening for individuals of average risk starting at age 50 include FOBT yearly, *or* flexible sigmoidoscopy every 5 years, *or* FOBT yearly with flexible sigmoidoscopy every 5 years, *or* double-contrast barium enema examination with flexible sigmoidoscopy every 5 years, *or* colonoscopy every 10 years.
C. Persons with one or more polyps larger than 1 cm should undergo colonoscopy. There are more extensive recommendations for cancer surveillance in certain high-risk groups; please see other medical texts for details.
XIII. **Screening for cervical cancer.** Routine screening for cervical cancer with Papanicolaou (Pap) testing is recommended for all women who are or have been sexually active and who have a cervix.
A. Pap smears should begin at age 18 or with the onset of sexual activity and should be repeated yearly until results are normal on three consecutive tests; thereafter, the test should be performed at least every 3 years (yearly testing should be continued for all except women with low risk).
B. There is insufficient direct evidence to recommend for or against an upper age limit for Pap testing, but recommendations can be made on other grounds to discontinue regular testing after age 65 in women who have had regular previous screenings in which the smears have been consistently normal (per USPSTF).
XIV. **Screening for ovarian cancer.** Ovarian cancer has the highest mortality of all gynecologic cancers. Survival is improved when disease is detected before widespread dissemination, but unfortunately, few cases are diagnosed when the cancer is confined to the ovary. Routine screening for ovarian cancer by ultrasonography, the measurement of serum tumor marker levels, or pelvic

examination is not recommended. Whether measurement of cancer antigen 125 (CA-125) levels as a component of a multimodality screening program may be useful requires further evaluation in controlled clinical trials, as none of these methods is of proven benefit for the early detection of ovarian cancer. A National Cancer Institute multicenter trial is ongoing to test the usefulness of transvaginal ultrasonography and CA-125 measurement in reducing the mortality from ovarian cancer.

A. Women with two or more family members affected by ovarian cancer have a 3% chance of having a hereditary ovarian cancer syndrome and should be counseled by a qualified geneticist regarding their individual risk. The Cancer Genetics Studies Consortium has recommended annual or semiannual screening by transvaginal ultrasonography and measurement of serum CA-125 levels beginning at age 25–35 years for *BRCA1* mutation carriers.

B. Risk factors: The most significant risk factor for ovarian cancer is a positive family history. The lifetime risk of developing ovarian cancer is 7% for a woman with two or more first-degree relatives with ovarian cancer. This risk increases 17- to 50-fold if a heritable cancer syndrome is identified, such as hereditary breast or ovarian cancer (*BRCA1*) or Lynch family syndrome II. Advanced age is also associated with increased risk, whereas increased parity, oral contraceptive use, tubal ligation, and hysterectomy decrease one's risk.

XV. **Screening for depression.** Major depressive episodes affect 20 million American adults yearly. The lifetime risk for women of developing a major depressive disorder is 10–25%; depression is two to three times more common in women than in men. However, nearly 80% of cases of depression are undiagnosed. Factors that may predispose women to depression include perinatal loss, infertility, or miscarriage; physical or sexual abuse; socioeconomic deprivation; lack of support, isolation, and feelings of helplessness; family history of mood disorders; loss of a parent during childhood (before age 10); history of substance abuse; and menopause.

A. The following are the **criteria for diagnosing** a major depressive episode. At least five of the following nine symptoms must be present for at least 2 weeks to fulfill the definition of major depressive episode, and at least one of the symptoms must be either depressed mood or loss of interest or pleasure. The symptoms must represent a change from the patient's previous level of functioning.
1. Depressed mood most of the day, nearly every day
2. Markedly decreased interest or pleasure in activities
3. Significant appetite or weight change
4. Insomnia or hypersomnia nearly every day
5. Observable psychomotor retardation or agitation nearly every day
6. Fatigue or loss of energy nearly every day
7. Feelings of worthlessness or inappropriate guilt nearly every day
8. Diminished ability to think, concentrate, or make decisions
9. Recurrent thoughts of death or suicide

B. **Diagnostic categories**
1. **Major depressive episode.** One episode; symptoms may develop over days to weeks and may be either experienced by the patient or observed by others.
2. **Major depressive disorder.** One or more major depressive episodes.
3. **Dysthymic disorder.** Chronically depressed mood on most days for 2 or more years, plus at least two of the symptoms from the list defining a major depressive episode.
4. **Depressive disorder not otherwise specified.** This category includes such diagnoses as premenstrual dysphoric disorder.

C. There is insufficient evidence to recommend for or against the routine use of **standardized questionnaires** to screen for depression in asymptomatic primary care patients. Clinicians should maintain an especially high index of suspicion for depressive symptoms in those persons at increased risk for depression (see earlier). There are many screening tools available to help identify patients who are most likely to be depressed; these tools are designed to rate the severity of depression. Screening is recommended when depression is suspected. Commonly used patient self-report screens that are symptom-oriented include the General Health Questionnaire, the Beck Depression Inventory, the Symptom Checklist, the Inventory of Depressive Symptoms, and the Zung Depression Scale. If scores are above a predetermined cutoff, patients should have a more comprehensive evaluation for depression.

D. **Treatment.** Treatable causes of depression should be identified first; for example, depression may be related to menstruation, pregnancy, the perinatal period, or the perimenopausal period. There can also be a relationship between depression and medications such as birth control pills or agents used in hormone replacement therapy (particularly the progesterone component).

1. **Psychosocial treatment.** Commonly used therapies include psychotherapy to correct interpersonal conflicts and to help women develop interpersonal skills; cognitive-behavioral therapy to correct negative thinking and associated behavior; and couples therapy to reduce marital conflicts. For patients with mild to moderate depression, psychosocial therapies may be used alone, or they may be used in conjunction with antidepressant medication.

2. **Pharmacologic treatment.** A large percentage of women experience significant improvement or even complete remission with medication. Factors to consider for treatment with medications include severe symptoms, recurrent episodes (two or more prior episodes), chronicity, presence of psychotic features such as hallucinations or delusions, presence of melancholic symptoms, family history, prior response to medication, incomplete response to psychotherapy alone, and patient preference.

ACKNOWLEDGMENT

Special thanks to Gail L. Sawyer, MD, for her advice and proofreading.

2. BREAST DISEASES

Sven Becker and Michael Choti

For many women, the gynecologist serves as the primary care physician, so that an understanding of a variety of issues related to women's health is required. Therefore it is crucial that the gynecologist be able to adequately evaluate and treat breast disease. In addition, breast cancer is an important women's health issue. This chapter can instruct practicing gynecologists in the understanding, screening, diagnosis, and treatment of this common malignancy.

I. **Anatomy.** The adult breast lies between the second and sixth ribs in the cervical axis and between the sternal edge and midaxillary line in the horizontal axis. Breast tissue projects into the axilla, also called the *axillary tail of Spence*.

The breast is comprised of three major tissues: skin, subcutaneous tissue, and breast tissue consisting of both parenchyma and stroma. The parenchyma is divided into 15–20 segments that converge at the nipple in a radial arrangement. Between five and ten major collecting ducts open into the nipple. Each duct drains a lobe made up of 20–40 lobules. Each lobule consists of 10–100 alveoli. The major blood supply to the breast is from the internal mammary and thoracic arteries. The lymphatic drainage is typically unidirectional from the superficial to deep lymphatic plexus, draining toward the axillary (97%) and internal mammary nodes (3%).

II. **Methods for screening and diagnosis of breast disease**

A. **Breast examination.** A complete breast examination by a physician should be performed once a year and should be performed as part of every routine examination by the gynecologist. A thorough examination requires some time, yet it is greatly appreciated by the patient as an indicator of the quality of care received.

1. **Inspection** should first be performed with the patient sitting with her arms relaxed at her sides. The contour and symmetry of the breasts as well as skin changes or scars, position of the nipples, and appearance of any mass should be observed. Erythema or edema should be noted. Skin dimpling and nipple retraction sometimes can be seen when the patient is asked to lift her hands above her head and then press her hands on her hips, thereby contracting the pectoralis muscles.

2. **Palpation** is best performed with the flat portion of the fingers. The patient's breast should be palpated in a methodical fashion either in concentric circles or by quadrant until the entire breast is palpated (Fig. 2-1).

The entire axilla and supraclavicular areas should be palpated to detect adenopathy. The entire breast from the clavicle to the costal margin should be examined in both the upright and supine positions. Nodes close to the chest wall, in particular, are best appreciated with the patient lying supine.

Any distinct tumor or mass must be evaluated and biopsy performed, regardless of the mammographic appearance, to rule out malignancy and to make a definitive diagnosis. Many patients have a normally nodular breast parenchyma that can make the detection of a dominant mass difficult. Breast cancer that presents as a mass is often nontender and firm with indistinct borders. It may be fixed to the skin or underlying fascia. The optimal time for breast examination is during the first 10–14 days after menses when the hormonal influence is the least. The nipple should also be checked for nipple discharge, as well as examined for skin changes, including retraction, erythema, and scaling. All positive findings should be well documented in writing and with a drawing.

B. **Breast self-examination** is recommended for all women after age 20 on a monthly basis. This skill should be demonstrated and taught to the patient.

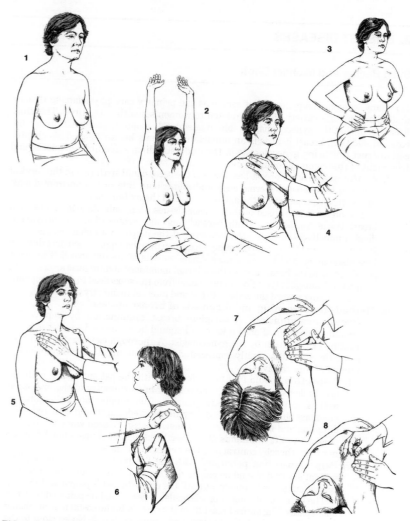

FIG. 2-1. Breast examination. (From Scott JR, et al. *Danforth's obstetrics and gynecology*, 7th edition. Philadelphia: Lippincott Williams & Wilkins, 1994, with permission.)

The patient should begin the examination with inspection in front of a mirror in a well-lit room (Fig. 2-2). She should inspect her breasts with her hands held along her sides and then raised above her head. She should look for abnormalities in breast contour, asymmetry, skin changes, nipple alterations, and discharge. The patient should be instructed to palpate supraclavicular and axillary locations for masses or nodes. Then she should lie in the supine position with a pillow beneath her back on the side of the breast being examined to rotate her chest so that the breast being examined is symmetrically flattened against the chest wall. The patient should then systematically palpate each quadrant of her breast, including the area beneath the nipple. The nipples should be compressed for evidence of dis-

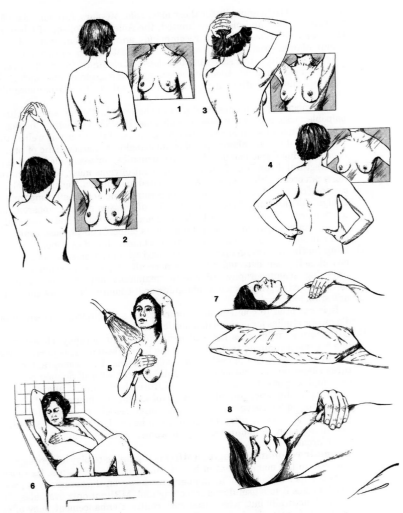

FIG. 2-2. Breast self-examination. (From Scott JR, et al. *Danforth's obstetrics and gynecology*, 7th edition. Philadelphia: Lippincott Williams & Wilkins, 1994, with permission.)

charge. The patient should feel for masses or other changes from previous examinations. If there are any findings of concern, she should contact her physician.

C. **Screening mammography** is perhaps the most useful method of detecting early breast cancer. In randomized controlled trials, screening mammography has been shown to reduce the mortality from breast cancer by up to 30% in women between the ages of 50 and 69. However, less than 40% of women, even in this group, undergo mammography as recommended. Although the data for younger women are less clear, the American College of Obstetricians and Gynecologists and the American Cancer Society recommend screening mammography every 1–2 years for all women aged 40–

49 years and then annually for those older than 50 years. Although data for women 70 years and older are limited, the American College of Obstetricians and Gynecologists also recommends annual screening in this age group. Mammography detects only 90% of breast cancers in asymptomatic women. Therefore, this screening tool does not eliminate the need for careful breast examination. Adequate screening mammography must include at least two views of both breasts: a mediolateral side view and a craniocaudal view.

Mammography is an essential part of the examination of women with a palpable mass, even when cancer is obvious. In such a situation the mammogram is most useful in evaluating other areas of the breast as well as the contralateral breast. Mammographic abnormalities characteristic of breast cancer include spiculated soft tissue densities, microcalcifications, and architectural distortion of the breast without obvious mass. Microcalcifications can occur with or without an associated mass lesion. Suspicious calcifications occur in clusters and are often pleomorphic and small compared to benign calcifications. Approximately 15% of cancers are not apparent on mammogram. This is true for both small and large lesions and is especially true in younger patients. Even if a lesion is palpable on physical examination but not apparent on a mammogram, a biopsy should be done.

D. **Diagnostic mammography** is often used when the presence of a lesion has already been detected either as a result of physical examination or screening mammography. Diagnostic mammography includes a more sophisticated approach such as obtaining spot compression views and magnification images.

It is essential to compare all mammograms with previous screening or diagnostic studies for optimal diagnostic yield.

E. **Ultrasonography** does not substitute for mammography. However, it has become a common tool in evaluating breast lesions. It is particularly useful in distinguishing cystic from solid lesions. Ultrasonographic features suspicious for cancer include solid masses with ill-defined borders or complex cystic lesions. Posterior diffuse shadowing is another hallmark of malignancy on ultrasonography. The evaluation of Doppler ultrasonography curves in the perilesional vessels is currently being studied. On occasion, ultrasonography can be used as a regular screening tool in addition to mammography in women with particularly dense or cystic breasts.

F. **Magnetic resonance imaging (MRI)** is beginning to play a more significant role in the management of breast cancer in select patients. Its sensitivity is superior to that of mammography; however, the specificity is poor, which makes it less useful as a screening tool. MRI not only evaluates the lesion structurally but, when used with contrast enhancement, may offer improved characterization regarding blood flow in the lesion. Larger studies are being conducted to better define the role of MRI in diagnosis of breast disease and to determine whether this imaging modality can improve detection and clinical outcomes in a cost-effective manner.

G. **Breast biopsy**
1. **Fine-needle aspiration biopsy** has traditionally been used to obtain material from a breast abnormality for cytologic evaluation. This method is quick and less invasive than other methods. It involves introduction of a narrow-gauge (22-gauge) needle into a lesion under suction, typically with multiple passes. It is important to be aware that this procedure, although accurate at detecting malignant cells, often cannot distinguish between invasive and noninvasive carcinomas.
2. **Core biopsy.** In the era of breast-conserving surgery, accurate preoperative diagnosis is essential to allow the patient to weigh her options in the case of malignancy before the definitive therapy is undertaken. For palpable lesions, core biopsy reveals better, more reliable, and clinically

more useful information than fine-needle aspiration biopsy. When core biopsy is performed, a large-bore needle is used to obtain the specimen, which consists of cylindric fragments or cores of tissue that are sent for histologic evaluation. Both frozen and permanent sections can be done. Often, four or five core biopsies are taken. This procedure can be performed under mammogram guidance, under ultrasonographic guidance, or directly on a palpable mass. Newer techniques for obtaining larger tissue samples have been developed. These include the Mammotome and Abby devices. These methods use image guidance and suction methodology to achieve more accurate and complete tissue acquisition for diagnostic purposes.

During these procedures, if there is any question that the mammographic abnormality has been removed or distorted, which potentially impacts subsequent management, a small metallic clip or marker can also be inserted.

3. **Excisional biopsy** is typically performed under local anesthesia. With this approach, the abnormality is completely removed. Excisional biopsy can be performed for both palpable and nonpalpable lesions. To excise a nonpalpable mammographically identified abnormality, needle localization and wire are used, termed **needle localization breast biopsy**. With this technique, a needle or wire (or both) is first placed in the area of the lesion under mammographic guidance. In addition, a vital dye can be injected to aid in complete surgical extirpation. The patient is then brought to the operating room, where the area around the tip of the needle is excised. Specimen radiography should always be performed during surgery to confirm complete removal of the original suspicious lesion.

H. **Evaluation of the palpable breast mass** requires a careful history, including family history, physical examination, and radiologic examination. In the majority of these cases, the mass is painless. The presence of pain should not lead to a false reassurance, however, because as many as 10% of patients with cancer may present with breast pain. Less common associated symptoms include nipple discharge, nipple rash or ulceration, diffuse erythema of the breast, adenopathy, or symptoms associated with distant metastatic disease. Enlargement of the breast with or without presence of a distinct mass, erythema, and *peau d'orange* are the hallmarks of locally advanced breast cancer that can sometimes be confused with mastitis. Early breast cancer can also be associated with a breast abscess or mastitis. Any nonlactating woman with an infection of the breast must be closely followed. A biopsy should be performed sooner rather than later, particularly if the "infection" does not promptly resolve.

Ultrasonography with needle aspiration is useful in distinguishing between cystic and solid lesions. Any mass that does not disappear on aspiration, yields bloody aspirate, or does not completely resolve on ultrasonography is an indication for core or excisional biopsy.

I. **Evaluation of a mammographic abnormality.** There are multiple radiologic findings that usually require surgical consultation and consideration of breast biopsy even when the physical examination is unremarkable (Table 2-1).

When a woman's screening mammogram is ambiguous, diagnostic mammography with special views should be performed and a decision made whether to perform a diagnostic biopsy. If the mammographic studies are inconclusive, a short-term follow-up study at 3–6 months can be considered. Biopsy techniques for mammographically identified nonpalpable lesions include needle localization excision biopsy and stereotactic core biopsy.

III. **Common benign breast problems**

A. **Mastalgia** is the most common breast symptom causing women to consult a physician. Although the vast majority of patients with pain have a benign

TABLE 2-1. RADIOLOGIC FINDINGS OF CONCERN ON MAMMOGRAPHY

Soft tissue density, especially if the borders are not well defined radiographically
Clustered microcalcifications in one area of the breast
Calcifications within or closely associated with a soft tissue density
Asymmetric density or parenchymal distortion
New abnormality compared with previous mammogram

cause, up to 10% of patients with cancer complain of pain, often with an associated mass. Benign breast pain can be either cyclic or noncyclic. Cyclic pain usually is maximal premenstrually and relieved with the onset of menses and can be either unilateral or bilateral. Noncyclic breast pain can have various causes, including hormonal fluctuations, firm adenomas, duct ectasia, and macrocysts. Noncyclic pain may also arise from musculoskeletal structures, such as soreness in the pectoral muscles from exertion or trauma. Costochondritis is another possible cause of breast pain. With most noncyclic breast pain, however, no definite cause is determined. Although breast cancer can present only as pain, this is very uncommon. The evaluation in a patient with breast pain should include a complete history and physical examination as well as mammography in women older than 35 years of age to exclude a suspicious density as the source of the pain. Patients who do not have a dominant mass can be reassured. In most patients, mastalgia remits spontaneously, although sometimes only after many months or years. Restriction of methylxanthine-containing substances (coffee, tea) has not been shown to be superior to placebo in large studies, but might produce relief in some individual patients. If therapy is indicated, oral contraceptive pills (estrogen plus progestin combination oral contraceptive pills) are one option. Alternatives include danazol (100–400 mg/day for 3–6 months) or tamoxifen citrate (10 mg/day for 3–6 months).

B. **Nipple discharge** is a common presenting complaint. Not all nipple discharge is pathologic, and an attempt should be made to classify the discharge as physiologic, pathologic, or galactorrheic based on history, physical examination, and guaiac testing.

1. **Physiologic discharge** is nonspontaneous and usually bilateral. It arises from multiple ducts and is usually serous in character. It can be caused by use of exogenous estrogens or tranquilizers, or nipple stimulation. This type of discharge is not associated with underlying breast disease and requires no further evaluation. Reassurance is sufficient treatment.

2. **Galactorrhea** is a typically bilateral, multiduct discharge with a milky character. Galactorrhea may have a variety of causes, including chest wall trauma or use of oral contraceptives, phenothiazines, antihypertensives, or tranquilizing drugs. Several endocrine abnormalities give rise to galactorrhea, including amenorrhea syndromes, pituitary adenomas, and hypothyroidism. An evaluation for endocrine abnormality should be performed with measurement of prolactin level and thyroid function tests. Hyperprolactinemia should be evaluated with a CT scan and visual field testing.

3. **Pathologic discharge** is typically localized to a single duct. It is usually a spontaneous discharge that is intermittent. It may be greenish-gray, serous, or bloody. The most common cause of pathologic discharge is benign breast disease, even if the discharge contains blood. The quadrant of the breast in which pressure results in discharge should be noted to localize the duct. Testing the fluid for occult blood is useful to identify subtle bloody discharge. Cytologic study can also be performed.

A mammogram should be part of the evaluation of any patient with a pathologic discharge. Biopsy should be performed if an associated mammographic abnormality or palpable mass is present. Also, in cases of persistent pathologic discharge or discharge that is bloody, biopsy should be undertaken using a surgical procedure called *terminal duct excision*. Benign causes for pathologic nipple discharge include intraductal papilloma, duct ectasia, and fibrocystic changes. Carcinoma accounts for only 5% of pathologic discharge, and 3–11% of women with cancer have an associated nipple discharge.

C. **Breast infections**
   1. **Puerperal mastitis** is an acute cellulitis of the breast in a lactating woman. If treatment is not begun promptly, puerperal mastitis can progress to abscess formation. Mastitis usually occurs during the early weeks of nursing. On inspection, there is often cellulitis of a wedge-shaped pattern over a portion of the breast skin. The affected tissue is red, warm, and very tender. Usually, there is no purulent drainage from the nipple because the infection is around rather than within the duct system. High fevers and chills as well as flu-like body ache are common and not infrequently precede the local erythema. *Staphylococcus aureus* is the most common causal organism, and any antibiotic therapy should cover this organism. The antibiotic therapy usually recommended is dicloxacillin, 500 mg by mouth four times daily for 10 days. More important than antibiotic therapy, however, is aggressive emptying of the affected breast of milk. The patient should be encouraged to continue to breast feed or pump milk to promote drainage from the affected segments. Warmth and manual pressure to engorged areas is also beneficial. If puerperal mastitis is not treated promptly or fails to respond to therapy, an abscess may form. Fluctuance may be absent, and it could be difficult to detect because of the numerous fibrous septa within the breast. If the puerperal mastitis does not resolve quickly with treatment, incision and drainage with culturing is indicated.
   2. **Nonpuerperal mastitis** is uncommon. This type of infection is often subareolar with an area of tenderness, erythema, and induration. The patient is generally not systemically ill. Nonpuerperal mastitis is usually a polymicrobial infection including anaerobes. Antibiotic coverage should be appropriate, typically including clindamycin or metronidazole in addition to a beta-lactam antibiotic covering penicillinase-resistant organisms. All breast inflammation must raise concern for inflammatory breast cancer, and the threshold for performing a skin biopsy should be low, particularly in the elderly population. Skin biopsies can be easily done using the same punch biopsy instrument used in the vulvar area. If a suspected nonpuerperal mastitis does not respond promptly to antibiotic treatment, mammography and skin biopsy are indicated.

D. **Fibrocystic conditions** are a common benign breast complaint. They occur mostly in the premenopausal period. Common complaints are bilateral pain and tenderness, most often localized in the subareolar or upper outer regions of the breast. These symptoms are noted most often during the 7–14 days before menses. The pain is likely due to stromal edema, ductal dilation, and some degree of inflammation, but the true etiology is unclear. This condition should be considered a normal variation and not a disease, although some women can be significantly debilitated by persistent symptoms. Management should include regular examinations and imaging if indicated. Oral contraceptives suppress symptoms in 70–90% of patients. Analgesics, such as acetaminophen, aspirin, and nonsteroidal anti-inflammatory drugs, are also helpful. Often, reassurance that the symptoms are not related to a disease or serious pathologic condition is enough for the patient. Histologically, nonproliferative fibrocystic changes can be distinguished from proliferative changes. **Nonproliferative fibrocystic**

changes include microcysts, which can progress to form macrocysts that can present as palpable masses. **Proliferative fibrocystic changes** can involve hyperplasia of the ductal epithelium, which leads to layering of the epithelial lining. This is a histologic and not a clinical diagnosis.

When accompanied by cellular atypia, fibrocystic disease is associated with a fivefold increase in the risk of breast cancer. Intraductal proliferation can lead to intraductal papillomas, the most common cause of serosanguineous nipple discharge.

E. **Benign breast masses**

1. **Fibroadenoma** is the most common mass lesion found in women younger than 25 years. Growth is generally gradual, and there may be occasional cyclic tenderness. If the lesion is palpable, increasing in size, or psychologically disturbing, core or excisional biopsy should be considered. Conservative management may be appropriate for small lesions that are nonpalpable and have been identified as fibroadenomas by mammography, ultrasonography, or core biopsy. Careful follow-up is essential. Carcinoma within a fibroadenoma is a very rare occurrence. A rare malignant variation of fibroadenoma called *cystosarcoma phylloides* is treated by wide resection. Local recurrence is common and distant metastasis very rare.

2. **Breast cysts** can be found in pre- or postmenopausal women. Physical examination often cannot distinguish cysts from solid masses. Ultrasonography and cyst aspiration are often diagnostic. In these cases, no further therapy is required. If a cyst does not resolve with aspiration, yields a sanguineous aspirate, recurs within 6 weeks, or is complex on ultrasonography, surgical consultation should be obtained.

3. **Fat necrosis** is frequently associated with breast trauma resulting in a breast mass. It has also been reported to occur after breast biopsy, infection, duct ectasia, and reduction mammoplasty as well as after lumpectomy and radiotherapy for breast carcinoma. Fat necrosis may occur anywhere, but it is most common in the subareolar region. This process can be difficult to distinguish from breast cancer on both physical examination and mammography. Even if fat necrosis is suspected, the lesion needs to be evaluated like any other palpable breast lesion. Only a benign histologic appearance affords reassurance.

IV. **Breast cancer** in the United States is the most common malignancy and the second leading cause of death due to cancer in women (lung cancer being the first). There are approximately 180,000 new cases diagnosed each year and an estimated 45,000 deaths from this disease annually. Breast cancer is a common and devastating disease, and the cumulative lifetime risk of developing this cancer is approximately 12%. The risk of developing breast cancer increases with age (Table 2-2).

A. **Risk factors** associated with breast cancer include both genetic and environmental factors.

1. **Genetic predisposition and family history.** Although most breast cancers occur in women with no clear family history, breast cancer risk in an individual with breast cancer in first-degree relatives, such as mother, sister, or daughter—particularly when these individuals were affected at a young age—is clearly elevated. The risk is further increased when more than one first-degree relative is affected. Only 5–10% of breast cancers have a clear hereditary association. Of these cases, 30–60% are believed to be the consequence of *BRCA1* and *BRCA2* germ-line mutation. Currently, different molecular tests are commercially available to detect known mutations in these genes. Significant mutations are found at a rate of 1:800 (0.1%) in the general population. In Jewish patients of Eastern European descent (Ashkenazi), this rate increases to 20:800 (2.5%). The precise biological role of *BRCA1* and *BRCA2* remains unclear.

TABLE 2-2. A WOMAN'S CHANCE OF BEING DIAGNOSED WITH BREAST CANCER BY AGE

30 yrs	1 : 2212
40 yrs	1 : 235
50 yrs	1 : 54
60 yrs	1 : 23
70 yrs	1 : 14
80 yrs	1 : 10
Lifetime	1 : 8

2. **Gynecologic history.** Early menarche (younger than 12 years) and late natural menopause (older than 55 years) are associated with a mildly increased risk of developing breast cancer. Multiparity confers a somewhat decreased risk, as does an age at first childbirth of younger than 30 years.

3. **Diet and lifestyle.** The impressive differences in the incidence of breast cancer in different geographical and cultural areas have long raised the suspicion that there are underlying dietary risk factors. High-fat diets have been implicated in particular. The data presently available, however, are insufficient to provide firm dietary advice for reduction in breast cancer risk. Neither a low-fat diet, nor a high-fiber diet, nor the use of vitamins A, C, and E has been shown to lead to a risk reduction in large trials. Alcohol consumption, particularly in large amounts, appears to confer an increased risk, whereas exercise appears to lower the overall risk.

4. **Hormones.** The existing scientific evidence does not support a clinically significant or physiologically rational relationship between oral contraceptive pills and breast cancer. There is, however, a clear protective effect of oral contraceptives on the risk of ovarian cancer, with many studies showing a 40–50% reduction in risk. The question of whether hormone replacement therapy (HRT) in postmenopausal women increases the incidence of breast cancer is currently being debated. The same study that identified a slightly increased risk did not demonstrate an increased mortality due to breast cancer. Many other studies have shown no relationship.

The role of HRT in breast cancer remains one of the most controversial areas in gynecology. Fear of breast cancer is the number one reason why women who are candidates for HRT do not take it. Our practice is to discuss what is known with the patient and to determine if there are other risk factors for breast cancer, on the one hand, versus risk factors for cardiovascular disease or osteoporosis, on the other.

Another area of controversy is the use of HRT in postmenopausal survivors of breast cancer. Women with a history of breast cancer have a clearly increased risk of contralateral breast cancer as well as of local recurrence. Whether HRT increases this risk further is unclear. It is important to note that a history of breast cancer is not an absolute contraindication for HRT. The decision should be made on an individual basis after appropriate counseling.

B. **Prevention**
1. Prophylactic **mastectomy**, usually with breast reconstruction, is an option for high-risk patients. The procedure has been shown to decrease the risk of breast cancer in such groups by up to 90%.

2. **Screening for *BRCA1* and *BRCA2* mutations** is an option that can be considered in patients with a significant family history who are consid-

ering prophylactic mastectomy. A clearer delineation of the specific risk (e.g., higher than 80%) can make consideration of such an aggressive strategy easier. It is important to stress that any genetic screening should be preceded by extensive genetic counseling by a qualified individual. This is because the implications of genetic testing can be significant, with effects on insurability, job security, and other family members.

3. **Hormone chemoprevention** is another area of current controversy.

A recent study, the Breast Cancer Prevention Trial (BCPT), has evaluated the use of tamoxifen for preventive purposes in a population at high risk for developing invasive breast cancer. Tamoxifen is a nonsteroidal compound with antiestrogenic and estrogenic effects on specific tissues and has been used in the treatment of breast cancer for decades. In that context, studies had shown that tamoxifen-treated women had a significantly lower incidence of contralateral breast cancer.

The BCPT, evaluating a collective of 13,000 patients, demonstrated a risk reduction for breast cancer of 44% in a selected high-risk population with no prior history of breast cancer. High risk was defined by a combination of variables, including number of first-degree relatives with breast cancer, age at first childbirth, age at menarche, nulliparity, and so on. After review of the data, the U.S. Food and Drug Administration approved tamoxifen as a preventive medication for breast cancer. *High risk* was defined as a 5-year predicted risk of breast cancer of at least 1.67% as determined by the Gail model, a computerized risk calculator that includes most of the variables mentioned earlier.

This impressive beneficial effect needs to be weighed against the thromboembolic side effects and the increased incidence of endometrial cancer in the treatment group. Tamoxifen belongs to the family of selective estrogen receptor modulators (SERMs). Another SERM, raloxifene hydrochloride, has recently been shown not to increase the risk of endometrial cancer in osteoporosis prevention trials. A National Cancer Institute trial is currently evaluating tamoxifen and raloxifene for breast cancer prevention in postmenopausal women.

C. **Premalignant conditions**

1. **Atypical hyperplasia** is a proliferative lesion of the breast that possesses some, but not all, of the features of carcinoma in situ. Atypical hyperplasia can be categorized as either ductal or lobular in type. Atypical hyperplasia should be considered a premalignant finding and is associated with a four- to fivefold increased risk of breast cancer, usually in the ipsilateral breast. Women with proliferative breast disease but without atypical hyperplasia, such as sclerosing adenosis, ductal epithelium hyperplasia, and intraductal papillomas, have less risk of developing breast cancer. These proliferative changes, however, do increase the breast cancer risk to approximately twice that of women with no proliferative breast lesions.

   a. **Atypical ductal hyperplasia (ADH)** is a lesion that has some features of ductal carcinoma in situ, including nuclear monomorphism, regular cell placement, and round, regular spaces in at least part of the involved duct. The histologic features do not meet the criteria for ductal carcinoma in situ; therefore, ADH is considered a benign lesion. However, because of the concern for malignant potential and the possibility of associated malignancy in proximity to ADH, complete excision is recommended.

   b. **Atypical lobular hyperplasia** is characterized by changes similar to those of lobular carcinoma in situ but lacks the complete criteria for that diagnosis.

2. **Lobular carcinoma in situ** is a proliferative premalignant condition associated with a general increased risk of developing breast cancer. It is usually an incidental finding on biopsy not associated with a palpable mass or mammographic abnormality. It can, however, be seen in associ-

ation with or adjacent to a palpable or visible cancer. It is usually multi-centric and is associated with a *bilateral* increased risk of breast cancer. Any accompanying palpable or mammographically detected abnormality must be fully evaluated to rule out associated intraductal or invasive carcinoma. Patients with evidence of lobular carcinoma in situ are considered at high risk of cancer and should be followed carefully.

D. **Histologic subtypes of breast cancer**
1. **Ductal carcinoma in situ (DCIS)**, also called *intraductal cancer*, refers to a proliferation of cancer cells within the ducts without invasion through the basement membrane into the surrounding stroma. Histologically, DCIS can be divided into multiple histologic subtypes: solid, micropapillary, cribriform, and comedo. DCIS can also be graded as low, intermediate, or high. DCIS is the early, noninfiltrating form of breast cancer with minimal risk of metastasis and an excellent prognosis with local therapy alone.

   With the increased use of mammography, DCIS is being diagnosed with increased frequency. Often, diffuse microcalcifications on mammography lead to biopsy and the diagnosis of DCIS. Current recommendations are based on the completeness of the resection, the margin status, and the histologic subtype.

2. **Infiltrating ductal carcinoma** is the most common histologic type of invasive carcinoma, accounting for 60–75% of all tumors. These tumors can be associated with varying degrees of carcinoma in situ.
   a. **Mucinous and tubular cancers** are well-differentiated variants of infiltrating ductal carcinoma. These cancers account for approximately 5% of breast cancers, are often more circumscribed, have a lower risk of lymph node involvement, and have a better prognosis.
   b. **Medullary carcinoma**, which accounts for approximately 5% of all breast cancers, can present as a grossly well-defined lesion that is microscopically poorly differentiated with intense infiltration of lymphocytes or plasma cells.

3. **Infiltrating lobular carcinoma** is a variant of invasive cancer associated with microscopic lobular architecture. These cancers account for 5–10% of breast cancer and are more often multifocal and less evident on mammography.

E. **Staging and prognostic factors.** The American Joint Committee on Cancer TNM staging system for breast cancer uses tumor size, axillary nodal status, and metastasis status (Table 2-3). Most clinical trials use the stage I to IV system that combines different TNM stages with similar clinical prognoses (Table 2-4). Prognosis is most strongly correlated with tumor size and the status of the axillary lymph nodes. Another factor that predicts survival is the estrogen receptor (ER) and progesterone (PR) status. Hormone (ER/PR) status, in addition to providing prognostic information, can predict response to hormone therapy. Other prognostic factors include tumor grade, S phase, DNA ploidy and expression of the Her-2 receptor.

F. **Local treatment of primary breast cancer.** In the treatment of breast cancer, early detection is the key to improved survival. Treatment options for invasive breast cancer include modified radical mastectomy (with or without breast reconstruction) and breast conservation therapy. Only in selected cases are nonsurgical options such as primary radiation or chemotherapy considered.
1. **Mastectomy**
   a. **Modified radical mastectomy** includes the complete removal of the breast tissue with axillary lymph node dissection. In this operation, the pectoralis muscles are preserved. The original *radical mastectomy* first described by Halsted over 100 years ago included removal of the pectoralis muscles as well. This procedure is cur-

TABLE 2-3. TNM CLASSIFICATION OF BREAST CANCER

TX	Primary tumor cannot be assessed
T0	No evidence of primary tumor
Tis	Carcinoma in situ: intraductal carcinoma, lobular carcinoma in situ, or Paget's disease of the nipple with no tumor
T1	Tumor ≤2 cm in greatest dimension
T1a	Tumor ≤0.5 cm in greatest dimension
T1b	Tumor >0.5 cm but ≤1 cm in greatest dimension
T1c	Tumor >1 cm but ≤2 cm in greatest dimension
T2	Tumor >2 cm but ≤5 cm in greatest dimension
T3	Tumor >5 cm in greatest dimension
T4	Tumor of any size with direct extension to chest wall or skin
T4a	Extension to chest wall
T4b	Edema (including *peau d'orange*) or ulceration of the skin of the breast or satellite skin nodules confined to the same breast
T4c	Both T4a and T4b
T4d	Inflammatory carcinoma
NX	Regional lymph nodes cannot be assessed (e.g., previously removed)
N0	No regional lymph node metastasis
N1	Metastasis to movable ipsilateral axillary lymph node(s)
N2	Metastasis to ipsilateral axillary lymph node(s), fixed to one another or other structures
N3	Metastasis to ipsilateral internal mammary lymph node(s)
M	Presence of distant metastasis cannot be assessed
M0	No distant metastasis
M1	Distant metastasis [including metastasis to ipsilateral supraclavicular lymph node(s)]

rently used only in cases of locally advanced disease when the tumor directly invades into the muscle.

The modified radical mastectomy can be performed with or without immediate reconstruction. When no reconstruction is performed, skin flaps are closed primarily over the pectoralis muscles. Various types of reconstruction can be used, including autologous muscle reconstruction (pedicle transverse rectus abdominis myocutaneous, or TRAM, flap; free TRAM or latissimus dorsi flaps) or reconstruction using an expander and prosthetic implant.

b. **Total, or simple, mastectomy** is removal of the entire breast tissue without an axillary dissection. This operation is typically reserved for patients with DCIS or those undergoing prophylactic mastectomy. As with modified radical mastectomy, patients undergoing total mastectomy may have the option of immediate reconstruction.

Chest wall radiation therapy is sometimes recommended after mastectomy. It is typically indicated for patients with large, locally advanced tumors or those with large numbers of involved lymph nodes. More recently, studies have demonstrated the potential benefit of postoperative chest wall radiation even in earlier stage disease.

TABLE 2-4. CLINICAL STAGES BY TNM CATEGORIES

Stage	Tumor size	Lymph node metastases	Distant metastases
0	Tis	N0	M0
I	T1	N0	M0
IIa	T0	N1	M0
	T1	N1	M0
	T2	N0	M0
IIb	T2	N1	M0
	T3	N0	M0
IIIa	T0	N2	M0
	T1	N2	M0
	T2	N2	M0
	T3	N1, N2	M0
IIIb	T4	Any N	M0
	Any T	N3	M0
IV	Any T	Any N	M1

2. **Breast conservation therapy (BCT)** for infiltrating cancer has the advantage of preserving the breast. It requires complete resection of the tumor with sufficient margins (lumpectomy), axillary lymph node sampling, and radiation treatment to the remaining breast tissue. If the disease is multifocal or large or if negative margins cannot be achieved, BCT is not recommended. With this approach, typically two incisions are used. Axillary sampling or dissection is often performed through a separate small incision in the axillary region.

   With BCT, radiation therapy is delivered postoperatively to the entire breast and may include the supraclavicular and axillary regions. In some cases, additional radiation, called a *boost*, is also administered to the lumpectomy site. BCT, when used in appropriate patients, results in survival rates similar to those for mastectomy. Recurrence within the breast typically ranges from 0.5% to 1.0% per year.

3. **Axillary node sampling.** Assessment of the regional lymph nodes in infiltrating breast cancer provides important prognostic information as well as help in determining subsequent treatment planning. Although axillary node dissection is considered standard treatment for infiltrating ductal carcinoma, there is an increasing trend for its selective use. In some cases, patients with very small cancers may be offered no axillary dissection. In addition, lymphatic mapping and sentinel lymph node biopsy are being offered more commonly. In the lymphatic mapping technique, a specific, or **"sentinel," lymph node(s)** is identified using a radioactive tracer or dye injected into the region of the cancer. Only this node is then removed, which eliminates the need for axillary node dissection. Although the technique is promising, further clinical trials demonstrating accuracy of sentinel lymph node biopsy are necessary before it can be recommended routinely instead of axillary node dissection.

G. **Reconstructive surgery.** For women who are not candidates for BCT, breast reconstruction after mastectomy offers an excellent alternative. Breast reconstruction can be **autologous**, as in use of a pedicled TRAM flap or latissimus dorsi flap. Such myocutaneous flaps use the original blood supply of the muscle moved to a new location. Alternatively, free flaps created using microvascular surgical techniques are being employed with greater frequency. In this technique the flap is completely detached from its original site (e.g., free TRAM). This approach offers advantages in some cases, including fewer complications at the donor site.

Nonautologous reconstruction techniques rely on the placement of fluid-filled pouches or implants. Typically, an expander that can be accessed and gradually filled through a subcutaneous valve is first placed in the subpectoral location. The expander is then later replaced with a permanent implant.

H. **Treatment of ductal carcinoma in situ.** Patients who have DCIS can similarly be offered the options of mastectomy or BCT. Unlike for infiltrating cancer, for DCIS, in which the risk of nodal involvement is less than 1%, lymph node sampling is not recommended and only total mastectomy is performed. The patient may elect mastectomy or undergo lumpectomy followed by radiation therapy. In some cases of microscopic DCIS, lumpectomy alone can be considered. As with infiltrating cancer, lumpectomy must achieve complete negative margins. In some cases of multifocal disease, BCT is contraindicated.

I. **Systemic therapy.** Patients with a higher risk of developing systemic recurrence are often offered further treatment.

1. **Adjuvant systemic therapy** is typically recommended to patients when lymph node findings are positive or when the tumor size is large. Systemic therapy consists of chemotherapy or hormonal therapy or both. In most studies, adjuvant chemotherapy has been shown to reduce the odds of death by 25% in selected patients. Chemotherapy is typically administered postoperatively over 3–6 months. The original standard regiment is cyclophosphamide, methotrexate sodium, and 5-fluorouracil (CMF). More recently, doxorubicin hydrochloride (Adriamycin) and cyclophosphamide (AC) have been used as a potentially slightly more effective alternative. Other alternatives include drug combinations containing paclitaxel (Taxol).

   If a patient is undergoing BCT, chemotherapy can be administered either before or after radiation therapy. In rare cases, including cases of inflammatory breast carcinoma or locally advanced disease, chemotherapy is administered as neoadjuvant therapy before surgical treatment.

2. **Hormonal therapy** is the most frequently recommended adjuvant systemic therapy, most commonly using tamoxifen. As with chemotherapy, hormone therapy has been shown to result in a 26% annual reduction in the risk of recurrence and a 14% annual reduction in the risk of death from breast cancer. Tamoxifen, administered at 20 mg/day, has been shown to be more effective in patients whose tumors are ER/PR positive. Typically, tamoxifen therapy is administered for 5 years, after which its maximal effect is reached. This treatment is well tolerated, and side effects are rare. Most important for the gynecologist is the stimulatory effect tamoxifen has on the endometrium. Bleeding while taking tamoxifen—most often in the postmenopausal setting—is a common problem, as is thickening of the endometrial stripe on ultrasonography. Overall, tamoxifen use increases the risk of endometrial cancer by a factor of two. Other potential side effects include deep venous thrombosis and ophthalmologic complications. Patients on therapy should be monitored accordingly.

J. **Treatment of metastatic disease.** Although breast cancer is uncommonly found to be metastatic at the time of presentation, approximately one-third of patients subsequently develop distant metastatic disease. Median survival for patients with metastatic disease is 2 years, but fewer than 5% live beyond 5 years. Visceral metastases to brain, liver, or lung have a worse prognosis than skeletal metastases. Patients can be offered systemic therapy, either with chemotherapy or hormonal therapy. Patients whose tumors are ER/PR positive are more likely to respond to hormone therapy.

In addition to tamoxifen, other hormonal agents used are the progestins, including megestrol acetate (Megace) or aminoglutethimide.

High-dose chemotherapy with bone marrow or stem cell rescue was initially met with enthusiasm for the treatment of patients with metastatic disease. However, recent reports have not substantiated a significant survival benefit. Further clinical trials demonstrating efficacy and cost effectiveness are necessary before its use can be justified.

A novel therapeutic approach relies on the fact that approximately 30% of breast cancers express the oncoprotein Her-2 on their cell surfaces; this expression generally correlates with worse prognosis. Although the exact function of Her-2 is unknown, the oncoprotein appears to be important in regulating the growth of the breast cancer cells. A monoclonal antibody has been developed as a medication [trastuzumab (Herceptin)] that blocks the effect of the Her-2 protein. It is currently being offered to patients as salvage therapy. Ongoing clinical studies are evaluating its expanded use. Its long-term benefits remain to be evaluated, as does its role in adjuvant therapy.

K. **Pregnancy and breast cancer.** Breast cancer is the most common cancer in pregnancy, with an incidence of 1 in 3000 gestations. The average patient age is 32–38 years. Breast cancer can be especially difficult to diagnose during pregnancy and lactation. Pregnant patients do as well as their nonpregnant counterparts at a similar disease stage. Treatment during pregnancy is generally the same as that for nonpregnant patients. The tumor can usually be fully excised or mastectomy performed during pregnancy. There is no evidence that aborting the fetus or interrupting the pregnancy leads to improved outcome. Radiotherapy should be avoided until after delivery. Even though there are no teratogenic effects of chemotherapy in the third trimester, most physicians delay treatment until after delivery because there is little evidence that this delay has any significant impact on prognosis.

3. CRITICAL CARE

Alice W. Ko and Pamela Lipsett

I. **Respiratory failure, oxygen therapy, and mechanical ventilation**
   A. **Acute respiratory failure.** In general, two types of respiratory failure can occur: hypoxic respiratory failure [arterial partial pressure of oxygen (PaO_2) less than 60 mm Hg or arterial oxygen saturation (SaO_2) less than 90%] and hypercapnic respiratory failure [arterial partial pressure of carbon dioxide ($PaCO_2$) higher than 46 mm Hg and pH less than 7.35]. An adequate saturation does *not* rule out hypercapnic respiratory failure. When a patient with hypoxia or hypercapnia is evaluated, it is important to keep in mind that blood gas levels can vary in a clinically stable patient and that these variations do not necessarily reflect a significant change.
   1. **Evaluation.** The approach to identifying the source of hypoxemia and hypercapnia should begin with calculation of the alveolar-arteriolar (A-a) partial pressure of oxygen (PO_2) gradient. If the A-a gradient is normal or unchanged, calculation of the maximum inspiratory pressure helps in discerning a central hypoventilation source from a neuromuscular disorder. If the A-a gradient is increased in hypoxemia or hypercapnia, calculation of the mixed venous PO_2 or the rate of CO_2 production, respectively, helps in discerning a ventilation-perfusion ratio ($\dot{V}/\dot{Q}$) abnormality from other disorders.
      a. The **A-a gradient** is the difference between alveolar PaO_2 and arterial blood PaO_2. This can be calculated using arterial blood gas values in the following equation:

      A-a gradient = $148 - 1.2(PaCO_2) - PaO_2$

      This equation presumes the patient is breathing room air at sea level, at which fraction of inspired oxygen (FIO_2) = 0.21. The A-a gradient is influenced by age and inspired oxygen. The normal A-a gradient range rises with age and can be as high as 25–35 mm Hg for patients older than age 40. *For patients being given supplemental oxygen, the normal A-a gradient increases 5–7 mm Hg for every 10% increase in FIO_2.*
      b. **Maximum inspiratory pressure (PImax)** is calculated by having a patient make a maximal inspiratory effort from functional residual capacity against a closed valve. This value for most adults is higher than 80 cm H_2O; however, it can vary depending on age and sex. When the PImax is less than 40% of normal values, CO_2 retention results.
      c. **Mixed venous PO_2 ($P\bar{v}O_2$)** is ideally measured from pulmonary artery blood, but superior vena cava blood can be used as well. This value can be derived for patients with indwelling pulmonary artery catheters.
      d. **The rate of CO_2 production (VCO_2)** can be measured by a metabolic cart, which is an instrument that uses infrared light to measure CO_2 in expired gas. The normal VCO_2 range is 90–130 L/minute/m².
   2. **Hypoxic respiratory failure** should be suspected when a significant reduction in the arterial PO_2 is encountered (PO_2 less than 60 mm Hg or SaO_2 less than 90%). This type of respiratory failure is usually associated with tachypnea and hypocapnia; thus, the SaO_2 may be normal or elevated during the initial period. When hypoxemia is encountered, three main disorders should be considered.

a. **Hypoventilation** allows for increased alveolar CO_2 that displaces oxygen. In hypoventilation, the A-a gradient is normal or unchanged. If the PImax is normal, the most likely problem is a drug-induced central hypoventilation. If the PImax is low, the hypoventilation is due to a neuromuscular disorder. Oxygen therapy usually improves the hypoxemia but may exacerbate the degree of hypoventilation in patients with airflow obstruction. Hypoventilation as a source of hypoxic ventilatory failure in a patient without prior CO_2 retention is an unusual and critical cause of respiratory failure.

b. **Cardiopulmonary disorder.** If the A-a gradient is increased in hypoxemia, a cardiopulmonary disorder ($\dot{V}/\dot{Q}$ abnormality) or a systemic oxygen delivery/uptake imbalance ($DO_2/\dot{V}O_2$ imbalance) is present. A normal $P\bar{v}O_2$ in this setting suggests a $\dot{V}/\dot{Q}$ abnormality. A $\dot{V}/\dot{Q}$ abnormality can be a result of increased dead space ventilation ($\dot{V}/\dot{Q}$ greater than 1; pulmonary embolism, heart failure, emphysema, overdistended alveoli from positive pressure ventilation) or an intrapulmonary shunt ($\dot{V}/\dot{Q}$ less than 1; asthma, bronchitis, pulmonary edema, pneumonia, atelectasis). Generally, delivery of supplemental oxygen improves the PaO_2. Intrapulmonary shunt can be classified into two types: (1) true shunt in which $\dot{V}/\dot{Q} = 0$ and (2) venous admixture in which $\dot{V}/\dot{Q}$ is higher than 0, but lower than 1. The fraction of cardiac output that represents the intrapulmonary shunt is known as the shunt fraction. Normally, the shunt fraction is less than 10%. When the shunt fraction is above 50%, the PaO_2 is not improved by supplemental oxygen delivery.

c. **$DO_2/\dot{V}O_2$ imbalance** is suggested by a low $P\bar{v}O_2$ in the setting of an increased A-a gradient. Improving oxygen delivery by increasing hemoglobin or cardiac output improves $P\bar{v}O_2$ and PaO_2.

3. **Hypercapnic respiratory failure** should be suspected when the $PaCO_2$ is higher than 46 mm Hg and the pH is lower than 7.35. The three major sources of this type of failure are the following.

a. **Increased CO_2 production** can result from overfeeding (especially carbohydrate loads), fever, sepsis, and seizures.

b. **Hypoventilation** can result from respiratory muscle weakness (from shock, multiorgan failure, prolonged neuromuscular blockade, electrolyte imbalances, cardiac surgery) or central hypoventilatory processes (opiate or benzodiazepine respiratory depression, obesity).

c. **Increased dead space ventilation** as noted earlier.

B. **Oxygen therapy** is still used rather liberally despite evidence that oxygen is the primary culprit in cell injury in the critically ill patient. Oxygen can reduce systemic blood flow by acting as a vasoconstrictor in all vessels except the pulmonary vessels (where oxygen acts as a vasodilator) and by acting as a negative inotropic agent on the heart, thus reducing cardiac output. For patients who are hypoxemic or hypercapnic, oxygen therapy can facilitate improved oxygen supply to the peripheral tissues. When this is not achievable, plans for endotracheal intubation should be made. Oxygen delivery systems can be classified into low-flow and high-flow systems. Low-flow systems (nasal cannulae, face masks with and without bags) provide variable FIO_2 whereas high-flow systems provide a constant FIO_2.

1. **Nasal prong systems (nasal cannulae)** are well tolerated by most patients and use the oro- and nasopharynx together as an oxygen reservoir (capacity approximately 50 mL). The FIO_2 varies according to the patient's ventilatory pattern. As a loose guideline, in a patient with a normal ventilatory pattern (tidal volume of 500 mL, respiratory rate of 20 breaths/minute, and an inspiratory/expiratory time ratio of 1:2), 1 L/minute of nasal cannulae oxygen flow is equivalent to an FIO_2 of 24%. With each increase in flow of 1 L, the FIO_2 increases by approximately 4%. *The FIO_2 is significantly reduced in patients who are tachypneic or*

hyperventilatory. Oxygen flow rates beyond 6 L/minute do not improve FIO_2, and this level should not be exceeded.

2. **Face masks without reservoir bags.** Low-flow face masks have an oxygen reservoir capacity of 100–200 mL. To clear exhaled gas, a minimum oxygen flow rate of 5 L/minute is needed. The flow rate can range from 5 to 10 L/minute with a maximum FIO_2 of 0.6. Face masks without reservoir bags improve slightly on nasal prong systems by providing a slightly higher FIO_2.

3. **Face masks with a reservoir bag** improve the oxygen reservoir to 600–1000 mL. There are two types of reservoir mask devices: (1) partial rebreathers and (2) nonrebreathers. The partial rebreather can attain an FIO_2 of 70–80%, whereas the nonrebreather can permit inhalation of pure oxygen (FIO_2 of 100%). This device requires a tight seal during its use, so that it does not permit oral feeding. Also, a nebulizer treatment cannot be administered with this system. The partial rebreather achieves a higher FIO_2 by using the initial portion of exhaled air that comes from the upper airways (anatomic dead space). This air is exhaled at a higher rate than the oxygen flow rate and is returned to the reservoir bag. Toward the end of exhalation, the flow rate decreases below that of the oxygen flow rate and this air (which contains more CO_2) cannot return to the reservoir bag. Thus, in a partial rebreather the reservoir bag has a high oxygen content. In a nonrebreather, none of the expired air is allowed to return to the bag, so the reservoir bag can attain a content of 100% oxygen.

4. **High-flow oxygen masks** deliver a constant FIO_2 regardless of changes in ventilatory patterns. In patients with chronic hypercapnia ("CO_2 retainers") an increase in FIO_2 can result in more CO_2 retention; therefore, delivering a *constant* FIO_2 is desirable in this setting. The problem with high-flow oxygen masks is the inability to deliver a high FIO_2.

5. **Toxicity of oxygen therapy.** The lungs are protected by a concentrated supply of endogenous antioxidants; however, when there is too much oxygen or not enough of the antioxidants, the lungs may be damaged as in the acute respiratory distress syndrome (ARDS). An FIO_2 of less than 0.6 is considered a safe concentration of inhaled oxygen (*Crit Care Clin*, 6/749, 1990). **Oxygen therapy with an FIO_2 above 0.6 for longer than 48 hours is considered toxic.** If such therapy is used, mechanical ventilation or positive end-expiratory pressure (PEEP) should be considered to reduce FIO_2. One must keep in mind that, in critically ill patients, levels of protective endogenous antioxidants may be depleted. In this population, any FIO_2 higher than 0.21 (room air level) may be toxic. To prevent oxygen toxicity, the following guidelines can be observed.

   a. Oxygen therapy should be used only when indicated. Indications include arterial PaO_2 of less than 55 mm Hg, evidence of tissue dysoxia (i.e., blood lactate levels higher than 4 mmol/L), and increased risk of tissue dysoxia (i.e., cardiac index of less than 2 L/minute/m² or mixed venous oxygen saturation (SvO_2) of less than 50%).

   b. The lowest tolerable FIO_2 below 0.60 should be used.

   c. Antioxidant protection should be maintained by evaluating and supplementing the selenium and vitamin E supply.

C. **Modes of positive pressure mechanical ventilation.** Mechanical ventilation should be considered for a patient when the thought arises during evaluation of a patient exhibiting respiratory distress. More specific indicators that can be used to help decide whether a patient should be intubated are a respiratory rate higher than 35 breaths/minute, PaO_2 less than 60 mm Hg, $PaCO_2$ higher than 46 mm Hg with a pH less than 7.35, and absent gag reflex. The standard ventilator type is a volume-cycled device that delivers a preset volume of air.

1. **Assist-control ventilation (ACV).** In this mode of ventilation, each patient-initiated breath is "assisted" by a ventilator-delivered breath; when the patient cannot initiate a breath, the ventilator delivers a breath at a preset "controlled" rate and volume. Disadvantages of ACV arise in tachypneic patients and include respiratory alkalosis (from overventilation) and lung hyperinflation. An intrinsic form of PEEP called auto-PEEP can accompany hyperinflation.

2. **Intermittent mandatory ventilation (IMV)** was designed to address the disadvantages of ACV. IMV delivers a breath at a preset rate and volume, but allows the patient to breathe at a spontaneous rate and volume between machine breaths without machine assistance. In synchronized IMV, machine breaths are synchronized to occur with spontaneous respirations to avoid "stacking" of breaths and thus avoid respiratory alkalosis and lung hyperinflation. Asynchronous IMV is less favored as it delivers machine breaths at any time (during patient exhalation). Contrary to popular belief, the diaphragm does not rest during mechanical ventilation. Instead, the diaphragm, directed by brainstem neurons, contracts throughout a respiration. In IMV, the increased resistance created by ventilator tubing results in increased work of breathing by the diaphragm. *The work of breathing can be reduced by adding pressure support.* ACV should be chosen when a patient has respiratory muscle weakness or a history of left ventricular dysfunction, and IMV should be selected to avoid respiratory alkalosis or hyperinflation. Otherwise, there is no proven superiority of IMV over ACV, or vice versa. One mode is usually more popular in a given ICU based on personal preference.

3. **Pressure-controlled ventilation (PCV)** is pressure-cycled breathing that delivers controlled breaths at a constant pressure by decreasing the inspiratory flow rate as the breath progresses. Large inflation volumes in volume-controlled ventilation modes of ACV and IMV can result in lung injury. PCV minimizes this form of lung injury; however, the disadvantage of PCV is that inflation volumes vary with changes in the mechanical properties of the lungs. PCV is well suited for patients with neuromuscular disease, as their lung mechanics remain constant.

4. **Inverse-ratio ventilation (IRV)** results from setting a prolonged inflation time in PCV. The inspiratory to expiratory ratio during a normal inspiration is 1:2 to 1:4. In IRV, the inspiratory to expiratory ratio reverses to 2:1. Although the prolonged inflation time prevents alveolar collapse, there is an increased risk of hyperinflation and auto-PEEP, which lead to a reduced cardiac output. The main indication for IRV is refractory hypoxemia or hypercapnia in patients with ARDS with conventional modes of mechanical ventilation.

5. **Pressure-support ventilation (PSV)** allows the patient to breathe spontaneously and keeps the inflation pressure constant (preset pressure is usually from 5 to 10 cm H_2O) by adding inspired gas to augment the patient's inspiration. Pressure support is usually used to augment respirations in IMV by providing just enough pressure to overcome the added resistance of ventilatory tubes. PSV is commonly used as a weaning mode of ventilation. The degree of PSV required to support a tidal volume is dependent on the compliance of the patient's lungs and chest wall, as well as neuromuscular strength. PSV can be used as a noninvasive method of mechanical ventilation through specialized face masks or nasal masks with inflation pressures of 20 cm H_2O.

D. **Ventilator management**
   1. **Fraction of inspired oxygen.** Although it has been stressed that oxygen therapy can be toxic, in the acute phase of respiratory distress, hypoxemia is more detrimental than high levels of oxygen. The initial FIO_2 should be 100%, and it should then be brought down to the mini-

mum level needed to keep the PaO_2 above 60 mm Hg or the SaO_2 above 90%. In severe cases of ARDS, a lower saturation (88%) and PaO_2 (55 mm Hg) may be tolerated.

2. **Minute ventilation** is determined by the respiratory rate and tidal volume (TV). Normal minute ventilation is usually 6–8 L/minute, but it depends on the patient's size and metabolic state. Inflammatory conditions, infection, and acid-base disorders are common reasons for large variations in minute ventilation.

3. **Positive end-expiratory pressure** is the maintenance of positive airway pressure (alveolar pressure above atmospheric pressure) at the end of respiration. PEEP prevents end-expiratory alveolar collapse, which results in improved gas exchange and increased lung compliance.

   a. **Extrinsic PEEP** is created by a device that stops exhalation at a preselected pressure. PEEP reduces the risk of oxygen toxicity by improving gas exchange that increases the PaO_2 and ultimately allows a reduction in the inspired FIO_2.

   b. **Intrinsic PEEP (auto-PEEP)** is created by increasing minute ventilation or shortening expiratory time enough to promote hyperinflation. Auto-PEEP is also commonly seen in conditions that require a prolonged expiratory effort, such as asthma. In this patient population, sudden cardiovascular collapse may occur with auto-PEEP, and, irrespective of whether it is intrinsic or extrinsic auto-PEEP, the patient should be immediately disconnected from the ventilator and allowed to exhale. This may take 30–60 seconds, but it is life-saving.

   Patients with PEEP higher than 10 cm H_2O should not be weaned suddenly, as this can result in distal lung collapse. Instead, weaning should be done in PEEP increments of 3 to 5 cm H_2O.

   On morning rounds, the specific ventilatory settings, actual patient respiratory rate, spontaneous TV, minute ventilation, and most recent arterial blood gas values should be presented. Ventilatory settings reported should include mode, rate, TV, PEEP, FIO_2, and pressure support.

E. **Weaning from mechanical ventilation.** After intubation, the goal is to wean the patient from mechanical ventilation. Weaning is generally considered the process of removing an individual from mechanical ventilation. Although extubation is the removal of the endotracheal tube or its equivalent, no uniform weaning process is accepted across all disciplines as an optimal method. Today, T-piece weaning, pressure support, and synchronous intermittent mandatory ventilation weaning are all used in certain patient populations. T-piece trials and weaning per a respiratory care protocol are currently the most popular methods. Once a patient is on minimal ventilatory settings (i.e., FIO_2 less than 50%, IMV 2, pressure support less than 5, PEEP less than 5, or a T-piece), then a decision to proceed with extubation should be made promptly. Time on mechanical ventilation and intubation is directly related to complications, especially ventilator-associated pneumonia. Extubation parameters follow.

1. **General.** The patient should be clinically well, on a path to recovery with a defined and treated illness. For instance, the patient should not be in the midst of a myocardial infarction, be hemodynamically unstable from sepsis, or require significant ongoing volume supplementation to maintain hemodynamic stability. The patient should be warm (above 35°C) and should have undergone reversal of any neuromuscular blockade.

2. **Neurologic status.** The patient should be asked if he or she would like to be extubated. Is the patient alert, oriented, and cooperative? Can the patient follow commands?

3. **Airway.** If the patient has facial edema or there is a concern about the patency of the supraglottic airway, it is usually advisable to perform the

"cuff test": The tube cuff is deflated, the endotracheal tube is occluded, and the patient is asked to breathe in and out around the tube. This test allows one to assess the diameter of the airway around the tube. The normal-sized patient should be able to breathe both in and out around a normal-sized tube. One should consider advanced methods of extubation if the patient fails a cuff test and one wishes to proceed with extubation.

4. **Arterial blood gases.** The patient should maintain normal arterial blood gas levels on supplemental oxygen at an FIO_2 of less than 60%. The patient should have a PaO_2 of greater than 60 mm Hg, a PCO_2 of between 35 and 45 mm Hg, and a pH of between 7.35 and 7.45. Patients with known pulmonary disease, especially those who have chronic obstructive pulmonary disease and require oxygen at home, may require low FIO_2 and may have an elevated partial pressure of carbon dioxide (PCO_2) at baseline. For anyone with baseline disease, values should be assessed on an individual basis.

5. **Respiration mechanics**
   a. **Forced vital capacity (FVC)** should be **at least** 10 mL/kg. In most normal patients FVC should be 1000 mL. This measurement is effort dependent and can vary widely depending on the patient as well as on the individual measuring the FVC. A patient who cannot cooperate for FVC testing or who cannot understand the directions may also be unable to follow good pulmonary care when extubated.
   b. **Negative inspiratory force (NIF).** Although the range of "acceptable" NIF is –20 to –30, a generally accepted NIF is –25. This measurement is *not* effort dependent when done as an "occlusion NIF." It is a measure of the patient's ability to suck in a deep breath. NIF may also be a proxy for the ability to cough.
   c. **Rapid shallow breathing index (RSBI, Tobin index).** The RSBI or Tobin index is a measure of the patient's ability to remain extubated for 24 hours after extubation. The measurement is obtained by placing the patient on continuous positive airway pressure of 5 for 1 minute (from *any* vent setting) and then assessing the patient's respiratory rate (f) and the patient's TV in liters:
   RSBI = f/TV.
   If the RSBI is less than 80, the patient is eight to nine times more likely to remain extubated than not. If the RSBI value is above 100, the patient is eight to nine times more likely to require reintubation. Values between 80 and 100 do not contribute additional information beyond the bedside clinical judgment regarding the suitability of the patient to be extubated.

6. **Secretions and cough.** Although no guide exists to the assessment of secretions and cough, the practitioner should be aware of the presence of a large amount of secretion and should assess the patient's ability to clear these secretions when present, from both a strength and sensorium standpoint. Once a patient is extubated, a humidified oxygen-delivering face mask should be given. The patient should also be instructed to take deep breaths and cough regularly. If a patient requires reintubation, extubation should not be attempted for 24–72 hours. A complete assessment of the reason for failure of extubation should be made, and issues identified should be corrected before another attempt at extubation.

II. **Postoperative care**
A. **Routine postoperative care**
   1. The **formula for fluid administration** for any individual who has no intake is the **4-2-1 rule.** For the first 10 kg of weight, 40 mL/hour of intravenous (IV) fluid should be given. For the next 10 kg of weight, 20 mL/hour of IV fluid should be given. Therefore, for the first 20 kg of

weight, 60 mL/hour of IV fluid should be administered. For the next 1 kg of weight, 1 mL/hour of fluid should be given. *Although maintenance fluid is theoretically considered to be 5% dextrose, 0.25% normal saline, and 20% KCl, based on sodium needs, postoperative hormonal stress states cause universal hyponatremia if hypotonic fluids are used. This finding is especially prominent in young women having gynecologic surgery. Therefore, a strong preference exists for the administration of isotonic fluids, certainly for resuscitation.*

2. **Patient evaluation.** All inpatients undergoing a surgical procedure should be seen and evaluated after surgery. The time interval of this assessment should be determined in part by the severity of illness, and more than one assessment may be required. All patients, however, should be seen at least once. In this evaluation, recovery from anesthesia, control of pain, assessment of respiratory effort and adequacy, and hemodynamic assessments should be made. This evaluation should be documented in the medical record. Special attention should be given to the adequacy of intravascular volume, with pulse, BP, and fluid intake and output as basic determinants of satisfactory volume. Adequacy of intraoperative fluid administration should be assessed and a special note should be made of any ascites drained. *On-going cardiac output and intravascular volume are commonly considered adequate if the urine output is higher than 0.5 mL/kg [ideal body weight for women = 45 kg + (2.3 kg × each inch of height over 5 ft) in the absence of glucosuria].* If the urine output is low, the patient should be assessed for the possibility of bleeding or insensible third space losses. Intraoperative insensible losses can be approximated as 250 mL/hour per quadrant, on the assumption that the abdomen/pelvis is divided into four quadrants. An isotonic fluid bolus of 10 mL/kg can be administered to test the volume status of a patient who is not hypotensive, whereas 20 mL/kg is generally preferred in a hypotensive hypovolemic patient.

3. **Daily weight measurements** should be recorded for patients who are at higher risk of postoperative fluid imbalances (i.e., patients with cardiovascular, pulmonary, or renal problems, patients in prolonged cases, or patients in whom fluid losses may be in question).

4. **Incentive spirometry** should be used as a way to encourage the patient to take deep breaths and cough.

5. **Prophylaxis for deep venous thrombosis (DVT)** should be considered. The minimum for medium- and high-risk patients is the use of thromboembolic disease stockings and sequential compression devices. In some patients at risk for postoperative DVT, anticoagulation with heparin sodium is advised. These patients include those with underlying malignancy, a history of DVT or pulmonary embolism, obesity, hypercoagulable states, and prolonged abdominal or pelvic surgery.

6. **Prophylactic antibiotics** are indicated *before* and *during* the operation. They are of *no incremental benefit* when used for prophylaxis outside of the operating room. Use of antibiotics beyond this time period, and certainly beyond 24 hours after a surgical procedure, should be *strongly* discouraged. Of course, patients to whom antibiotics are administered for a proven or suspected infection (i.e., as therapy) are exempt from this policy.

B. **Common postoperative problems**
1. **Postoperative hypertension.** A systolic BP more than 40 mm Hg above the baseline or a mean arterial pressure more than 15 mm Hg above baseline is often considered significant hypertension. The ill effects of hypertension are based on long-term effects and not short-term consequences, except, of course, in patients who are at risk of hypertension, that is, those with coronary artery disease, and so on.

a. The cause of hypertension should be assessed carefully.
   (1) Inadequacy of pain control. The patient is awake, usually alert, and complaining of pain. This cause should be treated with aggressive pain management, especially with narcotics.
   (2) Hypercarbia may be the cause, especially when the patient is somnolent, hypertensive, and tachycardic. **Caution:** Administration of additional narcotics to these patients or failure to consider hypercarbia as the cause can lead to respiratory arrest.
   (3) A full bladder should be considered as a possible cause of hypertension in patients without a urinary catheter.
b. In patients in whom hypertension is considered to be a specific danger (i.e., those with coronary artery disease, recent myocardial infarction, etc.), specific treatment may be rendered. The physician should consider whether the need is immediate and continuous and should therefore be treated with sodium nitroprusside, nitroglycerin, nicardipine hydrochloride, or esmolol hydrochloride or whether intermittent IV medications such as alpha- and beta-blockers or other medications the patient may have been taking previously are sufficient.

2. **Hypotension and shock**
   a. **Shock** is a clinical syndrome in which the patient shows signs of decreased perfusion of vital organs, including possible alterations in mental status with somnolence and oliguria with an output of 0.5 mL/kg/hour (with weight determined according to the formula given earlier). No absolute value is used to define hypotension in shock, but patients generally display a decrease in BP of 50–60 mm Hg or a BP of less than 100 mm Hg. In approaching a patient with shock, management begins with defining the class of shock exhibited, with the goal being fluid resuscitation and treatment of the underlying disease process. In patients with a gynecologic malignancy, the most common causes of shock in the perioperative period are hemorrhage, sepsis, postoperative myocardial infarction, and pulmonary embolus.
      Providing oxygen and insuring adequacy of ventilation are always the first step in treating a patient with shock. Shock can be classified into four varieties:
      (1) **Hypovolemic shock** secondary to bleeding or other causes of fluid loss (i.e., nasogastric suction or diarrhea)
      (2) **Distributive shock** secondary to increased venous pooling (i.e., early septic shock, peritonitis, anaphylaxis, and neurogenic shock)
      (3) **Cardiogenic shock** secondary to decreased myocardial contractility and function (as in myocardial infarction)
      (4) **Obstructive shock** or hypoperfusion state secondary to mechanical obstruction (i.e., cardiac tamponade, massive pulmonary embolism, thrombosed prosthetic valve)
   b. **Hypovolemic or hemorrhagic shock.** Acute blood loss has been classified by the American College of Surgeons based on volume of blood lost and other parameters (Table 3-1). When blood loss exceeds 30–40%, hypovolumic shock ensues, and expedient volume resuscitation is necessary. Repletion with crystalloid is at least as important as replacement of red cell losses. Volume replacement to improve BP, filling pressures, and urine output is essential. In the setting of massive hemorrhage, fresh red cells are preferred over red cells stored for longer than 1 week, as the fresh product is better at oxygen delivery due to higher levels of 2,3-DPG. For more than 25 years there has been ongoing debate over the type of solution best suited for volume replacement. The duration and rigor of the debates suggest that there is no substantial benefit to the use of one type of solution

TABLE 3-1. CLASSIFICATION OF HEMORRHAGE BASED ON EXTENT OF BLOOD LOSS

Parameter	Class I	Class II	Class III	Class IV
Blood volume lost (%)	<15	15–30	30–40	>40
Pulse rate (beats/min)	<100	>100	>120	>140
Supine blood pressure	Normal	Normal	Decreased	Decreased
Urine output (mL/hr)	>30	20–30	5–15	<5
Mental status	Anxious	Agitated	Confused	Lethargic

From Committee on Trauma. *Advanced trauma life support student manual.* Chicago: American College of Surgeons, 1989:57, with permission.

over another. In the current practice of medicine, however, one must also consider the costs of various products. All colloidal solutions are substantially more expensive than crystalloid solutions and were found to offer no substantial benefit in any of the three recent meta-analyses published on this subject. Administration of human albumin solution has been suggested in one meta-analysis to be harmful (increase in mortality when used to treat hypovolemia, low serum albumin, or burns) and has been withdrawn from general practice in England. In young patients, a hematocrit as low as 20% can be well tolerated. In older adults, however, individual assessment of the need, risks, and benefits of transfusion should be considered. In a recent large Canadian trial examining "transfusion trigger," patients who were allowed to maintain a hemoglobin level in the range of 7–9 g/dL were not harmed and in fact perhaps did better. This study has been criticized, however, for a possible selection bias in entering patients into the trial. Nonetheless, patients with the lower hemoglobin group, including those with coronary heart disease, did not suffer adverse consequences. Certainly a patient who has ongoing signs of myocardial ischemia or impaired oxygen delivery should have a hemoglobin level of 10 g/dL or above. In addition to the listed circumstances, other conditions may warrant special consideration with regard to maintaining a higher hemoglobin level. For example, it is common practice to keep the hemoglobin above 10 g/dL in a gynecologic oncologic patient who is about to undergo chemotherapy. The benefit of this strategy, however, has not been rigorously studied. What has been shown to be efficacious is a hemoglobin level above 11.5 g/dL for patients undergoing radiotherapy.

(1) **Crystalloid therapy** has the advantage of being more readily available and less costly than colloid therapy. Ringer's lactate is less acidic than normal saline (pH 6.7 versus 5.7) and can ameliorate the hyperchloremic metabolic acidosis that results when large volumes of saline are administered. Ringer's lactate does contain potassium and has less sodium than serum (130 mEq/L). There is no physiologic difference in the degree of resuscitation with each solution (Table 3-2).

(2) **Colloid therapy** is more costly in all cases than crystalloid therapy. Depending on the type and amount of solution, a colloid solution may in the short term provide more volume expansion than crystalloids. This effect, however, may not last more than 60 minutes.

TABLE 3-2. COMPOSITION OF INTRAVENOUS CRYSTALLOID FLUIDS

Preparation	Na (mEq /L)	Cl (mEq /L)	K (mEq /L)	Ca (mEq /L)	Mg (mEq /L)	Buffers	pH	Osmolality (mOsm/L)
Plasma	141	103	4–5	5	2	Bicarbonate	7.4	289
0.9% NaCl	154	154	0	0	0	0	5.7	308
7.5% NaCl	1283	1283	0	0	0	0	5.7	2567
Lactated Ringer's	130	109	4	3	0	Lactate	6.74	273
Normosol/ Plasma-lyte	140	98	5	0	3	Acetate, gluconate	7.4	295

From Marino PL. *The ICU book*, 2nd ed. Baltimore: Williams & Wilkins, 1998, with permission.

(3) **Vasoactive agents** can be used in conjunction with fluid resuscitation. Their use requires invasive monitoring (i.e., pulmonary artery catheter).

(a) **Dopamine.** The theoretical dosages and effects of dopamine are given in the following paragraphs. It should be noted, however, that there is a wide variation and overlap both within and between patients.

(i) In dosages of 2–3 µg/kg/minute, dopamine acts on renal, splanchnic, and other vascular bed receptors, causing vasodilation and increasing blood flow to these areas. These dosages are no longer commonly used for this reason. In fact, the major effect of dopamine at these dosages is to serve as a natriuretic, with sodium loss and a definite but unpredictable salt wasting.

(ii) In dosages of 4–5 µg/kg/minute, dopamine acts on cardiac beta$_1$-receptors, which results in increased cardiac contractility and cardiac output.

(iii) In dosages higher than 10 µg/kg/minute, dopamine acts on peripheral alpha-receptors and causes vasoconstriction, which results in increased BP.

(b) **Dobutamine** is a powerful inotropic agent and acts principally on beta$_1$- and beta$_2$-receptors. It causes peripheral vasodilation with only small increases in heart rate and, because of this, is generally considered as a drug to enhance cardiac performance.

(c) **Epinephrine** is chosen for anaphylactic shock and has marked alpha- and beta-adrenergic activity. Epinephrine is also useful in low doses to support cardiac performance, especially in right heart failure (i.e., from pulmonary embolus, pulmonary hypertension), because it has vasodilating effects on the pulmonary bed.

(d) **Norepinephrine** is a potent alpha and beta agent that is most frequently used in profound sepsis because it causes vasoconstriction and also enhances cardiac output. Norepinephrine provides better renal blood flow in severe sepsis when the patient is adequately resuscitated with volume than does dopamine.

    c. **Septic shock**

      (1) **Pathophysiology.** Septic shock involves the release of vasoactive kinins with vasodilation, activation of complement with increased vascular permeability, activation of the intrinsic clotting cascade with disseminated intravascular coagulation, and induction of a fibrinolytic state with bleeding. In the early stages, septic shock is a form of distributive shock. In the later stages, septic shock can demonstrate aspects of both distributive and cardiogenic shock, with myocardial depression from ischemia associated with hypotension, acidosis, and possibly myocardial depressant factors produced by the infecting organisms.

      (2) **Management.** Treatment is with aggressive fluid replacement, administration of vasopressor and inotropic agents, use of broad-spectrum antibiotics, and removal of the infectious source.

    d. **Cardiogenic shock** can also occur in the setting of septic shock or hemorrhagic shock, especially in patients who have baseline cardiovascular disease. Management requires invasive monitoring and treatment of the underlying disorder.

III. **Invasive hemodynamic monitoring**

  A. **Pulmonary artery catheter (Swan-Ganz catheter, PA catheter)**

    1. **Design.** The basic PA catheter, originated by Dr. H. J. C. Swan, is 110 cm long, 2.3 cm in diameter (7 French), and has two adjacent lumens. One lumen extends the entire length of the catheter and has its opening at the tip (distal port). The other lumen has its opening 30 cm from the catheter tip (proximal port) and is positioned in the superior vena cava or right atrium. The catheter tip has a 1.5-cc capacity balloon that, when inflated, encompasses the tip and protects surrounding tissue from contact with the tip. A thermistor is located 4 cm from the catheter tip and calculates blood flow rate (equivalent to cardiac output) by measuring the flow of cold fluid from the proximal to the distal tip.

    2. **Placement.** The PA catheter is placed in the subclavian or internal jugular vein (preferred) and its tip advanced after the balloon is inflated. The balloon acts as a sail that is "blown" by the flow of blood to guide the tip through the right atrium, right ventricle, and into the pulmonary artery. The pressure waveforms should be analyzed continuously. Once the balloon has "wedged" into a branch of the pulmonary artery, the waveform should be relatively flat, which results in a pressure reading known as the pulmonary capillary wedge pressure (PCWP). Normal PCWP is 6–12 mm Hg. At this point, the balloon should be deflated. Fatal complications can occur after placement of a PA catheter, such as PA rupture secondary to overinflation of the balloon in a distal PA branch. Ventricular tachycardia is seen commonly during insertion, and the physician placing the PA catheter should be prepared to recognize and treat this common complication.

    3. **Indications.** The PA catheter provides information on a large number of hemodynamic variables that allow assessment of cardiac performance (compliance), fluid status, and oxygen transport. It may be placed to assess fluid status in patients with high perioperative risk (i.e., those with cardiac, pulmonary, or renal disease) and those with shock, renal failure, and unexplained acidosis. The PA catheter is also helpful in distinguishing cardiogenic and noncardiogenic pulmonary edema.

  B. **Hemodynamic parameters**

    1. **Cardiovascular performance.** A parameter expressed relative to **body surface area (BSA)** is termed an **index.** BSA (m^2) = [height (cm) + weight (kg) – 60]/100. Average BSA is 1.6–1.9 m^2.

    a. **Central venous pressure (CVP)** normally ranges from 1 to 6 mm Hg. CVP reflects right atrial pressure (RAP). CVP is recorded from the proximal port of the PA catheter as this is positioned in the superior vena cava or right atrium. When there is no obstruction between the right atrium and ventricle, CVP = RAP = right ventricular end-diastolic pressure. CVP can be measured via a PA catheter as noted earlier or via a central line with its tip in the superior vena cava. For the CVP to be measured accurately, the patient should be lying on the back and not in any lateral position. The transducer should be held at the level of the right and left atria, the phlebostatic axis, the fourth intercostal space along the midaxillary line. Spontaneous variations in CVP of 4 mm Hg are not clinically significant.

b. **Pulmonary capillary wedge pressure**

(1) **Normal values.** PCWP normally ranges from 6 to 12 mm Hg. PCWP reflects left atrial pressure. PCWP is recorded when the PA catheter balloon is inflated and wedged in a branch of the pulmonary artery. When there is no obstruction between the left atrium and ventricle, PCWP = left atrial pressure = left ventricular end-diastolic pressure. Left ventricular end-diastolic pressure is considered a reflection of left ventricular preload only when ventricular compliance is normal.

(2) **ARDS versus cardiogenic pulmonary edema.** ARDS is generally diagnosed by a group of criteria that include presence of diffuse infiltrates in more than two of four quadrants on chest radiograph, most often bilateral; an impaired FIO_2/PaO_2 ratio (less than 200); and a PCWP of less than 18 if a PA catheter is in place. If the patient is a candidate for CHF and has poor oxygenation and infiltrates, a PA catheter is helpful in distinguishing between ARDS and CHF.

PCWP ≤ 18 mm Hg = ARDS
PCWP > 18 mm Hg = cardiogenic pulmonary edema

c. **Cardiac index (CI)** ranges from 2.4 to 4.0 L/minute/m². Cardiac output is measured by the thermodilution technique: A volume of cold fluid is injected through the proximal port of the PA catheter and the flow rate is detected by the thermistor. CI = cardiac output/BSA.

d. **Stroke volume index (SVI)** ranges from 40 to 70 mL/beat/m². SVI is the volume ejected by the ventricles during systole. SVI = CI/heart rate.

e. **Right ventricular ejection fraction (RVEF)** normally is 46–50%.

f. **Right ventricular end-diastolic volume (RVEDV)** ranges from 80 to 150 mL/m². RVEF is the fraction of ventricular volume ejected during systole. RVEF = stroke volume/RVEDV. Likewise, RVEDV = stroke volume/RVEF.

g. **Left ventricular stroke work index (LVSWI)** ranges from 40 to 60 g-m/m². LVSWI is the work performed by the left ventricle to eject the stroke volume into the aorta. LVSWI = [mean arterial pressure (MAP) – PCWP] × SVI × 0.0136.

h. **Right ventricular stroke work index (RVSWI)** ranges from 4 to 8 g-m/m². RVSWI is the work performed by the right ventricle to eject the stroke volume across the pulmonary vessels. RVSWI = [pulmonary artery pressure (PAP) – CVP] × SVI × 0.0136.

i. **Systemic vascular resistance index (SVRI)** ranges from 1600 to 2400 dynes-sec-m²/cm⁵. SVRI = (MAP – CVP) × 80/CI.

j. **Pulmonary vascular resistance index (PVRI)** ranges from 200 to 400 dynes-sec-m²/cm⁵. PVRI = (PAP – PCWP) × 80/CI.

2. **Oxygen transport parameters**

a. **Arterial oxygen delivery (DO_2)** ranges from 520 to 570 mL/minute-m² and is the rate of oxygen transport in arterial blood. DO_2 = CI × 13.4 × hemoglobin level × SaO_2.

b. **Mixed venous oxygen saturation** ranges from 70% to 75%. SvO_2 is the oxygen saturation in pulmonary arterial blood. It can be measured from a blood sample drawn from the distal port or as a continuous reading from a specialized PA catheter.

c. **Oxygen uptake ($\dot{V}O_2$)** ranges from 110 to 160 mL/minute-m². $\dot{V}O_2$ = CI × 13.4 × hemoglobin level × ($SaO_2 - SvO_2$).

d. **Oxygen extraction ratio (O_{2ER})** ranges from 20% to 30%. O_{2ER} is the ratio between O_2 delivery and uptake. $O_{2ER} = \dot{V}O_2/DO_2$ (× 100).

3. **Hemodynamic profiles**

a. **Right heart failure:** high CVP and RAP, low CI, high PVRI

b. **Left heart failure:** high PCWP, low CI, high SVRI

c. **Hypovolemic hypotension:** low CVP, low CI, high SVRI

d. **Cardiogenic hypotension:** high CVP, low CI, high SVRI

e. **Vasogenic hypotension:** low CVP, high CI, low SVRI

f. **Heart failure versus cardiogenic shock**

(1) Heart failure: high CVP, low CI, high SVRI, normal $\dot{V}O_2$

(2) Cardiogenic shock: high CVP, low CI, high SVRI, low $\dot{V}O_2$

IV. Fluid management and common electrolyte disorders

A. **General guidelines**

1. In a patient with no preexisting renal disease, normal size, and no disorder of water or electrolyte metabolism, a reasonable fluid maintenance regimen is 3 L/day of one-half normal saline with 20 mEq of KCl in each liter. (This is an average of 125 mL/hour.) The 4-2-1 rule as described earlier may be applied here as well.

2. In patients with significant renal impairment (glomerular filtration rate less than 25 mL/minute), potassium therapy should be given only based on serially determined potassium levels.

3. In patients who may have a defect in free water excretion due to hyponatremia or the presence of predisposing causes such as ascites, edematous disorders, or pulmonary or brain metastases, the free water content of IV fluids should be decreased by using normal saline solution.

4. Patients undergoing nasogastric suctioning should also have fluid replacement with 1 mL of hypotonic saline solution (half normal saline) for every milliliter of nasogastric suction output.

B. **Hyponatremia**

1. **Definition.** Serum sodium level of less than 135 mEq/L.

2. **Types.** Hyponatremia is the most common disorder occurring in critically ill patients and can be classified into three types (Fig. 3-1).

a. Hyponatremia associated with diminished total body sodium content and hence extracellular volume depletion

b. Hyponatremia with normal or slightly expanded extracellular volumes

c. Hyponatremia with increased total body sodium and increased extracellular volume

3. **Management** is based on appropriate diagnosis of type, treatment of the underlying condition, and correction of the sodium deficit. The major complication of hyponatremia is a metabolic encephalopathy resulting from cerebral edema and increased intracranial pressure. If the hyponatremia is corrected too rapidly, the development of a demyelinating encephalopathy or **central pontine myelinolysis** can occur. Therefore, sodium replacement must be approached with care. *The goal is to correct the plasma sodium to 130 mEq/L.* Determination of the rate of correction can be calculated as follows.

a. **Calculate the total body water and sodium deficit.**

Total body water (TBW) (L) = 50% of lean body weight (kg) in women.

$$\text{Sodium deficit (mEq)} = \text{normal TBW} \times \left[130 - \left(\begin{array}{c} \text{current plasma} \\ \text{sodium level} \end{array} \right) \right]$$

(That is, for a 60-kg woman with a sodium level of 120 mEq/L, the sodium deficit is 300 mEq.)

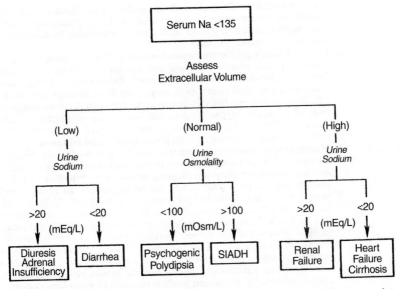

FIG. 3-1. Diagnostic approach to hyponatremia. SIADH, syndrome of inappropriate secretion of antidiuretic hormone. (From Marino PL. *The ICU book*, 2nd ed. Baltimore: Williams & Wilkins, 1998, with permission.)

b. **Calculate the volume of hypertonic saline needed** to correct the calculated sodium deficit.

Three percent NaCl solutions contain 513 mEq/L of sodium. Isotonic saline contains 154 mEq/L.

$$\text{Volume of 3\% NaCl needed} = \frac{\text{Sodium deficit (mEq)}}{513 \text{ mEq/L}}$$

(That is, the 60-kg woman in the earlier example with a deficit of 300 mEq requires 585 mL of 3% NaCl.)

$$\frac{\text{Volume of 0.9\%}}{\text{normal saline}} = \frac{\text{Sodium deficit (mEq)}}{154 \text{ mEq/L}} \left(\begin{array}{c} \text{or just multiply volume} \\ \text{of 3\% NaCl needed by 3.3} \end{array} \right)$$

c. Calculate the rate of infusion for the volume needed. The rate of infusion should be no greater than 0.5 mEq/L/hour.

$$\frac{\text{Number of hours needed}}{\text{for correction}} = \frac{[130 - (\text{current plasma sodium level})]}{0.5}$$

(That is, for the example given earlier, 20 hours will be required for correction.)

$$\text{Fluid rate} = \frac{(\text{volume of hypertonic solution needed})}{(\text{number of hours needed})}$$

(That is, the rate required for the earlier example is 29 mL/hour.)

C. **Hypokalemia**
   1. **Definition.** Serum potassium level of less than 3.5 mEq/L.

2. **Causes** include artifactual result of dilution of the blood sample (i.e., sample is drawn over an IV site), decreased dietary potassium, insufficient replacement in a patient with a nasogastric tube, laxative abuse, diarrhea, or diuretic therapy.

3. **Clinical findings.** Severe hypokalemia (less than 2.5 mEq/L) may be associated with muscle weakness and mental status changes. Milder forms of hypokalemia can be asymptomatic. Other findings include ileus mimicking intestinal obstruction, and tetany. ECG findings are nonspecific for hypokalemia but can demonstrate flattened T waves and presence of U waves. Hyperglycemia can occur from diminished insulin secretion. Chronic hypokalemia can result in renal tubular disorders with concentrating abnormalities, phosphaturia, and azotemia.

4. **Management** involves treating the underlying cause and replenishing potassium. Unless potassium levels are severely depleted, the patient is also on digoxin, or there are ongoing arrhythmias, repletion of potassium is not emergent and should not be aggressive. In these special cases, the goal is to bring the potassium level to 4.0 mEq/L. In general, for each 10 mEq of KCl given either orally or IV, there is a rise in serum KCl by 1 mEq/L. *Rapid increases in serum potassium levels can result in fatal myocardial depression; therefore, patients should not receive more than 40 mEq/hour IV, and IV administration should be performed cautiously only in those patients with a documented need.* In patients who are taking a potassium-sparing diuretic or who have renal failure, close monitoring of potassium levels is required to avoid hyperkalemia. Magnesium depletion promotes urinary potassium losses and can cause a refractory hypokalemia; therefore, magnesium should be replenished in all hypokalemic patients with normal renal function. Magnesium levels do not reflect active levels of the element (ionized), and their measurement is generally not helpful unless the patient has impaired renal function or is receiving a magnesium infusion.

D. **Hyperkalemia** is not as well tolerated as hypokalemia and can be life-threatening.

1. **Definition.** Serum potassium level of more than 5.5 mEq/L.

2. **Causes** include an artifactual result from a hemolyzed specimen (reported in 20% of blood samples with an elevated K^+ level), redistribution associated with acidosis (i.e., diabetic ketoacidosis), renal insufficiency, adrenal insufficiency, and cellular breakdown due to hemolysis or rhabdomyolysis.

3. **Clinical findings.** The majority of patients, even those with dangerous levels, have no signs or symptoms of hyperkalemia. ECG changes can be found when the serum potassium level reaches 6 mEq/L. The earliest ECG finding is peaked T waves, followed by P-wave flattening, prolonged PR intervals, P-wave disappearance, widened QRS complexes, and ultimately ventricular fibrillation or asystole. Hyperkalemia is a medical emergency.

4. **Management.** An unexpected finding of hyperkalemia in an asymptomatic patient warrants an immediate repeat measurement, because hemolysis of specimens is not uncommon. If the level is elevated on a reliable repeat sample, acute management of hyperkalemia should be guided by the serum potassium level and ECG findings (Table 3-3).

E. **Hypercalcemia**

1. **Definition.** Total serum calcium level of more than 12 mg/dL or ionized calcium level of more than 3.0 mmol/L.

2. **Causes.** In 90% of cases the underlying cause is hyperparathyroidism or malignancy, with malignancy the most common cause of severe hypercalcemia (total serum calcium level above 14 mg/dL or ionized calcium level above 3.5 mmol/L). In gynecologic oncology patients, the most common mechanism is increased osteoclastic bone resorption without direct bone involvement by tumor.

TABLE 3-3. MANAGEMENT OF HYPERKALEMIA

Clinical findings	Management
K < 6 mEq/L and *no* ECG changes	Treatment of the underlying cause and careful monitoring of K levels and ECG changes.
K 6.0–7.0 and no ECG findings, OR after acute phase	Sodium polystyrene sulfonate (Kayexalate):
	30 g PO in 50 mL of 20% sorbitol (oral dosing preferred).
	Sodium polystyrene sulfonate should *never* be administered rectally due to the possibility of colonic necrosis.
K > 6.0 and *any* ECG findings (i.e., peaked T waves, QRS widening and loss of P waves)	Calcium gluconate (10%) 10 mL IV over 3 mins; usual effect lasts 20 mins, can repeat in 20–30 mins. Calcium stabilizes the myocardium and should be the first medication given to a hyperkalemic patient with ECG changes. (A third dose is not effective if there was no response to the second dose.)
	To facilitate the movement of potassium into cells:
	IV glucose and insulin (10 U regular insulin in 500 mL of 20% dextrose; infuse over 1 hr. (This treatment should lower the serum K by 1 mEq/L for 1–2 hrs.)
	Sodium bicarbonate (44–88 mEq); this should not be given in the same IV as calcium, however, because it binds calcium and forms calcium carbonate precipitates.
	To enhance urinary excretion, loop diuretics and furosemide can be used but are ineffective in renal failure.
ECG changes and circulatory compromise	Calcium chloride (10%) one ampule (10 mL) IV over 3 mins. It contains three times more elemental calcium than calcium gluconate.
Atrioventricular block refractory to calcium treatment	IV insulin and glucose, 10 U regular insulin in 500 mL of 20% dextrose, infuse over 1 hr. (This treatment should lower the serum K by 1 mEq/L for 1–2 hrs.)
	Transvenous pacemaker.
Digitalis cardiotoxicity	**Do not use calcium for hyperkalemia related to digitalis toxicity**.
	Magnesium sulfate, 2-g IV bolus.
	Digitalis-specific antibodies if necessary.
Renal failure	Hemodialysis is the most effective treatment for these patients.

3. **Clinical findings** are usually nonspecific and can appear when total serum calcium level is above 12 mg/dL or ionized calcium level is above 3.0 mmol/L. GI findings include nausea, vomiting, constipation, ileus, abdominal pain, pancreatitis, and elevations in serum amylase levels. Cardiovascular findings include hypovolemia and hypotension, but some patients have hypertension, prolonged PR, and shortened QT intervals. Renal findings include polyuria, polydipsia, and nephrocalcinosis. Neurologic findings include lethargy, confusion, depressed consciousness, and coma.
4. **Management** in the acute phase includes the following.
   a. **Hydration with isotonic saline to promote renal calcium excretion,** because hypercalciuria can produce an osmotic diuresis

TABLE 3-4. EXPECTED CHANGES IN ACID-BASE DISORDERS

Primary disorder	Expected changes
Metabolic acidosis	$P_{CO_2} = 1.5 \times HCO_3 + (8 \pm 2)$
Metabolic alkalosis	$P_{CO_2} = 0.7 \times HCO_3 + (21 \pm 2)$
Acute respiratory acidosis	$\Delta pH = 0.008 \times (P_{CO_2} - 40)$
Chronic respiratory acidosis	$\Delta pH = 0.003 \times (P_{CO_2} - 40)$
Acute respiratory alkalosis	$\Delta pH = 0.008 \times (40 - P_{CO_2})$
Chronic respiratory alkalosis	$\Delta pH = 0.017 \times (40 - P_{CO_2})$

Δ pH, change in pH.
From Marino PL. *The ICU book*, 2nd ed. Baltimore: Williams & Wilkins, 1998, with permission.

leading to hypovolemia. Administration of isotonic saline allows for natriuresis, which promotes renal calcium excretion. One should be sure to replace the urine output with isotonic saline.

b. **Furosemide** (40–80 mg IV every 2 hours) should be given to promote further urinary calcium excretion, with the goal of 100–200 mL/hour of urine output. This output must be replaced with isotonic saline or hypovolemia will result, which defeats the purpose of hydration and diuresis.

c. **Calcitonin** (salmon calcitonin 4 U/kg subcutaneously or intramuscularly every 12 hours) inhibits bone resorption and thus addresses the underlying issue of bone resorption. The onset of action is a few hours and the effect is not profound: only a maximal drop in serum calcium of 0.5 mmol/L.

d. **Hydrocortisone** (200 mg IV daily in two or three divided doses) inhibits lymphoid neoplastic tissue growth and enhances vitamin D action.

e. **Pamidronate disodium** (90 mg IV continuous infusion over 24 hours) is more potent than calcitonin in inhibiting bone resorption. The peak effect is 4–5 days, and the dose can be repeated then if necessary.

f. **Plicamycin** (25 µg/kg IV over 4 hours, repeated in 24–48 hours if necessary) is an antineoplastic agent that inhibits bone resorption and is more potent than calcitonin. This agent is not commonly used as it has a potential for bone marrow suppression and other adverse affects. Pamidronate is favored over plicamycin.

g. **Dialysis** (hemodialysis or peritoneal dialysis) is effective in patients with renal failure.

V. **Acid-base disorders.** To assess acid-base disorders, values for interpretation are obtained from arterial blood gas measurements. Normal values are as follows:

pH = 7.36–7.44, P_{CO_2} = 36–44 mm Hg, HCO_3 = 22–26 mEq/L (Table 3-4).

A. **Approach to interpretation: assessment of pH and P_{CO_2}.**

1. A **primary metabolic disorder** is present if the pH is abnormal and the change in pH and P_{CO_2} are in the same direction.

a. In **primary metabolic acidosis,** the pH is less than 7.36 and the P_{CO_2} is decreased. In **primary metabolic alkalosis,** the pH is higher than 7.44 and the P_{CO_2} is increased.

b. **Calculate the expected P_{CO_2} with full respiratory compensation.**

2. A **primary respiratory disorder** is present if the P_{CO_2} is abnormal and the change in pH and P_{CO_2} are in opposite directions.

a. In **primary respiratory acidosis,** the P_{CO_2} is higher than 44 mm Hg and the pH is decreased. In **primary respiratory alkalosis,** the P_{CO_2} is less than 36 mm Hg and the pH is increased.

b. **Calculate the expected change in pH.** In **acute (uncompensated) respiratory acidosis or alkalosis,** the change in pH is 0.008 times the change in P_{CO_2}. In **chronic (fully compensated) respiratory acidosis or alkalosis,** the change in pH is 0.003 times the change in P_{CO_2}. When the change in pH is 0.003–0.008 times the change in P_{CO_2}, then the respiratory disorder is **partially compensated.** If the change in pH is more than 0.008 times the change in P_{CO_2}, then a superimposed metabolic disorder is present (i.e., **a superimposed metabolic acidosis in the setting of a primary metabolic acidosis**).

3. A **mixed (acidosis and alkalosis) disorder** is present in two circumstances:
   a. The P_{CO_2} is abnormal and the pH is unchanged or normal
   b. The pH is abnormal and the P_{CO_2} is unchanged or normal

4. **Calculation of the anion gap in metabolic acidosis** permits distinguishing the cause of metabolic acidosis as an accumulation of hydrogen ions or a loss of bicarbonate ions.

   Anion gap = $[Na^+ + K^+] - [Cl^- + HCO_3^-]$ (normal range is 10–14 mEq/L).

   Of note, a 50% reduction in the level of plasma proteins can result in a 75% reduction in the anion gap.

   a. **Causes of normal anion gap acidosis** (mnemonic **USEDCAR**) include: **U**terosigmoidostomy, **S**aline administration (in the face of renal dysfunction), **E**ndocrine disorder (Addison's disease; treatment with spironolactone, triamterene, amiloride hydrochloride; primary hyperparathyroidism), **D**iarrhea, **C**arbonic anhydrase inhibitors, **A**mmonium chloride, and **R**enal tubular acidosis.

   b. **Causes of increased anion gap acidosis** (mnemonic **MUDPIILES**) include: **M**ethanol, **U**remia, **D**iabetes (ketoacidosis), **P**araldehyde, **I**soniazid, **I**nfection, **L**actic acidosis, **E**thylene glycol, **S**alicylates.

B. **Treatment** is based on the severity of the process. In most situations, treatment of the underlying cause is the only therapy necessary. In patients with profound disturbances, pH less than 7.2 or bicarbonate levels less than 10 mEq/L, bicarbonate therapy should be considered. This therapy should be approached carefully, as there is a theoretical risk of causing a transient worsening of the cerebrospinal fluid pH level or of inducing fluid overload and rebound metabolic alkalosis.

VI. **Oliguria** is the most frequently encountered acute renal problem in critical care medicine.

A. **Definitions**
   1. **Oliguria** is defined as a urine output of less than 400 mL/day. Although low urine output is generally defined as less than 25–30 mL/hour, many clinicians do not take into account the fact that urine output is dependent on body weight. Therefore, minimal adequate urine output should be calculated by the following formula:

$$\text{Urine output} = 0.5 \text{ mL/kg} \left[\substack{\text{ideal body} \\ \text{weight for women}} = 45 + \left(2.3 \times \substack{\text{height in inches} \\ \text{above 5 ft}} \right) \right]$$

   2. **Acute oliguric renal failure (AORF)** is identified by oliguria, as defined by the formula given earlier, accompanied by any of the following:
      a. An increase in serum creatinine of at least 50% over baseline
      b. An increase in serum creatinine of at least 0.5 mg/dL above baseline
      c. A reduction in calculated creatinine clearance of at least 50%
      d. Severe renal dysfunction requiring some form of renal replacement therapy

B. **Differential diagnoses of AORF** can be classified into prerenal, renal, and postrenal causes.

1. **Prerenal disorders** account for approximately 50% of cases of AORF and result from decreased renal perfusion. In gynecology, the most common prerenal cause of oliguria is volume depletion from either inadequate fluid repletion or hemorrhage. Other causes include hypotension, heart failure, renal vasoconstriction (i.e., from nonsteroidal anti-inflammatory drugs), and reduced glomerular filtration pressure (i.e., from angiotensin-converting enzyme inhibitors). A prerenal cause of AORF is supported by an elevated specific gravity, a fractional excretion of sodium (FE_{Na}) of less than 1%, a BUN/creatinine ratio of 20 or more, a urinary sodium ($urine_{Na}$) level of less than 20 mEq/L, or some combination of these.

2. **Intrinsic renal disorders,** as the name implies, result from injuries to and dysfunction of the renal parenchyma. They can be classified into three types of disorders: acute tubular necrosis (ATN), acute glomerulonephritis, and acute interstitial nephritis. Of these, ATN is the most common intrinsic renal cause of AORF. The most common causes of ATN are sepsis, shock, and exposure to toxins (i.e., radiocontrast dye, aminoglycosides, pigments, and uric acid). In ATN, there is damage to the renal tubules and surrounding parenchyma without damage to the glomeruli from ischemia and inflammatory cell injury. Of note, necrosis of the tubes may not necessarily exist. Injured tubular epithelial cells that have been shed off block the proximal tubular lumen, which reduces the net glomerular filtration pressure and results in a decreased glomerular filtration rate. Laboratory evidence for ATN includes an FE_{Na} of more than 2% or $urine_{Na}$ higher than 40 mEq/L. Consideration should be given to the fact that ATN can be seen as part of multiorgan failure, and therapy should be directed at the primary cause rather than the kidneys alone in this situation.

3. **Postrenal disorders** rarely give rise to oliguria unless only a single functioning kidney exists. Postrenal disorders result from obstruction of the urinary tract distal to the renal tissue: collecting system (i.e., papillary necrosis), ureters (i.e., transection, compression, clot, calculus, tumor, sloughed papillae), bladder (i.e., calculus, neurogenic bladder, carcinoma, clot), and urethra (i.e., calculus, stricture, clot). Early treatment can prevent permanent renal damage. Assessment usually involves bladder catheterization and urinary tract ultrasonography. Postobstructive diuresis is the significant increase in urinary flow after resolution of bilateral postrenal obstruction. This diuresis can result in electrolyte depletion and intravascular volume contraction. In an over-distended obstructed bladder, sudden emptying may cause capillary bleeding, hematuria, and even hemorrhage. This is not common but does occur, and one should be cautious and watch expectantly when decompressing a bladder containing more than 500 mL and certainly for one containing more than 1000 mL.

C. **Laboratory assessment**

1. **Urinalysis and urine microscopy.** The specific gravity of urine (normal range, 1.003–1.030) is elevated in the setting of dehydration and is a reflection of the concentrating ability of the kidneys. False elevations in specific gravity can result from administration of mannitol, glucose, and radiocontrast dye. Urine microscopy is not helpful in identifying prerenal causes of AORF; however, it is helpful in distinguishing intrinsic disorders. The presence of large amounts of tubular epithelial cells and epithelial cell (granular) casts is pathognomonic for ATN (ischemic damage). White cell casts suggest interstitial nephritis (pyelonephritis). Red blood cell casts suggest glomerulonephritis. Pigmented casts suggest myoglobinuria. In postrenal cases involving collection system disorders, sloughed papilla from papillary necrosis can be seen.

2. **Urinary sodium level** is best calculated by means of a 24-hour urine collection; however, a randomly obtained specimen of 10 mL may be

used as well. A urine$_{Na}$ of less than 20 mEq/L suggests a prerenal disorder. In renal hypoperfusion, sodium reabsorption increases and sodium excretion decreases. Urine$_{Na}$ higher than 40 mEq/L suggests impaired sodium reabsorption and thus an intrinsic renal disorder. However, a level higher than 40 mEq/L does not rule out a prerenal disorder. An elevated urine$_{Na}$ level can be seen in cases of coexisting prerenal and renal disorders as well as in the setting of diuretic therapy. In elderly patients, there is an obligatory sodium loss that can elevate the urine$_{Na}$ level in prerenal states.

3. **Fractional excretion of sodium** is the fraction of sodium filtered at the glomerulus that is excreted in the urine. Normally, FE$_{Na}$ is less than 1%. Calculation of this value in the setting of oliguria is one of the most reliable tests for distinguishing prerenal causes from renal causes of AORF. A 10-mL randomly collected urine specimen is taken for assay of sodium and creatinine (urine$_{Cr}$) levels. A blood sample is also taken for assay of sodium (plasma$_{Na}$) and creatinine (plasma$_{Cr}$) levels. FE$_{Na}$ is then calculated by the following formula:

$$\frac{Urine_{Na}/Plasma_{Na}}{Urine_{Cr}Plasma_{Cr}} \times 100$$

When a patient is oliguric, an FE$_{Na}$ lower than 1% suggests a prerenal disorder and an FE$_{Na}$ higher than 2% suggests an intrinsic renal disorder.

4. **Creatinine clearance (Cl$_{Cr}$)** is best measured from values obtained from a 24-hour urine collection, according to the following formula:

$$Cl_{Cr}(ml/min) = \frac{Cr_{urine}(mg/dl) \times volume\ of\ urine(mL)}{Cr_{serum}(mg/dl) \times time(min)}$$

where Cr$_{urine}$ is the urinary level of creatinine and Cr$_{serum}$ is the serum creatinine level.

A 24-hour urine collection is best accomplished by discarding the first void and then collecting the voids thereafter for 24 hours. The specimen should be refrigerated during the collection at 4°C. Cl$_{Cr}$ reference range for women is 72–110 mL/minute (at the Johns Hopkins Central Laboratories). Renal impairment is considered at a Cl$_{Cr}$ level of 50–70 mL/minute, renal insufficiency at a level of 20–50 mL/minute, and renal failure at a level of 4–20 mL/minute. Of note, a serum creatinine level of 1.2 mg/dL in a pregnant patient indicates an approximately 50% reduction in glomerular filtration rate.

D. **Clinical assessment.** In approaching the assessment of oliguria, the patient should always be evaluated first. Subjective symptoms including those for hypovolemia (dizziness, chest pain, shortness of breath, palpitations), infection, and obstruction (pain, bloating) as well as signs (tachycardia, orthostatic hypotension, elevated temperature, hypertension) should be assessed, and total fluid input and output should be calculated. In the setting of oliguria, if the output exceeds the input (the patient is in negative fluid balance), hypovolemia should be considered. If the patient's fluid input exceeds the output (the patient is in positive fluid balance), inadequate cardiac output is suggested. Serum and urine laboratory tests should be performed *before* initiation of any fluid challenges or diuretic therapy. Mechanical problems with the urinary drainage catheter should be addressed (i.e., displaced bulb, obstruction that may be cleared by flushing the catheter). When testing is necessary in a low-risk patient with postoperative oliguria, if the patient has a negative fluid balance, the most cost-effective test for hypovolemia is to measure urine specific gravity. In this setting, if the specific gravity is elevated (and in the absence of substances that falsely elevate specific gravity), the patient should be given a fluid challenge. The healthy patient should tolerate a fluid challenge of 10 mL/kg of normal saline or lactated Ringer's solution run over 30 minutes. Lack of response may necessitate another fluid challenge or consideration of administering furosemide, depending on the patient's fluid status.

E. **Management.** The management of acute oliguria in a patient with invasive hemodynamic monitoring involves optimizing central hemodynamics (cardiac filling pressures and cardiac output) and increasing glomerulotubular flow. Cardiac filling pressures are measured by the CVP and PCWP. First CVP and PCWP should be assessed. If CVP is less than 4 mm Hg and PCWP is less than 8 mm Hg, volume should be infused until CVP is between 6 and 8 mm Hg and PCWP is between 12 and 15 mm Hg. Next, cardiac output should be assessed, with a CI above 3 L/minutes/m² as the goal. If the cardiac output is low, volume should be infused until CVP is 10–12 mm Hg and PCWP is close to 20 mm Hg. If the cardiac output is still low after these measures, inotropic support should be initiated. If BP is normal, a dobutamine hydrochloride drip (starting at 5 µg/kg/minute) for inotropic support should be started. If BP is low, a dopamine drip (starting at 5 µg/kg/minute) should be given for inotropic and pressure support. If oliguria persists after these measures are taken, the probable cause of renal failure is an intrinsic disorder. Although low-dose dopamine (2 µg/kg/minute) and furosemide are common treatment attempts when arriving at this situation, neither therapy has been shown to be effective. In fact, administration of low-dose dopamine may increase the risk of bowel ischemia. In patients with CHF or borderline BP, a furosemide drip (1–9 mg/hour) has a greater diuretic effect than an IV bolus. Use of furosemide in this setting may convert an oliguric renal failure into a nonoliguric renal failure and assist in fluid management. Conversion to a nonoliguric state does not influence the outcome of renal failure; however, it certainly makes the care of a critically ill patient easier. Rarely, a patient is encountered who is "furosemide dependent." Although this condition is commonly discussed, it is in fact uncommon, and most perioperative patients with oliguria, especially in the first 48 hours after surgery, are hypovolemic. If a patient is believed to be diuretic dependent, every effort should be made to ensure that volume and cardiac output are adequate before assuming that the patient is indeed diuretic deficient. *Patients who have undergone extensive gynecologic surgery involving drainage of ascites are at increased risk for oliguria, as the intravascular volume tends to be drawn into the abdominal cavity to replace the removed ascitic fluid.* Special attention should be given to following the urine output in these patients. Replacement fluids should be comprised of isotonic solutions.

4. PRECONCEPTION COUNSELING AND PRENATAL CARE

Pascale Duroseau and Karin Blakemore

I. **Preconception care and counseling** are important because they may identify women who can benefit from early intervention, such as those with diabetes mellitus or hypertension, and may help to reduce birth defects. The risk of major birth defects (with or without chromosomal abnormalities) in the general population is approximately 3%. Because organogenesis begins 17 days after fertilization, it is important to provide the optimal environment for the developing conceptus. Preconception care and education can be incorporated into any visit with a woman of childbearing age. The following issues should be discussed with both prospective parents.

   A. **Reproductive history.** Diagnosis and treatment of conditions such as uterine malformations, maternal autoimmune disease, and genital infection may lessen the risk of recurrent pregnancy loss. Review of an obstetric history when the woman is not pregnant may allow prospective parents to explore their fears, concerns, and questions. Recording the menstrual history provides an opportunity to evaluate a woman's knowledge of menstrual physiology and offer counseling about how she might use such knowledge to plan a pregnancy.

   B. Preconception assessment of **family history** for genetic risks offers a number of advantages.

      1. **Carrier screening** based on family history or the ethnic background of the couple allows relevant counseling before the first potentially affected pregnancy. Preconception recognition of carrier status allows women and their partners to be informed of autosomal recessive risks outside the emotional context of pregnancy. Knowledge of carrier status also allows both informed decision making about conception and planning for desired testing should pregnancy occur.

         a. **Tay-Sachs** disease mainly affects families of Ashkenazi Jewish and French-Canadian ancestry.

         b. **Canavan's disease** also affects families of Ashkenazi Jewish ancestry.

         c. **Beta-thalassemia** mainly affects families of Mediterranean, Southeast Asian, Indian, Pakistani, and African ancestry.

         d. **Alpha-thalassemia** mainly affects families of Southeast Asian and African ancestry.

         e. **Sickle cell anemia** mainly affects families of African, Mediterranean, Middle Eastern, Caribbean, Latin American, and Indian descent.

         f. **Cystic fibrosis** screening should be offered to patients with a family history of the disease. New recommendations suggest that all white and Jewish women be offered carrier screening.

      2. Family history can reveal risks for other genetic diseases such as **muscular dystrophy**, **fragile X syndrome**, or **Down syndrome** for which genetic counseling should be offered. Information about appropriate diagnostic tests such as chorionic villus sampling or amniocentesis can be introduced. In some instances, genetic counseling may result in a decision to forgo pregnancy or to use assisted reproductive technologies that may obviate the risk.

   C. **Medical assessment** (Tables 4-1 and 4-2). Preconception care for women with significant medical problems should include an assessment of potential risks not only to the fetus but also to the woman, should she become pregnant. Appropriate care may require close collaboration with other specialists. Risk assessment includes the following.

TABLE 4-1. PRECONCEPTION RISK ASSESSMENT: LABORATORY TESTS RECOMMENDED FOR ALL WOMEN

Hemoglobin level or hematocrit

Rh factor

Rubella factor

Urine dipstick testing (protein and sugar)

Pap smear test (for cervical cancer)

Gonococcal/chlamydial screen and pap screen

Syphilis test

Hepatitis B virus screen

Human immunodeficiency virus screen (offer)

Illicit drug screen (offer)

Adapted from U.S. Department of Health and Human Services. *Caring for our future: the content of prenatal care. A report of the PHS Export Panel.* Washington: U.S. Department of Health and Human Services, 1989, with permission.

1. **Infectious disease screening**
   a. Rubella-nonimmune women can be identified by preconception screening, and **congenital rubella syndrome** can be prevented by vaccination. No case of congenital rubella syndrome has ever been reported after rubella immunization within 3 months before or after conception.
   b. Universal screening of pregnant women for **hepatitis B virus** (HBV) has been recommended by the Centers for Disease Control and Prevention since 1988. Women with social or occupational risks for exposure to HBV should be counseled and offered vaccination.
   c. Patients at risk for **tuberculosis** should be tested if their histories of bacille Calmette-Guérin vaccination do not meet the guidelines for screening or preventive therapy.

TABLE 4-2. PRECONCEPTION RISK ASSESSMENT: LABORATORY TESTS RECOMMENDED FOR SOME WOMEN

Tuberculosis screen

Rubella IgG screen

Varicella IgG screen

Toxoplasmosis IgG screen

Cytomegalovirus IgG screen

Parvovirus B19 IgG screen

Genetic carrier screening for hemoglobinopathies, Tay-Sachs disease, Canavan's disease, or other genetic diseases

Screening for parental karyotype for habitual spontaneous abortion

IgG, immunoglobulin G.

Adapted from U.S. Department of Health and Human Services. *Caring for our future: the content of prenatal care. A report of the PHS Export Panel.* Washington: U.S. Department of Health and Human Services, 1989, with permission.

    d. **Cytomegalovirus (CMV)** screening should be offered preconceptually to women who work in neonatal ICUs, child care facilities, or dialysis units.

    e. **Parvovirus B19 IgG** may be offered preconceptually to schoolteachers and child care workers.

    f. **Toxoplasmosis** is of most concern to cat owners and people who eat or handle raw meat. Routine toxoplasmosis screening to determine antibody status before conception mainly provides reassurance to those who are already immune. Patients' cats can also be tested. Routine testing of **pregnant** women without known risk factors is **not** recommended.

    g. Screening for **varicella** antibody should be performed if a positive history cannot be obtained. The varicella zoster virus vaccine is now recommended for all nonimmune adults.

    h. **Human immunodeficiency virus (HIV)** counseling and testing should be offered confidentially and voluntarily to all women.

    i. Testing for *Neisseria gonorrhea, Chlamydia trachomatis,* and *Treponema pallidum* is often performed routinely in sexually active patients.

  2. **Evaluation of exposure to medications** includes exposure to over-the-counter and prescribed drugs. Drug use should be ascertained and information provided on the safest choices. A genetic counselor may be helpful.

    a. **Isotretinoin (Accutane),** an oral treatment approved by the U.S. Food and Drug Administration for severe cystic acne, should be avoided before conception. Isotretinoin is highly teratogenic, causing craniofacial defects (microtia, anotia).

    b. **Warfarin sodium (Coumadin),** an anticoagulant, and its derivatives have been associated with warfarin embryopathy. Because heparin sodium does not cross the placenta, women requiring anticoagulation should be encouraged to switch to heparin therapy before conception.

    c. The offspring of women treated with **anticonvulsants** for epilepsy are at increased risk for congenital malformations. Debate continues as to whether the disease process, the medication, or a combination of both causes the malformations. The patient's neurologist may feel it is appropriate to attempt withdrawal from anticonvulsants for women who have not had a seizure in at least 2 years. For women who are not candidates for anticonvulsant withdrawal, drug regimens that have the fewest teratogenic risks may be attempted.

    d. No evidence exists of teratogenicity from **oral contraceptive or contraceptive implant** use.

    e. **Vaginal spermicides** are not teratogenic to the offspring of women who conceive while using them or immediately after discontinuing their use.

D. **Nutritional assessment**

  1. The **body mass index,** defined as [weight in kilograms/(height in meters)^2], is the preferred indicator of nutritional status. Very overweight and very underweight women are at risk for poor pregnancy outcomes. Women with a history of anorexia or bulimia may benefit from both nutritional and psychological counseling before conception.

  2. **Eating habits** such as fasting, pica, eating disorders, and the use of megavitamin supplementation should be discussed. Excess use of multivitamin supplements containing vitamin A should be avoided because the estimated dietary intake of vitamin A for most women in the United States is sufficient. Vitamin A is teratogenic in humans at dosages of more than 20,000–50,000 IU daily, producing fetal malformations like those seen with isotretinoin, a synthetic derivative of vitamin A.

  3. Periconceptual intake of **folic acid** reduces the risk of neural tube defects (NTDs). The U.S. Public Health Service recommends daily sup-

plementation with 0.4 mg of folic acid for all women capable of becoming pregnant. Unless contraindicated by the presence of pernicious anemia, women who have previously carried a fetus with an NTD should take 4.0 mg of folic acid daily.

E. **Social assessment.** A social and lifestyle history should be obtained to identify potentially risky behaviors and exposures that may compromise a good reproductive outcome and to identify social, financial, and psychological issues that could affect pregnancy planning.

Assistance in answering questions about **reproductive toxicology** is available through the online database REPROTOX (http://reprotox.org). The Reproductive Toxicology Center at Columbia Hospital for Women Medical Center, one of the sponsors of REPROTOX, also offers a clinical inquiry program. Many states have teratogen hotlines or state-funded programs; the local March of Dimes is a good source for information about these and other resources.

Maternal use of **alcohol, tobacco, and other mood-altering substances** may be hazardous to a fetus. Alcohol is a known teratogen, and a clear dose-response relationship exists between alcohol use and fetal effects. Increasing evidence suggests that cocaine is a teratogen as well as a cause of prematurity, abruptio placentae, and other complications. Tobacco use has been identified as the leading preventable cause of low birth weight. Although many women understand the risks of substance exposures after confirmation of pregnancy, they may be unaware of the risks of exposure during the earliest weeks of pregnancy. If substance addiction is present, structured recovery programs are needed to effect behavioral change. All patients should be asked about use of alcohol, tobacco, and illicit drugs. The preconception interview enables timely education about drug use and pregnancy, informed decision making about the risks of using these substances at the time of conception, and the introduction of interventions for women who abuse substances.

Victims of **domestic violence** should be identified before they conceive, because they are more likely to be abused during pregnancy than at other times. Approximately 37% of obstetric patients are physically abused during their pregnancies. Such assaults can result in abruptio placentae; antepartum hemorrhage; fetal fractures; rupture of the uterus, liver, or spleen; and preterm labor. Information about available community, social, and legal resources should be made available to women who are abused and a plan for dealing with the abusive partner devised.

The preconception interview is an appropriate time to discuss insurance coverage and **financial difficulties.** Many women and couples do not know the eligibility requirements or amount of maternity coverage provided by their insurance carriers. Some women may have no medical insurance coverage. Also, many women are unaware of their employers' policies regarding benefits for complicated and uncomplicated pregnancies and the postpartum period. Facilitating enrollment in medical assistance programs should be part of preconception care for eligible women.

II. **Prenatal care.** Table 4-3 lists the tests to perform during routine prenatal care, along with the recommended times for conducting them.

A. **Pregnancy dating**

1. **Clinical dating**

   a. The average duration of human pregnancy is 280 days from the first day of the last menstrual period (LMP) until delivery. The 40-week gestational period is based on menstrual weeks (not conceptual weeks), with an assumption of ovulation and conception on the fourteenth day of a 28-day cycle.

   b. The most reliable clinical indicator of gestational age is an accurate LMP date. Using Nägele's rule, the estimated date of delivery is calculated by subtracting 3 months from the first day of the LMP, then adding 1 week.

TABLE 4-3. ROUTINE PRENATAL TESTING

Timing	Tests
Initial OB visit	Blood type, Rh type, antibody screen, CBC, rubella, VDRL/STS/RPR, HBsAg, HIV, Hgb electrophoresis, urine culture and sensitivity, Pap smear, gonorrhea and chlamydiosis testing; dating sonogram if questionable dating criteria.
16–18 wks' gestation (range: 15–22 wks)	MSAFP/triple screen.
16–20 wks' gestation	Sonogram to rule out abnormalities.
28 wks' gestation	Blood type, Rh type, antibody screen, CBC, VDRL/STS/RPR, glucose screen. If high-risk OB patient, repeat HBsAg, HIV, gonorrhea, and chlamydia cultures.
36 wks' gestation	Group B streptococci culture (optional).

CBC, complete blood cell count; HBsAg, hepatitis B surface antigen; Hgb, hemoglobin; HIV, human immunodeficiency virus; MSAFP, maternal serum alpha-fetoprotein; OB, obstetric; RPR, rapid plasma reagin; STS, serologic test for syphilis.

    c. A Doppler ultrasonography device allows detection of fetal heart tones by 11–12 weeks' gestation.
    d. A fetoscope can enable detection of heart tones at 19–20 weeks' gestation.
    e. Quickening is noted at approximately 19 weeks in the first pregnancy; in subsequent pregnancies, quickening usually is noted approximately 2 weeks earlier.
    f. The uterus reaches the umbilicus at 20 weeks.
  2. **Ultrasonographic dating** is most accurate from 7 to 11-6/7 weeks of pregnancy. If LMP dating is consistent with ultrasonographic dating within the established range of accuracy for ultrasonography (Table 4-4), the estimated date of delivery is based on LMP. Before 22 weeks' gestation, if LMP dating is outside the range of accuracy, then ultrasonographic dating is used.
B. **Nutrition and weight gain**
  1. **Balanced nutrition**
    a. Pregnant women should avoid uncooked meat because of the risk of toxoplasmosis.

TABLE 4-4. RANGE OF ACCURACY OF PREGNANCY DATING BY ULTRASONOGRAPHY ACCORDING TO GESTATIONAL AGE

Gestational age	Ultrasonographic measurements	Range of accuracy
<8 wks	Sac size	±10 days
8–12 wks	CRL	±7 days
12–14 wks	CRL or BPD	±14 days
15–20 wks	BPD/HC/FL/AC	±10 days
20–28 wks	BPD/HC/FL/AC	±2 wks
>28 wks	BPD/HC/FL/AC	±3 wks

AC, abdominal circumference; BPD, biparietal diameter; CRL, crown-rump length; FL, femur length; HC, head circumference.

    b. Pregnant women require 15% more kilocalories than nonpregnant women, usually 300–500 kcal more per day, depending on the patient's weight and activity.

    c. Dietary allowances for most minerals and vitamins increase with pregnancy. All of these nutrients, with the exception of iron, are supplied adequately by a well-balanced diet. Increased iron is needed both for the fetus and for the mother, whose blood volume increases. Therefore, consumption of iron-containing foods should be encouraged. Iron is found in liver, red meats, eggs, dried beans, leafy green vegetables, whole-grain enriched breads and cereals, and dried fruits. Some physicians choose to give 30 mg of elemental ferrous iron supplements to pregnant women daily. The 30-mg iron supplement is contained in approximately 150 mg of ferrous sulfate, 300 mg of ferrous gluconate, or 100 mg of ferrous fumarate. Taking iron between meals on an empty stomach or with orange juice facilitates its absorption. For calcium, the prenatal requirement is 1200 mg daily.

2. The total **weight gain** recommended for pregnancy is based on the prepregnancy body mass index. The total weight gain recommended is 25–35 lb for women who fall within the normal range of prepregnancy weight.

    a. Underweight women may gain 40 lb or more, whereas overweight women should limit weight gain to less than 25 lb.

    b. Three pounds to 6 lb is gained in the first trimester and 0.5–1.0 lb per week is gained in the last two trimesters of pregnancy.

    c. If a patient has not gained 10 lb by midpregnancy, her nutritional status should be carefully evaluated.

    d. Inadequate weight gain is associated with an increased risk of low birth weight in infants. Inadequate weight gain seems to have the greatest effect in women whose weight is low or normal before pregnancy.

    e. Patients should be warned against weight loss during pregnancy. Total weight gain in an obese patient can be as low as 15 lb, but weight gains of less than 15 lb are associated with a lack of expansion of plasma volume and a risk of intrauterine growth restriction.

3. **Nausea and vomiting**

    a. **Nonpharmacologic** recommendations for controlling nausea and vomiting in early pregnancy include the following:

      (1) Greasy or spicy foods should be avoided.

      (2) Some food should be kept in the stomach at all times by consumption of frequent small meals or snacks.

      (3) A protein snack should be eaten at night; crackers should be kept at the bedside for consumption before rising in the morning.

    b. **Pharmacologic** therapy is discussed in Chap. 16.

C. **Exercise.** In the absence of obstetric or medical complications, women who engage in a moderate level of physical activity can maintain cardiovascular and muscular fitness throughout pregnancy and the postpartum period. No data suggest that moderate aerobic exercise is harmful to mother or fetus. Women who engage in regular non–weight-bearing exercise (cycling or swimming) are more likely to maintain their regimens throughout their pregnancies than women whose regular exercise before pregnancy is weight bearing. Women who wish to maintain body conditioning during their pregnancies may consider switching to non–weight-bearing exercise.

1. Pregnancy induces alterations in **maternal hemodynamics,** including increases in blood volume, cardiac output, and resting pulse, and a decrease in systemic vascular resistance.

2. Because of **increased resting oxygen requirements** and the increased work of breathing brought about by the physical effects of an

enlarged uterus on the diaphragm, a decreased amount of oxygen is available for the performance of aerobic exercise during pregnancy.

3. For women who do not have any obstetric or medical contraindications, the following **exercise recommendations** may be made:

a. Mild to moderate exercise routines are encouraged. Regular exercise (at least three times per week) is preferable to intermittent activity.

b. Pregnant women should avoid exercise in the supine position after the first trimester. This position is associated with decreased cardiac output in most pregnant women, and the cardiac output is preferentially distributed away from splanchnic beds (including the uterus) during vigorous exercise; therefore, exercises performed supine are best avoided during pregnancy. Prolonged periods of stationary standing should also be avoided.

c. Because of the decrease in oxygen available for aerobic exercise during pregnancy, pregnant women should modify the intensity of their exercise in response to symptoms of oxygen depletion such as shortness of breath. Pregnant women should stop exercising when fatigued and should not exercise to exhaustion.

d. Physical maneuvers involving a shift in the physical center of gravity that may result in a loss of balance are contraindicated during pregnancy. Any type of exercise with the potential for even mild abdominal trauma should be avoided.

e. Because pregnancy requires an additional 300 kcal/day to maintain metabolic homeostasis, women who exercise during pregnancy must be careful to ensure an adequate diet.

f. Pregnant women who exercise should augment heat dissipation by maintaining adequate hydration, wearing appropriate clothing, and ensuring optimal environmental surroundings during exercise.

g. Many of the physiologic and morphologic changes of pregnancy persist for 4–6 weeks postpartum. Therefore, prepregnancy exercise routines should be resumed gradually, based on a woman's individual physical capability.

4. The following conditions are **contraindications** to exercise during pregnancy:

a. Pregnancy-induced hypertension

b. Preterm rupture of membranes

c. Preterm labor during a prior pregnancy, the current pregnancy, or both

d. Incompetent cervix or cerclage

e. Persistent second- or third-trimester bleeding

f. Intrauterine growth restriction

5. Women with certain other conditions, including chronic hypertension or active thyroid, cardiac, vascular, or pulmonary disease, should be carefully evaluated to determine whether an exercise program is appropriate.

D. **Smoking**

1. Carbon monoxide and nicotine are believed to be the main ingredients in cigarette smoke responsible for adverse fetal effects. Compared to nonsmoking, smoking is associated with increased rates of occurrence of the following events:

a. Spontaneous abortion (risk is 1.2–1.8 times greater in smokers than in nonsmokers)

b. Abortion of a chromosomally normal fetus (39% more likely in smokers than in nonsmokers)

c. Abruptio placentae, placenta previa, and premature rupture of membranes

d. Preterm birth (risk is 1.2–1.5 times greater in smokers than in nonsmokers)

e. Low infant birth weight

f. Sudden infant death syndrome

2. **Smoking cessation** during pregnancy improves the birth weight of the infant, especially if cessation occurs before 16 weeks' gestation. If all pregnant women stopped smoking, it is estimated that a 10% reduction in fetal and infant deaths would be observed.

3. Prospective, randomized, controlled clinical trials have shown that intensive smoking reduction programs with frequent patient contact and close supervision aid in smoking cessation and result in increased infant birth weights. Successful interventions emphasize ways to stop smoking rather than merely providing antismoking advice.

4. **Nicotine replacement therapy** (chewing gum or transdermal patch). The package inserts of these therapies suggest that pregnant women should not use them because nicotine is considered an important cause of the adverse effects of smoking on mothers and fetuses. Nicotine, however, is only one of the toxins absorbed from tobacco smoke; cessation of smoking with nicotine replacement reduces fetal exposure to carbon monoxide and other toxins. For women who smoke more than 20 cigarettes per day and who are unable to reduce their smoking otherwise, it may be reasonable to advise nicotine replacement as an adjunct to counseling during pregnancy.

E. **Alcohol consumption**
1. Ethanol freely crosses the placenta and the fetal blood–brain barrier. Ethanol is a known teratogen. Fetal ethanol toxicity is dose related, and the exposure time of greatest risk is the first trimester; however, fetal brain development may be affected throughout gestation. Although an occasional drink during pregnancy has not been shown to be harmful, patients should be counseled that the threshold for adverse effects is unknown.

2. **Fetal alcohol syndrome** is characterized by three findings: growth retardation (prenatally, postnatally, or both), facial abnormalities, and CNS dysfunction. Facial abnormalities include shortened palpebral fissures, low-set ears, midfacial hypoplasia, a smooth philtrum, and a thin upper lip. CNS abnormalities of fetal alcohol syndrome include microcephaly, mental retardation, and behavioral disorders such as attention deficit disorder. Skeletal abnormalities and structural cardiac defects are also seen with greater frequency in the children of women who abuse alcohol during pregnancy than in those of women who do not. The most common cardiac structural anomaly is ventricular septal defect, but a number of others occur.

F. **Illicit drug use**
1. **Marijuana.** The active ingredient is tetrahydrocannabinol. No evidence exists that marijuana is a significant teratogen in humans. Cannabinoid metabolites can be detected in the urine of users for days to weeks after use, much longer than for alcohol and most other illicit drugs. The presence of cannabinoid metabolites in the urine may identify patients who are likely to be current users of other illicit substances as well.

2. **Cocaine. Adverse maternal effects** include profound vasoconstriction leading to malignant hypertension, cardiac ischemia, and cerebral infarction. Cocaine may have a direct cardiotoxic effect, leading to sudden death. **Complications** of cocaine use in pregnancy include spontaneous abortion and fetal death in utero, premature rupture of membranes, preterm labor and delivery, intrauterine growth restriction, meconium-staining of amniotic fluid, and abruptio placentae. Cocaine is teratogenic, and its use has been associated with cases of in utero fetal cerebral infarction, microcephaly, and limb reduction defects. Genitourinary malformations have been reported with first trimester cocaine use. Infants born to women who use cocaine are at risk for neurobehavioral abnormalities and impairment in orientation, motor, and state-regulation neurobehaviors.

3. **Opiates.** Opiate use has been associated with increased rates of stillbirth, fetal growth retardation, prematurity, and neonatal mortality, perhaps due to risky behaviors in opiate substance abusers. Opiates are not known to be teratogenic. Treatment with methadone is associated with improved pregnancy outcomes. The newborn narcotic addict is at risk for a severe, potentially fatal, narcotic withdrawal syndrome. Although the incidence of clinically significant withdrawal is slightly lower among methadone-treated addicts, its course can be just as severe. Neonatal withdrawal is characterized by a high-pitched cry, poor feeding, hypertonicity, tremors, irritability, sneezing, sweating, vomiting, diarrhea, and, occasionally, seizures. Frequent sharing of needles has resulted in extremely high rates of HIV infection (greater than 50%) and hepatitis among narcotic addicts.

4. **Amphetamines.** Crystal methamphetamine, a potent stimulant administered intravenously, has been associated with decreased fetal head circumference and increased risk of abruptio placentae, intrauterine growth restriction, and fetal death in utero. There is, however, no proven teratogenicity.

5. **Hallucinogens.** No evidence has shown that lysergic acid diethylamide (LSD) or other hallucinogens causes chromosomal damage, as was once reported. Few studies exist on the possible deleterious effects of maternal hallucinogen use during pregnancy. There is no proven teratogenicity to LSD.

6. **Prenatal care for the substance abuser.** Intensive prenatal care to address the multiple problems of substance abusers, involving a multidisciplinary team of health care and social service providers, has been shown to ameliorate the maternal and neonatal complications associated with substance abuse. At each prenatal visit, substance abuse treatment should be offered to substance abusers who have not quit. All substance abusers should be counseled about the potential risks of preterm delivery, fetal growth restriction, fetal death, and possible long-term neurobehavioral effects in the child. HIV testing should be encouraged. Periodic urine toxicologic testing should be offered. The reliability of urine toxicologic testing is limited by the rapid clearance of most substances. Overaggressive urine testing may be perceived by the patient as threatening and thus decreases patient compliance. Early ultrasonographic confirmation of gestational age is necessary, because growth restriction is a frequent finding among fetuses of substance abusers, and accurate assessment of gestational age is important in the management of intrauterine growth restriction. A fetal anatomic survey is indicated because of the increased frequency of structural anomalies among offspring of substance abusers. Antepartum testing is appropriate when a reason to suspect fetal compromise exists (e.g., size small for date, decreased fetal movement, suspected growth restriction). When normal growth and an active fetus are present, no evidence shows that regular antepartum testing is associated with improved perinatal outcome in substance-abusing patients. All patients should be screened for substance abuse (including use of alcohol and tobacco) at the time of their first prenatal visit. Several screening questionnaires have been developed to detect problem drinking (e.g., the T-ACE questions and the CAGE questionnaire) and substance abuse.

G. **Immunizations.** Preconception immunization of women to prevent disease in their offspring is preferred to vaccination of pregnant women; only live-virus vaccines, however, carry any risk to the fetus.

1. All women of childbearing age should be immune to measles, rubella, mumps, tetanus, diphtheria, poliomyelitis, and varicella through childhood natural or vaccine-conferred immunization.

2. Rubella infection during pregnancy is associated with congenital infection; measles, with high risk of spontaneous abortion, preterm birth,

and maternal morbidity; tetanus, with transplacental transfer of toxin, which causes neonatal tetanus; and varicella, with fetal CNS and limb defects and severe maternal pneumonia.

3. All pregnant women should be screened for hepatitis B surface antigen. Pregnancy is not a contraindication to the administration of an HBV vaccine or hepatitis B immune globulin. Women at high risk of HBV infection who should be vaccinated during pregnancy include those with histories of the following: intravenous drug use, acute episode of any sexually transmitted disease, multiple sexual partners, occupational exposure in a health care or public safety environment, household contact with an HBV carrier, occupational exposure or residence in an institution for the developmentally disabled, occupational exposure or treatment in a hemodialysis unit, or receipt of clotting factor concentrates for bleeding disorders.

4. Combined tetanus and diphtheria toxoids are the only immunobiological agents routinely indicated for susceptible pregnant women.

5. There is no evidence of fetal risk from inactivated-virus vaccines, bacterial vaccines, or tetanus immunoglobulin, and these agents should be administered if appropriate.

6. Measles, mumps, and rubella single-antigen vaccines, as well as the combined vaccine, should be given at a preconception or postpartum visit. Despite theoretical risks, no evidence has been reported of congenital rubella syndrome in infants born to women inadvertently given rubella vaccine while pregnant. Women who undergo immunization should be advised not to become pregnant for 3 months afterward. Measles, mumps, and rubella vaccines can be given to children of pregnant women, as there is no evidence that the viruses can be transmitted by someone who has recently been vaccinated.

7. Immune globulin or vaccination against poliomyelitis, yellow fever, typhoid, or hepatitis may be indicated for travelers to areas where these diseases are endemic or epidemic.

8. Influenza and pneumococcal vaccines are recommended for women with special conditions that put them at high risk of infection. Women in their second or third trimester should be given influenza vaccine during influenza season. This is especially true for women who work at chronic care facilities that house patients with chronic medical conditions or who themselves have cardiopulmonary disorders, including asthma, are immunosuppressed, or have diabetes mellitus. Women who have undergone splenectomy should be given pneumococcal vaccine.

9. Immune globulin or a specific immune globulin may be indicated after exposure to measles, hepatitis A or B, tetanus, chickenpox, or rabies.

10. Varicella zoster immune globulin (VZIG) should be administered to any newborn whose mother developed chickenpox within 5 days before or 2 days after delivery. No evidence shows that administration of VZIG to mothers reduces the rare occurrence of congenital varicella syndrome. VZIG can be considered for treating a pregnant woman to try to prevent the maternal complications of chickenpox (see Chap. 11, sec. **III.D.1.b**).

H. **Sexual intercourse**
1. Generally, no restriction of sexual activity is necessary for pregnant women.
2. Patients should be instructed that pregnancy may cause changes in physical comfort and sexual desire.
3. Increased uterine activity after intercourse is common.
4. For women at risk of preterm labor placenta or vasa previa or women with histories of previous pregnancy loss, avoidance of sexual activity may be recommended.

I. **Employment**
1. Most patients are able to work throughout the entire pregnancy.
2. Heavy lifting and excessive physical activity should be avoided.

   3. Modification of occupational activities is rarely needed, unless the job involves physical danger.
   4. Patients should be counseled to discontinue an activity whenever they experience discomfort.
   5. Jobs that involve strenuous physical exercise, standing for prolonged periods, work on industrial machines, or other adverse environmental factors should be modified as necessary.
 J. **Travel.** The following are general recommendations for all pregnant women:
   1. Prolonged sitting should be avoided because of the increased risk of venous thrombosis and thrombophlebitis during pregnancy.
   2. Patients should drive a maximum of 6 hours a day and should stop at least every 2 hours and walk for 10 minutes.
   3. Support stockings should be worn for prolonged sitting in cars or airplanes.
   4. A seat belt should always be worn; the belt should be placed under the abdomen as the pregnancy advances.
 K. **Carpal tunnel syndrome.** In pregnancy, weight gain and edema can compress the median nerve, producing carpal tunnel syndrome. The syndrome consists of pain, numbness, or tingling in the thumb, index finger, middle finger, and radial side of the ring finger on the palmar aspect. Compressing the median nerve and percussing the wrist and forearm with a reflex hammer (Tinel's maneuver) often exacerbates the pain. The syndrome most often occurs in primigravidas over the age of 30 during the third trimester and usually recedes within 2 weeks of delivery. Treatment is conservative, with splinting of the wrist at night. Local injections of glucocorticoids may be necessary in severe cases.
 L. **Back pain**
   1. Back pain may be aggravated by excessive weight gain.
   2. Exercises to strengthen back muscles and loosen the hamstrings can help alleviate back pain.
   3. Pregnant women should maintain good posture and wear low-heeled shoes.
 M. **Round ligament pain.** These very sharp groin pains are caused by spasm of round ligaments associated with movement. The spasms are generally unilateral and are more frequent on the right side than the left because of the usual dextroversion of the uterus. Patients sometimes awaken at night with round ligament pain after having suddenly rolled over in their sleep.
 N. **Hemorrhoids** are varicose veins of the rectum.
   1. Patients with hemorrhoids should avoid constipation, because straining during bowel movement aggravates hemorrhoids.
   2. Good hydration and certain fruits like prunes and apricots help to soften the stool.
   3. Patients should avoid prolonged sitting.
   4. Hemorrhoids often regress after delivery but usually do not disappear completely.
 O. **Genetic screening and testing.** A summary of the indications for genetic counseling is provided in Table 4-5.
   1. **Triple screen**
      a. The maternal serum triple screen is performed at 15–20 weeks of pregnancy (ideally 16–18 weeks) and measures three substances in maternal serum:
         (1) Maternal serum alpha-fetoprotein (MSAFP) [average is 0.7 multiples of the median (MoM) for women carrying a fetus with Down syndrome].
         (2) Human chorionic gonadotropin (hCG): Levels decline after approximately 10 weeks and throughout much of the second trimester. It is the most sensitive second trimester maternal serum screening marker for detection of fetal Down syndrome (average is 2.1 MoM for women carrying a fetus with Down syndrome).

TABLE 4-5. INDICATIONS FOR GENETIC COUNSELING

Older maternal age
  Mother 35 yrs of age or older at her estimated date of delivery
Fetal anomalies detected via ultrasonography
Abnormal triple screen or abnormal alpha-fetoprotein test results
Parental exposure to teratogens
  Drugs
  Radiation
  Infection
Family history of
  Genetic disease (includes chromosome, single gene, and multifactorial disorders)
  Birth defects
  Mental retardation
  Cancer, heart disease, hypertension, diabetes, and other common conditions (especially when onset occurs at an early age)
Membership in ethnic group in which certain genetic disorders are frequent when appropriate screening for or prenatal diagnosis of the disease is available (e.g., sickle cell anemia, Tay-Sachs disease, Canavan's disease, thalassemia)
Consanguinity
Reproductive failure
  Infertility
  Repeated spontaneous abortions
  Stillbirths and neonatal deaths
Infant, child, or adult with
  Dysmorphic features
  Developmental and/or growth delay
  Mental or physical retardation
  Ambiguous genitalia or abnormal sexual development

---

      (3) Unconjugated estriol (average is 0.7 MoM with fetal Down syndrome). It is important to realize that the three serum marker results are combined with maternal age to generate a risk of Down syndrome.

    b. The maternal serum triple screen has a different profile for fetal trisomy 18 (Edward's syndrome). A typical triple screen result for this chromosome abnormality is low for AFP, low for estriol, and very low for hCG.

  2. **First trimester screening.** First trimester maternal serum screening for Down syndrome and trisomy 18 is being evaluated using levels of hCG and pregnancy-associated plasma protein A (PAPP-A). The hCG level is elevated, whereas the PAPP-A level is lower than average in women carrying a fetus with Down syndrome. When these measurements are combined with maternal age and a standard measurement of the thin skin fold behind the fetal neck (nuchal translucency) at 10–14 weeks' gestation, the detection rate for Down syndrome in the first trimester is predicted to approach 85–90%.

3. **Maternal serum alpha-fetoprotein** is a fetal glycoprotein that is synthesized sequentially in the embryonic yolk sac, GI tract, and liver. Normally, AFP crosses the fetomaternal circulatory interface within the placenta to appear in the mother's serum. In addition, a small amount of AFP enters the amniotic fluid via fetal urination, GI secretions, and transudation from exposed blood vessels. The concentration of AFP in amniotic fluid is highest at the end of the first trimester and slowly declines during the remainder of pregnancy. MSAFP concentrations, on the other hand, rise until approximately 30 weeks' gestation. In the second trimester, the level of AFP in fetal blood is approximately 100,000 times that in maternal serum, whereas the level of AFP in amniotic fluid is 100 times that in maternal serum. With an open fetal NTD or an abdominal wall defect, more AFP will be present in the amniotic fluid and more will cross the membranes and lead to an elevated level in the mother's blood in 85% of cases.

4. **Screening for neural tube defects.** NTDs result from a failure of the neural tube to close or attain its normal musculoskeletal coverings in early embryogenesis. Among the most common major congenital malformations, NTDs include the fatal condition of anencephaly as well as spina bifida (meningomyelocele and meningocele); most have the potential for surgical correction.

   a. The incidence of NTDs in the United States is 1–2:1000 live births.

   b. A family history of NTD in either parent generally signifies an increased risk of an NTD in the offspring. If one partner has an NTD, this risk is 2–3%. In a couple with a prior affected child, the risk of recurrence is 2%. Ninety percent of NTDs, however, occur in families without such histories. Therefore, all pregnant women in the United States are currently offered MSAFP screening.

   c. Prenatal diagnosis of an NTD allows for termination of pregnancy or preparation for the birth of an affected infant. The potential exists for in utero repair of spina bifida.

5. **Significance of elevated alpha-fetoprotein level**

   a. Diagnostic ultrasonography should be performed on patients with abnormal MSAFP screening results to determine gestational age, as well as to visualize the placenta, detect multiple pregnancies, and detect any fetal anomalies. Amniocentesis is generally offered to patients found to have a single living fetus of the expected gestational age without anomalies.

   b. Elevated AFP levels are usually found in maternal serum (80% of cases) and amniotic fluid (over 95% of cases) with open NTDs (elevated value for MSAFP of 2.5 MoM or higher). Closed defects, however, including those associated with hydrocephalus, are not associated with abnormal AFP findings. In addition to open NTDs, elevated MSAFP levels can also occur with multiple pregnancies, abdominal wall defects such as omphalocele or gastroschisis, congenital nephrosis, Turner's syndrome with cystic hygroma, fetal bowel obstruction, and some teratomas.

   c. Fetal growth retardation, fetal death, and other adverse outcomes are also associated with elevated MSAFP levels.

   d. Assignment of incorrect gestational age may lead to incorrect interpretation of AFP levels, because both MSAFP and amniotic fluid AFP levels change in relation to gestational age.

   e. MSAFP measurement alone is performed for fetal NTD screening. Most women, however, have AFP testing performed as part of the triple screen. An elevated MSAFP level is often defined as 2.5 MoM or higher. The first MSAFP screen specimen is drawn at 15–18 weeks' gestation after informed consent and counseling. A second MSAFP screen specimen is drawn only from patients with a slightly high initial test result. A second screening is not recommended if the first is higher than 3.0 MoM.

f. The normal range of AFP values is established by each reference laboratory. Laboratories should provide interpretations of results and risk assessments that take into account race, maternal weight, multiple pregnancy, and the presence of insulin-dependent diabetes mellitus. Results are reported in multiples of the median to standardize interpretation of values among different laboratories.

6. **Maternal age screening for fetal aneuploidy**
   a. There are normally 46 chromosomes in every cell of the body. *Aneuploidy* refers to the condition in which there is an additional or missing chromosome that results in, for example, a total of 47 or 45 chromosomes altogether. The way that a cytogenetics laboratory would convey a diagnosis of Down syndrome, the most common aneuploid condition in liveborns, is as 47,XX,+21 or 47,XY,+21. Down syndrome, or trisomy 21, most often results from meiotic nondisjunction during maternal chromosomal replication and division.
   b. Down syndrome is characterized by mental retardation, cardiac defects, hypotonia, and characteristic facial features.
   c. Incidence increases with maternal age (Table 4-6).
   d. Prenatal diagnosis by chromosomal analysis currently is offered to women who will be 35 or older at the time of delivery. This approach detects only approximately 30% of cases of Down syndrome; 70% of cases occur in women younger than 35 years.
   e. The risk of recurrence for a couple who are both chromosomally normal and have had a prior child with Down syndrome is often cited to be 1%.

7. **Amniocentesis**
   a. **Procedure.** Amniocentesis involves withdrawal of a small sample of the fluid that surrounds the fetus. Amniotic fluid contains cells that are shed primarily from the fetal bladder, skin, GI tract, and amnion. These cells can be used for karyotyping or other genetic diagnostic tests. Amniocentesis is most commonly performed at 15–18 weeks' gestation.
   b. **Indications.** In the United States, the current standard of care is to offer chorionic villus sampling (CVS) or amniocentesis to women who will be 35 years or older when they give birth, because older women are at increased risk for giving birth to infants with Down syndrome and other types of aneuploidy. Patients with a positive obstetric history of NTD should be appropriately counseled about the 2–3% risk of recurrence of NTD and offered second trimester amniocentesis for amniotic fluid AFP testing; detailed ultrasonographic evaluation of the fetus for NTD at 18–20 weeks' gestation should also be offered. If the amniotic fluid AFP results and the ultrasonographic findings are normal, the likelihood of an open NTD is minimal. The amniocentesis site should be selected carefully; the placenta should be avoided to reduce the risk of contaminating the amniotic fluid specimen with fetal blood, which obviously will result in falsely elevated amniotic fluid AFP levels. False-positive results due to contamination of amniotic fluid with fetal blood can be identified by the absence of acetylcholinesterase in amniotic fluid. After fetal blood contamination of the amniotic fluid has been excluded, elevated amniotic fluid AFP levels not accompanied by elevated acetylcholinesterase levels should be investigated by performing detailed ultrasonographic examination.
   c. **Risks and complications.** The miscarriage rate from amniocentesis is 0.25–0.50% (1:400 to 1:200). Unsensitized Rh⁻ women are given Rh⁻ immune globulin after amniocentesis.

8. **Chorionic villus sampling**
   a. **Procedure.** CVS uses either a catheter or a needle to biopsy placental tissue derived from the same fertilized egg as the fetus. CVS is

TABLE 4-6. CHROMOSOMAL ABNORMALITIES IN LIVEBORNS[a]

Maternal age	Risk of Down syndrome	Total risk of chromosomal abnormalities[b]
20	1:1667	1:526
21	1:1667	1:526
22	1:1429	1:500
23	1:1429	1:500
24	1:1250	1:476
25	1:1250	1:476
26	1:1176	1:476
27	1:1111	1:455
28	1:1053	1:435
29	1:1000	1:417
30	1:952	1:385
31	1:909	1:385
32	1:769	1:322
33	1:602	1:286
34	1:485	1:238
35	1:378	1:192
36	1:289	1:156
37	1:224	1:127
38	1:173	1:102
39	1:136	1:83
40	1:106	1:66
41	1:82	1:53
42	1:63	1:42
43	1:49	1:33
44	1:38	1:26
45	1:30	1:21
46	1:23	1:16
47	1:18	1:13
48	1:14	1:10
49	1:11	1:8

[a]Because sample size for some intervals is relatively small, 95% confidence limits are sometimes relatively large. Nonetheless, these figures are suitable for use in genetic counseling.

[b]Karyotype 47,XXX was excluded for ages 20–32 (data not available).

Adapted from Hook EB, Cross PK, Schreinemachers DM. Chromosomal abnormality rates at amniocentesis and in live-born infants. *JAMA* 1983;249:2034–2038, with permission. Copyright 1983, American Medical Association from Hook EB. Rates of chromosomal abnormalities at different maternal ages. *Obstet Gynecol* 1981;58:282–285. Copyright 1981, American College of Obstetricians and Gynecologists.

usually performed at 10–12 weeks' gestation but may be performed throughout the second or third trimester. CVS may be more acceptable than amniocentesis to some women because of the psychological and medical advantages provided by early diagnosis of abnormalities and first trimester termination.

b. **Risks and complications.** When adjusted for confounding factors such as gestational age, the CVS-related miscarriage rate has not been shown to be statistically different from that for second trimester amniocentesis. Unsensitized Rh⁻ women are given Rh⁻ immunoglobin after CVS.

c. Cytogenetically ambiguous results caused by maternal cell contamination or mosaicism are reported more often after CVS than after amniocentesis. In such instances, follow-up amniocentesis may be required to clarify results, which increases both the total cost of testing and the risk of miscarriage.

d. Reports of clusters of infants born with limb deficiencies after CVS were first published in 1991. Data from studies of CVS suggest that this outcome is associated with the specific time of CVS exposure. Therefore, CVS is not recommended before 10 weeks' gestation.

9. **A midtrimester ultrasonographic evaluation** should include a systematic search of the fetal anatomy, in addition to establishment of the usual fetal growth parameters. One should routinely conduct a search of the entire spinal column for any dorsal effects of the canal or abnormal vertebrae, as well as perform an evaluation of the intracranial anatomy. The cord insertion site on the fetal ventral wall is examined carefully, and the remainder of the fetal anatomy is visualized to detect structural anomalies. Presence of an increased nuchal fold is being used as a screening test for Down syndrome at 15–21 weeks, and a slightly short humerus (and femur) also has been associated with Down syndrome, although the positive predictive value of this sign is poor. Ultrasonography cannot rule out Down syndrome with certainty. The woman's age and maternal serum triple screen results are often evaluated in combination with sonographic findings to improve Down syndrome screening in a noninvasive way. Assessment of the fetal karyotype (by amniocentesis or CVS) is necessary, however, to make the diagnosis or to rule it out with complete certainty. Ultrasonography is better at detecting aneuploidies other than Down syndrome such as trisomy 18 or trisomy 13, which are associated with much higher incidence of major structural anomalies.

Section Two. OBSTETRICS

5. NORMAL LABOR AND DELIVERY, OPERATIVE DELIVERY, AND MALPRESENTATIONS

Amy E. Hearne and Rita Driggers

I. **Labor** is defined as repetitive uterine contractions of sufficient frequency, intensity, and duration to cause cervical effacement and dilation.

II. **Stages and phases of labor**

A. The **first stage** begins with the onset of labor and ends with full cervical dilation. It is further subdivided into latent and active phases.

1. The **latent phase** begins with the initial perception of regular contractions and ends when the rate of cervical dilation increases (usually at 3–4 cm of dilation). Uterine contractions typically begin as mild and irregular, becoming more intense, frequent, and regular as the latent phase progresses. Cervical dilation progresses slowly. The latent phase is considered to be prolonged if it exceeds 20 hours in a nulliparous patient and 14 hours in a multiparous patient.

2. The **active phase** is characterized by an increased rate of cervical dilation with descent of the presenting fetal part. This phase is further subdivided into an acceleration phase, a phase of maximum slope, and a deceleration phase.

   a. **Acceleration phase.** A gradual increase in dilation initiates the active phase (usually beginning at 3 to 4 cm of dilation) and leads to a period of rapid dilation.

   b. The **phase of maximum slope** is defined as the period of active labor when the rate of cervical dilation is maximal. Once established, this rate tends to be constant for each individual until the deceleration phase is reached. Primary dysfunctional labor is defined as an active-phase dilation at a rate less than the fifth percentile. This value is 1.2 cm/hour for nulliparas and 1.5 cm/hour for multiparas (Table 5-1).

   c. **Deceleration phase.** During the terminal portion of the active phase, rate of dilation sometimes slows, with termination at full cervical dilation.

B. The **second stage** of labor is the interval between full cervical dilation and delivery of the infant. The average duration is 50 minutes for nulliparas and 20 minutes for multiparas. Descent of the fetal presenting part begins in the late active phase and continues during the second stage. The second stage is considered prolonged after 2 hours in nulliparous patients or 1 hour in parous patients. An additional hour may be allowed if epidural anesthesia is used. Studies show that duration of the second stage of labor is unrelated to perinatal outcome in the absence of a nonreassuring fetal heart rate pattern or traumatic delivery. Therefore, a prolonged second stage alone usually is not considered an indication for operative intervention, provided steady descent of the presenting part continues.

C. The **third stage** is the interval between delivery of the infant and delivery of the placenta, umbilical cord, and fetal membranes. This stage averages 10 minutes and is considered prolonged if it lasts longer than 30 minutes. Placental separation occurs along Nitabuch's layer and is the result of continued uterine contractions. Continued contractions control blood loss by compression of spiral arteries and also result in migration of the placenta into the lower uterine segment and then through the cervix.

D. The **fourth stage,** or puerperium, follows delivery and concludes with resolution of the physiologic changes of pregnancy, usually by 6 weeks postpartum. During this time, the reproductive tract returns to the nonpregnant state, and ovulation may resume.

TABLE 5-1. STAGES AND PHASES OF LABOR

Parameter	Nulliparas	Multiparas
Total labor		
Mean	10.1 hrs	6.2 hrs
Fifth percentile	25.8 hrs	19.5 hrs
First stage of labor		
Mean	9.7 hrs	8.0 hrs
Fifth percentile	24.7 hrs	18.8 hrs
Second stage of labor		
Mean	50 mins	20 mins
Prolonged (without epidural)	2 hrs	1 hr
Prolonged (with epidural)	3 hrs	2 hrs
Third stage of labor		
Mean	10 mins	10 mins
Prolonged	30 mins	30 mins
Duration of latent phase		
Mean	6.4 hrs	4.5 hrs
Fifth percentile	20.0 hrs	14.0 hrs
Rate of maximal dilation		
Mean	3.0 cm/hr	5.7 cm/hr
Fifth percentile	1.2 cm/hr	1.5 cm/hr
Rate of descent		
Mean	3.3 cm/hr	6.6 cm/hr
Fifth percentile	1.0 cm/hr	2.1 cm/hr

III. **Mechanisms of labor,** or seven cardinal movements of labor, refer to the changes in position of the fetal head during passage through the birth canal in the vertex presentation.

   A. **Engagement** is descent of the biparietal diameter of the fetal head below the plane of the pelvic inlet. Clinically, if the lowest portion of the occiput is at or below the level of the maternal ischial spines (station 0), engagement has usually taken place. Engagement can occur before the onset of true labor, especially in nulliparas. Patients may experience a change in the shape of the abdomen and a decreased sense of shortness of breath, referred to as lightening.

   B. **Descent** of the fetal head to the pelvic floor is an important event of labor. The highest rate of descent occurs during the deceleration phase of the first stage and during the second stage of labor.

   C. **Flexion** of the fetal head onto the chest is a passive movement that permits the smallest diameter of the fetal head (suboccipitobregmatic diameter) to be presented to the maternal pelvis.

   D. **Internal rotation.** The fetal occiput rotates from its original position (usually transverse) toward the symphysis pubis (occiput anterior) or, less commonly, toward the hollow of the sacrum (occiput posterior).

   E. **Extension.** The fetal head is delivered by extension from the flexed position, rotating around the symphysis pubis.

   F. **External rotation.** The fetus resumes its face-forward position, with the occiput and spine lying in the same plane.

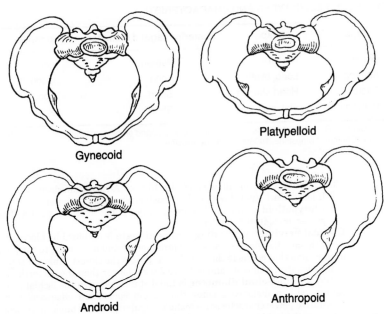

FIG. 5-1. Four pelvic types. (From Beckmann CR, et al. *Obstetrics and gynecology,* 2nd ed. Baltimore: Williams & Wilkins, 1995:36,with permission.)

    G. **Expulsion.** Further descent brings the anterior shoulder of the fetus to the level of the symphysis pubis. After the shoulder is delivered under the symphysis pubis, the rest of the body is usually expelled quickly.

IV. **Pelvimetry and labor**

    A. **Pelvic shapes, planes, and diameters.** Four pelvic planes are commonly described.

        1. The **pelvic inlet** (obstetric conjugate) is bordered anteriorly by the posterior border of the symphysis pubis, posteriorly by the sacral promontory, and laterally by the linea terminalis. The pelvic inlet separates the false pelvis from the true pelvis. Measurement of the inlet's transverse diameter is taken at its widest point.

        2. The **plane of greatest diameter** is bordered by the midpoint of the pubis anteriorly, the upper part of the obturator foramina laterally, and the junction of the second and third vertebrae posteriorly.

        3. The **plane of least diameter** (midplane) is bordered anteriorly by the lower margin of the symphysis, posteriorly by the sacrum (S4 or S5), and laterally by the inferior margins of the ischial spines.

        4. The **pelvic outlet** is bordered anteriorly by the lower margin of the symphysis, laterally by the ischial tuberosities, and posteriorly by the tip of the sacrum.

    B. Based on the general bony architecture, pelvises may be classified into four basic **types** (Fig. 5-1). Gynecoid and anthropoid pelvises are most amenable to childbirth (Table 5-2).

        1. **Gynecoid** (40–50% of women). Inlet is rounded, side walls are straight, and sacrum is well curved.

        2. **Anthropoid** (20% of all women, 40% of African-American women). Inlet is oval, long, and narrow; side walls are straight; sacrum is long and narrow; and sacrosciatic notch is wide.

TABLE 5-2. PELVIC TYPES AND CHARACTERISTICS

Type	Shape	Posterior sagittal diameter	Prognosis
Gynecoid	Round	Average	Good
Anthropoid	Long, oval	Long	Good
Android	Heart shaped	Short	Poor
Platypelloid	Flat, oval	Short	Poor

From Gabbe SG, Niebyl JK, Simpson JL. *Obstetrics: normal and problem pregnancies*, 3rd ed. New York: Churchill Livingstone, 1996:433, with permission.

3. **Android** (30% of all women, 10–15% of African-American women). Inlet is heart shaped with a short posterior sagittal diameter.
4. **Platypelloid** (2–5% of all women). Inlet is flat and oval with a short posterior sagittal diameter.

C. **Clinical pelvimetry.** The **diagonal conjugate** is obtained by placing the tip of the middle finger at the sacral promontory and measuring to the point on the hand that contacts the symphysis. This is the closest clinical estimate of the obstetric conjugate and is 1.5 to 2.0 cm longer than the obstetric conjugate. The **bi-ischial diameter** is the distance between the ischial tuberosities, with a distance greater than 8 cm considered adequate. Other qualitative pelvic characteristics include angulation of the pubic arch, prominence of the ischial spines, size of the sacrospinous notch, and curvature of the sacrum and coccyx.

D. **Radiologic pelvimetry**
   1. **Radiographic pelvimetry.** Indications for performing radiographic pelvimetry to obtain more precise pelvic measurements include clinical evidence or obstetric history suggestive of pelvic abnormalities, history of pelvic trauma, and breech presentation for which a vaginal delivery is being contemplated. The most commonly used measurements are the anteroposterior and transverse diameters of the inlet and midplane (Table 5-3). A high likelihood of cephalopelvic disproportion exists if measurements are less than the established critical values.
   2. **Pelvimetry by other modalities.** CT pelvimetry is superior to radiographic pelvimetry for assessing the exact position of the fetal head relative to the maternal pelvis. MRI has also been used successfully to assess maternal pelvic structure and has the advantage of better definition of soft tissue structures, given that soft tissue dystocia is a more frequent cause of fetopelvic disproportion than bony dystocia. Unlike radiography and CT, MRI does not require the use of ionizing radiation.

V. **Management of normal labor and delivery**
   A. **Initial assessment** of labor includes an appropriate history taking, physical examination, review of the prenatal data, and necessary laboratory testing. The time of onset of contractions, status of the fetal membranes, presence or absence of vaginal bleeding, fetal activity, maternal allergies, time of last food or fluid intake, and use of any medications should be noted. The admitting physical examination should include assessment of the patient's initial vital signs; fetal presentation; fetal heart rate; and frequency, duration, and character of uterine contractions. If rupture of membranes is suspected, a sterile speculum examination should be performed to look for evidence of ruptured membranes (gross vaginal pooling of fluid, positive results on Nitrazine and fern testing of vaginal secretions) and evidence of meconium. If clinically indicated, genital specimens for culture and wet preparation may be obtained. If membranes are intact, a digital examination can be performed to determine the amount of cervical dilation,

TABLE 5-3. AVERAGE AND CRITICAL LIMIT VALUES FOR PELVIC MEASUREMENTS BY RADIOGRAPHIC PELVIMETRY

Diameter	Average value	Critical value
Inlet		
Anteroposterior (cm)	12.5	10.0
Transverse (cm)	13.0	12.0
Total (cm)	25.5	22.0
Area (cm^2)	145.0	123.0
Midplane		
Anteroposterior (cm)	11.5	10.0
Transverse (cm)	10.5	9.5
Total (cm)	22.0	20.0
Area (cm^2)	125.0	106.0

From Gabbe SG, Niebyl JK, Simpson JL. *Obstetrics: normal and problem pregnancies,* 3rd ed. New York: Churchill Livingstone, 1996:434, with permission.

effacement, and nature and position of the presenting part. If premature rupture of membranes has occurred, digital examination may be deferred until active labor to reduce the risk of chorioamnionitis.

B. **Leopold's maneuvers** are a series of four abdominal palpations of the gravid uterus to ascertain fetal lie and presentation.
   1. The fundus is palpated to ascertain the presence or absence of a fetal pole (vertical versus transverse lie) and the nature of the fetal pole (cranium versus breech).
   2. The lateral walls of the uterus are examined using one hand to palpate and the other to fix the fetus. In vertical lies, the lateral uterus is usually occupied by the fetal spine (long, firm, and linear) and small parts or extremities.
   3. The nature and station of the presenting part is determined by palpating above the symphysis pubis.
   4. If the presentation is vertex, the cephalic prominence is palpated to determine the position of the fetal head. Provided the head is not too deep in the pelvis, the chin will be prominent if the head is neither flexed nor extended, as in a military presentation. If the head is not flexed, as in face presentation, the occiput will be felt below the spine. If the head is well flexed, neither chin nor occiput will be prominent.
C. **Cervical examination.** Three main components constitute a complete cervical examination.
   1. **Dilation** (or dilatation) is the degree of patency of the cervix. The diameter of the *internal* os of the cervix is measured in centimeters, from closed to 10 cm, with 10 cm corresponding to complete cervical dilation.
   2. **Effacement** is shortening and thinning of the cervix. Effacement is expressed as a percentage, ranging from 0% (no reduction in length) to 100% (minimal cervix palpable below the fetal presenting part).
   3. **Station** is a measure of descent of the presenting fetal part through the birth canal and is the estimated distance in centimeters between the leading bony presenting part and the level of the ischial spines. The level of the spines is defined as station 0. The stations below the spines are +1 for 1 cm below the spines to +5 at the perineum. The stations above the spines are –1 for 1 cm above the spines to –5 at the level of the pelvic inlet.

D. **Standard admission procedures.** For patients who have not received prenatal care, samples should be drawn for prenatal laboratory tests, including rapid plasma reagin, screening for hepatitis B virus and human immunodeficiency virus, determination of ABO blood group, antibody screening, urine culture and toxicology, screening for rubella IgG, and CBC. Patients with prenatal laboratory test results on record and an uncomplicated prenatal course require only urine testing (for protein and glucose), CBC, and drawing of a blood bank sample to be available for crossmatching if needed. Decisions regarding perineal hair shaving, enemas, showers, intravenous (IV) catheters, and positioning during labor and delivery should be based on the wishes of the patient and her family, and informed and prudent guidelines set forth by her health care team. Signed informed consent for management of labor and delivery should be obtained.

E. **Management of labor in low-risk patients.** The quality of uterine contractions should be regularly assessed. Cervical examinations should be kept to the minimum required to detect abnormalities in the progression of labor. Maternal BP and pulse should be recorded every hour during the first stage of labor and every 10 minutes during the second stage of labor.

1. Well-controlled studies have shown that, when performed at specific intervals with a 1:1 nurse-to-patient ratio, intermittent auscultation of the fetal heart is equivalent to continuous electronic monitoring in assessment of fetal well-being. The fetal heart rate should be recorded immediately after a contraction at least every 30 minutes during the active phase of the first stage of labor and at least every 15 minutes during the second stage.

2. Gastric emptying time increases in pregnant women, which results in an increased risk of regurgitation and subsequent aspiration. Aspiration pneumonitis is a major cause of anesthesia-related maternal mortality and is related to the acidity of gastric contents. The use of an antacid such as sodium citrate (30 mL of 0.3 mol/L solution orally) during the course of labor as well as restriction of the patient to NPO has been recommended by many authors.

3. For low-risk patients, delivery may take place in birthing rooms or traditional delivery areas. The lithotomy position is most frequently assumed for vaginal delivery in the United States, although alternative birthing positions, such as the lateral or Sims position or the partial sitting or squatting positions, are preferred by some patients, physicians, and midwives.

F. **Management of labor in high-risk patients.** Monitoring is intensified in high-risk labors. The fetal heart rate should be assessed according to the following guidelines.

1. During the active phase of the first stage of labor, if intermittent auscultation is used, the fetal heart rate should be recorded after a contraction at least every 15 minutes. If external continuous electronic fetal monitoring is used, the tracing should be evaluated every 15 minutes.

2. During the second stage of labor, either the fetal heart rate should be auscultated and recorded every 5 minutes or, if continuous monitoring is used, the tracing should be evaluated every 5 minutes.

G. **Induction of labor**

1. **Indications.** Induction of labor is indicated when the benefits of delivery to the mother or fetus outweigh the benefits of continuing the pregnancy.

2. An assessment of **fetal lung maturity** is necessary before elective induction of labor before 39 weeks' gestation based on standard dating criteria. Amniocentesis is not necessary if the induction is medically indicated and the risk of continuing the pregnancy is greater than the risk of delivering a baby before lung maturity.

3. The **state of the cervix** at the time of induction can be related to the success of labor induction. When the Bishop score (Table 5-4) exceeds 8,

TABLE 5-4. BISHOP SCORE

	Rating			
Factor	0	1	2	3
Dilation	Closed	1–2 cm	3–4 cm	5+ cm
Effacement	0–30%	40–50%	60–70%	80%+
Station	–3	–2	–1, 0	> +1
Consistency	Firm	Medium	Soft	—
Position	Posterior	Middle	Anterior	—

the likelihood of vaginal delivery after labor induction is similar to that with spontaneous labor. Induction with a lower Bishops score has been associated with a higher rate of failure, prolonged labor, and cesarean delivery. Cervical ripening may be helpful in a patient with a low Bishop score.

H. **Cervical ripening** is a complex process that ultimately results in physical softening and distensibility of the cervix. Some degree of spontaneous cervical ripening usually precedes spontaneous labor at term. In many postterm pregnancies, however, the cervix is unripe. Acceptable methods for cervical ripening include pharmacological methods, such as synthetic prostaglandins (prostaglandin E_1, prostaglandin E_2, prostaglandin $F_2\alpha$) or mechanical methods, such as *Laminaria japonicum* (osmotic dilator), 24 French Foley balloon, hygroscopic dilators, and double-balloon device (Atad Ripener device).

1. **Prostaglandin E_2.** Studies show that prostaglandin E_2 is superior to placebo in promoting cervical effacement and dilation. Prostaglandin E_2 also enhances sensitivity to oxytocin.
   a. **Prepidil** (prostaglandin E_2) gel contains 0.5 mg of dinoprostone in a 2.5-mL syringe; the gel is injected intracervically up to every 6 hours for up to three doses in a 24-hour period.
   b. **Cervidil** (prostaglandin E_2) is a vaginal insert containing 10 mg of dinoprostone. It provides a lower rate of release of medication (0.3 mg/hour) than the gel but has the advantage that it can be removed should hyperstimulation occur.
2. **Cytotec (misoprostol)** (prostaglandin E_1) is available in 100 µg tablets, which are divided into the desired dose. Dosing regimens range from 25 to 50 µg every 3–4 hours. The use of misoprostol for cervical ripening is an off-label use.
3. **Side effects.** The major complication associated with the use of prostaglandins is uterine hyperstimulation, which is usually reversible with administration of a beta-adrenergic agent (e.g., terbutaline sulfate). Maternal systemic effects such as fever, vomiting, and diarrhea are possible but infrequent.
4. **Contraindications.** Candidates for prostaglandin administration should not have an allergy to prostaglandins or active vaginal bleeding. Caution should be exercised when using prostaglandin E_2 in patients with glaucoma or severe hepatic or renal impairment. Prostaglandin E is a bronchodilator, so it is safe to use in asthmatic patients.

I. **Oxytocin administration**
1. **Indications.** Oxytocin is used for both induction and augmentation of labor. Augmentation should be considered for slow progression through the latent phase, protraction or arrest disorders of labor, or the presence of a hypotonic uterine contraction pattern. In general, starting dosages of 2.0–4.0 mIU/minute, with incremental increases of 1.0–2.0 mIU/minute

every 20–30 minutes, are reasonable. Cervical dilation of 1 cm/hour in the active phase indicates that oxytocin dosing is adequate. If an intrauterine pressure catheter is in place, calculation of more than 180 Montevideo units/period also indicates that oxytocin dosing is adequate.

2. **Complications.** Adverse effects of oxytocin are primarily dose related. The most common effect is fetal heart rate deceleration due to uterine hyperstimulation and resultant uteroplacental hypoperfusion. Hyperstimulation is usually reversible with terbutaline. Hypotension can result from rapid IV infusion. Natural and synthetic oxytocins structurally resemble antidiuretic hormone; therefore, water intoxication and hyponatremia can develop with prolonged administration.

J. Examination of **fetal heart rate patterns** can give clues to fetal conditions. Normal baseline heart rate at term is between 120 and 160 beats/minute. The presence or absence of variability (variation in the timing of successive beats) is a useful indicator of CNS integrity. The fetal CNS is very sensitive to hypoxia. In some instances of decreased oxygenation, the pattern of deceleration of the fetal heart rate can identify the cause.

1. **Variable decelerations** may start before, during, or after the uterine contraction starts (hence the designation variable). They usually show an abrupt onset and return, which gives them a characteristic V shape. Variable decelerations are caused by umbilical cord compression.

2. **Early decelerations** are shallow and symmetric and reach their nadir at the peak of the contraction. They are caused by vagus nerve–mediated response to fetal head compression.

3. **Late decelerations** are U-shaped decelerations of gradual onset and gradual return, reach their nadir after the peak of the contraction, and do not return to the baseline until after the contraction is over. They result from uteroplacental insufficiency and fetal hypoxia.

K. **Management of nonreassuring fetal heart rate patterns.** Studies have shown that abnormal fetal heart rate patterns do not predict long-term adverse neurologic outcomes such as cerebral palsy, and electronic fetal heart rate monitoring has resulted in an increased cesarean delivery rate without decreasing long-term adverse neurologic outcomes. Nevertheless, such monitoring is the best tool currently available for ensuring an optimal perinatal outcome.

1. **Noninvasive management**
   a. **Oxygen.** Administration of supplemental oxygen to the mother results in improved fetal oxygenation, assuming that placental exchange is adequate and umbilical cord circulation is unobstructed.
   b. **Maternal position.** Left lateral positioning releases vena caval compression by the gravid uterus, which allows increased venous return, increased cardiac output, increased BP, and therefore improved uterine blood flow.
   c. **Oxytocin** should be discontinued until fetal heart rate and uterine activity return to acceptable levels.
   d. **Vibroacoustic stimulation** (VAS) or fetal scalp stimulation may be used to induce accelerations when the fetal heart rate lacks variability. Heart rate acceleration in response to these stimuli indicates the absence of acidosis. An acceleration of greater than 10–15 beats/minute lasting at least 10 or 15 seconds in response to 5 seconds of VAS correlates with a mean pH value of 7.29 ± 0.07. Conversely, about a 50% chance of acidosis exists in a fetus who fails to respond to VAS in the setting of an otherwise nonreassuring heart rate pattern.

2. **Invasive management**
   a. **Amniotomy.** If the fetal heart rate cannot be adequately monitored externally, an amniotomy should be performed if necessary to allow access for internal monitoring. The amount and character of fluid should be noted. After amniotomy, examination should be performed to verify that the cord is not prolapsed.

b. **Fetal scalp electrode.** Direct application of a fetal scalp electrode records the fetal ECG and thus allows the fetal heart rate to be determined on a beat-by-beat basis. This greater physiologic detail is useful when trying to evaluate effects of intrapartum stress on the fetus.

c. **Intrauterine pressure catheter and amnioinfusion.** A catheter is inserted into the chorioamnionic sac and attached to a pressure gauge. Accurate pressure readings provide quantitative data on the strength, or amplitude, and duration of contractions. Amnioinfusion through the catheter of room-temperature normal saline can be used to replace amniotic fluid volume in the presence of variable decelerations in patients with oligohydramnios, or to dilute meconium. Studies have shown a decrease in newborn respiratory complications in fetuses with moderate to heavy meconium-stained fluid with amnioinfusion, probably due to the dilutional effect of amnioinfusion. Either bolus infusion or continuous infusion can be used, with care taken to avoid overdistention of the uterus.

d. **Tocolytic agents.** Beta-adrenergic agonists (e.g., terbutaline, 0.25 mg subcutaneously or 0.125 to 0.25 mg IV) can be administered to decrease uterine activity in the presence of uterine hyperstimulation. Potential side effects of beta-adrenergic agonists include both elevated serum glucose levels and increased maternal and fetal heart rates.

e. **Management of maternal hypotension.** Maternal hypotension, as a complication of the sympathetic blockade associated with epidural anesthesia, can lead to uteroplacental insufficiency and fetal heart rate decelerations. Management of hypotension includes IV fluid administration, left uterine displacement, and ephedrine administration.

f. **Fetal scalp blood pH.** Determination of fetal scalp blood pH can clarify the acid-base state of the fetus. A pH value of 7.25 or higher is normal. A pH range of 7.20–7.24 is a preacidotic range. A pH of less than 7.10–7.20 on two collections 5–10 minutes apart is thought to indicate sufficient fetal acidosis to warrant immediate delivery.

g. **Other procedures.** Newer techniques, such as continuous fetal pulse oximetry to monitor fetal oxygenation, may become more popular, but current data do not support a role for this.

L. The goals of **assisted spontaneous vaginal delivery** are reduction of maternal trauma, prevention of fetal injury, and initial support of the newborn.

1. **Episiotomy** is an incision into the perineal body to enlarge the outlet area and facilitate delivery. Episiotomy may be necessary in cases of vaginal soft tissue dystocia or as an accompaniment to forceps or vacuum delivery. The role of prophylactic episiotomy, however, is debated.

a. **Technique.** An incision is made vertically in the perineal body (midline episiotomy) or at a 45-degree angle off the midline (mediolateral episiotomy). The incision should be approximately half the length of the perineal body. The incision should extend into the vagina 2–3 cm. Excessive blood loss can result from performing the episiotomy too early. The episiotomy can be performed either before or after the application of forceps or a vacuum.

b. Midline episiotomies are classified by degree. A first-degree episiotomy involves the vaginal mucosa, a second-degree episiotomy involves the submucosa, a third-degree involves the anal sphincter, and a fourth-degree involves the rectal mucosa.

2. **Delivery of the head.** The goal of assisted delivery of the head is to prevent excessively rapid delivery. If extension of the head does not occur easily, a modified Ritgen maneuver can be performed by palpating the fetal chin through the perineum and applying pressure upward. After delivery of the head, external rotation is possible, which allows the occiput to be in line with the spine. If a nuchal cord is present, it is

looped over the head or double-clamped and cut. Mucus and amniotic fluid are aspirated from the infant's mouth and nose using bulb suction, or a DeLee suction catheter in the presence of meconium.

3. **Delivery of the shoulders and body.** After the fetal airway has been cleared, two hands are placed along the parietal bones of the fetal head, and the mother is asked to bear down. The fetus is directed posteriorly until the anterior shoulder has passed beneath the pubic bone. The fetus is then directed anteriorly until the posterior shoulder passes the perineum. After the shoulders are delivered, the fetus is grasped with one hand supporting the head and neck and the other hand along the spine. Delivery is completed spontaneously or with a maternal push. Once delivered, the infant is dried off, and any remaining mucus is suctioned from the airway.

4. **Cord clamping.** After delivery, a net transfer of blood from the placenta to the infant occurs via the umbilical vein, which permits passage of blood for up to 3 minutes after birth. Lowering the height at which the infant is held allows gravitational forces to increase the postnatal transfusion. The cord is generally double-clamped and cut shortly after delivery of the infant. After the cord is cut, a vigorous infant can be placed on the maternal abdomen and chest for bonding.

5. **Delivery of the placenta.** As a result of continued uterine contractions after delivery of the fetus, placental separation occurs within 15 minutes in 95% of all deliveries. While placental separation is awaited, a thorough inspection of the cervix, vagina, and perineum is performed. Classic signs of placental detachment are increased bleeding; descent of the umbilical cord; a change in shape of the uterine fundus from discoid to globular; and an increase in the height of the fundus as the lower uterine segment is distended by the placenta. After separation, the placenta, cord, and membranes are delivered by gentle traction on the cord and maternal expulsive efforts. The placenta and membranes are examined for integrity. The cord is examined for length, presence of knots, and number of vessels. If retained tissue is suspected or excessive uterine bleeding is present, intrauterine exploration is necessary.

VI. **Shoulder dystocia**

A. Shoulder dystocia occurs in 0.15–1.70% of all vaginal deliveries. It is defined as impaction of the fetal shoulders after delivery of the head and is associated with an increased incidence of fetal morbidity and mortality secondary to brachial plexus injuries and asphyxia.

B. **Macrosomia** is strongly associated with shoulder dystocia. Compared to average-sized infants, the risk of shoulder dystocia is 11 and 22 times greater for infants weighing more than 4000 g and 4500 g, respectively. Up to 50% of cases, however, occur in infants weighing less than 4000 g. Postterm and macrosomic infants are at risk because the trunk and shoulder growth is disproportionate to growth of the head in late pregnancy.

C. Other risk factors include maternal obesity, previous macrosomic infant, diabetes mellitus, and gestational diabetes. Shoulder dystocia should be suspected in cases of prolonged second stage of labor or prolonged deceleration phase of first stage of labor.

D. **Management**

1. Anticipation and preparation are important. Help should be called; extra hands will be needed during the delivery. A pediatrician should be notified. The clock should be checked when the dystocia occurs, and the time elapsed should be followed. If necessary, an attempt should be made to intubate the fetus while the head is still on the perineum.

2. **First-line measures**

a. A generous episiotomy is performed. One should not hesitate to extend it to a fourth-degree, a mediolateral, or even two mediolateral incisions.

b. McRoberts maneuver is performed by hyperflexion of the maternal hips, a maneuver that results in flattening of the lumbar spine and ventral rotation of the pelvis to increase the posterior outlet diameter.

c. Suprapubic pressure is applied. Fundal pressure should *not* be applied, as it only presses the fetal shoulder into the pubic symphysis and may lead to uterine rupture.

d. Pressure is applied to the fetal sternum to decrease shoulder diameter.

3. **Second-line measures**

a. A hand is placed into the vagina behind the fetal occiput, and the anterior shoulder pushed to oblique.

b. The Wood corkscrew maneuver is performed. The posterior shoulder is rotated 180 degrees forward and an attempt made to deliver it first.

c. The posterior arm is flexed and swept across the fetal chest, then the arm is delivered.

d. One or both clavicles is fractured. A thumb should be used to fracture the clavicle outward to avoid lung or subclavian injury.

4. **Third-line measures**

a. Symphysiotomy is performed.

b. A Zavanelli maneuver is performed. The fetal head is returned to the uterus and cesarean section is undertaken.

VII. **Forceps delivery**

A. **Classification is by station** of the fetal head at the time the forceps are applied.

1. **Mid forceps.** Head is engaged but above the level of +2 station.

2. **Low forceps.** Station is +2 or greater.

3. **Outlet forceps.** Scalp is visible without separating the labia, skull has reached pelvic floor, head is at or on perineum, and the occiput is either directly anterior-posterior in alignment or does not require more than 45 degrees of rotation to accomplish this.

B. **Indications.** No indication is absolute. Indications include prolonged second stage of labor, maternal exhaustion, fetal distress, or a maternal condition requiring a shortened second stage.

C. **Prerequisite criteria.** Before forceps delivery is performed, the following criteria should be met.

1. The fetal head must be engaged in the pelvis.

2. The cervix must be fully dilated.

3. The exact position and station of the fetal head should be known.

4. Maternal pelvis type should be known, and the pelvis must be adequate. Cephalopelvic disproportion is a contraindication for forceps delivery.

5. If time permits, the patient should be given adequate anesthesia.

6. If forceps delivery is done for fetal distress, someone who is able to perform neonatal resuscitation should be available.

7. The operator should have knowledge about, and experience with, the appropriate instrument and its proper application, and should be aware of possible complications.

D. **Complications**

1. **Maternal.** Uterine, cervical, or vaginal lacerations, extension of the episiotomy, bladder or urethral injuries, and hematomas.

2. **Fetal.** Cephalohematoma, bruising, lacerations, facial nerve injury, and, rarely, skull fracture and intracranial hemorrhage.

VIII. **Soft cup vacuum delivery.** Indications, contraindications, and complications are largely the same as for forceps delivery. The suction cup is applied to the head away from the fontanelles. Vacuum pressure to 0.7–0.8 kg/cc is reached, and traction is applied with one hand on the vacuum while the other hand maintains fetal flexion and supports the vacuum cup. Traction should be applied only during contractions. The vacuum pressure can be reduced between contractions and should not be maintained for longer than 30 minutes.

IX. **Cesarean section**
  A. **Indications.** Absolute indications for cesarean section are marked with an asterisk.
    1. **Fetal** indications include
      a. Fetal distress or nonreassuring fetal heart tracing
      b. Nonvertex or breech presentation
      c. Active maternal herpes simplex virus infection
      d. Fetal anomalies, such as hydrocephalus, that would make successful vaginal delivery unlikely
    2. **Maternal** indications include
      a. Obstruction of the lower genital tract (e.g., large condyloma)
      b. *Abdominal cerclage
      c. *Conjoined twins
      d. Previous cesarean section
      e. Previous uterine surgery involving the contractile portion of the uterus (classical cesarean, myomectomy)
    3. **Maternal and fetal** indications include
      a. *Placenta previa and vasa previa
      b. Abruptio placentae
      c. Labor dystocia or cephalopelvic disproportion
  B. **Risks.** The patient should be counseled about the standard risks of surgery, such as discomfort, bleeding that may require transfusion, infection, and damage to nearby organs.
  C. **Procedure**
    1. The **abdominal incision** should be of sufficient length to allow for delivery and may be vertical or transverse.
      a. Vertical incisions are faster and can be extended above the umbilicus if more room is needed. Less dead space is present in the wound, which decreases the risk of infection. The resulting wound, however, is weaker than that from a transverse incision. The skin and subcutaneous tissue are dissected sharply down to the fascia. The fascia can be incised vertically with the knife, or a window can be created and then the incision extended with Mayo scissors. The rectus and pyramidalis muscles are then separated in the midline, which exposes the peritoneum. The peritoneum can be entered bluntly or tented between two instruments and entered sharply, after transillumination demonstrates no underlying bowel or omentum. The peritoneal incision is extended superiorly and inferiorly, with care taken to avoid the bladder and bowel.
      b. A sufficient transverse or Pfannenstiel incision is made approximately 2 finger breadths above the pubic symphysis. The tissue is divided sharply down to the fascia, which is transversely incised in a curvilinear fashion, either with the scalpel or with scissors. The superior and then the inferior edge of the fascia is grasped and elevated, and the fascia is either bluntly or sharply separated from the underlying rectus muscles. Dissection is continued superiorly to the level of the umbilicus and inferiorly to the pubic symphysis. The peritoneum is entered in the manner described earlier.
    2. **Bladder flap.** The vesicouterine serosa is grasped, elevated, and sharply incised above the upper border of the bladder in the midline. Metzenbaum scissors are used to extend the serosal incision in a curvilinear fashion, then opened in each direction to undermine the serosa before sharply incising it. The bladder and lower portion of the peritoneum are then bluntly dissected off the lower uterine segment, and a bladder blade may be replaced between the bladder and lower uterine segment.
    3. **Uterine incision**
      a. Low transverse. The transverse incision is used most commonly. A curvilinear incision is made transversely in the lower uterine seg-

ment at least 1–2 cm above the upper margin of the bladder. The uterine cavity is entered carefully in the midline, with care taken to avoid injury to the fetus. The incision is then extended bilaterally and cephalad, either bluntly or with bandage scissors, with care taken to avoid the uterine vessels laterally. This type of incision is associated with less blood loss, fewer extensions into the bladder, decreased time of repair, and lower risk of rupture with subsequent pregnancies than other types of incisions. Disadvantages are the limitation in length and greater risk of extension into the uterine vessels.

b. Low vertical. The advantage of the low vertical incision is that it can be extended if more room is needed; in so doing, however, the active segment of the uterus may be entered. Such an occurrence should be recorded in the operative notes, and the patient should be informed and counseled that vaginal birth trial is contraindicated thenceforth, as the risk of uterine rupture is as high as 9%. Low vertical incisions are associated with extensions into the active segment more frequently than transverse incisions. In addition, to avoid injury, the bladder must be dissected further for low vertical incisions than for transverse incisions.

c. Classical. The classical type of incision extends from 1 to 2 cm above the bladder vertically up into the active segment of the uterus. Classical incisions are associated with more bleeding, longer repair time, greater risk of uterine rupture with subsequent pregnancy (4–9%), and greater incidence of adhesion of bowel or omentum. In cases of fetal prematurity, lower uterine segment fibroids, malpresentations, or fetal anomalies, however, it may be necessary to make this type of incision to provide adequate room for delivery.

d. T and J extensions. If a low transverse incision is made, it may extend, or need to be extended, in a T or J fashion. If the active segment of the uterus is entered, the event should be recorded in the operative notes, and the patient should be informed and counseled that vaginal birth trial is contraindicated thenceforth, as risk of uterine rupture is 4–9%. The J extension results in a stronger wound than the T extension, but neither type of extension is compatible with a subsequent trial of labor if the active segment is entered.

4. **Delivery of the fetus**
   a. **Term, cephalic presentation.** Retractors are removed and a hand is inserted around the fetal head. The head is elevated through the incision. The remainder of the fetus is delivered using gentle traction on the head as well as fundal pressure. The infant's nose and mouth are suctioned, the cord clamped and cut, and the infant delivered to the resuscitation team. If the head is deeply wedged in the pelvis, it may be necessary to insert a sterile gloved hand into the vagina to elevate and disengage the head.
   b. **Breech presentation.** The fetal position should be confirmed before surgery. If the fetus lies transverse, back down, or is preterm with a poorly developed maternal lower uterine segment, a classical cesarean section should be performed. Alternatively, in cases of transverse, back down position, the fetus may be shifted to vertex or breech position by direct manipulation through the uterus. The surgical assistant can manually maintain the fetus in the new position until delivery.
   c. **Preterm delivery.** If the lower uterine segment is inadequately developed, a low vertical or classical uterine incision should be made. Making a transverse incision under such circumstances risks injury to the uterine vessels, bladder, cervix, and vagina resulting from extension of the incision.

d. **Vacuum extraction or forceps use in cesarean delivery.** If the fetus is difficult to bring down to the low transverse incision and is in the vertex presentation, a vacuum extractor or forceps may be applied to assist in delivery without altering the uterine incision.

5. **Uterine repair.** After delivery of the placenta, oxytocin is administered. The uterus may be removed through the abdominal incision or left in its anatomic position. The incision is inspected for extensions, and the angles and points of bleeding are clamped with ring or Allis clamps. The uterine cavity is wiped with a laparotomy pad to remove retained membranes or placental fragments, and the uterus is wrapped in a moist laparotomy pad.

   a. Repair begins lateral to the angle of the incision, with care taken to avoid the uterine vessels. A running or running locking stitch is placed. The entire myometrium should be included. A second imbricated stitch, either horizontal or vertical, may then be placed if hemostasis is not obtained with the initial suture. The incision is inspected, and further areas of bleeding may be controlled with figure-of-eight sutures or electrocautery.

   b. In classical cesarean sections, two or three layers of sutures may be required to close the myometrium. The serosa should then be closed with an inverting baseball stitch to decrease formation of adhesions of bowel and omentum to the uterine incision.

6. **Abdominal closure.** The tubes and ovaries are inspected. The posterior cul-de-sac and gutters are cleaned of blood and debris. The uterus is returned to the anatomic position in the abdominal cavity and the incision reinspected to assure hemostasis with the tension off the vessels. The fascia is then closed with running delayed-absorption sutures. The subcutaneous tissue is inspected for hemostasis, and dead space may be closed with interrupted absorbable sutures. The skin is closed with subcuticular stitches or staples.

D. **Intraoperative complications**

1. Uterine vessel, ureteral, bowel and bladder injuries are discussed in Chapter 23.

2. In cases of **atony,** the fundus should be massaged. Oxytocin (20–40 U/L), methylergonovine maleate (Methergine) (0.2 mg intramuscularly or IV), 15-methyl prostaglandin $F_2\alpha$ (Hemabate) (250 µg in successive doses up to 1.0–1.5 mg intramuscularly or intramyometrially) may be given if contraindications do not exist. Methylergonovine should not be used in patients with hypertension and 15-methyl prostaglandin $F_2\alpha$ should be avoided in patients with asthma. If pharmacologic treatment fails, uterine or hypogastric artery ligation, uterine compression sutures, or hysterectomy may be necessary.

X. **Cesarean hysterectomy**

A. The **indications** for cesarean hysterectomy include uterine atony unresponsive to conservative measures; laceration of major vessels; severe cervical dysplasia or carcinoma in situ; and abnormal plantation.

B. **Risks** include increased operative time, blood loss, rate of infection, and higher incidence of damage to the bladder and ureters than in nongravid hysterectomy or cesarean section alone. In addition, the cervix is not easily identified in a labored uterus and may not be completely excised at the time of cesarean hysterectomy.

XI. **Vaginal birth after cesarean section (VBAC).** Provided no contraindications exist, a patient may be offered VBAC. Success rates are higher for patients with nonrecurring conditions, such as malpresentation or fetal distress (60–80%), than for those with a prior diagnosis of dystocia (50–70%).

A. **Contraindications** include prior classical T- or J-shaped incision or other transfundal uterine surgery, contracted pelvis, medical or obstetric con-

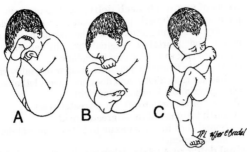

FIG. 5-2. Breech presentations. **A:** Frank breech. **B:** Complete breech. **C:** Incomplete breech, single footling. (From Beckmann CR, et al. *Obstetrics and gynecology,* 2nd ed. Baltimore: Williams & Wilkins, 1995:194, with permission.)

traindications to vaginal delivery, and inability to perform emergency cesarean delivery.

   B. **Management.** When VBAC is attempted, epidural anesthesia and oxytocin may be used. Appropriate staffing, fetal monitoring, blood products, and facilities that can accommodate an emergency cesarean section should be available. The most common sign of uterine rupture is a nonreassuring fetal heart rate pattern with variable decelerations evolving into late decelerations, bradycardia, and undetectable fetal heart rate. Other findings include uterine or abdominal pain, loss of station of the presenting part, vaginal bleeding, and hypovolemia.

XII. **Malpresentations**

   A. A **normal presentation** is defined by a longitudinal lie, cephalic presentation, and flexion of the fetal neck. All other presentations are malpresentations. Occurring in approximately 5% of all deliveries, malpresentations may lead to abnormalities of labor and endanger the mother or fetus.

   B. **Risk factors** are conditions that decrease the polarity of the uterus, increase or decrease fetal mobility, or block the presenting part from the pelvis.

      1. **Maternal** factors include grand multiparity, pelvic tumors, pelvic contracture, and uterine malformations.

      2. **Fetal** factors include prematurity, multiple gestation, poly- or oligohydramnios, macrosomia, placenta previa, hydrocephaly, trisomy, anencephaly, and myotonic dystrophy.

   C. **Breech** presentation occurs when the cephalic pole is in the uterine fundus. Major congenital anomalies occur in 6.3% of term breech presentation infants compared to 2.4% of vertex presentation infants.

      1. **Incidence.** Breech presentation occurs in 25% of pregnancies at less than 28 weeks' gestation, 7% of pregnancies at 32 weeks' gestation, and 3–4% of term pregnancies in labor.

      2. There are **three types** of breech presentation (Fig. 5-2).

         a. **Complete** breech (5–12%) occurs when the fetus is flexed at the hips and flexed at the knees.

         b. **Incomplete,** or footling breech (12–38%), occurs when the fetus has one or both hips extended.

         c. **Frank** breech (48–73%) occurs when both hips are flexed and both knees extended.

      3. **Risks**

         a. The breech presentation is associated with risk of cord prolapse and head entrapment. The risk of cord prolapse is 15% in footling breech, 5% in complete breech, and 0.5% in frank breech. If the fetal neck is hyperextended, a risk of spinal cord injury exists.

b. **Risks of vaginal breech delivery.** Patients with fetuses in a complete or frank breech presentation may be considered for vaginal delivery. Cesarean section poses the risk of increased maternal morbidity and mortality. Vaginal breech delivery, however, poses increased risk to the fetus of the following:

(1) Mortality (three to five times greater mortality rate if the fetus is heavier than 2500 g and does not have a lethal anomaly)

(2) Asphyxia (3.8 times greater risk)

(3) Cord prolapse (5 to 20 times greater risk)

(4) Birth trauma (13 times greater risk)

(5) Spinal cord injuries (occur in 21% of vaginal deliveries if deflexion is present)

4. **Vaginal delivery.** A trial of labor may be attempted if the following circumstances exist: breech is frank or complete; the estimated fetal weight is less than 3800 g; pelvimetry results are adequate; the fetal head is flexed; anesthesia is immediately available and a prompt cesarean section may be performed; the fetus is monitored continuously; and two obstetricians experienced with vaginal breech delivery and two pediatricians are present. A cesarean section should be performed in the event of any arrest of labor.

a. The goal in vaginal breech delivery is to maximize cervical dilatation and maternal expulsion efforts to maintain flexion of the fetal vertex.

b. In breech presentation, the fetus usually emerges in the sacrum transverse or oblique position. As crowning occurs (the bitrochanteric diameter passes under the symphysis), an episiotomy should be considered. One should not assist the delivery yet.

c. When the umbilicus appears, one should place fingers medial to each thigh and press out laterally to deliver the legs (Pinard maneuver). The fetus should then be rotated to the sacrum anterior position, and the trunk can be wrapped in a towel for traction.

d. When the scapulae appear, fingers should be placed over the shoulders from the back. The humerus should be followed down, and each arm rotated across the chest and out (Lovsett's maneuver). To deliver the *right* arm, the fetus is turned in a *counterclockwise* direction; to deliver the *left* arm, the fetus is turned in a *clockwise* direction.

e. If the head does not deliver spontaneously, the vertex must be flexed by placing downward traction and pressure on the maxillary ridge (Mauriceau-Smellie-Veit maneuver). Suprapubic pressure may also be applied. Piper forceps may be used to assist in delivery of the head.

f. For delivery of a breech second twin, ultrasonography should be available in the delivery room. The operator reaches into the uterus and grasps both feet, trying to keep the membranes intact. The feet are brought down to the introitus, then amniotomy is performed. The body is delivered to the scapula by applying gentle traction on the feet. The remainder of the delivery is the same as that described earlier for a singleton breech.

g. Entrapment of the head during breech vaginal delivery may be managed by one or more of the following procedures.

(1) Dührssen's incisions are made in the cervix at the 2, 6, and 10 o'clock positions. Either two or three incisions can be made. The 3 and 9 o'clock positions should be avoided due to the risk of entering the cervical vessels and causing hemorrhage.

(2) Cephalocentesis can be performed if the fetus is not viable. The procedure is performed by perforating the base of the skull and suctioning the cranial contents.

5. **External cephalic version**
   a. **Indication** for performing external cephalic version is persistent breech presentation at term. Version is performed to avoid breech presentation in labor.
   b. **Risks** include cord accident, placental separation, fetal distress, fetal injury, premature rupture of membranes, and fetomaternal bleeding (overall incidence is 0–1.4%). The most common "risk" is failed version.
   c. **Success rate** for external cephalic version ranges from 35% to 86%, but in 2% of cases the fetus reverts back to breech presentation.
   d. **Technique.** A gestational age of at least 36 weeks and reactive non-stress test must be established before the procedure, and informed consent must be obtained. Version is generally accomplished by applying a liberal amount of lubrication, then transabdominally grasping the fetal head and fetal breech and manipulating the fetus through a forward or backward roll. This can be achieved by one or two operators. Ultrasonographic guidance is an important adjunct to confirm position and monitor fetal heart rate. Tocolysis and spinal or epidural anesthesia may be used. After the procedure, the patient should be monitored continuously until the fetal heart rate is reactive, there are no decelerations, and there is no evidence of regular contractions. Rh-negative patients should receive Rh_0 (D) immune globulin (RhoGAM) after the procedure because of the potential for fetomaternal bleeding.
   e. **Factors associated with failure** include obesity, oligohydramnios, deep engagement of the presenting part, and fetal back posterior. Nulliparity and an anterior placenta may also reduce the likelihood of success.
   f. **Contraindications** to external cephalic version include conditions in which labor or vaginal delivery would be contraindicated (placenta previa, prior classical cesarean section, etc.). Version is not recommended in cases of ruptured membrane, third trimester bleeding, oligohydramnios, or multiple gestations, or if labor has begun.

D. **Abnormal lie.** "Lie" refers to the alignment of the fetal spine in relation to the maternal spine. Longitudinal lie is normal, whereas oblique and transverse lies are abnormal. Abnormal lie is associated with multiparity, prematurity, pelvic contraction, and disorders of the placenta.
   1. **Incidence** of abnormal lie is 1 in 300, or 0.33%, of pregnancies at term. At 32 weeks' gestation, incidence is less than 2%.
   2. **Risk.** The greatest risk of abnormal lie is cord prolapse, because the fetal parts do not fill the pelvic inlet.
   3. **Management.** If abnormal lie persists beyond 35–38 weeks, external version may be attempted. An ultrasonographic examination should be performed to rule out major anomalies and abnormal placentation. If an abnormal axial lie persists, mode of delivery should be cesarean section, with careful thought regarding type of uterine incision. A low segment transverse incision is still possible. However, 25% of transverse incisions will require an extension to allow for access to and atraumatic delivery of the fetal head. An intraoperative cephalic version may be attempted but should not be tried if ruptured membranes or oligohydramnios exists. A vertical incision may be prudent in cases with back down transverse or oblique lie with ruptured membranes or poorly developed lower uterine segment.

E. **Abnormal attitude and deflexion.** Full flexion of the fetal neck is considered normal. Abnormalities range from partial deflexion to full extension.
   1. **Face** presentation results from extension of the fetal neck. The chin is the presenting part.

a. **Incidence** is between 0.14% and 0.54%. In 60% of cases, face presentation is associated with a fetal malformation. Anencephaly accounts for 33% of all cases.

b. **Diagnosis.** Face presentation may be diagnosed by vaginal examination, ultrasonography, or palpation of the cephalic prominence and the fetal back on the same side of the maternal abdomen when performing Leopold's maneuvers.

c. **Risk.** Perinatal mortality ranges from 0.6% to 5.0%.

d. **Management.** The fetus must be mentum (chin) anterior for a vaginal delivery to be performed.

2. **Brow** presentation results from partial deflexion of the fetal neck.

a. **Incidence** is 1 in 670 to 1 in 3433 pregnancies. Causes of brow presentation are similar to those of face presentation.

b. **Risks.** Perinatal mortality ranges from 1.28% to 8.00%.

c. **Management.** The majority of cases spontaneously convert to a flexed attitude. A vaginal delivery should be considered only if the maternal pelvis is large, the fetus is small, and labor progresses adequately. Forceps delivery or manual conversion is contraindicated.

3. **Compound** presentation occurs when an extremity prolapses beside the presenting part.

a. **Incidence** is 1 in 377 to 1 in 1213 pregnancies; compound presentation is associated with prematurity.

b. **Diagnosis.** Suspicion of compound presentation should be aroused if active labor is arrested or if the fetus fails to engage, as well as if the prolapsing extremity is palpated directly.

c. **Risks.** Fetal risks are associated with birth trauma and cord prolapse. Cord prolapse occurs in 10–20% of cases. Neurologic and musculoskeletal damage to the involved extremity can occur.

d. **Management.** The prolapsing extremity should not be manipulated. Continuous fetal monitoring is recommended because compound presentation can be associated with occult cord prolapse. Spontaneous vaginal delivery occurs in 75% of vertex/upper extremity presentations. Cesarean section is indicated in cases of nonreassuring fetal heart tracing, cord prolapse, and failure of labor to progress.

XIII. **Cerclage**

A. **Indication.** Cervical incompetence.

B. **Risks** include premature rupture of membranes, chorioamnionitis, and fibrous scarring of the cervix, which may result in abnormal dilatation or rupture at the time of labor. Before the cerclage is placed, cervical culture results should be obtained and any infections treated. An ultrasonographic examination should be performed to rule out any anomalies (if longer than 16 weeks' gestation) and confirm cardiac activity.

C. **Procedures**

1. The **McDonald cerclage** is the most commonly performed and recommended technique. It involves placing a purse-string suture through the cervix as close as possible to the internal os. Care should be taken to avoid the vessels at the 3 and 9 o'clock positions on the cervix. Permanent suture material, such as Mersilene tape or nylon, is used. A second stitch may be placed above the first. The knot usually is tied anteriorly to facilitate removal. The cerclage is removed at the time of labor, in the event of premature rupture of membranes, if infection is suspected, or at 37 weeks.

2. In the **Shirodkar cerclage,** the suture is buried beneath the cervical mucosa, after the bladder is dissected off the anterior cervix. The suture may be left permanently in place, which necessitates cesarean section for delivery, or may be removed to allow for a vaginal delivery.

This type of cerclage is associated with more blood loss during placement than the McDonald cerclage and has not been proven to be more effective.

3. In cases in which a McDonald or Shirodkar cerclage has failed, an **abdominal** cerclage may be performed before the next pregnancy. Delivery via cesarean section is required after placement of this type of cerclage.

D. **Follow-up** of the patient with a cerclage includes frequent cervical examinations either digitally or with ultrasonography. Reduced activity or bed rest as well as abstinence from sexual intercourse may be considered.

6. FETAL ASSESSMENT

Dana Gossett and Karin Blakemore

I. **The purpose of fetal testing** is to assess the well-being of the high-risk fetus, with the primary goal of preventing fetal death. Fetal testing may consist of simply monitoring the fetal heart rate, or it may include ultrasonography or Doppler ultrasonography evaluation. Indications for testing include a variety of maternal and fetal conditions, including diabetes mellitus, chronic hypertension, history of previous fetal demise, fetal growth restriction, and oligohydramnios.

A. **Methods of fetal assessment**

1. **Maternal assessment of fetal movement ("kick counts").** This is the least invasive, least expensive, and simplest of the various surveillance methods. The mother is asked to count the number of times she feels her fetus move within a certain period of time. It is usually recommended that this be done with the mother lying on her left side, after having eaten. Several different standards exist to define "reassuring" maternal assessment of fetal movement. One approach is to have the mother count fetal movements over the course of 1 hour. Four or more is considered reassuring; three or fewer should prompt further investigation. A second approach is to have the mother begin counting fetal movements when she wakes up in the morning and record the number of hours required to feel ten movements. On average, this takes 2–3 hours. Again, maternal reports of decreased movement should prompt further testing.

2. **Nonstress test (NST).** This is the next simplest to perform of the various methods of fetal assessment. The fetal heart rate is monitored with an external cardiotocometer, whereas uterine activity is monitored with an external tocodynamometer. A "reactive" NST is one that demonstrates at least two accelerations of the fetal heart rate in 20 minutes, associated with fetal movement as recorded by the mother (or detected electronically). Each of the two accelerations must last at least 15 seconds and reach a peak fifteen beats above the baseline level (Fig. 6-1). A reactive NST is highly predictive of low risk of fetal mortality in the subsequent 72–96 hours and is still predictive at 1 week. Fetuses do not routinely demonstrate reactivity before 28 weeks, and it may be normal to have a nonreactive tracing as late as 32 weeks' gestation. After 32 weeks, a nonreactive tracing should prompt further evaluation of fetal well-being, such as measuring a biophysical profile.

3. **Biophysical profile (BPP).** The BPP, like the NST, has an excellent negative predictive value for fetal mortality in the 72–96 hours after the test; in fact, the NST is an integral part of the BPP. The BPP has five components altogether, each scored 0 or 2 for a maximum score of 10; these are listed in Table 6-1. All of the sonographic criteria (i.e., not including the NST) must be observed within a 30-minute period. A score of 8 or 10 is reassuring, and routine surveillance and expectant obstetrical management may continue. A score of 6 raises concern, and the BPP should be repeated in 6–24 hours, especially in fetuses over 32 weeks' gestation. If the score does not improve, delivery should be considered, depending on gestational age and individual circumstances. Scores of 4 or below are worrisome, and delivery should be considered, again depending on gestational age and clinical context.

4. **Contraction stress test (CST) or oxytocin challenge test (OCT).** The most labor-intensive method of fetal surveillance, this method also

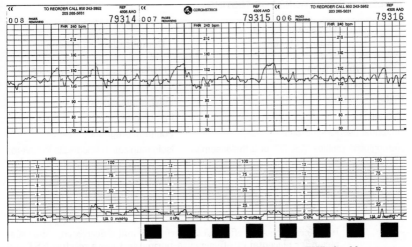

FIG. 6-1. Reactive nonstress test results. bpm, beats per minute; FHR, fetal heart rate.

has the highest specificity for detecting the compromised fetus. The mother is placed in dorsal supine position with a leftward tilt, and external monitors are applied. Contractions are induced either by nipple stimulation by the patient or by infusion of a dilute solution of oxytocin. Nipple stimulation is repeated, or the oxytocin infusion titrated up, until three contractions per 10-minute period are observed. A "positive" CST is one in which late decelerations occur with more than 50% of contractions. A "negative" CST is one in which no late decelerations occur. A CST with nonrepetitive late decelerations is considered equivocal, and further evaluation of the pregnancy is performed. An inadequate CST is one in which adequate contractions are not achieved. Relative contraindications to CST include preterm labor, preterm premature rupture of membranes, placenta previa, and high risk for uterine rupture. Prior low transverse cesarean section is not a contraindication.

5. **Nonstress test and amniotic fluid index (AFI).** In the third trimester, an AFI and NST are often used together to assess fetal well-being.

TABLE 6-1. BIOPHYSICAL PROFILE

	Score 2	Score 0
Nonstress test	Reactive	Nonreactive
Amniotic fluid (AF) volume	Single pocket of AF greater than 1 cm in two perpendicular planes	Largest pocket of AF less than 1 cm depth
Fetal tone	At least one extremity motion from flexion to extension and return to flexion	Extended position with no or slow return to flexion; absent movement
Fetal movement	At least three gross body movements	Two or fewer gross body movements
Fetal breathing	30 secs of sustained breathing effort (may contain pauses of up to 5 secs)	Less than 30 secs of fetal breathing; no breathing

TABLE 6-2. INDICATIONS FOR TESTING

Maternal conditions that may warrant testing	Complications of pregnancy
Chronic hypertension	Pregnancy-associated hypertension
Renal insufficiency	Oligohydramnios
Diabetes mellitus	Polyhydramnios
Cyanotic heart disease	Intrauterine growth restriction
Antiphospholipid syndrome	Postterm pregnancy
Hemoglobinopathies (SS, SC, or S thalassemia)	Isoimmunization (moderate to severe)
	Discordant twin gestation
	Decreased fetal movement

In general, the AFI reflects fetal perfusion, and if decreased, raises suspicion for placental insufficiency. A normal test has a reactive NST and an AFI greater than 5 (and less than 25); an abnormal test lacks one or both of these findings.

6. **Doppler ultrasonography** is a noninvasive method of assessing fetal vascular impedance. Umbilical artery Doppler ultrasonography has been used to assess fetal well-being, based on observations that growth-restricted fetuses have different Doppler characteristics than normal fetuses. The most frequently used measurement is the umbilical artery systolic to diastolic ratio (S/D ratio). The normal values vary depending on gestational age. Significant elevations in the S/D ratio have been associated with intrauterine growth retardation, fetal hypoxia or acidosis or both, and higher rates of perinatal morbidity and mortality. Absent and reversed end-diastolic flow are the more extreme examples of abnormal S/D ratio and may prompt delivery in some situations.

B. **Factors affecting test results**
   1. **Sleep cycles.** Fetuses may have sleep cycles 20–80 minutes in duration. During these periods, the long-term variability of the fetal heart rate is decreased, and the tracing is likely to be nonreactive. To rule out sleep cycle as a cause for a nonreactive NST, prolonged monitoring is often required (longer than 80 minutes at times).
   2. **Medications and illicit drugs** taken by the mother, such as narcotics and sedatives, betamethasone, dexamethasone, and beta-blockers, will also reach the fetus, resulting in decreased fetal heart rate variability and nonreactivity. Magnesium sulfate can also have this effect in high doses.
   3. **Maternal smoking** results in a transient decrease in fetal heart rate variability.
   4. **Maternal hypoglycemia** may reduce long-term fetal heart rate variability as well as fetal movement.
   5. **Prematurity.** The NST is not expected to be routinely reactive before 32 weeks. If fetal surveillance is required at earlier gestational ages, obtaining a biophysical profile may be helpful.

II. **Indications for fetal testing**
   A. **Maternal conditions and pregnancy complications** indicative of the need for testing are listed in Table 6-2.
   B. **Frequency of testing.** If the indication for fetal surveillance is temporary (e.g., decreased fetal movement or oligohydramnios that subsequently resolves), the surveillance need only continue as long as the indication is present. Chronic maternal or fetal conditions, however, require regular test-

ing. For many of the indications described in Table 6-2, weekly testing with one of the described modalities is adequate. For particularly high-risk conditions, however, such as moderate to severe fetal growth restriction, poorly controlled diabetes, or moderate to severe hypertension, twice-weekly testing may be performed. Decisions about the frequency of testing must take into account the full clinical picture. Deterioration of maternal or fetal status at any time should prompt reevaluation. Fetal testing results, when normal, have excellent negative predictive value; however, morbidity and mortality due to an acute event (such as abruptio placentae) cannot be predicted. Of note, the positive predictive value (i.e., the prediction of a compromised fetus) is low for all of these antepartum tests of fetal well-being.

7. COMPLICATIONS OF LABOR AND DELIVERY

Cynthia Holcroft and Ernest Graham

I. **Postpartum hemorrhage**
   A. **Incidence.** Defined as more than 500 mL of blood loss during the first 24 hours after a vaginal delivery or as more than 1 L of blood loss after a cesarean section, postpartum hemorrhage remains the third most common cause of maternal mortality in the United States and accounts for 30% of maternal mortality in the developing world. These statistics are difficult to interpret, however, because the blood loss during most deliveries is underestimated. When quantitatively measured, the average blood loss during a vaginal delivery is 500 mL, and the average blood loss during a cesarean section is 1 L.
   B. **Management.** When a patient develops postpartum hemorrhage, prompt action is crucial. The uterus of a pregnant woman at term has a blood supply of 600 mL/minute, and patients can rapidly become unstable. Signs of hemorrhage in young, healthy women tend to be masked until serious intravascular depletion has occurred, so the clinical picture may be falsely reassuring. Large-bore intravenous access must be obtained and aggressive fluid resuscitation used. In general, transfusion of blood products should be considered after 1–2 L of blood has been lost. Fresh frozen plasma (FFP) should be added after transfusion of 6 U of packed red blood cells to reduce the chances of dilutional and citrate-related coagulopathy. Platelet transfusion should also be considered. As soon as intravenous access is obtained, the physician must examine the patient to determine the cause of the hemorrhage and address the problem appropriately.
   C. **Causes** of postpartum hemorrhage include uterine atony, lacerations, retained products of conception, uterine dehiscence or rupture, abruptio placentae, coagulopathy, and uterine inversion.
      1. **Uterine atony** occurs in 90% of cases of postpartum hemorrhage. Postpartum uterine bleeding is typically controlled by compression of vessels by uterine contraction, so atony leads to rapid blood loss. Predisposing factors include overdistension of the uterus from multiple gestation, polyhydramnios, or macrosomia; rapid or prolonged labor; grand multiparity; chorioamnionitis; use of general anesthesia or tocolytic agents; and use of oxytocin (Pitocin) during labor.
         a. The first step in managing uterine atony is **bimanual massage** of the uterus with evacuation of clot from the lower uterine segment to allow the uterus to contract adequately.
         b. Next, **uterine contractile agents** such as oxytocin, methylergonovine maleate (Methergine), 15-methyl prostaglandin $F_{2\alpha}$ (Hemabate), dinoprostone (Prostin), or misoprostol (Cytotec) can be administered (Table 7-1).
            Methylergonovine is contraindicated for patients with hypertension or preeclampsia, and 15-methyl prostaglandin $F_{2\alpha}$ is contraindicated for patients with asthma.
         c. If uterine atony continues after administration of uterine contractile agents, **blunt curettage** may be performed to rule out retained products of conception. Large curettes and ultrasonographic guidance may be used to minimize the risk of uterine perforation.
         d. Persistent hemorrhage resulting from uterine atony warrants more **invasive measures**. If interventional radiology is readily available, embolization of pelvic vessels may be attempted; if not, the obstetrician must perform a laparotomy. To save the uterus, bilateral uter-

TABLE 7-1. UTERINE CONTRACTILE AGENTS

Agent	Dose	Frequency
Oxytocin (Pitocin)	10 U IM *or* 10–20 U/L NS IV	Initial dose may be followed by 10–20 U oxytocin in 1 L NS at 125 mL/hr
Methylergonovine maleate (Methergine)	0.2 mg PO/IM/IV	2–4 hrs
15-methyl prostaglandin $F_{2\alpha}$ (Hemabate)	125 μg IM	15–90 mins
Dinoprostone (Prostin)	20 mg PR	2 hrs
Misoprostol (Cytotec)	400–600 μg PO/ PR/buccally	4 hrs

NS, normal saline.

ine artery ligation, hypogastric artery ligation, or both may be attempted. Such measures decrease the pulse pressure to the uterus and help reduce blood loss and promote clot formation, but because of the extent of collateral blood flow to the uterus, arterial ligation does not stop all bleeding. As hypogastric artery ligation can be technically difficult, it may prove more prudent to proceed with hysterectomy instead of attempting arterial ligation. If hypogastric artery ligation is decided on, the hypogastric artery should be isolated and ligated approximately 2 cm distal to the origin of the posterior branch to avoid cutting off the blood supply to the gluteal muscles. Care should be taken to avoid injury to the hypogastric vein that lies beneath the artery. Permanent suture, such as silk, is traditionally used for ligation. Aortic pressure may be applied to control blood loss temporarily.

   e. The definitive measure for controlling intractable uterine bleeding remains **hysterectomy**. If the cervix is fully dilated at the time of hysterectomy, then a total abdominal hysterectomy must be performed, but if the cervix is not fully dilated, supracervical hysterectomy may be considered in an attempt to minimize blood loss. If total hysterectomy is performed, care must be taken not to shorten the vagina. This can be facilitated by palpating the cervix vaginally or by amputating the fundus and palpating the cervicovaginal junction through a dilated cervix. Often, patients must be monitored in an intensive care setting after peripartum hysterectomy because of massive blood loss and postoperative fluid shifts.

2. **Lacerations** cause approximately 6% of all postpartum hemorrhages and should be suspected particularly if an operative delivery or episiotomy was performed. Although lacerations often manifest as brisk vaginal bleeding, concealed pelvic hematomas, identified mainly by hypotension and pelvic pain, may also form.

   a. **Vulvar and vaginal hematomas** are particularly associated with operative deliveries. Nonexpanding hematomas may be managed conservatively, but expanding hematomas should be evacuated.

   b. **Retroperitoneal hematoma** is a potentially life-threatening condition that may present as hypotension, cardiovascular shock, or flank pain. If a retroperitoneal bleed is stable, it is safest to provide supportive care and allow the hematoma to tamponade itself in the retroperitoneum. If the hematoma continues to expand, however, then surgical exploration may be necessary. The retroperitoneum should be opened and bleeding vessels identified and ligated. Care should be taken to localize the ureter in retroperitoneal dissection. If necessary, the hypogastric arteries may also be ligated. The retroperitoneum should then be closed and the patient closely monitored.

3. **Retained products of conception** cause 3–4% of cases of postpartum hemorrhage. Risk factors include the presence of accessory lobes of the placenta and abnormal placentation such as placenta accreta, percreta, or increta. After the placenta is delivered it should be inspected carefully for missing cotyledons or vessels in the membranes that might indicate missing accessory lobes. Abnormal placentation should be suspected if the placenta fails to emerge spontaneously within 30 minutes after delivery of the infant. When the placenta is retained, manual exploration of the uterus is performed. If products of conception remain in the uterus after manual exploration, blunt curettage should be performed. Because of the high risk of perforation of the postpartum uterus during curettage, large curettes and ultrasonographic guidance should be used if available. In cases of abnormal placentation, it may be impossible to remove all of the placenta without injury to the uterus. In these cases, part of the placenta may be left in the uterus if the bleeding is adequately controlled with uterine contractile agents. Methotrexate sodium can also be administered to help speed resorption of the remaining placenta. If significant bleeding persists despite curettage of the uterus and the use of contractile agents, further invasive procedures such as embolization of the uterine arteries or laparotomy must be performed.

4. **Coagulopathy** can also lead to postpartum hemorrhage. Risk factors include severe preeclampsia, abruptio placentae, idiopathic thrombocytopenia, amniotic fluid embolism, and hereditary coagulopathies such as von Willebrand's disease. If a patient's bleeding is the result of coagulopathy, supportive measures to correct the coagulopathy are required; surgical treatment does not address the problem and only leads to further hemorrhage. If coagulation factors are depleted, FFP or cryoprecipitate should be given; platelets should be given if the platelet count falls below 20,000 or if the patient's platelets are malfunctioning, regardless of the platelet count. Dexamethasone has also been shown to improve both platelet number and function in patients with severe preeclampsia. Dexamethasone, 10 mg by mouth daily, should be administered for 2 days, followed by 5 mg by mouth daily for 2 days.

II. **Uterine dehiscence or rupture.** Uterine dehiscence is defined as separation of a lower uterine scar that does not penetrate the serosa and rarely causes significant hemorrhage. Rupture is defined as complete separation of the uterine wall and may lead to significant hemorrhage and fetal distress.

A. **Risk factors** include a history of prior uterine surgery, including cesarean section, myomectomy, and ectopic surgery involving the cornua. Other risk factors are hyperstimulation of the uterus, internal version or extraction, operative delivery, cephalopelvic disproportion, and cocaine use. Approximately 1% of patients with a history of a prior low-segment transverse cesarean section and 5% of patients with a history of a cesarean section extending to the active segment of the uterus experience rupture if allowed a trial of labor. One-third of women with a history of prior classic cesarean section who experience rupture do so before onset of labor.

B. If **rupture** occurs, severe hemorrhage can result, which leads to a nonreassuring fetal heart tracing. On examination, the station of the presenting part may rise with change in the fetal heart position. The patient should undergo laparotomy with delivery of the infant and repair of the uterine rupture.

III. **Uterine inversion**

A. **Incidence.** Uterine inversion occurs in 1 in 2000 deliveries and is diagnosed by partial delivery of the placenta that is followed by massive blood loss and hypotension. Inversion occurs most commonly with fundal placentas and is classified as incomplete if the corpus travels partially through the cervix, complete if the corpus travels entirely through the cervix, and prolapsed if the corpus travels through the vaginal introitus.

B. **Treatment** of uterine inversion consists of manually replacing the uterus after adequate intravenous access has been established.

1. If the uterus can be replaced easily without removing the placenta, less blood will be lost; if the bulk of the placenta prevents replacement of the uterus, however, the placenta should be removed to facilitate uterine replacement.

2. If the cervix has contracted around the corpus of the uterus, uterine relaxant agents may be used, including nitroglycerin; betamimetics such as terbutaline sulfate or ritodrine hydrochloride; magnesium sulfate; and halogenated general anesthetics such as halothane or isoflurane. If the patient is normotensive and has been given adequate analgesia, nitroglycerin is the preferred agent because it has a rapid onset of 30–60 seconds and a short half-life, which enables the uterus to contract again after it has been replaced and minimizes further blood loss. General anesthesia should be used if other agents are unsuccessful in freeing the uterus.

3. After the uterus is replaced, uterine contractile agents should be used.

4. If the obstetrician is unable to replace the uterus manually, laparotomy is performed. In addition to attempts to reduce the prolapse vaginally, traction can then be placed on the round ligaments. If traction is unsuccessful, a vertical incision can be made on the posterior lower uterine segment to enable replacement of the uterus.

IV. **Amniotic fluid embolism** occurs during 1 in 30,000 deliveries and carries a 50% mortality rate.

A. **Diagnosis and etiology.** Definitive diagnosis is made at postmortem autopsy, when fetal squames and lanugo are found in the maternal pulmonary vasculature. The term **embolism** is a misnomer because the clinical findings are probably a result of anaphylactic shock, not massive pulmonary embolism. In fact, fetal squames and lanugo have been found in the pulmonary vasculature of postpartum women who have died from reasons other than amniotic fluid embolism. Whatever its cause, amniotic fluid embolism is potentially catastrophic and should be suspected when sudden respiratory and cardiovascular collapse follows delivery of an infant. Cyanosis, hemorrhage, coma, and disseminated intravascular coagulation rapidly ensues.

B. **Management.** Aggressive supportive management is needed, and the patient should be intubated and monitored closely. Good intravenous access is essential, and invasive monitoring devices should be placed. Volume support, inotropic agents, and pressors should be given as needed to maintain adequate BP. Packed red blood cells and FFP should also be available, as these patients are at high risk for developing disseminated intravascular coagulation. Despite all efforts, approximately one-half of patients who develop amniotic fluid embolism die.

V. **Septic pelvic thrombophlebitis (SPT)** occurs in 1 in 2000 deliveries, most commonly after cesarean section.

A. **Diagnosis and etiology.** Thrombi form in the deep pelvic veins as a result of the hypercoagulability, increased predilection to injury, and relative venous stasis of pregnancy. The thrombi become superinfected and can cause septic emboli, particularly in the pulmonary system. SPT should be suspected when a patient's fever fails to respond to adequate antibiotic therapy for endomyometritis after 2–3 days. A pelvic examination should be performed to assess for masses or hematomas, and chest and abdominal radiographic studies should be obtained to rule out pneumonia or retained sponges. If such a workup is negative, pelvic ultrasonography, pelvic and abdominal CT, or pelvic and abdominal MRI should be performed to locate abscesses or obvious thrombi in the inferior vena cava or iliac vessels. Unfortunately, imaging studies miss the majority of septic pelvic thrombi, and SPT remains largely a diagnosis of exclusion.

B. **Management.** If no other explanation of the persistent fever is found, the patient should be given heparin sodium intravenously; patients with SPT treated with heparin typically experience fever reduction in 1–2 days and should be maintained on heparin for 7–14 days. Long-term anticoagulation therapy is unnecessary unless deep venous thrombus or pulmonary embolus is visualized. If the patient remains febrile despite appropriate antibiotic and heparin therapy, surgical exploration may be necessary to identify and treat the cause of febrile morbidity.

VI. **Chorioamnionitis** occurs in 0.5–2.0% of all full-term pregnancies. Risk factors include low socioeconomic status, poor nutrition, invasive procedures including vaginal examination and internal monitoring, prolonged rupture of membranes, preterm rupture of membranes, and infections such as gonorrhea and chlamydia.

A. **Diagnosis.** Chorioamnionitis is a polymicrobial infection and is usually diagnosed by clinical assessment. Signs and symptoms include maternal fever, tachycardia, leukocytosis, fundal tenderness, foul-smelling vaginal discharge, and fetal tachycardia. Chorioamnionitis should be suspected in patients in preterm labor who are unresponsive to tocolytic therapy, and the pediatrics caregiver should be informed of all patients with suspected chorioamnionitis. If a patient presents with fever and physical examination findings are inconclusive, amniocentesis may be performed to help distinguish chorioamnionitis from other causes of fever. The amniotic fluid is sent for glucose testing, Gram's stain, and bacterial culture. A glucose level less than or equal to 15 mg/dL is indicative of chorioamnionitis. Gram's stain is approximately 60% sensitive for this diagnosis.

B. **Management.** Definitive treatment of chorioamnionitis consists of delivery of the infant with antibiotic coverage during labor. Ampicillin, 2 g intravenously every 6 hours, and gentamicin sulfate, 120 mg intravenous loading dose followed by 80 mg intravenously every 8 hours, are administered during labor; if the patient is allergic to penicillins, clindamycin 600 mg intravenously every 8 hours may be given instead of ampicillin. If the patient is not in labor already, labor should be induced to help avoid sepsis in both the mother and infant. After delivery, a specimen may be sent for bacterial culture after separation of the chorion and amnion, and the placenta should be sent to the pathology department for examination for evidence of chorioamnionitis. No further antibiotic therapy is necessary after vaginal delivery. Patients who undergo cesarean section, however, should be given broad-spectrum antibiotics for prophylactic treatment of endomyometritis until the patient is afebrile for 24–48 hours.

VII. **Endomyometritis.** In addition to the risk factors for chorioamnionitis, risk factors for endomyometritis include cesarean section or pregnancy complicated by chorioamnionitis.

A. **Diagnosis.** Endomyometritis is mainly a clinical diagnosis based on presence of fever, fundal tenderness, and foul-smelling lochia accompanied by leukocytosis. Endometrial cultures tend to be unhelpful because they are usually contaminated by vaginal or cervical flora, and generally endomyometritis is a polymicrobial infection. If the patient's clinical picture is consistent with endomyometritis, blood cultures do not necessarily need to be obtained because they have a low yield and do not affect the choice of antibiotics.

B. **Management.** Broad-spectrum antibiotics, such as gentamicin and clindamycin, should be started. Ampicillin can also be added, particularly if the patient presents with a high fever within the first 24–48 hours after a delivery, because early temperature spikes are usually a result of streptococcal infection. Although gentamicin should be administered every 8 hours before delivery, daily doses may be administered after delivery. If daily dosing is chosen, gentamicin levels do not require monitoring. If the patient continues to be febrile 24–48 hours after appropriate antibiotics are initiated, further workup should be undertaken to establish the source of the fever.

C. **Further workup** includes urine and blood cultures, chest and abdominal radiography, pelvic examination, and, possibly, pelvic ultrasonography, CT, or MRI. Patients with endomyometritis usually show improvement in physical examination findings and temperature curves 24–48 hours after beginning antibiotics. If the patient's examination findings show improvement, antibiotic therapy can be stopped after the patient has remained afebrile for 48 hours, and no further antibiotic treatment is necessary. It is worth noting that patients with endomyometritis carry an increased risk of secondary infertility as a result of scarring from inflammation.

VIII. **Umbilical cord prolapse** occurs when the umbilical cord slips past the presenting fetal part and passes through the open cervical os. The blood supply to the fetus is cut off when the fetus compresses the umbilical cord against the cervix. Risk factors include rupture of membranes when the fetus is not yet engaged in the pelvis, footling breech presentation, transverse lie, oblique lie, and unstable fetal presentations. These factors may be influenced by cephalopelvic disproportion, abnormal placentation, multiple gestation, polyhydramnios, and fetal and uterine anomalies.

A. **Diagnosis.** Vaginal examination should be performed shortly after rupture of membranes to evaluate cervical dilatation and investigate the possibility of cord prolapse. Vaginal examination should also be performed promptly when fetal bradycardia occurs to rule out cord prolapse.

B. **Management.** If umbilical cord is palpated on vaginal examination the examiner should call for help and elevate the presenting fetal part to prevent compression of the umbilical cord. The examiner can assess the fetal pulse by palpating the umbilical cord, taking care not to confuse his or her own pulse with that of the fetus. While the examiner continues to elevate the presenting fetal part, the patient should be transported to an operating room where appropriate anesthesia is initiated and urgent cesarean section performed. If a patient presents with a prolapsed cord, viability of the fetus must be established before proceeding with cesarean section. Placing the patient in knee-chest position may be helpful in relieving cord compression with prolapse.

IX. **Meconium** complicates 8–16% of all deliveries and 25–30% of all postterm deliveries. Meconium passage by the fetus results from hypoxic stimulation of the parasympathetic system or triggering of a mature vagal reflex.

A. Uncommonly, meconium passage leads to **meconium aspiration syndrome**, which carries a mortality rate of 28%. Symptoms of meconium aspiration syndrome include tachypnea, chest retractions, cyanosis, barrel-shaped chest, and coarse breath sounds. Chest radiography shows coarse, irregular pulmonary densities with areas of decreased aeration. Persistent pulmonary hypertension also occurs. Amnioinfusion may be performed in an effort to reduce meconium aspiration.

B. **Management.** If meconium is present, a DeLee suction device should be used to aspirate the infant's oropharynx while the head is at the perineum. The infant should then be handed over to a pediatrician quickly with minimal stimulation. Ideally, the pediatrician performs laryngoscopy and suctions below the vocal cords if meconium is present; laryngoscopy is deferred, however, if the infant is crying or breathing vigorously. The placenta can be examined and sent for examination by a pathologist to help determine how recently meconium passage occurred.

X. **Fistulas**

A. **Vesicovaginal fistulas** occur when obstructed and prolonged labor causes pressure necrosis of the anterior vagina and vesicovaginal septum. The fistula usually becomes apparent by 1 week postpartum when the patient presents with continuous, painless leakage of urine from the vagina that is unrelated to position. Diagnosis is confirmed when methylene blue is instilled into the bladder and either is observed draining from the vagina or stains a tampon placed in the vagina. To evaluate possible damage to the ureters, IVP should be performed. An indwelling Foley catheter is placed to allow the fistula time to heal. If the fistula fails to heal despite placement of a urinary catheter, cystoscopy with biopsy of the tract margins should be performed to rule out other pathologic conditions. The fistula then can be closed in layers vaginally.

B. **Rectovaginal fistulas** usually involve the perineum, anal sphincter, anal canal, and distal rectum. Rectal examinations should be done after all vaginal deliveries in which rectal trauma is suspected to identify and repair occult damage. If a fourth-degree laceration is identified immediately after a delivery, it should be irrigated thoroughly and repaired directly after delivery. If a rectovaginal fistula presents later after delivery, the patient should be carefully examined. Fistulograms can delineate anatomy with instillation of a barium contrast agent into the vagina by Foley catheter. If the tissue appears inflamed or necrotic, dressing changes and débridement should be performed until the tissue appears healthy and granulated. The fistula may be repaired once the tissue is healthy and not inflamed. Before surgery the patient requires a thorough bowel preparation. The fistulous tract is then excised and closed in layers without tension with reconstruction of the anal sphincter and perineal body. Postoperatively, stool softeners are used to avoid excessive straining.

XI. **Postpartum depression.** Known colloquially as the **postpartum blues**, postpartum depression occurs after 10–15% of all deliveries. Manifestations range from transient tearfulness, anxiety, irritability, and restlessness to full-blown depression that can last up to 1 year. Risk factors include a prior history of depression, young age, and poor social support. Postpartum depression also tends to recur in future pregnancies. If a postpartum patient appears to be depressed, thyroid function tests should be performed and tricyclic antidepressants can be started. The patient should be questioned about suicidal and homicidal ideation, and psychiatric follow-up should be arranged. It may be necessary to involve social services to ensure that the baby is receiving adequate care. Postpartum psychosis can also occur, especially in patients with a prior history of psychiatric illness. Such patients require close psychiatric follow-up as well as antipsychotic drug therapy.

8. GESTATIONAL COMPLICATIONS

Dana Gossett and Edith Gurewitsch

I. **Amniotic fluid disorders**
   A. **Physiologic aspects of amniotic fluid.** The volume of amniotic fluid represents a balance between production, primarily from fetal urine and fetal alveolar fluid and removal, via fetal swallowing and absorption by the amniotic-chorionic surface. Amniotic fluid volume (AFV) increases from a mean of 250 mL at 16 weeks' gestation to approximately 800 mL at approximately 32 weeks' gestation. The average volume of amniotic fluid remains stable from 32 weeks' to 35 weeks' gestation, then declines to approximately 500 mL at term.
   B. **Technique for assessing amniotic fluid volume.** The vertical depth of the largest amniotic fluid pocket is measured (in centimeters) in each of four equal quadrants of the uterus. The abdominal ultrasonic transducer should be oriented vertically to the floor; all pockets containing loops of umbilical cord must be excluded. The sum of these measurements establishes the amniotic fluid index (AFI) in centimeters. AFI appears to be highly reproducible; it may be applied reliably after 24 weeks using normative values. The AFI cannot be reliably used in assessing multiple gestations; for these pregnancies, the largest single vertical pocket is measured (maximum vertical pocket depth).
   C. **Polyhydramnios** is the pathologic accumulation of amniotic fluid. It is defined as more than 2000 mL at any gestational age, more than the ninety-fifth percentile for gestational age, or an AFI greater than 20 cm at term. The incidence of polyhydramnios in the general population ranges from 0.2% to 1.6%. Mild increases in AFV are usually clinically insignificant. Larger increases in amniotic fluid volume are associated with increased perinatal morbidity, due to preterm labor, cord prolapse, and congenital malformations. In uncommon cases, abruptio placentae is associated with polyhydramnios at the time of rupture of membranes, due to rapid decompression of the overdistended uterus. Increased maternal morbidity results from postpartum hemorrhage due to uterine overdistension and atony.
      1. **Etiology.** Between 16% and 66% of cases of polyhydramnios are idiopathic. The remaining cases can be attributed to increased fetal urine production or decreased amniotic fluid absorption, either due to impaired swallowing or impaired absorption at the amnionic interface with the uterus (Fig. 8-1).
         a. **Fetal structural malformations.** In cases of CNS abnormalities such as acrania or anencephaly, the polyhydramnios is probably due to several factors: impairment of the swallowing mechanism, lack of antidiuretic hormone and resultant polyuria, and possibly transudation of fluid across the exposed fetal meninges. Obstructions of the GI tract, such as esophageal atresia, may also result in polyhydramnios due to decreased absorption (although swallowing in these fetuses is usually normal). In some cases, ventral wall defects may result in increased AFV due to transudation of fluid across the peritoneal surface or bowel wall.
         b. **Chromosomal and genetic abnormalities.** The prevalence of chromosomal abnormalities in cases of significant polyhydramnios (over 23) can be as high as 35%. The most common abnormalities are trisomies 13, 18, and 21; in these cases, the polyhydramnios may be due to impaired swallowing, although the pathophysiology is unclear. For this reason karyotype analysis should be offered in all cases of isolated severe polyhydramnios.

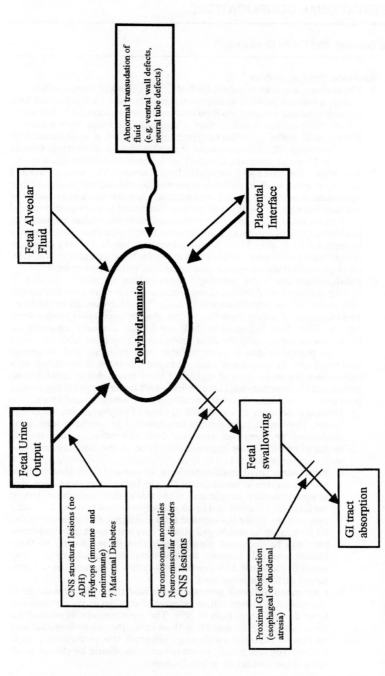

FIG. 8-1. Causes of polyhydramnios. ADH, antidiuretic hormone; GI, gastrointestinal.

    c. **Neuromuscular disorders** may also be manifested clinically as polyhydramnios; this is also probably due to impaired swallowing.

    d. **Diabetes mellitus.** Maternal diabetes is a common cause of polyhydramnios. In these cases, the etiology of polyhydramnios is unclear, but it is often associated with poor glycemic control or fetal malformations. The fetal hyperglycemia may increase oncotic pressure, which causes transudation of fluid across the placental interface to the amniotic cavity, as well increased glomerular filtration rate.

    e. **Other causes.** In the absence of any of the aforementioned factors, the detection of polyhydramnios should prompt further testing. Screening tests for toxoplasmosis and cytomegalovirus, syphilis, and isoimmunization should be performed. In the twin-to-twin transfusion syndrome, the recipient twin develops polyhydramnios and, occasionally, hydrops fetalis, whereas the donor twin develops growth retardation and oligohydramnios. Twin-to-twin transfusion syndrome is found in monozygotic twins with large arteriovenous anastomoses connecting their placentas.

2. **Diagnosis.** Polyhydramnios should be suspected in cases of uterine enlargement (size larger than normal for date) or difficulty in palpating fetal small parts or hearing fetal heart tones. Ultrasonographic examination is necessary both to quantify amniotic fluid volume and to identify multiple fetuses and fetal abnormalities. Amniocentesis is an indispensable tool for obtaining specimens for viral culture and, when indicated, karyotyping.

3. **Treatment.** Minor and moderate degrees of polyhydramnios with some discomfort can be managed expectantly until the onset of labor or spontaneous rupture of membranes. In more severe cases, or if the patient develops dyspnea, abdominal pain, or difficulty ambulating, treatment becomes necessary.

    a. **Amnioreduction** is the most common treatment. The purpose of amnioreduction is to relieve maternal discomfort, and to that end it is transiently successful. The volume of fluid removed is critical. Frequent removal of smaller volumes (removal at a rate of 500 mL/hour to a total of 1500–2000 mL) is less often associated with preterm labor than less frequent removal of larger volumes. Amnioreduction is repeated every 1–3 weeks as needed until the fetus has reached pulmonary maturity or delivery is required for another reason.

    b. **Pharmacologic treatment** involves manipulation of fetal urine flow. Fetal renal blood flow is maintained under normal conditions chiefly by prostaglandins. The cyclooxygenase inhibitor indomethacin has been used to decrease fetal renal blood flow and therefore fetal urine production. Data exist regarding treatment of polyhydramnios from 21 to 35 weeks' gestation with indomethacin (25 mg orally every 6 hours) for 2–11 weeks. The primary concern about the use of indomethacin is the potential closure of the fetal ductus arteriosus. Although closure of the ductus has not been described, ductal constriction has been detected as early as 48 hours after initiating therapy with indomethacin. Thus, close monitoring of amniotic fluid volume and ductal diameter is warranted, and therapy should be stopped if any decrease in ductal diameter is noted. Treatment for twin-to-twin transfusion is discussed later in sec. **III**, Multiple Pregnancy.

D. **Oligohydramnios** is defined as an AFI of less than the fifth percentile for gestational age or less than 5 cm at term. Oligohydramnios is associated with increased perinatal morbidity and mortality at any gestational age, but the risks are particularly high when it is detected during the second trimester. In these cases, perinatal mortality may approach 80–90%. Pulmonary hypoplasia can result from the lack of fluid available for inhalation into the terminal air sacs of the lungs, with lack of expansion and subsequent failure of growth (17%). Furthermore, prolonged oligohydramnios can lead to a deformation sequence in 10–15% of cases, characterized by cranial, facial, or skeletal abnormalities.

1. **Etiology.** The clinical conditions commonly associated with oligohydramnios are ruptured membranes, fetal urinary tract malformations, intrauterine growth restriction (IUGR), postdate pregnancy, and placental insufficiency. Possible rupture of membranes must be considered at any gestational age. Renal agenesis or urinary tract obstruction often becomes apparent during the second trimester of pregnancy, when fetal urine flow begins to contribute significantly to AFV. IUGR often is associated with oligohydramnios. This may be due to smaller fetal vascular volume with decreased glomerular filtration and urinary flow rates. The association of oligohydramnios and IUGR may also reflect the fact that placental insufficiency can cause both conditions. AFV also decreases in the postterm fetus; although the mechanism is unclear, the deterioration in placental function may cause a less efficient transfer of water from the mother to the fetus (Fig. 8-2).

2. **Diagnosis.** Clinical findings suspicious for oligohydramnios are a lag in fundal height measurements (size less than normal for date), a reduction in perceived fetal movements, or easy palpitation of fetal parts. Ultrasonographic examination is necessary to quantify amniotic fluid and to identify fetuses with IUGR or fetal abnormalities. If the diagnosis of ruptured membranes is being considered, a "tampon test" can be performed by instilling dye into the amniotic sac via amniocentesis techniques and observing for staining of a tampon placed in the vagina.

3. **Treatment.** Therapeutic options for the patient with oligohydramnios are limited. Maternal intravascular fluid status appears to be closely tied to that of the fetus; thus, hydrating the mother may have some transient effect on AFV. In cases in which oligohydramnios is caused by obstructive genitourinary defect, in utero surgical diversion of urine flow has produced promising results. To achieve optimal benefit, urinary diversion must be accomplished before the development of renal dysplasia and early enough in gestation to allow for lung development. Until term, oligohydramnios should be managed with frequent fetal surveillance; at term, it is an indication for induction of labor due to the increased risks of perinatal morbidity and mortality. Intrapartum, treatment with amnioinfusion may improve short-term fetal heart rate variability and lower rates of cesarean section for fetal distress.

II. **Intrauterine growth restriction**

A. **Description.** A diagnosis of IUGR is considered when the estimated fetal weight by sonogram falls below the tenth percentile for gestational age. The majority of these fetuses are simply constitutionally small, as would be expected from population-based nomograms. The incidence of pathologic IUGR varies according to the population under investigation; it is estimated to be 4–8% in developed countries and 6–30% in developing countries. These cases are the ones of concern to the obstetrician due to their increased perinatal morbidity and mortality.

1. **Symmetric growth restriction** has an earlier onset than asymmetric growth restriction, and all organs tend to be proportionally reduced in size. Factors associated with symmetric restriction include chromosomal abnormalities; anatomic (especially cardiac) malformations; congenital infection with rubella, cytomegalovirus, or *Toxoplasma*; severe chronic maternal malnutrition; and maternal smoking.

2. **Asymmetric growth restriction** has a later onset, and some organs are more affected than others. Abdominal circumference is the measurement to be first affected; femur length may be affected later; head circumference and biparietal diameter are usually spared. Asymmetric IUGR is attributed to placental insufficiency, which can be caused by a

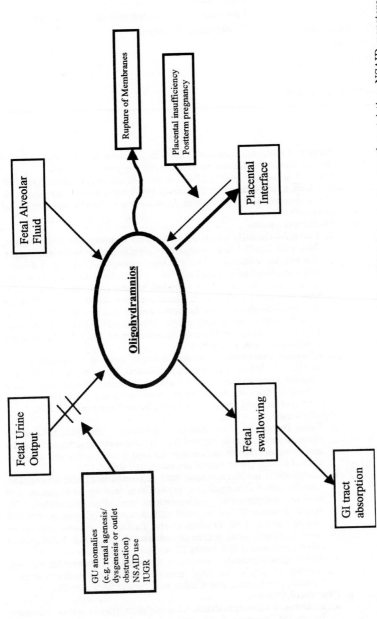

FIG. 8-2. Causes of oligohydramnios. GI, gastrointestinal; GU, genitourinary; IUGR, intrauterine growth restriction; NSAID, nonsteroidal anti-inflammatory drug.

TABLE 8-1. INFECTIOUS CAUSES OF INTRAUTERINE GROWTH RESTRICTION

Viral	Bacterial	Protozoan	Spirochetal
Rubella	Listeriosis	Toxoplasmosis	Syphilis
Cytomegalovirus infection	Tuberculosis	Malaria	
Hepatitis A, B			
Varicella			
Influenza			
Parvovirus B19 infection			

variety of maternal conditions, including chronic or pregnancy-induced hypertension and diabetes mellitus (typically pregestational).

B. **Etiology.** Approximately 75% of IUGR infants are constitutionally small; 15–20% have uteroplacental insufficiency resulting from various causes; 5–10% have impaired growth resulting from perinatal infection or congenital malformation.

1. **Maternal causes**
   a. **Constitutionally small mothers and inadequate weight gain.** Maternal familial factors appear to significantly affect birth weight. If a woman weighs less than 100 lb at conception, her risk of delivering a small-for-gestational-age infant is doubled. Inadequate weight gain during pregnancy or arrested weight gain after 28 weeks is also associated with IUGR; weight gain goal should be 20–25 lb for a normal-weight woman. An underweight woman should be encouraged to achieve ideal body weight plus an additional 20–25 pounds. For the overweight mother, on the other hand, low weight gain alone is unlikely to cause IUGR.
   b. **Chronic maternal disease.** Multiple medical conditions of the mother, including chronic hypertension, cyanotic heart disease, long-standing diabetes, and collagen vascular disease, can cause growth restriction. All of these conditions place the patient at risk for superimposed preeclampsia, which itself can lead to IUGR.

2. **Fetal causes**
   a. **Fetal infection.** Viral, bacterial, protozoan, and spirochetal infections all have been associated with fetal growth restriction. Rubella and cytomegalovirus are among the best-known infectious antecedents of IUGR. Other causes are listed in Table 8-1.
   b. **Congenital malformations and chromosomal abnormalities.** Chromosomal abnormalities, particularly trisomy or triploidy, and severe cardiovascular malformations are often associated with IUGR. Trisomy 18 is associated with severe, early, symmetric IUGR and polyhydramnios. Trisomy 13 and Turner's syndrome also can be associated with some degree of restricted fetal growth. Fetal growth restriction caused by trisomy 21 is usually minimal.
   c. **Teratogen exposure.** Any agent that causes a teratogenic injury is capable of producing fetal growth restriction. Anticonvulsants, tobacco, illicit drugs, and alcohol may impair fetal growth.

3. **Placental causes**
   a. **Placental abnormalities.** Chronic abruptio placentae, extensive infarction, chorioangioma, and velamentous insertion of the cord may cause growth restriction due to decreased perfusion of the fetus. A circumvallate placenta or placenta previa also may impair growth.

  b. **Multiple fetuses.** Pregnancy with two or more fetuses is complicated by appreciable impairment in growth of one or both fetuses in 12–47% of cases.
C. **Diagnosis.** Early establishment of gestational age and careful measurements of uterine height throughout pregnancy should help to identify most instances of abnormal fetal growth.
  1. **A history of risk factors,** such as a previously growth-restricted fetus, prior fetal or neonatal death, or chronic maternal illness, should alert the care provider to the possibility of IUGR.
  2. **Clinical diagnosis** of IUGR may be unreliable. If a lag in fundal height of more than 2 cm is found, growth restriction should be suspected and ultrasonographic examination performed.
  3. **Ultrasonographic diagnosis.** To determine if a fetus is growing appropriately, the gestational age must be established with certainty. The most reliable method of estimating gestational age is certain knowledge of the date of the patient's last menstrual period (LMP). Some 20–40% of pregnant women, however, fail to recall the exact date of their LMP. Therefore, sonography may be of help in dating a pregnancy. Once a fetus is suspected of being growth restricted on clinical examination, a sonographic estimate of fetal weight should be obtained. If this measurement confirms the presence of IUGR, further detailed sonography should be performed to look for structural abnormalities. (See Chap. 4, sec. **IIA-1** for information on clinical dating.)
  4. **Third trimester measurements** are the least reliable for determining gestational age because growth restriction may already have occurred. Transverse cerebellar diameter has been shown to correlate with gestational age in weeks up to 24 weeks and is not significantly affected by growth restriction. Abdominal circumference is the parameter that correlates best with fetal weight. In contrast to biparietal diameter, abdominal circumference is smaller in both symmetric and asymmetric types of IUGR; therefore, its measurement has high sensitivity for detecting IUGR. Abdominal circumference, however, is subject to more intraobserver and interobserver variation in measurement than either biparietal diameter or femur length. Variability in abdominal circumference may also result from fetal breathing movements, compression, or position of the fetus. Femur length generally is decreased in symmetrically growth-restricted fetuses but may be normal with asymmetric IUGR. An elevated femur length to abdominal circumference ratio raises suspicion for asymmetric IUGR.
  5. **Other associated findings.** An association between oligohydramnios and fetal growth restriction has long been recognized, in which IUGR is preceded by oligohydramnios. Detection of a grade III placenta before 34 weeks' gestation should alert the clinician to the possibility of impending IUGR.
D. **Management.** Because perinatal morbidity and mortality are increased two- to sixfold in patients with IUGR, careful surveillance is critical, and early delivery may be indicated in some cases.
  1. **IUGR at or near term.** The best outcome for these fetuses is achieved by prompt delivery.
  2. **IUGR remote from term.** Structural anomalies should be sought in these fetuses, and if a chromosomal abnormality is suspected then amniocentesis, chorionic villus sampling, or fetal blood sampling for karyotyping and viral studies should be recommended. The parents may decide to terminate the pregnancy based on this information; however, even in a pregnancy for which termination is not considered, the information gained from such studies may be important for parents, obstetricians, and pediatricians in planning delivery and newborn care. In cases such as trisomy 13 or 18 in which the neonate has a short life expectancy, cesarean section can be avoided.

   a. **General management.** After ruling out structural and chromosomal abnormalities and possible congenital infection as completely as possible, physical activity should be restricted, adequate diet ensured, and fetal surveillance started. If compliance with bed rest at home cannot be assured, hospitalization should be considered. Fetal assessment should include maternal assessment of fetal movement, sonographic assessment of fetal growth every 3–4 weeks, and performance of a nonstress test or measurement of BPP once or twice per week. Doppler flow studies of the umbilical artery are suggestive of a compromised fetus when they show elevated systolic to diastolic ratio or absent or reversed end-diastolic flow. (See Chap. 6 for more information on fetal assessment techniques.)

   b. **Treatment.** In most cases of fetal growth restriction remote from term, no specific treatment exists beyond the supportive care described earlier. Possible exceptions are cases of inadequate maternal nutrition or maternal heavy smoking, use of street drugs, or alcoholism. In women with a history of recurrent, severe fetal growth restriction, early antiplatelet therapy with low-dose aspirin (80 mg taken orally once a day) may prevent placental thrombosis, placental infarction, and fetal growth restriction.

   c. **Delivery.** For the severely growth-restricted fetus remote from term, the decision to deliver involves comparing the risks from further exposure to the intrauterine environment with the risks of preterm delivery. Confirmation of lung maturity by measurement of a lecithin to sphingomyelin ratio of 2 or more or by identification of phosphatidylglycerol in amniotic fluid is a clear indication for delivery. Close monitoring during labor to avoid further fetal compromise, cesarean delivery if fetal distress is identified, and excellent neonatal care are imperative for a successful neonatal outcome. The likelihood of fetal distress during labor is increased considerably, because fetal growth restriction is commonly the result of insufficient placental function, which is likely to be aggravated by labor. The association of IUGR with oligohydramnios also predisposes the fetus to cord compression and intolerance of labor as a result.

E. **Fetal outcome.** The growth-restricted fetus is at risk for perinatal hypoxia and meconium aspiration. It is essential that care of the newborn infant be provided by someone who is skillful at clearing the airway below the vocal cords of meconium. The severely growth-restricted newborn is also particularly susceptible to hypothermia and may develop other metabolic abnormalities, including severe hypoglycemia. In general, prolonged symmetrical IUGR is likely to be followed by slow growth after birth, whereas the fetus with asymmetric IUGR is more likely to recuperate with "catch-up" growth after birth. The subsequent neurologic and intellectual effects of IUGR cannot be predicted precisely. Some data show that fetal growth restriction has long-term negative effects on cognitive function, independent of other variables. One study found that almost 50% of children born small for gestational age were found to have learning deficits at 9–11 years of age.

III. **Multiple pregnancy**

A. **Epidemiology.** The incidence of multiple pregnancy in the United States is just over 2% of all births and has been increasing annually due to improved success rates of assisted reproductive technologies. Approximately one-third of spontaneous multiple gestations are monozygotic, the result of cleavage of a single fertilized ovum. The incidence of monozygotic twins is constant at approximately 4 in 1000 births and is unrelated to maternal age, race, or parity. The incidence of dizygotic twins, the result of two fertilized ova, is higher in certain families, is more common in African Americans and less common in Asians than in other races, and increases with maternal age, parity, weight, and height. Women taking medications to induce ovulation are at greatest risk. The incidence of multiple gestations after clomiphene citrate therapy is 5–10%, and it is significantly higher (10–30%) when gonadotropins are used. In the absence of fertility agent use, triplet pregnancies occur at a rate of approximately 1 in 8000 births, and births of higher order are more rare. Multiple gestations increase morbidity and mortality for both the mother and the fetuses; perinatal mortality rates in developed countries range from 50 to 100 per 1000 births for twins and from 100 to 200 per 1000 births for triplets.

B. **Clinical characteristics.** Clinical findings such as size larger than normal for gestation date, palpation of apparently multiple fetuses, and apparent auscultation of two fetal heart tones are insufficient to definitively diagnose multiple gestation. If multiple gestation is suspected, a sonogram should be obtained to confirm the diagnosis. Maternal serum alpha-fetoprotein levels are elevated (more than four times the median) in multiple pregnancies; many multiple gestations are identified after an abnormal serum screening result. Patients with multiple gestations should be referred to high-risk perinatal units early in their pregnancies.

C. **Zygosity, placentation, and mortality.** Multiple gestations that result from the fertilization of multiple ova (dizygotic) are termed **dichorionic** and **diamniotic**. Each fetus has its own placenta (although these may fuse during development), and the fetuses are each contained within a complete amniotic-chorionic membrane. Multiple gestations that result from the cleavage of a single fertilized ovum (monozygotic) may share an amnion, a chorion, a placenta, or some or all of these, depending on the timing of cleavage. Twins that divide in the first 3 days after fertilization are dichorionic, diamniotic, and may have distinct placentas (20–30% of cases). If cleavage occurs between the fourth and eighth days after fertilization, the twins are diamniotic, monochorionic (because the chorionic layer has already formed), and have a single placenta (70–80% of cases). If cleavage occurs after the eighth day, the twins are monoamniotic and monochorionic (because the amnion and chorion are formed before the embryos divide); they are contained in the same sac and have a single placenta (approximately 1% of cases). Later cleavage results in conjoined twins and is even more rare. Dichorionic twins have the lowest perinatal mortality rate (8.9%) of all placenta types. The mortality rate of diamniotic monochorionic twins is approximately 25%. Monoamniotic gestations have a 50–60% mortality rate, with death usually occurring before 32 weeks' gestation. The relationship of placentae among triplets, quadruplets, and higher-order multiple fetuses generally follows the same principles, except that monochorionic and dichorionic placentation may coexist and placental anomalies, particularly marginal and velamentous insertions of the cord and single umbilical artery, are more frequently found in higher-order multiples.

D. **Complications**

1. **Miscarriage** is at least twice as common in multiple pregnancies as in singleton pregnancies, and a continued pregnancy with resorption of one or more of the embryos may be even more common. Fewer than 50% of twin pregnancies diagnosed via ultrasonography during the first trimester result in delivery of twins. Some twins may be resorbed silently, whereas the demise of others is associated with bleeding and uterine activity.

2. **Congenital anomalies and malformations** are approximately twice as common in twin infants as in singleton infants and are four times as common in triplets. Monozygotic twins have a risk of 2–10% for developmental defects, which is twice the incidence of fetal abnormalities in dizygotic twins. Because the risk of chromosomal anomalies increases with each additional fetus, amniocentesis should be offered at a younger maternal age based on the number of fetuses (at 33 years for twins; at 28 years for triplets).

3. **Nausea and vomiting** are often worse in twin pregnancies than in singleton pregnancies. Although the cause is unclear, higher levels of human chorionic gonadotropin β-subunit have been implicated in stimulation of the chemoreceptor trigger zone.

4. **Preeclampsia** is more common, occurs earlier, and is more severe in multiple pregnancy than in singleton pregnancy. Approximately 40% of twin pregnancies and 60% of triplet pregnancies are affected.

5. **Polyhydramnios** occurs in 5–8% of multiple pregnancies, particularly with monoamniotic twins. Acute polyhydramnios before 28 weeks' gestation has been reported to occur in 1.7% of all twin pregnancies; the perinatal mortality in these cases approaches 90%.

6. **Preterm delivery.** Approximately 10% of preterm deliveries are twin gestations, which account for 25% of preterm perinatal deaths. The incidence of preterm delivery in twin gestations approaches 50%. Most neonatal deaths in multiple premature births are associated with gestations of less than 32 weeks and birth weight under 1500 g. The average gestational age at delivery is 36 weeks for twins and 32–33 weeks for triplets.

7. **Intrauterine growth restriction.** Although growth curves exist for twin and triplet gestations, nomograms for singletons are more commonly used. Because growth restriction is so common among multiple gestations, the use of a nomogram based on the normal range of twin and triplet birth weights might be insufficiently sensitive to detect IUGR. IUGR is common, and low-birth-weight has an additive effect with prematurity in increasing neonatal morbidity and mortality. Follow-up of growth-restricted twins shows a tendency for persistence of short stature and lower weight percentiles.

8. **Discordant twin growth** is defined as a discrepancy of more than 20% in the estimated fetal weights, expressed as a percentage of the larger twin's weight. Causes include twin-to-twin transfusion syndrome (see sec. **III.D.9**), chromosomal or structural anomalies of one twin, or discordant viral infection. When weight discordance exceeds 25%, the fetal death rate increases 6.5-fold and the neonatal death rate 2.5-fold.

9. **Twin-to-twin transfusion syndrome.** Approximately 15% of monochorionic twin pregnancies have some demonstrable vascular anastomoses. Single or multiple placental arteriovenous shunts may exist, some in opposing directions. When these anastomoses are not accompanied by artery-to-artery or vein-to-vein anastomoses, one fetus continuously donates blood into the other, which leads to hypervolemia, heart failure, and hydrops in the recipient twin, and anemia in the donor twin. This is referred to as *twin-to-twin transfusion syndrome* and is a rare but dangerous complication of monochorionic gestations. A common maternal symptom is rapid uterine growth between 20 and 30 weeks' gestation due to the polyhydramnios of the recipient twin, which frequently causes premature delivery. The severity and time of observable growth discrepancy probably depends on the size, number, and direction of arteriovenous shunts. Fetal hydrops is usually a terminal sign. Prenatal diagnosis of twin-to-twin transfusion syndrome can be made when sonography suggests single placentation and a single chorion, discordant fetal growth, polyhydramnios in the sac of the larger twin, and little or no fluid around the smaller fetus ("stuck twin" sign). If extreme prematurity prevents immediate delivery, several interventions can be considered in view of the high mortality associated with expectant management. Repeated decompression amniocentesis of the sac of the recipient twin has been shown to improve outcome in some cases. Intrauterine transfusion of the anemic (donor) twin is futile as there is ongoing loss; in addition, it risks congestive cardiac failure in the recipient twin, who is already polycythemic. Fetoscopically guided laser ablation of the anastomotic placental vessels is performed in some centers, but its efficacy remains highly controversial.

10. **Hemorrhage.** The risk of uterine atony and of postpartum hemorrhage is significantly increased in multiple pregnancies, probably due to overdistension of the uterus.

11. **Intrapartum complications,** including malpresentation, cord prolapse, cord entanglement, discoordinated uterine action, fetal distress, and need for cesarean delivery are more common during labor in multiple gestations than in single gestations. Locking of twins, which occurs with breech-vertex presentations only, is extremely rare.

E. **Antenatal management of multiple gestations**

1. **Clinical management** should include adequate nutrition (daily intake of approximately 300 kcal more per fetus than for a singleton pregnancy), restriction of physical activity, more frequent prenatal visits, ultrasonographic assessment of fetal growth (every 3–4 weeks), assessment of fetal well-being, and prompt hospital admission for preterm labor or other obstetric complications. The role of bed rest in prevention of preterm labor in women with multiple gestations remains controversial. Prophylactic use of tocolytic agents has not been shown to prevent preterm birth in twin gestations.

2. **Ultrasonographic assessments** should be conducted every 3–4 weeks from 23 weeks' gestation to delivery, to monitor the growth of each fetus and to detect evidence of discordant growth or twin-to-twin transfusion syndrome.

3. **Fetal surveillance.** Performance of a nonstress test before 34 weeks' gestation is not indicated unless clinical or ultrasonographic measurements suggest IUGR or discordant growth. Although the practice of routine cardiotocography after 34 weeks' gestation is debatable from a cost-efficiency point of view, cardiotocography certainly should be considered if any risk factors are present. A major therapeutic dilemma arises when the results of the nonstress test are discordant. Additional testing, such as measurement of a BPP, may be necessary to better ascertain fetal condition. The utility of a contraction stress test is debatable, as it might precipitate preterm delivery.

4. **Amniocentesis** should be performed in both sacs if indicated for prenatal diagnosis of a fetal condition, including genetic disorders or isoimmunization. As described earlier, the definition of *advanced maternal age* for genetic testing should take into account the number of fetuses (sec. **III.D.2**). To ensure aspiration from both sacs, 1–5 mL of indigo carmine is injected into the first sac. Recovery of blue-tinged fluid at the time of the second aspiration indicates that the first sac has been reentered, and another attempt is necessary. To establish lung maturity, a lecithin to sphingomyelin ratio of 2 or more obtained from one fetal sac is adequate. When twins are concordant, the lecithin to sphingomyelin ratio in one sac is usually similar to that obtained from the other. When twins are discordant, amniotic fluid should be obtained from the sac of the larger twin, who usually achieves pulmonary maturity later than the smaller twin.

5. **Death of one fetus,** once diagnosed, is managed based on the gestational age and condition of the surviving fetus. Until evidence of fetal lung maturity in the surviving fetus is exhibited, weekly fetal surveillance should be performed and weekly maternal clotting profiles measured. Delivery should be considered if fetal lung maturity is demonstrated or if compromise of the remaining fetus develops. In the setting of twin-to-twin transfusion syndrome, the death of one twin should prompt consideration of delivery, particularly after 28 weeks, given the high rates of embolic complications in the surviving twin.

F. **Intrapartum management.** The optimal route of delivery of twin gestations remains controversial and must be assessed on a case-by-case basis. Decisions about delivery must take into account the presentation of the twins, the gestational age, the presence of maternal or fetal complications, the experience of the obstetrician, and the availability of anesthesia and neonatal intensive care. Various presentations of twins and their incidence are twin A vertex, twin B vertex (43%); twin A vertex, twin B nonvertex (38%); and twin A nonvertex (19%).

1. **Vertex/vertex.** Successful vaginal delivery can be expected in 70–80% of cases of vertex-vertex twin presentations. Surveillance of twin B with real-time ultrasonography or continuous monitoring is advised during the time interval between vaginal delivery of the first and second twin. After the vertex of twin B is in the pelvic outlet, amniotomy is performed. If twin B is in jeopardy or shows evidence of distress before atraumatic vaginal delivery is possible, cesarean delivery is performed.

2. **Vertex/nonvertex.** Routine cesarean delivery is not always necessary for vertex-nonvertex twin presentation. If vaginal delivery is planned, external cephalic version of twin B may be attempted (with a success rate of approximately 70%). Vaginal delivery of twin B in nonvertex presentation (podalic extraction) is also reasonable to consider for infants with an estimated weight of more than 1500–2000 g. Insufficient data exist to advocate a specific route of delivery of a twin B whose birth weight is less than 1500 g. The relative weights of the twins must also be considered. For vaginal delivery of vertex/nonvertex twins, it is preferable if the weights are similar or if twin A is the larger of the two.

3. **Nonvertex twin A.** With this presentation, cesarean delivery of both twins appears to be preferable to vaginal delivery. Data documenting the safety of vaginal delivery for this group are insufficient to recommend it.

4. **Locked twins** is a rare condition that occurs in approximately 1 in 817 twin gestations. It occurs with breech/vertex twins, when the body of twin A delivers, but the chin "locks" behind the chin of twin B. Hypertonicity, monoamniotic twinning, or a reduced amount of amniotic fluid may contribute to the interlocking of the fetal heads.

G. **Multifetal pregnancy reduction.** The presence of three, four, or more fetuses in one pregnancy is associated with increased maternal and perinatal mortality and morbidity. Although moral, ethical, and psychological concerns exist about reducing the number of fetuses in early pregnancy, multifetal reduction is a reasonable option and should be offered to patients. The procedure usually is performed transabdominally at between 10 and 12 weeks' gestation by means of potassium chloride injection into the pericardia of the most accessible fetuses. Composite data from the centers with the most experience in reduction suggest an ultimate live birth rate after multifetal reduction of 75–80%. *Selective termination* refers specifically to the termination of one or more fetuses with structural or chromosomal anomalies.

IV. **Other complications of pregnancy**

A. **Postterm pregnancy,** by definition, extends beyond 294 days or 42 weeks from the first day of the LMP. Increased perinatal morbidity and mortality have been documented when pregnancy extends beyond 42 weeks' gestation. The incidence of congenital anomalies is also increased in postdate pregnancies.

1. **Epidemiology.** The incidence of postterm pregnancy has been reported to range between 7% and 12% of all pregnancies. Approximately 4% of all pregnancies extend beyond 43 weeks. Recurrence risk is 50% for subsequent pregnancies.

2. **Diagnosis** of postterm pregnancy must be based on an accurate estimate of gestational age. Obstetric dates should be considered valid if two or more of the following criteria are met: certain LMP; positive urine pregnancy test 6 weeks from the LMP; fetal heart tone detected with Doppler ultrasonographic testing at 10–12 weeks' gestation or with DeLee stethoscope at 18–20 weeks' gestation; fundal height at the umbilicus at 20 weeks' gestation; pelvic examination consistent with LMP before 13 weeks' gestation;

and ultrasonographic dating by crown–rump length between 6 and 12 weeks' gestation or by biparietal diameter before 26 weeks' gestation. The best estimates of gestational age are based on as many criteria as possible.

3. **Complications**
   a. **Postmature or dysmature neonates** exhibit some of the following findings, probably due to decreased placental reserve: wasting of subcutaneous tissue, failure of intrauterine growth, meconium staining, dehydration, absence of vernix caseosa and lanugo hair, oligohydramnios, and peeling of skin. Such findings are described in approximately 10–20% of true postterm fetuses.
   b. **Macrosomia** is far more common in postterm than term pregnancies because, under most circumstances, the fetus continues to grow in utero. Twice as many postterm fetuses as term fetuses weigh more than 4000 g, and the occurrence of birth injuries caused by difficult forceps deliveries and shoulder dystocia is increased in postterm pregnancy.
   c. **Oligohydramnios.** Amniotic fluid tends to decrease in postterm gestation, probably due to decreasing uteroplacental reserve. Low AFV is associated with increased rates of intrapartum fetal distress and cesarean delivery.
   d. **Meconium.** Most studies of postterm gestations report a significantly increased incidence of meconium-stained amniotic fluid, and an increased risk of meconium aspiration syndrome. Oligohydramnios also increases the risks of meconium-stained amniotic fluid, because the meconium is not diluted.

4. **Management.** After 40 weeks' gestation, patients may keep daily fetal motion charts. It is generally accepted that careful fetal monitoring can reduce the risk of perinatal mortality of the postterm fetus to virtually that of the term fetus. It remains controversial which method of fetal testing provides the greatest prognostic accuracy, and whether the patient who reaches 41–42 weeks' gestation with an unripe cervix is better managed by cervical ripening and induction or by continued testing.
   a. The use of the nonstress test as a single technique to evaluate the postterm gestation is not recommended, based on reports of poor outcome after a reactive nonstress test in this situation. In contrast, the contraction stress test, although more time consuming to perform, appears to be an earlier and more sensitive indicator of fetal hypoxia.
   b. Many experts recommend twice-weekly BPP testing beginning at 41 weeks, with delivery if oligohydramnios or a BPP score of 6 or lower is observed.
   c. Despite the fact that antenatal monitoring can almost entirely eliminate perinatal mortality in the postterm gestation, concern about morbidity persists. One alternative approach to fetal testing is to achieve cervical ripening and induction of labor with prostaglandin gel at 41 weeks' gestation.
   d. The data from studies of routine induction of labor rather than antenatal monitoring between 41 and 42 weeks' gestation remain the subject of some controversy. It seems appropriate, in evaluating and managing the postterm gestation, to perform weekly cervical examinations starting at 41 weeks and to induce labor if the Bishop score is 5 or higher. If the cervix is unfavorable, the decision regarding induction versus further testing must be based on an assessment of fetal well-being, risk factors for poor prognostic outcome, and the patient's concerns and desires.

B. **Fetal demise in utero** describes the antenatal diagnosis of the stillborn infant.
   1. **Diagnosis.** Fetal demise in utero should be suspected if the mother reports an absence of fetal movement for more than a few hours. Inabil-

ity to detect a fetal heartbeat via Doppler ultrasonography is suggestive, but definitive diagnosis is made by observing the absence of fetal heartbeats with real-time ultrasonography.

2. **Epidemiology.** Approximately 50% of perinatal deaths are stillbirths. In the past few years, the recorded incidence of fetal death (death at 28 or more weeks' gestation) has fallen from 9.2 to 7.7 per 1000. Of all fetal deaths in the United States, the majority occur before 32 weeks' gestation, 22% occur between 36 and 40 weeks' gestation, and approximately 10% occur beyond 41 weeks' gestation. With improvement in prenatal care and proper hospitalization, some of these deaths are preventable.

3. **Etiology.** Fetal deaths may be divided into those that occur during the antepartum period and those that occur during labor (intrapartum stillbirths). The antepartum fetal death rate in an unmonitored population is approximately 8 in 1000 and represents 86% of fetal deaths. Antepartum death can be divided into four broad categories: chronic hypoxia of diverse origin (30%); congenital malformation or chromosomal anomaly (20%); superimposed complication of pregnancy, such as Rh isoimmunization, abruptio placentae (25%), and fetal infection (5%); and deaths of unexplained cause (25% or more).

4. **Management.** Studies have been performed to identify any avoidable factors contributing to antepartum fetal death. Failure of the medical team to respond appropriately to problems detected during pregnancy and labor, such as abnormal fetal growth assessments or intrapartum fetal monitoring results, significant matzwernal weight loss, or reported reduction in fetal movements, constituted the largest group of avoidable factors. Extensive clinical experience has shown that antepartum fetal assessment can have a significant impact on the frequency and causes of antenatal fetal deaths. Among the inclusion criteria for selecting the population of patients for antepartum fetal assessment are uteroplacental insufficiency such as in prolonged pregnancy, diabetes mellitus, hypertension, previous stillbirth, IUGR, decreased fetal movement, and Rh disease (see Chap. 17).

9. PRETERM LABOR AND PREMATURE RUPTURE OF MEMBRANES

Andrea C. Scharfe and Jude P. Crino

I. **Preterm labor (PTL)** is traditionally defined as contractions that result in cervical change at less than 37 weeks' gestation. In clinical practice, however, the utility of this criterion has been called into question. An alternative definition is six to eight contractions per hour even in the absence of cervical change. It is a difficult diagnosis to make, because the signs and symptoms of PTL are seen in normal pregnancies and because of the cervical examination can be inaccurate. The incidence of PTL has remained at 9–11% of all live births despite the use of tocolytic agents.

   A. **Neonatal consequences.** There are numerous possible neonatal consequences of preterm delivery, which include respiratory distress syndrome, hypothermia, hypoglycemia, jaundice, bronchopulmonary dysplasia, patent ductus arteriosus, necrotizing enterocolitis, intraventricular hemorrhage, neurologic impairment, apnea, retrolental fibroplasias, and neonatal sepsis. In addition, preterm birth is the cause of at least 75% of neonatal deaths that are not attributable to congenital malformations. The survival of infants is directly related to their gestational age. Approximate survival rates are listed in Table 9-1. For newborns of extremely early gestational age (younger than 24 weeks) there is much controversy concerning the value of resuscitation due to the complications mentioned earlier, which may have lasting effects on child development. It is imperative that the family be fully counseled by a neonatologist once PTL is diagnosed so that an informed decision can be made concerning neonatal management.

   B. **Risk factors**
   1. **Infection** is an important cause of PTL. Ascending infection from the genital tract stimulates an inflammatory reaction that releases cytokines, including interleukin-1, interleukin-6, and tumor necrosis factor-α, from endothelial cells. These cytokines then stimulate a cascade of prostaglandin production, which heralds the onset of PTL. Pathogens commonly involved are *Gonorrhea, Chlamydia, Ureaplasma, Trichomonas,* organisms causing bacterial vaginosis, *Treponema pallidum,* and *Mycoplasma*. However, systemic infections, including pyelonephritis, have also been associated with PTL.
   2. **Uterine malformations**, due to overdistension of the smaller intrauterine cavity (i.e., bicornuate uterus or myoma) can cause PTL. Similarly, polyhydramnios and multiple gestation are known risk factors.
   3. **Antepartum hemorrhage** including placenta previa and abruptio placentae may instigate PTL.
   4. **Other risk factors** include low socioeconomic status; nonwhite race; low prepregnancy weight; diethylstilbestrol exposure; maternal age of less than 18 years or more than 40 years; smoking, cocaine use; lack of prenatal care; history of PTL (recurrence rate is 17–37%); cervical incompetence; premature rupture of membranes (PROM); congenital anomalies of the fetus; and medical problems, including severe hypertension or diabetes mellitus. In most cases, however, the cause of PTL is unknown.

   C. **Prevention.** A number of approaches to prevention have been advocated; none, however, has been proven effective. Education about PTL remains integral to prevention. Weekly cervical examinations have no demonstrated beneficial effect. In fact, numerous cervical examinations may cause harm by introducing pathogens, which may increase the risk of ascending infec-

TABLE 9-1. SURVIVAL BY GESTATIONAL AGE AMONG INBORNS ADMITTED TO THE NEONATAL INTENSIVE CARE UNIT AT JOHNS HOPKINS HOSPITAL, 1995–1999

Gestational age in wks	Survival rate (%)
22 wks	10
23 wks	50
24 wks	70
25 wks	85
26 wks	95
27 wks	90
28 wks	99
29 wks	95
30 wks	98
Greater than 30 wks	Approaches 100

tions. The benefits of home uterine monitoring and daily nurse contact are subjects of controversy, except in cases of multiple gestation. Prophylactic oral tocolytic therapy also has no demonstrated beneficial effect overall. Because of their side effects, tocolytic agents should be avoided before the onset of true PTL. Decreased activity or bed rest in the late second trimester and early third trimester commonly is recommended, although no studies demonstrating the efficacy of these measures have been done. Likewise, no studies demonstrating the efficacy of sexual abstinence have been completed. Cervical cerclage is recommended only for women who have been diagnosed with cervical incompetence and is not an appropriate treatment for cervical dilation due to preterm labor.

D. **Investigation.** Any evaluation of suspected PTL should include a thorough history, physical examination, laboratory studies, ultrasonography, and evaluation of the continuous fetal heart tracing.

1. **History.** The history taking should elicit previous occurrences of PTL, preterm delivery, or both; infections during the present pregnancy or symptoms of current infection, including upper respiratory tract or urinary tract infection; recent intercourse; physical abuse or recent abdominal trauma; and recent drug use.

2. **Examination.** Physical examination should include attention to vital signs (fever, maternal tachycardia, and fetal tachycardia), any potential source of infection (culture of cervical specimens and wet preparation), uterine tenderness, and contractions, as well as a sterile speculum examination of the cervix.

   a. **Sterile speculum** examination should include a Nitrazine and fern test to rule out membrane rupture, and procurement of specimens for cervical cultures, including cultures for *Chlamydia trachomatis*, *Neisseria gonorrhea* (GC), and group B β-hemolytic streptococci (GBS) and wet preparations for organisms causing bacterial vaginosis and *Trichomonas*. The advisability of obtaining cultures for *Ureaplasma* and *Mycoplasma* is a subject of controversy.

   b. **Bimanual** examination may be performed if there is no evidence of membrane rupture. The examination should be repeated at appropriate intervals to determine whether cervical change has occurred. If rupture has taken place, treatment for premature rupture of membranes should be initiated as outlined in the second half of this chapter.

3. **Laboratory studies.** It is important to include a blood sample for complete cell counts; cervical specimens for culture; urine specimens for a

toxicology screen, urinalysis, microscopic evaluation, and culture; and specimens for sensitivity studies. One should consider performing amniocentesis, especially if the patient does not respond well to tocolytic agents or is febrile without an obvious source of infection. If amniocentesis is performed, specimens should be designated for Gram's stain, cell count, glucose testing, culture, and fetal lung maturity studies if gestational age is between 30 and 35 weeks. The presence of fetal fibronectin from cervicovaginal secretions is a marker for decidual disruption, which is thought to be a potential diagnostic indicator. When found in secretions between 24 and 36 weeks' gestation, it can be a predictor of PTL; however, its presence usually precedes the event by more than 3 weeks, and therefore it cannot be used to diagnose PTL.

4. **Ultrasonography** is performed to assess fetal position, calculate amniotic fluid index, estimate fetal weight, determine placental location, detect evidence of abruptio placentae (a rare finding on ultrasonography even when abruptio placentae is the correct diagnosis), identify fetal or uterine anomalies, and determine a biophysical profile if indicated.

5. **Continuous fetal heart monitoring** should be performed until the patient is stable and the rate of contractions is less than six per hour for an extended period.

E. **Management**

1. **Intravenous hydration** is often used as an initial approach to treatment. Administration of a bolus of 500 mL of isotonic crystalloid solution is of great benefit for patients who are dehydrated. Excessive hydration should be avoided because of its association with pulmonary edema during tocolytic therapy. Maintenance fluid should be Ringer's lactated solution or 0.9 N saline, with or without dextrose, to minimize the risk of pulmonary edema.

2. **Strict bed rest** is recommended at least initially with continuous fetal monitoring.

3. **Antibiotic therapy.** All specific infections implicated by positive culture findings should be treated appropriately. Prophylaxis against GBS infection should be initiated while the patient is in active PTL, as a preterm neonate is highly susceptible to neonatal sepsis from these organisms. Penicillin or ampicillin is recommended unless the patient is allergic to penicillin, in which case clindamycin is recommended. Currently, antibiotic therapy is not indicated to prolong pregnancy in women with PTL and intact membranes, as this has been shown to increase neonatal mortality in these cases.

4. **Corticosteroids** accelerate the appearance of pulmonary surfactant from type II pneumocytes and decrease the incidence of neonatal deaths, intracerebral hemorrhage, and necrotizing enterocolitis. The current recommended dose of betamethasone is 12.0 mg intramuscularly, with a repeat dose in 24 hours. This should be administered to induce lung maturity in fetuses of between 24 and 34 weeks' gestation if no obvious signs of infection are present. Optimal benefit is achieved 24 hours after the second dose. The beneficial effects of corticosteroid therapy in PTL and PROM are significant. Concerns about corticosteroid therapy include the increased risk of infection for both baby and mother as well as impaired maternal glucose tolerance. The antenatal glucose screen test should be delayed for 1 week while administering steroids. Weekly doses of steroids are no longer recommended as recent studies have shown they may cause the fetus potential harm. A new area of controversy has arisen regarding the use of corticosteroids in cases of less than 23 weeks' gestation. Recently, a protective effect has been demonstrated in relation to intraventricular hemorrhage. Administration of steroids at this early gestational stage is not likely to aid in respiratory status, as most fetuses at this age have not yet formed the type II pneumocytes required to produce surfactant.

5. **Home management** of PTL is reserved for patients who have had stable cervical examination findings while taking no oral tocolytics with at least bathroom privileges in the hospital. Candidates for home management must be able to comply with bed rest and pelvic rest instructions. Kick count charts should be used. Antenatal testing should be ordered as indicated. If intrauterine growth retardation (IUGR) is present, sonograms to track growth should be performed every 3–4 weeks.

6. **Tocolytic therapy.** In the assessment of whether a patient is a candidate for tocolysis, gestational age should be confirmed and fetal anomalies ruled out.

   a. **Indications.** Tocolytic therapy is usually indicated when regular uterine contractions are present with cervical change documented. Cervical dilation of at least 3 cm is associated with a decreased success rate for tocolytic therapy. Tocolytic therapy is appropriate in some such cases, however, to allow time for transfer to a tertiary medical center or treatment with a corticosteroid. It is reasonable to begin treatment with tocolytic agents until 34 weeks' gestation. Analysis of data from neonatal centers reveals that the survival rate of infants delivered at 34 weeks is within 1% of the survival rate of those delivered at 37 weeks' gestation. No studies have convincingly demonstrated an improvement in survival or in any index of long-term neonatal outcome with tocolytic therapy alone.

   b. **General contraindications.** If there is evidence of acute fetal distress, acute chorioamnionitis, eclampsia, or severe preeclampsia, tocolytic agents should not be administered. Other contraindications include fetal demise (singleton), fetal maturity, and maternal hemodynamic instability. Finally, each tocolytic agent has its own specific contraindications.

   c. **Goals of tocolysis.** Primarily, tocolysis should decrease uterine contractions and arrest cervical dilation when the lowest effective dose is used. The drug should be decreased or stopped if significant side effects develop. If intravenous or subcutaneous therapy has been used and has produced sustained clinical improvement for 12–24 hours, the agent should be discontinued. Although many practitioners advocate the use of oral tocolytics immediately after parenteral tocolytics, this practice has not been shown to prolong pregnancy.

   d. **Inpatient management.** Once tocolysis has been achieved and maintained, the patient should be kept in the hospital for observation, initially on strict bed rest (which may be liberalized according to individual patient tolerance). A physical therapy consult should be considered if the possibility exists that bed rest will be prolonged. Fetal well-being is another major consideration. Therefore, fetal heart tones should be obtained at least every 8 hours and fetal testing used as needed (i.e., determined by evidence of IUGR or oligohydramnios, or by maternal factors). If cultures for GBS are positive, it is important to treat with penicillin for 7 days.

7. **Tocolytic agents**

   a. **Terbutaline sulfate** is a phenylethylamine derivative with β_2-mimetic properties. It may be used as a first-line tocolytic. The dosage of terbutaline is 0.25 mg given subcutaneously every 20 minutes. The drug should be withheld if maternal heart rates are higher than 120 bpm or fetal heart rates are higher than 160 bpm. Terbutaline may also be given orally. The total dose should not exceed 5 mg every 3–4 hours. The use of oral terbutaline has not been associated with prolongation of pregnancy past 72 hours. Finally, the terbutaline pump has been advocated by some clinicians for long-term management of PTL. The efficacy of this therapy is controversial.

b. **Magnesium sulfate.** The action of magnesium sulfate is thought to occur at neuronal levels. By influencing the amplitude of the motor plate potentials and interfering with calcium function at the myometrial neuronal junction, it is thought to decrease uterine contractility. The initial loading dose is 4–6 g intravenously over 20 minutes followed by a continuous infusion of 2–4 g/hour. The dose should be titrated to stop contractions, but usually 6 g/hour is not exceeded. Magnesium sulfate should be continued until the patient has had fewer than six contractions per hour for 12 hours and no cervical change. It is not essential to check magnesium levels; the patient's examination record can be followed and the dose titrated accordingly to stop contractions. Therapeutic levels of magnesium sulfate are between 6 and 8 mg/dL.

(1) **Absolute contraindications.** Myasthenia gravis and recent myocardial infarction are the most notable contraindications to magnesium sulfate therapy. Careful attention should be paid to patients with renal impairment, as magnesium is excreted by the kidneys and in such patients its effects can last longer and levels can become toxic at lower dosages.

(2) **Maternal side effects** include respiratory depression, pulmonary edema, cardiac arrest, tetany, nausea, and vomiting. Other notable effects are flushing, muscle weakness, hypotension, and hyporeflexia. Decreased variability is the only notable fetal side effect. Terbutaline and magnesium sulfate should not be administered together as the risk of side effects increases. Because of the side effects, close monitoring is essential. Flow sheets with hourly documentation of symptoms, lung examination findings, deep tendon reflexes, and total intake and outputs are often helpful. Intravenous fluids should be limited to 100 mL/hour.

c. **Indomethacin.** The method of action of indomethacin is inhibition of the synthesis of prostaglandins, primarily prostaglandin $F_{2\alpha}$, from fatty acid precursors. The recommended dosage is a loading dose of 100 mg per rectum, and therapeutic levels are maintained with doses of 25 mg orally or 50 mg per rectum every 4–6 hours for a maximum of 48–72 hours.

(1) **Contraindications.** Maternal contraindications include peptic ulcer disease, renal disease, coagulopathy, and oligohydramnios. Indomethacin should not be given when the estimated gestational age of the fetus is greater than 32 weeks as it may interfere with fetal circulation.

(2) **Side effects.** Oligohydramnios and irreversible constriction of the fetal ductus arteriosus are the most worrisome fetal side effects. Just as any nonsteroidal anti-inflammatory drug, indomethacin can affect the fetal kidneys; hence, amniotic fluid volume may decrease. An amniotic fluid index should be established before beginning therapy and should be checked after 48 hours. The effect of indomethacin on the fetal kidneys is reversible. Headache, dizziness, GI discomfort, fluid retention, nausea, vomiting, and pruritus are the primary maternal side effects.

d. **Nifedipine.** By inhibiting intracellular calcium entry, nifedipine blocks contraction of smooth muscle and inhibits uterine contraction. The recommended dosage is 10–20 mg every 6 hours orally. Nifedipine has been administered in a loading dose of 10 mg sublingually every 20 minutes for up to three doses.

(1) **Contraindications.** Concomitant use with magnesium sulfate is not recommended as it may illicit severe hypotension. Other contraindications include congestive heart failure and aortic stenosis.

(2) **Side effects.** The following are noted side effects of nifedipine: hypotension, flushing, nasal congestion, tachycardia, dizziness, nausea, nervousness, bowel changes, and, in one case report, skeletal muscle blockade.

F. **Chorioamnionitis** is an infection of the fetal membranes, usually from an ascending infection. It is a frequent cause of PTL and should always be excluded before one embarks on prolonged tocolytic therapy. Hallmarks of this infection are maternal and fetal tachycardia, maternal fever, leukocytosis, uterine tenderness, and uterine contractions. Premature rupture of membranes is frequently associated with this diagnosis. It is primarily a clinical diagnosis. However, amniocentesis may provide helpful information. Polymorphonuclear neutrophil leukocytes in amniotic fluid are suggestive but not diagnostic of chorioamnionitis, as is a glucose level of less than 14 mg/dL; bacteria on Gram's stain is specific but not sensitive, and culture results may take more than 1 week to return. The usual treatment is ampicillin and gentamicin sulfate intravenously and delivery of the fetus. Acetaminophen (Tylenol) is administered to reduce maternal fever after the diagnosis of chorioamnionitis has been made.

G. **Delivery**
1. **Timing.** It is important to proceed with delivery if signs or symptoms of chorioamnionitis or fetal distress are present. Anesthesia issues should be addressed early in the delivery process.
2. **Management.** Preterm infants are fragile and can easily experience asphyxia and birth trauma. These can be decreased by controlling the second stage of labor. Episiotomy is indicated only when perineal resistance is present. Forceps should be used for obstetrical indications.

   Management of a nonvertex presentation is dependent on gestational age and estimated fetal weight. If the fetus is older than 26 weeks' gestation, most obstetricians opt for delivery by cesarean section. Similarly, some have advocated performing a cesarean section if the estimated weight is greater than 1000 g. A vaginal delivery should be considered for fetuses with a nonvertex presentation weighing less than 1000 g.

   For attempted vaginal deliveries with both vertex and nonvertex presentations of fetuses of less than 26 weeks' gestation, it is imperative to discuss with patients the possible need for a classical cesarean section in case of fetal distress. At these early gestational ages, some mothers may not opt for cesarean section. They should be clearly informed of the risks and benefits of this procedure for an infant for whom survival may be limited. These can be difficult decisions that should be handled with the help of both the neonatologist and the obstetrician.

II. **Premature rupture of membranes (PROM)** is the rupture of the amnion and chorion 1 hour or more before the onset of labor. If this event occurs before 37 weeks' gestation, it is referred to as preterm PROM (PPROM). It becomes prolonged PPROM when ruptured longer than 12 hours before the onset of labor.

A. **Etiology.** Possible causative factors include local amniotic membrane defect; infection, including vaginal, cervical, or intra-amniotic infection; colonization, especially with GBS; history of PROM; incompetent cervix; hydramnios; multiple gestation; trauma; fetal malformations; abruptio placentae; and placenta previa.

B. **Investigation.** Similar to PTL, the investigation of PPROM includes history taking, examination, laboratory investigations, and ultrasonography.
1. **History.** It is important to note the time of the rupture and the color of the fluid. In addition, the patient should be asked about blood or discharge per vagina as well as any cramping.
2. **Examination.** Only a sterile speculum examination is performed. There should be no digital cervical examination performed unless delivery is anticipated within 24 hours. Nitrazine and fern tests can be used to confirm rupture. Both tests commonly have false-positive results. Nitrazine testing can be falsely positive in the presence of Trichomonas, blood,

semen, cervical mucus, and urine. Ferning is falsely positive in the presence of cervical mucus and falsely negative in the presence of blood. Cervical specimens should also be obtained for culture. Testing of vaginal pool fluid for fetal lung maturity should be considered (the Amniostat test is a rapid test used to detect the presence of phosphatidylglycerol). If phosphatidylglycerol is present, there is a higher likelihood of fetal lung maturity, and delivery is recommended as the risk of maternal infection is higher than the risk of fetal respiratory distress. All of the commercially available methods of detecting fetal lung maturity using vaginal pool collections of fluid have been shown to be affected by the vaginal environment. These results should be interpreted cautiously when there is evidence of maternal or intra-amniotic infection.

C. **Management.** Conservative management is usually the rule in PPROM. Before 34 weeks' gestational age, most obstetricians wait for signs or symptoms of infection or fetal distress to appear before intervening. Severe oligohydramnios, fetal tachycardia, and cessation of fetal breathing are associated with chorioamnionitis.

1. **Fetal well-being.** A neonatologist should be consulted to inform patients concerning survival rates and long-term outcomes of preterm infants with PROM. In cases of PROM, it is often important to assess the gestational age, weight, and position of the fetus by ultrasonography. Betamethasone may be given between 24 and 34 weeks' gestation. Prophylaxis against GBS infection with penicillin G is recommended (clindamycin is used if the patient is allergic to penicillin) until negative culture results are received. Positive culture results should prompt appropriate treatment. Evidence of fetal heart tones should be obtained at least every 8 hours. Recommendations for fetal testing vary from daily nonstress tests and weekly biophysical profile measurement to semiweekly testing. If IUGR is identified, sonograms to track growth should be performed every 3–4 weeks. If the fetus is not growing appropriately, delivery may be necessary.

2. **Maternal care.** Use of tocolytics generally is reserved for cases in which transport is necessary or a delay in delivery is desired, in some cases for 48 hours, so that steroid therapy can produce a maximal effect on pulmonary maturation. If the patient is not in labor and the fetal heart rate tracing is stable, the patient may be managed expectantly. Strict bed rest should be used due to the risk of cord prolapse, especially if the fetus is breech in presentation. The patient should receive physical therapy while confined to bed. Therapy with antithromboembolic agents and prophylactic subcutaneous heparin sodium should be considered as these patients are at increased risk for deep vein thrombosis.

3. **Antibiotic therapy.** Unlike in PTL, it has been shown that antibiotic therapy can prolong pregnancies in PPROM. Many regimes have been proposed. One common regime first described by Mercer et al. includes ampicillin 2 g intravenously every 6 hours coupled with intravenous erythromycin for 48 hours. After this, the intravenous medication may be converted to oral amoxicillin 250 mg every 8 hours and oral erythromycin 333 mg every 8 hours. The regimen should be continued for a total of 7 days (*JAMA*, 09/24, 1997).

4. **Delivery indications** are identical to those for PTL.

5. **Cerclage.** Management of PROM in the setting of a cerclage is the subject of some controversy. Most obstetricians remove the cerclage and proceed with expectant management.

D. **Consequences of PROM** include increased risk of maternal and fetal infection, fetal limb contracture formation, and pulmonary hypoplasia.

10. THIRD TRIMESTER BLEEDING

Fiona Simpkins and Cynthia Holcroft

I. **Introduction.** Third trimester bleeding occurs in 2–6% of all pregnancies. The amount of bleeding can range from spotting to massive hemorrhage. Because third trimester bleeding can lead to emotional and physical stress, as well as maternal and fetal morbidity and mortality, it remains important to make a diagnosis. The differential diagnosis of common causes includes abruptio placentae, placenta previa, vasa previa, labor (bloody show), cervicitis, trauma (including sexual intercourse), uterine rupture, and carcinoma. Because of the potential severe sequelae, this chapter focuses on abruptio placentae, placenta previa, and vasa previa.

II. **Abruptio placenta** (AP) is the premature separation of the implanted placenta from the uterine wall.

A. **Epidemiology.** The incidence varies from 1 in 86 to 1 in 206 births. AP has a recurrence rate of 5–17% after an episode in one previous pregnancy and 25% after episodes in two previous pregnancies.

B. **Etiology.** Although many cases continue to be idiopathic, AP is associated with maternal hypertension, advanced maternal age, multiparity, cocaine use, tobacco use, chorioamnionitis, and trauma. Rarely, rapid contraction of an overdistended uterus may lead to abruption, such as with rupture of membranes with polyhydramnios or delivery of an infant in a multiple gestation.

C. **Clinical manifestation.** The amount of external bleeding can vary from none to massive hemorrhage. The presence of blood in the basalis stimulates uterine contractions, which results in abdominal pain. Fetal and maternal mortality rates vary depending on the location and size of the hemorrhage.

D. **Maternal complications**
1. Hemorrhagic shock leading to ischemic necrosis of distant organs
2. Disseminated intravascular hemorrhage
3. Couvelaire's uterus (extravasation of blood into uterine muscle) leading to uterine atony. Rarely, Couvelaire's uterus may lead to uterine atony and massive hemorrhage, which necessitates aggressive measures such as selective arterial embolization or cesarean hysterectomy to control the bleeding.

E. **Fetal complications** include hypoxia leading to fetal distress, death, growth restriction, prematurity, anemia, and major malformations.

F. **Diagnosis**
1. **History and physical examination.** Classically, AP presents with vaginal bleeding and acute onset of constant abdominal pain, whereas placenta previa presents with painless vaginal bleeding. A vaginal examination should not be performed unless both placenta previa and vasa previa have been ruled out. Maternal vital signs, fetal heart pattern, and uterine tone should be monitored. Fundal height can also be followed to look for concealed hemorrhage.
2. **Ultrasonography.** Although ultrasonography is relatively insensitive in diagnosing AP, a hypoechoic area between the uterine wall and placenta may be seen with large abruptions.
3. **Pelvic examination.** If placenta previa is ruled out, perform a speculum examination to look for vaginal or cervical lacerations and evaluate vaginal bleeding. If there is a discharge that is suspicious for infection or the cervix is friable, obtain a wet prep, potassium hydroxide (KOH), and cervical cultures for gonorrhea and chlamydia.

4. **Laboratory tests. If the clinical presentation is suspicious for AP, the following tests may be performed:** complete blood cell count with a hematocrit and platelet count, prothrombin/activated partial thromboplastin time, fibrinogen and fibrin degradation product levels, blood type and screen (type and crossmatch determination should be considered depending on severity of bleeding), and Betke-Kleihauer test.

In addition, two bedside tests can be performed. A "poor man's clot test" consists of placing a specimen of whole blood in a red-top tube. If a clot does not form within 6 minutes or forms and lyses within 30 minutes, a coagulation defect is most likely present. To determine if vaginal blood is maternal or fetal in origin, an Apt test may be performed at the bedside. This test consists of mixing vaginal blood with potassium hydroxide. If the blood is maternal in origin, it will turn brown. If it is fetal in origin, no changes will occur because fetal hemoglobin is more resistant to changes in pH. This may prove helpful in distinguishing between placenta previa and vasa previa.

G. **Management.** The management of AP depends on the fetus's gestational age and the hemodynamic status of both patient and fetus. Standard management for all patients includes establishment of intravenous access with two large-bore catheters, fluid resuscitation, blood type and crossmatch determination, and continuous fetal monitoring. $Rh_o(D)$ immunoglobulin should be administered to Rh-negative individuals. In addition, maternal vital signs should be recorded frequently. A Foley catheter should be placed to monitor urine output, which should be more than 0.5–1.0 mL/kg/hour.

1. **Term gestation, maternal and fetal hemodynamic stability.** One should plan for vaginal delivery with cesarean section reserved for the usual obstetrical indications. If the patient does not present in labor, induction of labor should be initiated.

2. **Term gestation, maternal and fetal hemodynamic instability.** Aggressive fluid resuscitation as well as transfusion of blood products and coagulation factors should be performed as appropriate. Once maternal stabilization is achieved, cesarean section should be performed unless vaginal delivery is imminent.

3. **Preterm gestation, maternal and fetal hemodynamic stability.** Eighty-two percent of patients who are at less than 20 weeks' gestation can be expected to have a term delivery despite evidence of placental separation. Only 27% of patients who present after 20 weeks' gestation, however, will have a term delivery.

   a. **Preterm, absence of labor.** These patients should be followed closely with serial ultrasonographic examination for fetal growth starting at 24 weeks' gestation. Steroids should be administered to promote fetal lung maturity. If at any time maternal instability arises, delivery should be performed after appropriate resuscitation. Otherwise, labor should be induced at term or if testing shows signs of fetal compromise.

   b. **Preterm, presence of labor.** If both maternal and fetal hemodynamic stability are established, tocolysis may be used in selective cases, particularly cases of extreme prematurity. Magnesium sulfate is preferred over the β-sympathomimetic agents (terbutaline sulfate) because it has fewer cardiovascular side effects. The β-sympathomimetics may mask the physiologic signs of shock. If maternal or fetal hemodynamic status is compromised, delivery should be performed after appropriate resuscitation.

4. **Preterm gestation, maternal and fetal hemodynamic instability.** Delivery should be performed after appropriate resuscitation.

H. **Abruptio placentae and abdominal trauma.** Whenever abdominal trauma has occurred, AP must be ruled out. In the absence of vaginal bleeding, uterine contractions, or uterine tenderness, 2–6 hours of continuous fetal heart monitoring may be adequate. If any of these signs are present, then 24 hours of observation is warranted. The laboratory studies mentioned earlier can be performed as well. $Rh_o(D)$ immunoglobulin should be administered within 72 hours of the trauma to Rh-negative unsensitized patients.

III. **Placenta previa (PP)** is defined as the implantation of the placenta over or near the cervical os. PP can be classified into four types based on the location of the placenta relative to the cervical os: **complete or total previa**, in which the placenta covers the entire cervical os; **partial previa**, in which the margin of the placenta covers part but not all of the internal os; **marginal previa**, in which the edge of the placenta lies adjacent to the internal os; and **low-lying previa**, in which the placenta is located near but not directly adjacent to the internal os.

   A. **Epidemiology.** In general, the incidence of PP is 1 in 250 pregnancies. The frequency varies with parity, however. For nulliparas, the incidence is only 1 in 1000 to 1500, whereas in grand multiparas, it may be as high as 1 in 20. The most important risk factor for PP is a prior cesarean section. PP occurs in 1% of pregnancies after a cesarean section. Note that the placenta covers the cervical os in 5% of pregnancies when examined at midpregnancy. The majority of these cases resolve as the uterus grows with gestational age; the upper third of the cervix develops into the lower uterine segment, and the placenta "migrates" away from the internal os.

   B. **Etiology.** The etiology of PP is unknown. Bleeding is thought to occur in association with the development of the lower uterine segment in the third trimester. Placental attachment is disrupted as this area gradually thins in preparation for labor. Bleeding then ensues as the thinned lower uterine segment is unable to contract adequately to prevent blood flow from the open vessels.

   C. **Clinical manifestations.** Patients present most commonly at 29–30 weeks' gestation with painless vaginal bleeding. The fluid is usually bright red, and the bleeding is acute in onset and starts abruptly. The number of bleeding episodes is unrelated to the degree of placenta previa or to the prognosis for fetal survival. Placenta previa is associated with a doubling of the rate of congenital malformations. These include malformations of the CNS, GI tract, cardiovascular system, and respiratory system. Abnormal growth of the placenta into the uterus can result in one of the following three complications:

      1. **Placenta previa accreta.** The placenta adheres to the uterine wall without the usual intervening decidua basalis. The incidence in patients with previa who have not had prior uterine surgery is approximately 4%. The risk is increased to 16–25% in patients who have had a prior cesarean section or uterine surgery.
      2. **Placenta previa increta.** The placenta invades the myometrium.
      3. **Placenta previa percreta.** The placenta penetrates the entire uterine wall, potentially growing into bladder or bowel.

   D. **Diagnosis**
      1. **History and physical examination.** PP presents with acute onset of painless vaginal bleeding. Any prior history of cesarean section should be ascertained, and maternal vital signs and fetal heart pattern should be monitored.
      2. **Ultrasonography** accurately confirms diagnosis in 95–98% of cases. The diagnosis may be missed, however, if the placenta lies in the posterior portion of the lower uterine segment, because ultrasonography may not adequately visualize the placenta in this location. Vaginal sonography can be helpful in these instances.
      3. **Pelvic examination.** *If PP is present, digital examination is contraindicated.* A speculum examination can be used to evaluate the presence and quantity of vaginal bleeding; however, in most cases these can be assessed without placing a speculum and potentially causing more bleeding.

4. **Laboratory studies.** The following laboratory studies should be done for a patient with PP with vaginal bleeding:
   a. Complete blood cell count with hematocrit and platelets
   b. Type and crossmatch determination
   c. Prothrombin time and activated thromboplastin time
   d. Betke-Kleihauer test to assess for fetomaternal hemorrhage
      The Apt test may be performed to determine if vaginal blood is maternal or fetal in origin (see explanation in sec. **II.F.4**).

E. **Management.** Standard management of patients with PP includes initial hospitalization with hemodynamic stabilization. Laboratory studies should be ordered as outlined earlier. Steroids should be given to promote lung maturity for gestations between 24 and 34 weeks. $Rh_o(D)$ immunoglobulin should be administered to Rh-negative mothers. Management of PP is then based on gestational age, severity of the bleeding, and fetal condition and presentation. The location of the placenta also plays an important role in management and route of delivery.

Fetal testing is controversial, but often semiweekly testing is instituted. Follow-up ultrasonographic examinations to assess growth are often recommended as PP has been linked with an increased risk of intrauterine growth retardation and congenital anomalies (CNS, CDV, respiratory tract, and GI tract).

Management of complications, such as placenta accreta or one of its variants (placenta percreta or placenta increta), can be challenging. In patients with PP and a prior history of cesarean section, cesarean hysterectomy may be required. However, in cases where uterine preservation is highly desired and no bladder invasion has occurred, bleeding has been successfully controlled with selective arterial embolization or packing of the lower uterine segment, with subsequent removal of the pack through the vagina in 24 hours.

1. **Term gestation, maternal and fetal hemodynamic stability.** At this point, management depends on placental location.
   a. **Complete previa.** Patients with complete previa at term require cesarean section.
   b. **Partial, marginal previa.** These patients may deliver vaginally; however, a double setup in the operating room is recommended. The patient should be prepared and draped for cesarean section. An anesthesiologist and the operating room team should be present. If at any point maternal or fetal stability is compromised, urgent cesarean section is indicated.

2. **Term gestation, maternal and fetal hemodynamic instability.** The first priority is to stabilize the mother with fluid resuscitation and administration of blood products if necessary. Delivery should then occur via cesarean section.

3. **Preterm gestation, maternal and fetal hemodynamic stability.**
   a. **Labor absent.** Patients at 24–36 weeks' gestation with PP who are hemodynamically stable can be managed expectantly until fetal lung maturity has occurred. The patient should be on strict bed rest with an active type and screen at all times. Maternal hematocrit should be maintained above 30%. $Rh_o(D)$ immunoglobulin should be administered to Rh-negative mothers within 72 hours of a bleeding episode. After initial hospital management, care as an outpatient may be considered if the following criteria are met: the patient is compliant, has a responsible adult present at all times who can assist in an emergency situation, and has ready transportation to the hospital. In general, once a patient has been hospitalized for three separate episodes of bleeding, she should remain in the hospital until delivery.
   b. **Labor present.** Twenty percent of patients with PP show evidence of uterine contractions; however, it is difficult to document preterm labor, as cervical examinations are contraindicated. Tocolysis with

magnesium sulfate is the recommended choice. The β-mimetics should be avoided as they cause tachycardia and mimic hypovolemia. If tocolysis is successful, amniocentesis can be performed at 36 weeks. If fetal lung maturity is established, the patient can be delivered.

4. **Preterm gestation, maternal and fetal hemodynamic instability.** Again, maternal stabilization with resuscitative measures is the priority. Once stable, the patient should be delivered by urgent cesarean section.

IV. **Vasa previa (VP)** can occur when the umbilical cord inserts into the membrane of the placenta instead of the central region of the placenta. When one of these vessels is located near the internal os, it is at risk of rupturing and causing fetal hemorrhage. VP can also occur when vessels leading to an accessory lobe cover the internal os.

A. **Epidemiology.** VP is rarely encountered. The incidence of vasa previa is between 0.1% and 1.8% of pregnancies. Fetal mortality has been reported to be as high as 50%.

B. **Etiology.** The etiology of VP is unknown.

C. **Clinical manifestations.** Although VP is a rare cause of third trimester bleeding, the physician must make the correct diagnosis because of the catastrophic consequences to the fetus. As the total fetal blood volume is small, even small amounts of blood loss result in fetal instability. The patient usually presents with an acute onset of vaginal bleeding. This is associated with an acute change in fetal heart pattern. Typically, fetal tachycardia occurs, followed by bradycardia with intermittent accelerations. Short-term variability is often maintained. Rupture of the membranes can result in catastrophic exsanguination and fetal distress.

D. **Diagnosis.** Transvaginal ultrasonography in combination with color Doppler ultrasonography is the most effective tool in antenatal diagnosis. In addition, the Apt test (see sec. **II.F.4**) can prove helpful.

E. **Management.** Third trimester bleeding caused by VP is usually accompanied by fetal distress, and emergency cesarean section is indicated. If VP is diagnosed antenatally, elective cesarean section should be scheduled at 37–38 weeks under controlled circumstances to reduce fetal mortality.

11. PERINATAL INFECTIONS

Dana Virgo and Gina Hanna

I. **Human immunodeficiency virus (HIV)**
   A. **Epidemiology.** Worldwide, UNAIDS (Joint United Nations Programme on HIV/AIDS) estimates that 2.3 million women were newly infected with HIV in 1999, adding their numbers to the 15.7 million women living with HIV/AIDS. Overall, 34.3 million persons worldwide currently are infected with HIV. In the United States, by the end of 1999, over 400,000 cases of HIV had been reported to the U.S. Centers for Disease Control and Prevention (CDC). Approximately 90% of women infected with HIV in the United States today are between the ages of 13 and 44. Eighty-seven percent of HIV-infected children in the United States had a mother with HIV or at risk for HIV as their only known risk factor for the virus. It is impossible to predict accurately who is infected with HIV. According to the CDC, 40% of infected American women report heterosexual contact as their only risk factor; an additional 38% report no known risk factor.
   B. **Perinatal transmission**
      1. Perinatal transmission rates of HIV in the absence of antiretroviral prophylaxis range from 14% to 33% in industrialized nations. In Africa, rates up to 43% have been reported.
      2. The **timing** of perinatal transmission is an important factor in its prevention. Data support HIV transmission during the intrauterine, intrapartum, and postpartum periods.
      3. **Intrauterine transmission** of HIV is most likely transplacental. Transmission later in pregnancy is more likely to be preventable with antiretroviral agents. Overall, 20–30% of perinatal transmission probably occurs in the intrauterine period.
      4. **Intrapartum transmission,** which accounts for up to 80% of perinatal transmission, may occur by transplacental maternal-fetal transfusion of blood during uterine contractions or by exposure to infected maternal blood and cervicovaginal secretions.
      5. **Breast feeding** is the primary mechanism of postnatal transmission. HIV has been isolated from cellular and noncellular fractions of breast milk.
      6. **Prevention strategies** for vertical transmission include decreasing maternal viral load, decreasing maternal-fetal transfusion and fetal exposure to maternal secretions, and avoidance of breast feeding when possible.
      7. The **risk** of vertical transmission is proportional to the maternal viral load (concentration of virus in maternal plasma). In a recent study of 141 mother-infant pairs in which maternal viral load was less than 1000 copies/mL, the observed incidence of vertical transmission was 0 with a 95% upper confidence limit of 2%.
   C. **Diagnosis** of HIV infection is based on a screening test for specific antibodies using enzyme-linked immunosorbent assay (ELISA), usually against core (p24) or envelope (gp44) antigens. Positive results are confirmed by Western blot test. In untreated patients, the average time between initial infection and the development of AIDS is 10 years. Clinical progression of the disease is monitored using the CD4 cell count.
      1. **At CD4 counts of more than 500/mL,** patients usually do not demonstrate clinical evidence of immunosuppression.
      2. **At CD4 counts of 200–500/mL,** patients are more likely to develop symptoms and require intervention than at higher counts.

3. **At CD4 counts less than 200/mL,** or at higher CD4 cell counts accompanied by thrush or unexplained fevers for 2 or more weeks, patients are at increased risk for developing complicated disease.

D. **Management.** HIV testing should be offered to all pregnant women as part of routine prenatal care. The care of the HIV-infected obstetric patient parallels that of the nonpregnant HIV-infected patient and includes monitoring of immune status, prophylaxis as indicated for opportunistic infections, and testing for other sexually transmitted diseases.

1. **Strategies to prevent perinatal transmission**

   a. In 1994, the AIDS Clinical Trials Group 076 showed that administration of zidovudine (ZDV, or AZT; Retrovir) during pregnancy and childbirth could reduce vertical transmission rates by two-thirds. Further studies have found that ZDV is efficacious in reducing transmission in the context of advanced disease, low maternal CD4 cell counts, and prior use of ZDV therapy. It is therefore vitally important to offer this regimen to all infected women.

   b. To decrease maternal-fetal transfusion, certain procedures should be avoided, including chorionic villus sampling, amniocentesis, fetal scalp blood sampling, and the use of fetal scalp electrodes in labor. Avoidance of labor also may decrease the risk of transmission. Some studies have shown a decrease in the risk of vertical transmission when scheduled cesarean delivery is performed as opposed to vaginal delivery or unscheduled cesarean delivery. Most of this evidence, however, was compiled before the use of highly active antiretroviral therapy and without obtaining data regarding maternal viral load. Whether scheduled cesarean delivery decreases vertical transmission rates in women on highly active antiretroviral therapy or in those with low viral loads is unknown. The impact of the length of labor or of rupture of membranes on vertical transmission in unscheduled cesarean deliveries is also unknown. Maternal morbidity is higher with cesarean delivery than with vaginal delivery; increases in maternal morbidity seem to be greatest in HIV-infected women with lower CD4 cell counts. For now, patients should be counseled regarding the existing evidence and offered a choice between vaginal delivery and scheduled cesarian delivery.

   c. Treatment during pregnancy should focus not only on prevention of vertical transmission but on effective treatment of the women themselves. Pregnancy is not a reason to defer aggressive treatment regimens that maximally suppress viral replication. Although ZDV prophylaxis alone has substantially decreased the risk of perinatal transmission, antiretroviral monotherapy is now considered suboptimal treatment. Combination antiretroviral therapy, usually consisting of two nucleoside analog reverse transcriptase inhibitors and a protease inhibitor, is the currently recommended standard for HIV-infected adults. Triple-drug therapy is associated with the disappearance of detectable viral burden and an increase in CD4 cell counts. Special considerations in pregnancy include changes in dosing regimens and potential short- and long-term effects of antiretroviral drugs on the fetus and newborn.

2. **Opportunistic infection prophylaxis**

   a. *Pneumocystis carinii pneumonia* (PCP) prophylaxis: When the CD4 count is less than 200/mL, trimethoprim-sulfamethoxazole double strength (TMP/SMX-DS), once daily, is recommended. Alternatively, dapsone may be used. In the first trimester of pregnancy, TMP/SMX should be avoided; aerosolized pentamidine isethionate may be substituted.

   b. *Mycobacterium avium complex* (MAC) prophylaxis: Azithromycin, 1200 mg once weekly, is recommended for MAC prophylaxis when the CD4 count is less than 100/mL.

c. Toxoplasmosis prophylaxis should be given when the CD4 count is less than 100/mL; it is provided adequately by TMP/SMX, as given for PCP prophylaxis.

d. Previously, patients who were started on prophylaxis for opportunistic infections were kept on their regimens even when their CD4 counts increased or viral loads decreased; it has been postulated that the risk of these illnesses remains high because less effective CD4 cells form after HIV infection. However, more recent studies have shown that it is probably safe to discontinue PCP and MAC prophylaxis in patients in whom CD4 cell counts are increased for at least 3–6 months. There is less evidence to support the safety of discontinuing toxoplasmosis prophylaxis, however, so it should be continued indefinitely.

e. Women with HIV may be taking systemic antifungal medications for candidiasis prophylaxis; this prophylaxis should be discontinued in pregnancy due to the potential for azole-induced teratogenicity. Similarly, cytomegalovirus (CMV) prophylaxis with ganciclovir is not recommended in pregnancy.

f. Women with positive results on tuberculin skin tests should be treated after a chest radiograph has been obtained to rule out active disease. Treatment may be deferred until the second trimester. Isoniazid, either daily or twice weekly, is the treatment of choice. Pyridoxine hydrochloride should be administered as well to minimize the risk of neuropathy.

3. Routine **vaccinations** include the hepatitis B virus (HBV) series, one-time pneumonia vaccine, and an annual influenza vaccine. Rubella vaccine may be safely administered as indicated. Severely immunocompromised patients may fail to mount an appropriate response to vaccines, however. Studies of nonpregnant adults have shown transient bursts of viremia after vaccination. The effect of transient postvaccination viremia on vertical transmission rates is unknown. It is reasonable to defer vaccination in pregnancy until antiretroviral therapy has been established.

4. **Serum monitoring** of HIV-infected patients includes obtaining a baseline CD4 count, HIV RNA polymerase chain reaction (PCR) quantification, CBC, and liver function tests, and assessing CMV infection and toxoplasmosis status.

a. If the CMV test results are positive, an ophthalmologic evaluation is indicated. The risk of CMV retinitis is present in patients with a CD4 count of less than 50/mL. Toxoplasmosis in HIV-infected patients usually is caused by reactivation of latent disease (seroprevalence of 10–30%). Toxoplasmosis risk is increased in patients with a CD4 count of less than 100/mL (75% of cases occur in those with a CD4 count of less than 50/mL); prophylaxis is provided by TMP/SMX-DS.

b. After a patient is started on antiretroviral therapy, a set of laboratory studies should be repeated on a monthly basis for 2 months, then every 2 or 3 months, or after any changes in her medical therapy, depending on her response to therapy. An effective therapeutic regimen should result in an increase in the patient's CD4 count and a substantial decrease in her viral load; undetectable viral levels are to be expected on the triple-drug regimen. Failure to achieve such an effect warrants a reevaluation of the regimen.

c. Patients requiring only ZDV for fetal indications must be informed of the possibility that their risk of drug resistance will increase with one-drug therapy. Pregnancy is the only indication for such therapy at this point. Our practice is to administer zidovudine in combination with lamivudine (3TC, Epivir) in an attempt to decrease the risk that resistant viral serotypes will arise.

5. **Drug toxicity**

a. **General.** GI upset, chiefly nausea, vomiting, and diarrhea, can occur with any of the commonly prescribed medications and is a significant problem in pregnancy.

TABLE 11-1. PEDIATRIC AIDS CLINICAL TRIAL GROUP PROTOCOL 076 (PACTG 076) ZIDOVUDINE (ZDV) REGIMEN

Time of ZDV administration	Regimen
Antepartum	PO administration of 100 mg ZDV five times daily; initiated at 14–34 wks' gestation and continued throughout pregnancy
Intrapartum	IV administration of ZDV with a 1-hr bolus of 2 mg/kg body weight, followed by a continuous infusion of 1 mg/kg body weight/hr until delivery
Postpartum	PO administration of ZDV to the newborn: ZDV syrup at 2 mg/kg body weight/dose every 6 hrs for the first 6 wks of life, beginning 8–12 hrs after birth

   b. **Nucleoside analog reverse transcriptase inhibitors.** Of the five approved, only ZDV and 3TC have been evaluated in clinical trials involving pregnant women.
     (1) Zidovudine [U.S. Food and Drug Administration (FDA) Category B] (Table 11-1) is associated with a high incidence of reversible GI intolerance, insomnia, myalgias, asthenia, malaise, and headaches. Bone marrow suppression resulting in anemia or neutropenia can be severe and occasionally necessitates the use of erythropoietin (U.S. FDA Pregnancy Category C), blood transfusions, dose reductions, or drug holidays. Macrocytosis is usually observed during the first month of therapy and has been used as a measure of patient compliance. A mild, reversible elevation of transaminase levels can be seen. Fingernail, skin, and oral mucosa discoloration may appear at 2–6 weeks of therapy. Rarely, nucleoside analog therapy is associated with lactic acidosis or severe hepatomegaly with steatosis, either of which necessitates discontinuance of the therapy. ZDV has been shown to be toxic in animals when given early in gestation, and the manufacturer has recommended that ZDV be administered only after 14 weeks' gestation. Long-term follow-up of children exposed in utero is not available for any antiretroviral drug, but short-term studies of ZDV (up to 4 years) have been reassuring. ZDV is excreted in breast milk.
     (2) 3TC (U.S. FDA Pregnancy Category C) has minimal toxicity. Side effects include abdominal pain; nausea, vomiting, and diarrhea; headache; fever; rash; malaise; insomnia; cough; nasal symptoms; and musculoskeletal pain. Rarely, peripheral neuropathy and pancreatitis have been reported. TMP-SMX-DS has been shown to decrease serum levels of 3TC; the therapeutic implications of this interaction are unclear. 3TC is excreted in breast milk.
     (3) Didanosine (dideoxyinosine, Videx) (U.S. FDA Pregnancy Category B) requires concomitant antacid administration. Severe side effects include peripheral neuropathy and pancreatitis. It is not known whether didanosine is excreted in breast milk.
     (4) Stavudine (didehydrodeoxythymidine, Zerit) (U.S. FDA Pregnancy Category C) is being studied now as treatment for pregnant women.
     (5) Abacavir sulfate (ABC) and zalcitabine (dideoxycytidine) have not been studied for use in pregnant humans.
   c. **Nonnucleoside analog reverse transcriptase inhibitors**
     (1) Nevirapine (Viramune) has adverse effects that include fatigue, headache, nausea and diarrhea, increases in hepatic enzyme levels,

hepatitis, and skin rashes. Rarely, Stevens-Johnson syndrome and toxic epidermal necrolysis have resulted, so the drug should be discontinued if a severe skin rash or a rash accompanied by fever, blistering, oral lesions, conjunctivitis, swelling, myalgias, or arthralgias is noted. Nevirapine is excreted in breast milk.

(2) Delavirdine mesylate (Rescriptor) (U.S. FDA Category C) can cause nausea, vomiting, rash, headache, and fatigue. As with nevirapine, severe skin reactions have occurred. It is not known whether delavirdine is excreted in breast milk.

(3) Efavirenz (EFV, Sustiva) is contraindicated in pregnancy because primate studies reveal a high rate of severe birth defects with its use, including anencephaly, anophthalmia, cleft palate, and microophthalmia. Its use has not been tested in human gestation, however, so is designated U.S. FDA Pregnancy Category C. It is unknown whether efavirenz is excreted in breast milk.

d. **Protease inhibitors.** As a class, these drugs interact with the hepatic cytochrome P-450 system. Drug-drug interactions between other antiretrovirals and other medications are a common problem. Hyperglycemia and an association with the onset or worsening of diabetes mellitus has occurred in patients taking protease inhibitors. It is not known whether this effect is influenced by pregnancy, but glucose levels should be closely monitored in pregnant patients taking protease inhibitors. Allergic reactions have been a problem for indinavir sulfate, saquinavir mesylate, and ritonavir. It is not known whether any of the protease inhibitors is excreted in human breast milk.

(1) Indinavir sulfate (IDV, Crixivan) (U.S. FDA Pregnancy Category C), a frequently prescribed protease inhibitor, carries the risk of nephrolithiasis and requires the consumption of an additional liter of fluid daily. Because indinavir crosses the placenta and the fetus cannot voluntarily increase its fluid intake, it is best to avoid use of this drug in pregnancy. Other side effects of indinavir include nausea, vomiting, diarrhea, reflux, and dyspepsia. Indinavir is also considered unsafe for use during lactation.

(2) Nelfinavir (Viracept) (U.S. FDA Pregnancy Category B) has the common side effects of diarrhea, nausea, and fatigue. It is the most commonly used protease inhibitor in pregnancy.

(3) Saquinavir (Invirase) (U.S. FDA Pregnancy Category B) is associated with asthenia, diarrhea, and abdominal pain. Photosensitivity and pancreatitis have been noted.

(4) Ritonavir (Norvir) (U.S. FDA Category B) is commonly associated with vasodilation, and syncope and orthostatic hypotension have been noted.

(5) Amprenavir (Agenerase) (U.S. FDA Category C) is the newest protease inhibitor. Its use has not been studied in humans.

e. **Hydroxyurea** (U.S. FDA Category D) has been examined in only limited human studies, but significant toxicities have been noted in multiple animal species. In addition, its role in HIV therapy is not well defined. Women are advised to avoid pregnancy while taking hydroxyurea.

II. **Cytomegalovirus**
   A. **Epidemiology.** CMV infection is the most common congenital infection, affecting 0.4–2.3% of neonates. CMV is a ubiquitous DNA herpesvirus. In the United States, approximately half of the population is CMV seropositive. The virus has been isolated from saliva, cervical secretions, semen, and urine. Infection can also be contracted by exposure to infected breast milk or blood products. Transmission can occur from mother to child both in utero and postpartum. An estimated 40,000 infants are born infected with CMV infection in the United States annually. By school age, 30–60% of children are infected.

B. **Clinical manifestations**
1. **Maternal infection.** In immunocompetent adults, CMV infection is silent; symptoms appear in only 1–5% of cases. These symptoms include low-grade fever, malaise, arthralgias, and, occasionally, pharyngitis with lymphadenopathy. As in other herpesvirus infections, after primary infection, cytomegalovirus becomes latent, with periodic episodes of reactivation and shedding of virus. Mothers determined to be seronegative for CMV before conception or early in gestation have a 1–4% risk of acquiring the infection during pregnancy, with a 30–40% rate of fetal transmission. Fetal infection also can result from recurrent maternal CMV infection. In fact, most fetal infections are due to recurrent maternal infection. These infections rarely lead to congenital abnormalities. Previously acquired immunity confers a decreased likelihood of clinically apparent disease, because partial protection to the fetus is provided by maternal antibodies. Acquired immunity does not impede transmission, but evidently prevents the serious sequelae that develop with primary maternal infection.
2. **Congenital infection.** Ten percent to 15% of infected infants have clinically apparent disease, with 90% developing sequelae. Of the remaining 85–90% with asymptomatic infection, 5–15% develop long-term sequelae. A higher risk of sequelae is seen in fetuses infected earlier in gestation than in those infected later. Preterm neonates are at greatest risk of infection. Manifestations of CMV in the neonate may include focal or generalized organ involvement. Common clinical findings in fetal infection include the presence of petechiae, hepatosplenomegaly, jaundice, microcephaly with periventricular calcifications, oligohydramnios, intrauterine growth retardation, premature delivery, inguinal hernias in boys, and chorioretinitis. Nonimmune hydrops has also been reported. The severely affected infant may present with purpura, "blueberry muffin skin," and "salt and pepper skin." Approximately one-third of neonates with symptomatic infection die from severe disease, generally with cerebral involvement. Infants who survive symptomatic CMV are at high risk of significant developmental and neurologic problems. Sixty percent to 70% of these survivors suffer hearing loss; visual disturbances, motor impairments, language and learning disabilities, and mental retardation are also common.

C. **Diagnosis**
1. **Maternal infection** currently can be detected reliably only by documenting maternal seroconversion using serial Immunoglobulin G (IgG) measurements during pregnancy. If seropositivity is detected at least several months before conception, symptomatic fetal infection is unlikely. In practice, however, this testing does not occur. Most primary infections are clinically silent, so the majority are undiagnosed. Screening of asymptomatic pregnant women for seroconversion is not recommended because distinguishing primary from secondary CMV infection is frequently difficult using CMV serology. The CMV IgM test result is positive in only 75% of primary infections and in 10% of secondary infections. Screening is also of limited value due to the lack of a CMV vaccine and the inability to predict severity of sequelae of primary infection.
2. **Fetal infection.** Ultrasonography may enable the detection of the fetal anomalies that characterize CMV infection. Amniocentesis and cordocentesis also have been used to diagnosis fetal infection using measurement of total and specific IgM antibodies and viral culture.

D. **Management.** Effective in utero CMV therapy for the fetus does not exist. Given the difficulty in distinguishing primary from secondary maternal CMV infection, counseling patients about pregnancy termination is problematic because most infected fetuses do not suffer serious sequelae. Breast feeding is discouraged in women with active infection.

III. **Varicella zoster virus**
   A. **Epidemiology.** The incidence of varicella in pregnancy is approximately 0.7:1000 pregnancies. Herpes zoster is also uncommon in women of child-bearing age.
      1. The major mode of transmission is respiratory, although direct contact with vesicular or pustular lesions also may result in disease. Nearly all persons are infected before adulthood, 90% before the age of 10.
      2. Varicella outbreaks occur most frequently during the winter and spring. The incubation period is 13–17 days. Infectivity is greatest 24–48 hours before the onset of rash and lasts 3–4 days into the rash. The virus is rarely isolated from crusted lesions.
   B. **Clinical manifestations**
      1. **Maternal infection.** Primary varicella infection tends to be more severe in adults than in children. Infection is especially severe in pregnancy. The risk of varicella pneumonia appears to increase in pregnancy, starting several days after the onset of the characteristic rash. When varicella pneumonia occurs in pregnancy, maternal mortality may reach 40% in the absence of specific antiviral therapy. Early signs and symptoms of varicella pneumonia should be managed aggressively. Herpes zoster infection, or reactivation of varicella, is more common in older and immunocompromised patients. Zoster is not more prevalent or severe in pregnancy.
      2. **Congenital infection.** Of fetuses born to mothers who had active disease during the first 20 weeks of pregnancy, 20–40% are infected. The risk of congenital malformation after fetal exposure to primary maternal varicella before 20 weeks' gestation is estimated to be approximately 5%. Fetal infection with varicella zoster virus can lead to one of three major outcomes: intrauterine infection, which infrequently causes congenital abnormalities; postnatal disease, ranging from typical varicella with a benign course to fatal disseminated infection; and shingles, appearing months or years after birth. The sequelae of congenital varicella syndrome have been attributed to the occurrence of infection before 20 weeks' gestation. Those afflicted may exhibit a variety of abnormalities, including cutaneous scars, limb-reduction anomalies, malformed digits, muscle atrophy, growth restriction, cataracts, chorioretinitis, microphthalmia, cortical atrophy, microcephaly, and psychomotor retardation. The risk of this syndrome is estimated to be around 2%. Infection after 20 weeks' gestation may lead to postnatal disease. If maternal infection occurs within 5 days of delivery, hematogenous transplacental viral transfer may cause significant infant morbidity, incurring infant mortality rates between 10% and 30%. Sufficient antibody transfer to protect the fetus apparently requires at least 5 days after the onset of the maternal rash. Women who develop chickenpox, especially near term, should be observed for and educated about signs and symptoms of labor; they should receive tocolytic therapy if labor begins before day 5 of the maternal infection. Neonatal therapy is also important when a mother develops signs of chickenpox less than 3 days postpartum.
         Herpes zoster is not associated with fetal sequelae.
   C. **Diagnosis**
      1. **Clinical.** The diagnosis of acute varicella zoster in the mother usually can be established by the characteristic clinical cutaneous manifestations described as chickenpox. The generalized vesicular rash of chickenpox usually appears on the head and ears, then spreads to the face, trunk, and extremities. Mucous membrane involvement is common. Lesions in different areas will be in different stages of evolution. Vesicles and pustules evolve into crusted lesions, which then heal and may leave scars. Herpes zoster, or shingles, demonstrates a unilateral vesicular eruption, usually in a dermatomal distribution.

2. **Laboratory studies.** Confirmation of the diagnosis may be obtained by examining scrapings of lesions, which may reveal multinucleated giant cells. For rapid diagnosis, varicella zoster antigen may be demonstrated in exfoliated cells from lesions by immunofluorescent antibody staining.

3. **Ultrasonography.** Detailed ultrasonographic examination is probably the best means for assessing a fetus for major limb and growth disturbances. Other abnormalities that have been detected before 20 weeks' gestation include polyhydramnios, hydrops fetalis, multiple hyperechogenic foci within the liver, limb defects, and hydrocephaly. Although ultrasonography can be offered in pregnancies with maternal varicella, it is less likely to be helpful in cases of zoster due to the very low risk of fetal sequelae.

D. **Management**

1. **Exposure of a previously uninfected woman during pregnancy**

a. An IgG titer should be obtained within 24–48 hours of a patient's exposure to a person with noncrusted lesions. The presence of IgG within a few days of exposure reflects prior immunity. Absence of IgG indicates susceptibility.

b. Varicella zoster immune globulin. To prevent maternal infection in patients without IgG, some advocate administering varicella zoster immune globulin (VZIG) within 96–144 hours of exposure, in a dosage of 125 U/10 kg up to a maximum of 625 units, or five vials, intramuscularly (IM). Because it is difficult to obtain serologic test results in a timely manner, and because no proven benefit results from administration of VZIG for the prevention of maternal-fetal transmission or amelioration of maternal symptoms and sequelae, many experts do not currently recommend VZIG administration to pregnant women who have been exposed to varicella. If the mother becomes infected, a risk exists of fetal infection and the potential sequelae. Pregnant women with varicella, however, may be advised to continue with the pregnancy because the risk of congenital varicella is small.

2. **Maternal illness.** Generally, the disease course in pregnant patients is similar to that in nonpregnant patients and requires no specific treatment. Most patients require only supportive care with fluids and analgesics. If evidence of pneumonia or disseminated disease appears, the patient should be admitted to the hospital for treatment with intravenous acyclovir. A decrease in maternal morbidity and mortality occurs in pregnant women afflicted with varicella pneumonia who are treated with acyclovir during the last two trimesters, and the drug is safe to use at this stage of gestation. The dosage of acyclovir is 10–15 mg/kg intravenously (IV) every 8 hours for 7 days, or 800 mg by mouth (PO) five times per day.

3. **Vaccination.** An attenuated live vaccine was approved by the FDA in 1995. One dose is recommended for all children between ages 1 and 12, which results in a 97% seroconversion rate. Two doses, given 4–8 weeks apart, are recommended for adolescents and adults without a history of varicella infection. Use of the vaccine during pregnancy is not recommended.

IV. **Parvovirus B19**

A. **Epidemiology.** Thirty percent to 60% of adults have acquired immunity to human parvovirus B19. Most clinical infections, which are known as *erythema infectiosum* or *fifth disease*, occur in school-aged children. The virus is spread primarily by the respiratory route. Outbreaks usually occur in the midwinter to spring months.

B. **Clinical manifestations**

1. **Maternal infection.** Adults may present with the typical clinical features of fifth disease, particularly a red, macular rash and erythroderma affecting the face, which gives a characteristic "slapped cheek" appear-

ance. Sixty percent of infected adults have acute joint swelling, usually with symmetrical involvement of peripheral joints; the arthritis may be severe and chronic. Some adults have completely asymptomatic infection. Parvovirus B19 may cause aplastic crises in patients with hemolytic anemia (i.e., sickle cell disease). The course of the infection is unchanged in pregnancy.

2. **Fetal infection.** Approximately one-third of maternal infections are associated with fetal infection. On transplacental transfer of the virus, fetal red blood cell precursors may be infected. Infection of fetal red blood cell precursors can result in fetal anemia, which, if severe, leads to nonimmune hydrops fetalis. The likelihood of severe fetal disease is increased if maternal infection occurs during the first 18 weeks of pregnancy, but the risk of hydrops fetalis persists even when infection occurs in the late third trimester. Fetal immunoglobulin M (IgM) production after 18 weeks' gestation probably contributes to the resolution of infection in fetuses who survive. Fetal demise may occur at any stage of pregnancy. Studies suggest that the overall risk of fetal death after maternal parvovirus B19 infection is lower than 10%, and the risk is lower still in the second half of pregnancy. Although no direct evidence exists that parvovirus B19 causes congenital anomalies, there is some evidence that possible damage to the fetal myocardium results from infection.

C. **Diagnosis**

1. The illness may be suspected on epidemiologic grounds if a regional outbreak is ongoing or if a family member is known to be affected.

2. Clinical. Children, the most common transmitters of parvovirus B19 infection, present with systemic symptoms such as fever, malaise, myalgia, and headaches as well as with a confluent, indurated facial rash that imparts the characteristic "slapped-cheek" appearance of fifth disease. The rash spreads over 1–2 days to other areas, especially exposed surfaces such as the arms and legs, and is usually macular and reticular in appearance.

3. A pregnant woman who has been exposed to a child with fifth disease, who presents with an unexplained morbilliform or purpuric rash, or who has a known history of chronic hemolytic anemia and presents with an aplastic crisis should be evaluated for parvovirus B19 virus by measuring IgG and IgM titers. For patients who have had contact with an infected individual, titers should be drawn 10 days after exposure. Parvovirus B19 IgM appears 3 days after the onset of illness, peaks in 30–60 days, and may persist for 4 months. Parvovirus B19 IgG usually is detected by the seventh day of illness and persists for years.

D. **Management.** No specific antiviral therapy exists for parvovirus B19 infection.

1. Prophylaxis. Intravenous gamma globulin should be administered on an empiric basis to immunocompromised patients with known exposure to parvovirus B19 and should be used for treatment of women in aplastic crisis with viremia.

2. Detection of fetal hydrops. When maternal infection is identified, serial sonographic studies should be performed. Although hydrops fetalis usually develops within 6 weeks of maternal infection, it can appear as late as 10 weeks after maternal infection. Weekly or biweekly ultrasonographic scans can be performed.

3. Intrauterine blood transfusion has been demonstrated to be a successful therapeutic measure for correcting the fetal anemia in fetal hydrops. Single or serial intrauterine transfusions may be undertaken.

V. **Rubella virus**

A. **Epidemiology.** Despite immunization programs in the United States, up to 20% of adults remain susceptible to rubella. This number is due to failure to immunize susceptible individuals, not to a lack of effectiveness of the vaccine. The number of reported cases of congenital rubella syndrome, however, is now at an all-time low. Transmission results from direct contact with the nasopharyngeal secretions of an infected person. The most contagious period is the few days before the onset of a maculopapular rash. The disease is communicable, however, for 1 week before and for 4 days after the onset of the rash. The incubation period ranges from 14 to 21 days.

B. **Clinical manifestations**

  1. **Maternal infection.** Rubella is symptomatic in 50–70% of those who contract the virus. The illness is usually mild, with a maculopapular rash that generally persists for 3 days; generalized lymphadenopathy (especially postauricular and occipital), which may precede the rash; and transient arthritis. Rubella follows the same mild course in pregnancy. The disease is often asymptomatic. Up to 50% of women with affected infants report no history of a rash during their pregnancies.

  2. **Fetal infection** after maternal viremia leads to a state of chronic infection. At least 50% of all fetuses are infected when primary maternal rubella infection occurs in the first trimester, when the greatest risk of congenital anomalies exists. Multiple organ system involvement can occur. Permanent congenital defects include ocular defects such as cataracts, microphthalmia, and glaucoma; heart abnormalities, especially patent ductus arteriosus, pulmonary artery stenosis, and atrioventricular septal defects; sensorineural deafness; occasional microcephaly; and encephalopathy that culminates in mental retardation or profound motor impairment. As many as one-third of infants asymptomatic at birth may develop late manifestations, including diabetes mellitus, thyroid disorders, and precocious puberty. The extended rubella syndrome (progressive panencephalitis and type 1 diabetes mellitus) may develop as late as the second or third decade of life. Infants born with congenital rubella may shed the virus for many months.

  3. **Mortality.** Spontaneous abortion occurs in 4–9% and stillbirth in 2–3% of pregnancies complicated by maternal rubella. The overall mortality of infants with congenital rubella syndrome is 5–35%.

C. **Diagnosis**

  1. **Serology.** Diagnosis is usually confirmed by serology because viral isolation is technically difficult; moreover, results from tissue culture may take up to 6 weeks to obtain. Many rubella antibody detection methods exist, including hemagglutination inhibition and radioimmunoassay, and latex agglutination. Specimens should be obtained as soon as possible after exposure, 2 weeks later, and, if necessary, 4 weeks after exposure. Serum specimens from both acute and convalescent phases should be tested; a fourfold or greater increase in titer or seroconversion indicates acute infection. If the patient is seropositive on the first titer, no risk to the fetus is apparent. Primary rubella confers lifelong immunity; protection, however, may be incomplete. Antirubella IgM can be found in both primary and reinfection rubella. Reinfection rubella usually is subclinical, rarely is associated with viremia, and infrequently results in a congenitally infected infant.

  2. **Prenatal diagnosis** is made by identification of IgM in fetal blood obtained by direct puncture under ultrasonographic guidance at 22 weeks' gestation or later. The presence of rubella-specific IgM antibody in blood obtained by cordocentesis indicates congenital rubella infection, because IgM does not cross the placenta.

D. **Management**

  1. Pregnant women should undergo rubella serum evaluation as part of routine prenatal care. A clinical history of rubella is unreliable. The rubella vaccine is an attenuated live virus, and if the patient is nonimmune, she should receive rubella vaccine after delivery. Contraception should be used for a minimum of 3 months after vaccination. There is a

theoretical risk of teratogenicity if the vaccine is used during pregnancy. The CDC has maintained a registry since 1971 to monitor fetal effects of vaccination, however, and there have been no reported cases of vaccine-induced malformations.

2. If a pregnant woman is exposed to rubella, immediate serologic evaluation is mandatory. If primary rubella is diagnosed, the mother should be informed about the implications of the infection for the fetus. If acute infection is diagnosed during the first trimester, the option of therapeutic abortion should be considered. Women who decline this option may be given immune globulin because it may modify clinical rubella in the mother. Immune globulin, however, does not prevent infection or viremia and affords no protection to the fetus.

VI. **Hepatitis A virus**
   A. **Epidemiology.** The hepatitis A virus (HAV) accounts for approximately one-third of all cases of acute hepatitis in the United States. It is transmitted primarily through fecal-oral contamination. Epidemics frequently result from contaminated food or water supplies. The virus's incubation period ranges from 15 to 50 days, with a mean of 28–30 days. The duration of viremia is short. The virus typically is not excreted in urine or other bodily fluids. Feces contain the highest concentration of viral particles. Obstetric patients at highest risk of developing HAV infection are those who have emigrated from, or traveled to, countries where the virus is endemic (Southeast Asia, Africa, Central America and Mexico, and the Middle East). It affects approximately 1:1000 pregnant American women.
   B. **Clinical manifestations**
      1. **Maternal infection.** Serious complications of HAV infection are uncommon. A chronic carrier state does not exist. Symptoms include malaise, fatigue, anorexia, nausea, and abdominal pain, typically right upper quadrant or epigastric. Physical findings include jaundice, upper abdominal tenderness, and hepatomegaly. In fulminant hepatitis, signs of coagulopathy and encephalopathy may be seen.
      2. **Fetal effects.** Perinatal transmission of HAV has not been documented.
   C. **Diagnosis.** A complete travel history suggests the diagnosis in a jaundiced patient. A marked increase in liver function indicators (ALT and AST) is seen; serum bilirubin concentration may be increased. Abnormalities in coagulation and hyperammonemia may be noted. Hepatitis serologic testing should be performed. The presence of IgM antibody to the virus confirms the diagnosis. IgG antibody will persist in patients with a history of exposure (Table 11-2).
   D. **Management**
      1. Administration of HAV immune globulin is recommended for those with close personal or sexual contact with affected individuals. A single IM dose of 1 mL should be given as soon as possible after exposure; the agent is ineffective if given more than 2 weeks after exposure. HAV immune globulin is safe in pregnancy.
      2. There is no antiviral agent available for the treatment of HAV. Most affected individuals can be treated as outpatients. Activity level should be decreased and upper abdominal trauma should be avoided. Those with encephalopathy or coagulopathy and debilitated patients should be hospitalized.
      3. The HAV vaccine (inactivated viral vaccine) may be used in pregnancy. Anyone traveling to an endemic area should receive the vaccine series (two injections 4–6 months apart).

VII. **Hepatitis B virus**
   A. **Epidemiology.** In North America hepatitis B virus (HBV) transmission occurs most commonly via parenteral exposure or sexual contact. Approximately 300,000 new cases of HBV are diagnosed annually in the United

TABLE 11-2. INTERPRETATION OF HEPATITIS SEROLOGY RESULTS

Significance	Anti-HAV IgM	HBsAg	HBeAg	Anti-HBcAg IgG	Anti-HBcAg IgM	Anti-HBsAg IgG	Anti-HCV IgM/IgG
Acute HAV infection	+	–	–	–	–	–	–
Acute HBV infection	–	+	+	–	+	–	–
Chronic HBV infection, active replication	–	+	+	+	–	–	–
Chronic HBV infection, quiescent	–	+	–	+	–	–	–
HBV infection, resolved	–	–	–	–	–	+	–
Post-HBV vaccine	–	–	–	–	–	+	–
Acute or chronic HCV infection	–	–	–	–	–	–	+

HAV, hepatitis A virus; HBcAg, hepatitis B core antigen; HBeAg, hepatitis B e antigen; HBsAg, hepatitis B surface antigen; HBV, hepatitis B virus; HCV, hepatitis C virus; IgG, immunoglobulin G; IgM, immunoglobulin M; +, positive; –, negative.

States. More than 1 million Americans are chronic carriers. Acute HBV occurs in 1–2:1000 pregnancies and chronic HBV in 5–15:1000. Mother-to-infant transmission appears to be a significant mode of maintenance and transmission of infection throughout the world. Possible sources of mother-to-infant infection are infected amniotic fluid and blood. Between 85% and 90% of cases of perinatal transmission appear to occur during delivery.

B. **Natural history.** The hepatitis B virus contains three principal antigens. HBV surface antigen (HBsAg) is present on the surface and also circulates in plasma. It is detectable in serum in almost all cases of acute and chronic HBV. HBV core antigen (HBcAg) compromises the middle portion (the nucleocapsid) of the virus. This antigen is found only in hepatocytes during active viral replication. HBV e antigen (HBeAg) is another product of the core gene that produces HBcAg; its presence in serum indicates active viral replication. Circulating antibodies against the viral antigens develop in response to infection.

C. **Clinical manifestations**

1. **Maternal infection.** The prodrome of HBV virus often is associated with nonhepatic symptoms such as rash, arthralgias, myalgias, and occasional frank arthritis. Jaundice occurs in a minority of patients. Eighty-five percent to 90% of acute cases completely resolve, and the patient develops protective levels of antibody. The other 10–15% of patients become chronically infected; they have detectable levels of HBsAg but are completely asymptomatic and have normal liver function test results. Fifteen percent to 30% of chronic carriers have continued viral replication (biochemically manifested by persistent presence of HBeAg) and are at risk of the development of chronic hepatitis, cirrhosis, and hepatocellular carcinoma. Acute hepatitis carries a 1% mortality. In otherwise healthy women, no worsening of the course of the disease occurs during pregnancy.

2. **Fetal infection.** Ten percent to 20% of women seropositive for HBsAg transmit the virus to their neonates in the absence of immunoprophylaxis. In women who are seropositive for both HBsAg and HBeAg, the vertical transmission rate increases to 90%. The frequency of vertical transmission is also affected by the timing of maternal infection. When maternal infection occurs in the first trimester, 10% of neonates are seropositive; when it occurs in the third trimester, 80–90% of neonates are infected. Whether infection occurs in utero or intrapartum, the presence of HBeAg in a fetus carries an 85–90% likelihood of development of chronic hepatitis B virus infection and the associated hepatic sequelae. No increases in sequelae such as malformation, intrauterine growth retardation, spontaneous abortion, or stillbirth appear to exist.

D. **Diagnosis** is confirmed by serology (Table 11-2).

1. HBsAg appears in the blood before clinical symptoms develop, and its presence implies carrier or infective status.

2. HBeAg is detected during active viral replication.

3. The disappearance of HBeAg and the appearance of anti-HBcAg IgG signals a decrease in infectivity.

4. The presence of anti-HBsAg IgG indicates immunity or recovery.

5. If a patient is tested during the period in which results for HBsAg are negative, HBV virus can be identified by the presence of anti-HBsAg IgM.

6. The risk of fetal transmission is highest in mothers who are HBeAg positive at the time of delivery.

E. **Management**

1. If significant GI symptoms develop, including hepatitis and an inability to tolerate oral intake, patients may require hospitalization for parenteral hydration. Administration of alpha interferon has been shown to alter the natural history of acute HBV infection but has multiple side effects (myelosuppression, autoantibody formation, thyroid dis-

turbances, and possible cardiotoxicity). Its use should be avoided in pregnancy.

2. The CDC recommends universal screening of pregnant women for HBV virus. Serum transaminase levels should be measured in seropositive patients to detect evidence of active chronic hepatitis. Recombinant HBV vaccine should be offered to all pregnant women deemed to be at high risk for contracting HBV, such as those with histories of sexually transmitted diseases or intravenous drug use. The vaccine results in 95% seroconversion rates if administered into the deltoid muscle. Lower seroconversion rates are seen with intragluteal and intradermal injections.

3. Women exposed to HBV should receive passive immunization with HBV immune globulin (HBIG) and should undergo active immunization with the recombinant HBV vaccine, preferably in the contralateral arm. The HBIG regimen is 75% effective in preventing maternal HBV infection. HBIG and HBV vaccines interrupt vertical transmission of the virus in 85–90% of cases. HBIG, 5 mL, is administered to adults for prophylaxis as soon as possible after exposure. HBIG, 0.5 mL, should be administered to neonates within 12 hours of birth to infected mothers. HBIG administration should be followed by the standard three-dose immunization series, with HBV vaccinations at the time of HBIG administration.

4. During labor, invasive fetal monitoring (fetal scalp electrodes or fetal scalp blood sampling) should be avoided in the context of HBV.

VIII. **Hepatitis C virus**
   A. **Epidemiology.** Transmission of the hepatitis C virus (HCV) appears to be similar to that of HBV, with an increased incidence among intravenous drug abusers, recipients of blood transfusions, and patients with multiple sex partners. Parenteral transmission occurs via blood and body fluids. Fewer transmissions from blood product transfusions occur now than in the past, however, as a result of blood bank screening. HCV may infect as much as 0.6% of pregnant American women.
   B. **Clinical manifestations**
      1. **Maternal infection.** Approximately 50% of patients with acute HCV develop chronic disease. Of these patients, at least 20% subsequently develop chronic active hepatitis or cirrhosis. Unlike HBV antibodies, antibodies to HCV are not protective. HCV causes acute hepatitis in pregnancy but may go undetected if liver function tests and HCV antibody tests are not performed. Several months may elapse before positive results are detected on HCV antibody tests. Vertical transmission is proportional to the titer of HCV viral RNA in the maternal serum. Vertical transmission is also more likely if the mother also is infected with HIV. Approximately 8% of HCV-positive women transmit the virus to their children.
      2. **Fetal infection.** Currently, there is no way to prevent prenatal transmission. If transmission occurs transplacentally, the neonate is at increased risk of acute hepatitis and of probable chronic hepatitis or carrier status. To date, however, no teratogenic syndromes associated with this virus have been defined. During labor, fetal scalp electrode use and fetal scalp blood sampling should be avoided. When possible, women with HCV should not breast feed, because the risk of transmission through breast milk is 2–3%.
   C. **Diagnosis.** Serum analysis is performed to detect antibody to HCV. Because it takes up to 1 year after infection for infected individuals to become seropositive, however, many cases may be missed by serum analysis. HCV viral RNA can be detected by PCR assay of serum soon after infection and in chronic disease (Table 11-2).
   D. **Management.** Because no known method to prevent vertical transmission exists, prevention of maternal infection by blood product screening has been the mainstay of management. Treatment with alpha interferon produced

clinical improvement in 28–46% of patients with chronic HCV, but approximately 50% of these patients experienced relapse within 6 months of cessation of therapy. Pregnant women have not been studied. Until more data are available, it is reasonable to administer immune globulin in a 0.5 mL dose to infants at risk for HCV infection immediately after birth and 4 weeks later, to prevent neonatal HCV acquisition from a mother positive for anti-HCV antibody.

IX. **Rubeola virus**

A. **Epidemiology.** Rubeola (measles) is highly contagious. Its incubation period is 10–14 days. Since the advent of the measles vaccine, rates have fallen 99%. Rubeola is extremely rare in pregnancy because of low susceptibility in adults.

B. **Clinical manifestations**

1. The **prodrome,** which consists of fever, cough, conjunctivitis, and coryza, lasts 1–2 days; Koplik spots (pinpoint gray-white spots surrounded by erythema) appear on the second or third day; a rash emerges on the fourth day. Patients remain contagious from the onset of symptoms until 2–4 days after the appearance of the maculopapular and characteristic semiconfluent rash. Measles may be complicated by pneumonia, encephalitis, or otitis media. Pneumonia occurs in 3.5–50.0% of adults who contract measles, and superinfection may occur. Superinfection should be suspected in patients who demonstrate clinical deterioration, an elevated WBC with a leftward shift, and a chest radiograph with evidence of multilobar infiltrates. Encephalitis occurs in 1:1000 cases of measles and may result in permanent neurologic impairment and a mortality rate of 15–33%. Another rare but serious sequela is subacute sclerosing panencephalitis, which occurs in 0.5–2:1000 cases. It typically develops 7 years after measles infection and is most common in children who contract measles before the age of 2. Subacute sclerosing panencephalitis usually has a fatal outcome.

2. **Maternal infection.** Higher rates of mortality have been observed in pregnant women with measles, primarily due to pulmonary complications. A small increase in spontaneous abortion and preterm labor also has been noted.

3. **Fetal infection.** No definitive evidence of a teratogenic influence exists. Infants born to infected mothers are at risk of neonatal infection resulting from transplacental viral transmission.

C. **Diagnosis**

1. **Maternal infection.** Clinical diagnosis is considered to be reliable. When the patient's presentation is atypical, laboratory confirmation of the diagnosis by serologic studies may be required. A pregnant woman with measles should be evaluated for preterm labor, volume depletion, hypoxemia, and secondary bacterial pneumonitis.

2. **Fetal infection.** Ultrasonographic evaluation of the fetus is sufficient; microcephaly, growth restriction, and oligohydramnios should be sought.

D. **Management.** Susceptible (nonimmune) women should receive a vaccine postpartum and should be advised to use contraception for 3 months after vaccination, because the vaccine is of the live, attenuated viral variety. Susceptible pregnant women who are exposed to measles should receive immune globulin, 0.25 mg/kg IM. Measles is not a contraindication for breast feeding. No specific therapy is available for measles other than supportive measures and close observation for the development of complications. Infants delivered to mothers who develop measles within 7–10 days of delivery should receive IM immune globulin (0.25 mg/kg) as well.

X. *Mycoplasma* and *Ureaplasma*

A. **Epidemiology.** *Mycoplasma* species are common inhabitants of genital mucous membranes. Colonization rates are higher among patients from lower socioeconomic groups. Women who do not use barrier methods of contraception are more likely to be colonized. The rate of colonization increases with number of sexual partners.

B. **Clinical manifestations**

1. **Maternal infection.** *Mycoplasma hominis* and *Ureaplasma urealyticum* are commonly identified in women with bacterial vaginosis. The exact impact of these organisms on human reproduction has yet to be clarified. They have been implicated in infertility, habitual abortion, and low birth weight. An association between chorioamnionitis and mycoplasmal infection has been reported.

2. **Fetal infection.** Studies have failed to demonstrate an association between adverse pregnancy outcomes and maternal mycoplasmal infection. In neonates with meningitis, however, *Mycoplasma* species were most frequently isolated from cerebrospinal fluid.

C. **Diagnosis** is confirmed by cervical culture.

D. **Management.** *Mycoplasma hominis* infections respond to treatment with clindamycin. Infection with *Ureaplasma* species usually responds to tetracyclines and to erythromycin, which is the appropriate antibiotic to use in pregnancy. No immunizations for these infections exist.

XI. *Toxoplasma*

A. **Epidemiology.** In the United States, the incidence of acute toxoplasmosis infection in pregnancy has been estimated to be 0.2–1.0%. Congenital toxoplasmosis occurs in 1–8:1000 live births. Transmission occurs primarily via ingestion of undercooked or raw meat containing cysts, ingestion of food or water contaminated by the feces of an infected cat, or handling of material contaminated by the feces of an infected cat. Approximately one-third of American women carry antibodies to *Toxoplasma*.

B. **Clinical manifestations**

1. **Maternal infection.** Specific symptoms signaling acute toxoplasmosis infection are uncommon in pregnant women. A mononucleosis-like syndrome, including fatigue, malaise, cervical lymphadenopathy, and atypical lymphocytosis, may occur. Placental infection and subsequent fetal infection occur during the spreading phase of the parasitemia. The overall risk of fetal infection is estimated to be 30–40%, and the rate of transmission increases with gestational age.

2. **Fetal infection.** During the first trimester, the rate of transmission is approximately 15%. The rate of second trimester transmission is approximately 30% and of third trimester transmission, 60%. Fetal morbidity and mortality rates are higher after early transmission. Infected neonates often have evidence of disease, including low birth weight, hepatosplenomegaly, icterus, and anemia. Sequelae such as vision loss and psychomotor and mental retardation are common. Hearing loss is demonstrated in 10–30% and developmental delay in 20–75%. Chorioretinitis often develops.

C. **Diagnosis.** Screening for toxoplasmosis is not routine in the United States. Because most women with acute toxoplasmosis are asymptomatic, the diagnosis is not suspected until an affected infant is born. For women who do present with symptoms of acute toxoplasmosis, both IgM and IgG titers should be measured as soon as possible. Interpretation of *Toxoplasma* serology is shown in Table 11-3.

1. A negative IgM finding rules out acute or recent infection, unless the serum has been tested so early that an immune response has not yet been mounted. A positive test finding is more difficult to interpret because IgM may be elevated for more than 1 year after infection.

2. Serologic tests generally used include the Sabin-Feldman dye test, the indirect fluorescent antibody test, and ELISA.

3. PCR testing can be performed on amniotic fluid specimens and a diagnosis obtained in 1 day.

TABLE 11-3. INTERPRETATION OF *TOXOPLASMA* SEROLOGY RESULTS

IgM*	IgG	Interpretation
+	–	Possible acute infection; IgG titers should be reassessed in several weeks
+	+	Possible acute infection
–	+	Remote infection
–	–	Susceptible; uninfected

IgG, immunoglobulin G; IgM, immunoglobulin M; +, positive; –, negative.
*IgM titers may remain elevated for up to 1 year.

D. **Management.** For women who elect to continue their pregnancies after a diagnosis of toxoplasmosis, therapy must be initiated immediately and continued in the infant for a year or more to decrease the risk of development of sequelae. Medical therapy is believed to decrease the risk of development of permanent sequelae by 50%.
  1. Spiramycin is available in the United States through the FDA (301-443-4280), or through the drug's manufacturer (Rhône-Poulenc Rover, Valley Forge, PA). Its use reduces the incidence of fetal infection but not necessarily the severity of fetal infection. It is recommended for the treatment of acute maternal infections diagnosed before the third trimester and should then be continued for the duration of the pregnancy. If amniotic fluid PCR results for *Toxoplasma* are negative, spiramycin is used as a single agent; if results are positive, pyrimethamine and sulfadiazine should be added. Spiramycin dosing is 500 mg PO five times daily, or 3g/day in divided doses.
  2. Pyrimethamine and sulfadiazine. These two agents act synergistically against *Toxoplasma gondii*. The dosing is pyrimethamine, 25 mg PO daily, or sulfadiazine, 1 g PO four times daily, for 28 days. Folinic acid, 6 g IM or PO, is administered three times per week to prevent toxicity. During the first trimester, pyrimethamine is not recommended due to a risk of teratogenicity. Sulfadiazine is omitted from the regimen at term.
XII. **Herpes simplex virus (HSV)**
  A. **Epidemiology.** Type 1 herpes simplex virus (HSV) is responsible for most nongenital herpetic infections and infrequently involves the genital tract. Type 2 HSV is usually recovered from the genital tract. Approximately 1:7500 live-born infants contracts HSV perinatally. Whether pregnancy alters the rate of recurrence or frequency of cervical shedding of virus is disputed. Surveys indicate that the incidence of asymptomatic shedding in pregnancy is 10% after a first episode and 0.5% after a recurrent episode.
    1. Primary maternal infection with HSV results from direct contact, generally sexual, with mucous membranes or intact skin infected with the virus.
    2. Fetal infection with HSV can occur via three routes. In utero transplacental transmission and ascending infection from the cervix both occur. The most common route, however, is direct contact with infectious maternal genital lesions during delivery.
  B. **Clinical manifestations**
    1. **Maternal infection.** Primary infections are often severe but may be mild or even asymptomatic. Vesicles appear 2–10 days after exposure on the cervix, vagina, or vulva. Swelling, erythema, and pain are common, as is lymphadenopathy near the affected region. The lesions generally persist 1–3 weeks, with concomitant viral shedding. Reactivation occurs in 50% of patients within 6 months of the initial outbreak and subsequently at irregular intervals. Recurrent outbreaks are generally

milder, with viral shedding for less than 1 week. In pregnancy, primary outbreaks are not associated with spontaneous abortion but may increase the incidence of preterm labor in late pregnancy.

2. **Fetal infection** is usually the result of a primary maternal infection. Congenital infections resulting from a recurrent maternal infection are rare, accounting for less than 1% of fetal infections. The transplacental passage of maternal IgG antibody is believed to account for the low rate of transmission. Overall, congenital infections are very rare. Few are asymptomatic. The majority ultimately produce disseminated or CNS disease. Localized infection is usually associated with a good outcome, but infants with disseminated infection have a mortality rate of 60%, even with treatment. At least half of infants surviving disseminated infection develop serious neurologic and ophthalmic sequelae.

C. **Diagnosis.** When HSV is suspected, a swab specimen may be obtained from the lesion or vesicle and sent for tissue culture. Seven to 10 days must be allowed for isolation of the virus via tissue culture, because 6 days may be required for low numbers of infective particles to produce the characteristic cytopathic changes in vitro. Tissue culture has 95% sensitivity and very high specificity. The use of HSV-specific ELISA allows preliminary diagnosis within 24–48 hours of culturing. Serology is of limited value in diagnosis because a single antibody titer is not predictive of the presence or absence of genital shedding of the virus. To reduce the likelihood of a false-negative result, the patient should point out the location of any lesions, as well as sites of prior outbreaks. A sample from the endocervical canal and exfoliated cells from all suspicious areas should be obtained. Smears of scrapings from the bases of vesicles may be stained using Tzanck or Papanicolaou techniques, which reveal multinucleated giant cells that implicate HSV infection. CMV cervical infection, however, is difficult to differentiate from HSV infection by smears.

D. **Management.** Patients with a history of genital herpes should undergo a careful perineal examination at the time of delivery. Active genital HSV in patients in labor or with ruptured membranes is an indication for cesarian section, regardless of the duration of rupture. There is evidence that HSV recurrences in the regions of the buttocks, thighs, and anus are associated with low rates of cervical virus shedding, so that vaginal delivery is allowed. Vaginal delivery is indicated if there are no signs or symptoms of HSV. Acyclovir may be used to treat HSV infection in pregnancy; however, valacyclovir hydrochloride (Valtrex) has been shown to be more effective and is more easily tolerated due to a twice-daily dosing schedule. Third trimester suppression with valacyclovir, 500 mg PO daily, should be considered in women with frequent outbreaks during their pregnancies.

XIII. **Group B *Streptococcus***

A. **Epidemiology.** Group B *Streptococcus* (GBS), primarily *S. agalactiae*, can be isolated from the vagina, rectum, or both in 10–30% of obstetric patients. Vaginal colonization presumably results from contamination by rectal flora rather than from sexual transmission. Although maternal colonization is common, invasive disease in term neonates is rare. Maternal-fetal transmission can occur via an ascending route in utero or during passage of the fetus through the vagina. The vertical transmission rate varies from 42% to 72%. No more than 1–2% of full-term infants delivered to colonized women, however, develop the serious sequelae of sepsis, pneumonia, or meningitis. In preterm infants, invasive disease is more common and is accompanied by significant morbidity and mortality.

B. **Clinical manifestations**

1. **Maternal infection** is occasionally a cause of asymptomatic bacteriuria and acute cystitis. Several complications occur with increased frequency in GBS-infected women, including the following:

   a. Premature rupture of membranes

   b. Preterm labor

   c. Chorioamnionitis

    d. Puerperal endometritis, especially after cesarean section
    e. Postoperative wound infections after cesarean section
    f. Increased risk of bacteremia in patients with endometritis
    g. Increased risk of preterm delivery in patients with GBS bacteriuria, but decreased risk after antibiotic therapy

2. **Fetal infection.** GBS is acquired in the immediate perinatal period as a result of contamination of the infant with the microorganism from the mother's genital tract. GBS is a leading cause of pneumonia, sepsis, and meningitis during the first 2 months of life.

3. **Neonatal morbidity and mortality.** The overall neonatal case fatality rate ranges from 5% to 20%, with low-birth-weight infants at higher risk. The fatality rate has fallen from a high of 15–50% in the 1970s, likely due to improvements in neonatal care. Early-onset GBS disease, which occurs before 7 days of life, has an incidence of 1.3–3.7:1000 live births. Late-onset GBS infection, which occurs 7 days or later after birth, affects 0.5–1.8:100 live births and carries a mortality rate of approximately 10%. Approximately 25% of affected infants are preterm. Meningitis occurs in 85%, but infants may also present with bacteremia without localizing symptoms. Other clinical syndromes include pneumonia, osteomyelitis, and cellulitis. **Neurologic sequelae develop in 15–30% of meningitis survivors.**

C. **Diagnosis.** Definitive diagnosis is made by culture, and the highest yield is found when samples are obtained from both the lower vagina and the rectum. These samples must be inoculated immediately into Todd-Hewitt broth or onto selective blood agar.

D. **Management.** In cases of lower urinary tract infection, the treatment is ampicillin or penicillin, 250 mg PO four times per day for 3–7 days. For pyelonephritis, hospitalization is required, and ampicillin, 1–2 g IV every 6 hours, is administered. When the patient has been afebrile and asymptomatic for 24–48 hours, she may be discharged, and an oral regimen of ampicillin or penicillin should be followed to complete a total of 7–10 days of therapy. The CDC recommends treating all patients with risk factors for GBS in the intrapartum period. Risk factors include a history of delivering an infant with invasive GBS; GBS bacteriuria; and labor before 37 weeks. Multiple gestation is not considered a risk factor for GBS independent of prematurity. Patients without risk factors may be screened with testing of lower vaginal and rectal swab specimens at 35–37 weeks' gestation. Patients with risk factors, with positive screening results, or with preterm premature rupture of membranes, preterm labor, rupture of membranes of longer than 18 hours' duration, or overt chorioamnionitis should all be treated for GBS during active labor. In cases of preterm premature rupture of membranes without labor, cultures should be sent; the patient may be treated empirically for GBS and the treatment discontinued if the culture results are negative, or treatment may be delayed pending positive culture results. The drug of choice for intrapartum treatment of GBS infection is penicillin, 5-million-U IV loading dose, followed by 2.5 million U IV every 4 hours. For patients with an allergy to beta-lactam antibiotics, clindamycin, 600 mg IV; erythromycin, 1–2 g IV; or vancomycin hydrochloride, 500 mg IV is administered every 6 hours (Fig. 11-1).

E. **Immunization.** Recent studies have found that neonatal susceptibility to GBS disease is caused by a deficiency of maternal anticapsular antibody. Maternal immunization may prevent peripartum maternal disease and neonatal disease by transplacental transfer of protective IgG anticapsular antibodies. Vaccines designed to induce anticapsular antibodies against GBS are being developed. These vaccines can potentially be used to prevent GBS disease in nonpregnant adults as well. The potential impact of effective vaccines may be limited because of reduced transplacental transport of protective antibody before 32–34 weeks' gestation and because of possible difficulty in making the vaccine available to pregnant women.

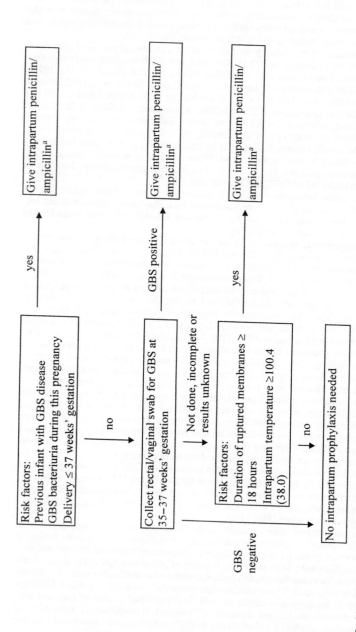

FIG. 11-1. Centers for Disease Control and Prevention algorithm for group B *Streptococcus* (GBS) testing and management. [a]Broader spectrum antibiotics may be considered at the physician's discretion, based on clinical indications.

12. CONGENITAL ANOMALIES

Dana Gossett and Edith Gurewitsch

I. **Introduction.** Congenital malformations and genetic disorders play an important role in neonatal morbidity and mortality. Two percent of all liveborn infants have a congenital malformation that has surgical or cosmetic significance. Birth defects or genetic disorders are caused by a multitude of conditions, including environmental agents, chromosomal abnormalities, single-gene abnormalities, and multifactorial causes. The etiologies of many disorders are still unknown. Some of the factors that should raise the clinician's suspicion include a positive family history of such disorders, advanced maternal age, exposure to teratogens during pregnancy, abnormal maternal serum marker levels, fetal growth restriction, and abnormal amniotic fluid volume.

II. **Methods of evaluation**

A. **Ultrasonographic examination** should be performed whenever there is a suspicion of an anomalous fetus based on the criteria described earlier. Given the relatively high incidence of congenital malformations in the general population, however, routine sonography for anatomic survey is advocated by many academicians. Sonography should evaluate fetal number, fetal presentation, fetal lie, placental location, amniotic fluid volume, and gestational age; confirm presence or absence of maternal pelvic mass and provide evaluation; and provide a gross survey of fetal anatomy. Ultrasonography to exclude many congenital anomalies should be deferred until mid-gestation (17 weeks' gestation or later). At this time, organogenesis is complete, and the structures of interest are large enough to permit accurate evaluation, but ossification is not yet complete (which allows better visualization than would be afforded later in pregnancy) and time remains for workup and exercise of all options should abnormalities be discovered. Structures to be evaluated include the following:

1. **Head.** The head can be measured using the biparietal diameter and head circumference. Intracranial anatomy should be examined at three levels to ascertain that midline structures are present (biparietal diameter level), and that the ventricular and posterior fossa anatomy is normal.

2. **Spine.** In a targeted examination for neural tube defects, the fetal spine should be examined in both longitudinal and transverse planes from the cranium to the sacrum.

3. **Heart.** A four-chamber image of the fetal heart and examination of the ventricular outflow tracts should be part of all examinations after 18–20 weeks' gestation.

4. **Abdomen.** Ventral wall defects of the abdomen can be excluded by the demonstration of an intact abdomen in the area of the umbilical cord insertion. Other normal structures that should be sought are the single cystic area representing the stomach on the left side of the abdomen and the umbilical vein, which hooks in a crescentic fashion toward the right within the liver. Kidneys can be visualized as early as 14 weeks' gestation. The fetal bladder is usually visible as a fluid-filled structure in the midline, low in the pelvis; in fact, the bladder may visibly fill and empty during the course of an examination.

5. **Skeleton.** When the extremities are examined, the four fetal limbs should be identified and measured routinely during any second or third trimester evaluation. Both bones of the distal extremities should be present. If possible, digits should be counted, feet should be assessed for normal positioning, and hands should be observed to open and close.

B. **Maternal alpha-fetoprotein (AFP) determination and triple screen** have been used to screen for neural tube defects, abdominal wall defects, and chromosomal abnormalities. A high AFP level is suggestive of neural tube defect or abdominal wall defect; triple screen results with a low level of AFP, low level of estriol, and high level of human chorionic gonadotropin are suggestive of trisomy 21. When all three values are low, the fetus is at risk for trisomy 18.

C. **Amniocentesis** for karyotyping and amniotic fluid analysis can be a critical part of antenatal diagnosis of congenital anomalies (see Chap. 8).

III. **Anomalies of the head and neck and CNS.** The most common abnormalities of these organ systems are neural tube defects and hydrocephalus.

A. **Neural tube defects** result from failure of the rostral neuropore (anencephaly) or caudal neuropore (spina bifida) to close during the third to fourth week of gestation.

1. The **etiology** of these disorders is multifactorial. In anencephaly, the cranial vault is absent, as well as the telencephalic and encephalic structures. Associated malformations are common, and polyhydramnios frequently is found. Spina bifida is characterized as occult (characterized by vertebral schisis covered by normal soft tissue) or open (characterized by a defect in the skin, underlying soft tissues, and vertebral arches that exposes the neural canal). Open spina bifida almost always is associated with a specific intracranial malformation (Arnold-Chiari, type II). Frontal cranial narrowing (the lemon sign) and abnormal convex configuration of the cerebellum (the banana sign), in addition to splaying of the vertebral arches, are consistently found in fetuses with spina bifida. Hydrocephalus occurs in 60–85% of low lumbar and sacral defects and in 96% of high lumbar and thoracic lesions. Predictors of poor outcome include high lumbar or thoracic defects, severe hydrocephalus (less than 1 cm of frontal cerebral mantle), other brain malformations, and other structural anomalies. The term **cephalocele** denotes a protrusion of intracranial contents through a bony defect of the skull. Cephalocele may occur either as an isolated defect or as a part of genetic syndromes (Meckel's syndrome) or nongenetic syndromes (amniotic band syndrome).

2. **Diagnosis.** The combined use of AFP determination and ultrasonography as a screening tool for the prenatal diagnosis of neural tube defects is a routine part of antenatal care. Targeted ultrasonographic examinations of patients at risk because of either family history or elevated AFP levels are recommended.

3. **Management.** Anencephaly is invariably fatal. Spina bifida is frequently complicated by birth injury due to traction on the exposed neural tissue, and although disagreement exists, cesarean delivery is commonly recommended. The outcome for infants with spina bifida is dictated by the site and extension of the lesion. The mortality rate has been reported to be as high as 40%, and many of the survivors suffer disability, mainly from lower limb paralysis, sexual dysfunction, or incontinence, or a combination of these. Recurrence of neural tube defects in offspring of women with prior affected infants can be decreased by preconception folic acid supplementation (4 mg daily), in accordance with the guidelines of the Centers for Disease Control and Prevention.

B. **Hydrocephalus** is characterized by dilation of the fetal cerebral ventricles (ventriculomegaly) and ultimately enlargement of the fetal head (macrocrania). It can be due to an obstructing lesion or it can be "communicating," usually due to nonresorption of cerebrospinal fluid. Possible causes include isolated aqueductal stenosis, intracranial hemorrhage, and other cerebral structural anomalies. Incidence ranges from 0.3 to 1.5 per 1000 births in different series. Both congenital infection and genetic factors are involved in the pathogenesis of aqueductal stenosis. Infectious antecedents include toxoplasmosis, syphilis, cytomegalovirus infection, mumps, and influenza.

Analysis of familial cases indicates an X-linked pattern of transmission that is thought to account for 25% of lesions occurring in male fetuses. A multifactorial etiology with a recurrence risk of 1–2% has also been suggested. The Dandy-Walker malformation consists of hydrocephalus, retrocerebellar cyst, and abnormal cerebellar vermis, and its cause is still unclear. Dandy-Walker malformation frequently is associated with other nervous system abnormalities and systemic anomalies such as congenital heart disease.

1. **Diagnosis** of hydrocephalus by sonography is based on measurement of an enlarged ventricular system. After hydrocephalus has been recognized, the site of obstruction may be determined by identifying the enlarged and normal portions of the ventricular system. The incidence of severe associated anomalies, both structural and chromosomal, is approximately 30%. Detailed sonographic examination of the entire fetal anatomy, fetal echocardiography, and karyotyping are strongly recommended.

2. **Management.** Fetuses with progressive hydrocephalus should be delivered as soon as fetal maturity is achieved, at a center able to provide prompt neurologic treatment, to maximize the chances of survival and normal development. A cesarean section is recommended in cases of hydrocephalus with associated macrocrania. Infants with aqueductal stenosis have been found to have normal intelligence after surgical correction in over 50% of those studied. Isolated communicating hydrocephalus carries a good long-term prognosis. Infants with Dandy-Walker deformity have a mortality risk of up to 44% and an intelligence quotient below 85 in up to 90% of cases.

C. **Large neck masses.** A variety of neck masses, such as fetal goiters, lymphoceles, and teratomas, can grow to proportions that interfere both with normal vaginal delivery and with resuscitative efforts for the newborn. When such a mass is identified on ultrasonography, an MRI should be performed to better evaluate the extent and the nature of the mass. If it is thought that the mass is large enough both to prevent successful vaginal delivery and to compromise the newborn's airway, an Ex-Utero Intrapartum Technique (EXIT) procedure may be performed. In this complex surgery, which involves both obstetric and pediatric surgeons, a hemostatic incision is made in the uterus using automatic staplers, with continuous uterine relaxation maintained; then only the head and neck of the fetus are delivered without compromising the fetal circulation, and the fetus is intubated or a tracheostomy performed before the delivery of the body and the clamping of the umbilical cord.

IV. **Fetal thoracic malformations.** The most common thoracic malformations are congenital diaphragmatic hernia (CDH) and cystic congenital adenomatoid malformation (CCAM).

A. **Congenital diaphragmatic hernia** is a diaphragmatic defect characterized by herniation of abdominal contents into the thoracic cavity. Despite optimal postnatal medical management and surgical repair, many infants with CDH die of pulmonary hypoplasia, secondary to compression of the developing fetal lungs in utero by the herniated abdominal viscera. Mortality rates for neonates with prenatally diagnosed CDH have been reported to range from 70% to 90%, especially if polyhydramnios is present. In contrast, the mortality rate for neonates diagnosed at or after birth is reported to be 50%.

1. **Diagnosis.** Prenatal sonographic evaluation reveals the presence of an echolucent mass or masses in the fetal chest, which represent the fetal stomach or small bowel. Poor prognostic indicators include diagnosis before 25 weeks' gestation, polyhydramnios, other structural anomalies, and the presence of stomach or liver in the chest.

2. **Management.** All fetuses with CDH diagnosed before 28 weeks' gestation should undergo detailed ultrasonography, karyotype determination, and fetal echocardiography to exclude other anomalies. If an isolated CDH with poor prognostic indicators is present, the fetus is placed in an early or severe category with poor prognosis. In these

cases, fetal surgical repair at a specialty center may be offered. When the fetal prognosis is equivocal according to the prognostic criteria, appropriate parental counseling should be provided to help parents choose between fetal surgery and expectant management. Fetuses in the less severe category are managed conservatively and undergo postnatal surgical correction.

B. **Congenital cystic adenomatoid malformation** represents a disease spectrum characterized by cystic lesions of the lung. Most cases of CCAM are diagnosed in infancy or early childhood; patients present with pulmonary masses causing either respiratory difficulty or recurrent pulmonary infections. The most severe lesions, however, can result in fetal hydrops, pulmonary hypoplasia, and fetal death.

   1. **Types of lesions.** CCAMs can be divided into macrocystic or microcystic types, based on the presence or absence of cysts larger than 5 mm in diameter. Macrocystic lesions usually are not associated with hydrops and have a more favorable prognosis. Microcystic, or solid, lesions more frequently induce fetal hydrops, which is caused by vena caval obstruction or cardiac compression from extreme mediastinal shift. Once this occurs, rapid fetal demise may ensue.

   2. **Management.** The majority of affected fetuses have isolated small lesions, without hydrops, that are best treated by surgical resection after term delivery. Fetuses diagnosed in early gestation with large CCAMs should undergo serial sonographic examinations to evaluate fetal growth and monitor for hydrops. If pulmonary maturity is documented and hydrops develops, the fetus should be delivered, and the lesion may immediately be resected ex utero. Between 28 and 34 weeks, the detection of hydrops should prompt an attempt at steroid-induced lung maturation and delivery for immediate surgical resection. Earlier than 28 weeks, the fetus with a large CCAM and hydrops should be considered as a candidate for in utero resection of the tumor (see sec. **IX**).

V. **Cardiovascular anomalies.** Congenital heart defects are the malformations most frequently observed at birth. Incidence has been estimated at 0.5–1.0%. Congenital heart defects probably result from a wide variety of causes. Chromosomal anomalies are found in 4–5% of cases; extracardiac structural abnormalities are present in 25–45% of these fetuses. In pregnancies affected by the following risk factors, fetal echocardiography should be performed: nonimmune hydrops, suspected cardiac abnormalities on screening sonogram, other structural anomalies, teratogen exposure, parental or sibling heart defects, aneuploidy, maternal diabetes mellitus, maternal phenylketonuria, and fetal arrhythmias.

A. **Diagnosis.** Cardiac malformations may be detected at screening sonogram by examining the four-chamber view of the heart and the ventricular outflow tracts. Any suspected abnormality should be further evaluated by echocardiography. Fetal echocardiography is performed by perinatologists and pediatric cardiologists with specialized training in this area. In all cases of prenatally diagnosed congenital heart disease, further evaluation should include karyotyping.

B. **Management.** Some cardiovascular anomalies are incompatible with life (those associated with severe nonimmune fetal hydrops), and parents should be given the option of terminating the pregnancy. For many cardiac diagnoses, however, accurate prenatal diagnosis allows for parental counseling and medical planning both for delivery and for neonatal medical and surgical management. Survival statistics for fetuses with severe congenital heart disease remain discouraging because prenatal diagnosis is more commonly made with severe forms of disease.

C. **Common cardiac defects**

   1. **Tetralogy of Fallot** is the association of a ventricular septal defect, infundibular pulmonic stenosis, aortic valve overriding the ventricular

septum, and hypertrophy of the right ventricle. Enlargement of the ascending aorta is usually present. Views of the right ventricular out-flow tract and pulmonary artery provide information about the degree of infundibular stenosis. Doppler ultrasonography is useful to establish the presence of blood flow in the pulmonary artery. Tetralogy of Fallot is compatible with intrauterine life but may result in severe cyanosis and hypoxia after birth. The treatment includes administration of prosta-glandins to maintain the ductus arteriosus, and surgical repair. The timing of this repair depends on the severity of the infundibular steno-sis and hence the amount of blood oxygenated by the lungs.

2. **Transposition of the great arteries (TGA)** has two anatomic forms: complete TGA (in which the aorta arises from the right ventricle and the pulmonary artery from the left ventricle) and corrected TGA (the association of atrioventricular and ventriculoarterial discordance). Fetal echocardiography can identify abnormalities of the ventriculoarte-rial connection, but meticulous scanning is required to identify the aorta and pulmonary artery and their relationships with each ventricle. Fetuses with uncomplicated complete transposition should not be sub-jected to hemodynamic compromise in utero; survival after birth depends on the persistence of fetal circulation. In cases of corrected transposition, ideally no hemodynamic imbalance should be present.

3. **Hypoplastic left heart syndrome (HLHS)** is characterized by a very small left ventricle, with mitral or aortic atresia or both. HLHS fre-quently is associated with intrauterine heart failure. Sonographic diag-nosis of HLHS in utero is suspected when a very small left ventricle, hypoplastic ascending aorta, and enlarged right ventricle, right atrium, and pulmonary artery are found. The prognosis is extremely poor; how-ever, palliative procedures and, recently, cardiac transplantation have been attempted, and long-term survivors have been reported.

4. **Fetal arrhythmia** denotes irregular patterns of fetal heart rhythm. Brief periods of tachycardia, bradycardia, and ectopic beats are a fre-quent finding and are not cause for concern. Therefore, clear differenti-ation between physiologic variations and pathologic alteration can be difficult but must be attempted. Sustained bradycardia (less than 100 beats per minute), sustained tachycardia (more than 200 beats per minute), and irregular rhythms occurring more than once in 10 beats should be considered abnormal. M-mode echocardiography of cardiac motion, pulsed Doppler ultrasonography, and color-encoded M-mode echocardiography can be used to assess irregular fetal heart rhythms.

   a. **Premature atrial and ventricular contractions** are the most frequent fetal arrhythmias. These are benign rhythms and usually disappear in utero or soon after birth. Serial monitoring of the fetal heartbeat during pregnancy is suggested because a theoretical possi-bility exists that a premature beat could trigger a reentrant tachy-arrhythmia.

   b. **Supraventricular tachyarrhythmias** include supraventricular paroxysmal tachycardia, atrial flutter, and atrial fibrillation. Diagno-sis of fetal tachyarrhythmia can be accomplished easily by direct auscultation or continuous Doppler ultrasonographic examination. M-mode or pulsed Doppler ultrasonography or both can identify the exact heart rate and the atrioventricular sequence of contraction. The association of fetal tachyarrhythmia with nonimmune hydrops is well established. The fast ventricular rate results in suboptimal filling of the ventricle, decreased cardiac output, right atrial over-load, and congestive heart failure (CHF). Intrauterine pharmaco-logic cardioversion of fetal tachyarrhythmia by intravenous or oral administration of drugs to the mother (digoxin, verapamil hydro-chloride, propranolol hydrochloride, quinidine, procainamide hydrochloride, amiodarone hydrochloride, flecainide acetate) has been attempted with success. Direct administration of medications to the fetus via umbilical venous puncture is also possible if no response to maternal treatment occurs. The optimal approach to treating these conditions is still uncertain.

c. **Atrioventricular (AV) block** can result from immaturity of the fetal conduction system, absence of connection to the AV node, or abnormal anatomical position of the AV node. AV block is classified into three types: first, second, and third degree. First- and second-degree AV blocks are not usually associated with significant hemodynamic perturbations. Third-degree AV block may lead to significant bradycardia, decreased cardiac output, and CHF in utero. In more than half of cases, third-degree AV block is accompanied by a structural anomaly. In cases without structural cardiac disease, testing should be performed for maternal antibodies against SSA and SSB antigens (anti-RO and anti-LA). Transplacental passage of these antibodies can lead to inflammation and damage of the cardiac conduction system. Anti-SSA antibodies have been reported in more than 80% of mothers who delivered infants with AV block, although only 30% of these women showed clinical evidence of connective tissue disease. In these women, treatment with dexamethasone may reduce the fetus's risk of heart block. Intrauterine ventricular pacing has also been attempted.

VI. **Gastrointestinal anomalies** are relatively common. Fetuses with isolated GI anomalies, which often allow a good quality of life after postnatal surgical correction, benefit greatly from prenatal diagnosis. Anomalies can be divided into two major groups: intestinal obstructions and ventral wall defects.

A. **Intestinal obstructions**

1. **Esophageal atresia** occurs in 1 in 3000–3500 live births. In the most common type (90–95%), the upper portion of the esophagus ends blindly, and the lower portion develops from the trachea near the bifurcation. Other severe structural anomalies are associated with esophageal atresia in nearly 50% of cases and include cardiac and genitourinary anomalies, skeletal deformity, cleft defects of the face, and CNS disorders (meningocele or hydrocephalus). Because the prognosis of affected newborns is worse if other severe congenital anomalies are present, sonographic evaluation of the entire fetal anatomy should be performed. Chromosomal anomalies, particularly trisomy 21, are also common in cases of esophageal atresia, so fetal karyotype should also be determined. Prenatal diagnosis is based on indirect findings: polyhydramnios, failure to visualize the stomach, and, rarely, presence of an enlarged upper mediastinal and retrocardiac anechoic structure (dilated proximal esophageal pouch). In the majority of cases, however, a fistula between the respiratory and the GI tracts distal to the obstruction allows ingestion of amniotic fluid, so both the polyhydramnios and the mediastinal anechoic structure may be absent.

2. **Duodenal atresia** occurs in 1 in 7500–10,000 live births. Nearly 30% of affected fetuses have trisomy 21; other common associated anomalies include structural cardiac anomalies (20%), malrotation of the colon (22%), and, less frequently, tracheoesophageal fistula or renal malformation. Detection of two echo-free areas inside the abdomen, which represent the dilated stomach and the first portion of the duodenum (double bubble sign), is the critical sonographic finding for diagnosis. Polyhydramnios is almost always an associated finding. Complete survey of fetal anatomy and determination of fetal karyotyping are indicated in these pregnancies. If the anomaly is isolated, a good quality of life may be anticipated after postnatal surgical correction. Premature labor resulting from polyhydramnios is a frequent complication. Prena-

TABLE 12-1. OMPHALOCELE AND GASTROSCHISIS

	Omphalocele	Gastroschisis
Physical findings	Defect covered by amnioperito- neal membrane; size variable; may contain few bowel loops or all abdominal contents.	Defect has no covering membrane; all bowel usually herniates, and other organs may as well.
Relationship to umbilical cord	Hernia sac enters umbilical cord.	Defect occurs to the right of the umbilical insertion.
Other structural anomalies	May occur in up to 45%.	No significant association.
Chromosomal anomalies	May occur in up to 5%.	No significant association.
Mortality	Approximately 34%.	Approximately 13%.
Antenatal complications	Liver evisceration and ectopia cordis can result in fetal demise.	Damage to and stricture of small and large bowel occurs due to exposure to amniotic fluid.
Long-term prognosis	Depends on size (very poor with giant omphalocele), presence of other anomalies, and chro- mosomal anomalies.	Excellent after surgical repair.

tal diagnosis can prevent neonatal vomiting and aspiration pneumonia caused by aspiration of gastric contents.

3. **Small or large bowel obstructions** occur in 1 in 300–1500 live births. Obstruction can be intrinsic or extrinsic. In cases of GI obstruction below the duodenum, multiple echo-free areas within the fetal abdomen are usually seen on ultrasonographic examination (dilated loops of small or large bowel or both). In these cases, associated structural and chromosomal anomalies are rare. Proximal bowel obstructions often are associated with a certain degree of polyhydramnios, whereas obstruction of the colon typically is associated with normal amniotic fluid volume. Bowel perforation is a possible consequence of impaired blood supply to the distended bowel; perforation should be suspected when ultrasonographic examination reveals ascites that was absent on previous examination. Because meconium begins to accumulate in the fetal bowel at 4 months' gestation, any perforation occurring after that time could cause meconium peritonitis. Fetuses with uncomplicated intestinal obstruction can be delivered vaginally at term. When perforation occurs and ascites is seen, early induction should be considered. In these cases, fetal paracentesis should be performed to decrease abdominal pressure on the diaphragm and thus allow expansion of the lungs at birth.

B. **Abdominal wall defects**

1. **Omphalocele** is a sporadic anomaly with an occurrence rate of 1 in 6000 live births (Table 12-1). A protrusion of intra-abdominal contents is covered by a translucent, avascular membrane, consisting of peritoneum inside and amniotic membrane outside. The skin defect may vary greatly in size, from a small opening through which only one or two loops of small intestine protrude to a large defect containing all abdominal contents. A dense, echogenic mass outside the abdomen and covered by amnioperitoneal membrane can be seen on ultrasonographic exami-

nation. In small defects, umbilical cord insertion is on the top of the mass, whereas in large lesions, the cord is attached to the lower border of the mass. Polyhydramnios may be present, and amniotic fluid levels of AFP are significantly elevated. Omphalocele is frequently associated with additional structural or chromosomal anomalies; the mortality rate for fetuses with omphalocele is therefore high. Thorough sonographic evaluation of the fetus anatomy should be performed and karyotype determined. The volume of the protruded viscera is a critical factor in fetal prognosis; giant defects frequently are associated with liver evisceration and ectopia cordis and have a worse prognosis. When giant omphalocele or multiple other malformations are diagnosed prenatally, termination of the pregnancy may be considered. In cases of ruptured omphalocele, preterm delivery to avoid the pathologic alterations of the bowel exposed to amniotic fluid should be considered. Delivery should be performed in a medical center with neonatal intensive care and pediatric surgery facilities.

2. **Gastroschisis** is caused by the herniation of some of the intra-abdominal contents through a paraumbilical defect of the abdominal wall (Table 12-1). The umbilical cord is inserted normally, and no covering sac is visible. The defect is on the right side of the abdomen. In most cases, all segments of the small and large intestine protrude. Stomach, gallbladder, urinary bladder, and adnexa may also prolapse. Chemical peritonitis is a serious complication that results from exposure of eviscerated abdominal contents to amniotic fluid. The intestine can show marked dilatation of the lumen and increased thickness of the wall, with single or multiple atretic sites. The extruded structures are not covered by amnioperitoneal membrane. Polyhydramnios and increased amniotic fluid AFP levels are common findings. Unlike omphalocele, gastroschisis often is associated with intrauterine growth retardation and oligohydramnios. As with omphalocele, a fetus affected by gastroschisis commonly is delivered in a medical center at which the neonate can receive intensive care and undergo prompt neonatal surgical correction. Long-term follow-up of survivors demonstrates excellent outcomes.

VII. **Urinary tract anomalies.** Congenital malformations of the genitourinary tract are classified as either primary renal dysgenesis (of variable types and severity) or obstructive disorders.

A. **Renal dysgenesis.** The most severe variant of renal dysgenesis is bilateral and is characterized by absence of recognizable renal tissue (bilateral renal agenesis), absent bladder, severe oligohydramnios or anhydramnios (invariably present after 16 weeks), and lethal pulmonary hypoplasia. Bilateral renal agenesis is incompatible with life; affected fetuses die in utero or soon after birth. Less severe variants of renal dysgenesis may manifest as unilateral (typically) or bilateral (less common) multicystic dysplasia, characterized by an increase in renal size; distortion of renal architecture; multiple, echolucent renal cysts of various sizes; and areas of increased echogenicity. Bilateral disease may be associated with oligohydramnios and is always fatal. Unilateral disease is associated with normal or increased amniotic fluid volume and evidence of contralateral renal function (bladder filling), and has a more favorable prognosis.

B. **Congenital urinary tract obstruction.** Genitourinary lesions are the most common cause of fetal abdominal masses, and obstruction may occur at several sites. The most common site of obstruction is the ureteropelvic junction; obstructions at this site produce renal pelvis dilatation in mild cases and renal calyceal dilatation (hydronephrosis) in more severe cases. In these instances, the disease typically progresses slowly, and early delivery is rarely indicated. Outlet obstruction may be due to posterior urethral valve syndrome, urethral atresia, or persistent cloacal syndrome. Outlet obstruction produces megalocystis, bilateral hydroureter, and bilateral hydronephrosis. Oligohydramnios is common. For the fetus for whom good renal function is predicted, management options depend on fetal lung maturity. Persistent outlet obstruction, particularly when caused by posterior urethral valve syndrome, can be treated with in utero diversion therapy. If the fetus's gestational age is 28 weeks or older but inadequate lung maturity is indicated, temporary decompression can be achieved with percutaneous placement of a fetal vesicoamniotic shunt catheter. Once lung maturity is established, however, the fetus with persistent outlet obstruction should be delivered.

VIII. **Fetal skeletal anomalies,** or skeletal dysplasias, are a complex group of anomalies with a variety of morphometric characteristics and prognoses. The diagnosis of skeletal dysplasia is based on objective data pertaining to limb length and growth and on subjective assessment of skeletal shape, density, and proportion. Nomograms for individual bone length and growth have been published.

A. **Thanatophoric dysplasia,** a fatal condition, manifests as extreme shortening of limbs, thoracic cage deformity, and relative cephalomegaly. It is frequently associated with cardiac anomalies and respiratory distress, and is usually lethal in the neonatal period.

B. **Camptomelic dysplasia** is characterized by limb reduction and extreme bowing of the long bones. Other features include cleft palate and generalized hypotonia. Perinatal death is the usual outcome.

C. **Diastrophic dysplasia,** an autosomal recessive condition, is characterized by scoliosis, severe limb shortening, and, frequently, radial displacement of the thumbs. After birth, these infants may have respiratory distress, as well as difficulty feeding and walking due to progressive joint contractures. Some may also have associated cardiac defects.

D. **Osteogenesis imperfecta** is a disease spectrum; characteristics range from mild bowing to extreme demineralization, fracture, and short limbs. Spontaneous intrauterine fracture, indicated by displacement of bone elements and seen most often in the ribs, is diagnostic of a severe form of disease. Types I and II are lethal; type III is compatible with life, but these patients are usually wheelchair or bed bound due to multiple fractures.

E. **Achondroplasia** is an autosomal dominant disorder. In the homozygous form, it manifests as short limbs with marked flaring and enlargement of the metaphyses, small thorax, and protruding abdomen. Malrotation and malflexion of the feet and various cranial abnormalities are also seen. Homozygous achondroplasia may be lethal in the neonatal period. Heterozygotic individuals have somewhat less severe deformities and a better prognosis overall; they frequently live to adulthood.

IX. **Fetal surgery** has been proposed for the treatment of a variety of structural anomalies. For fetal surgery to provide benefits, the anomaly must be one that can be reliably diagnosed via sonography, carries significant morbidity or mortality in the fetal or neonatal period, and for which in utero surgical correction would provide significant reduction in morbidity, mortality, or deformity compared with postnatal surgery. Trials of fetal surgery have been plagued with high rates of preterm delivery and neonatal mortality. Several centers, however, have had increasing success at treating a variety of conditions. These procedures include repairs of neural tube defects and diaphragmatic hernias, and excision of CCAMs and teratomas. In cases in which the neonatal outcome is bleak without intervention, or in which there is evidence of progressive tissue damage, referral to an academic center performing fetal surgery should be considered.

13. ENDOCRINE DISORDERS OF PREGNANCY

Janice Falls and Lorraine Milio

DIABETES MELLITUS

I. **General**

   A. In the United States, the most common medical complication of pregnancy is diabetes mellitus (DM).

      1. Three percent to 5% of pregnancies are associated with gestational diabetes mellitus (GDM), whereas 0.5% are complicated by pregestational diabetes mellitus (PDM).

      2. In 85–90% of all pregnancies complicated by diabetes, the DM is gestational.

   B. If carbohydrate intolerance occurs before or persists after pregnancy, the condition is classified as either type 1 or type 2 diabetes mellitus, or impaired glucose tolerance (Table 13-1).

   C. GDM is a state of carbohydrate intolerance that is first diagnosed during pregnancy.

   D. Of the women who develop GDM, more than 40% will later develop overt diabetes in the subsequent 15 years after the index pregnancy, and 50% will have recurrent GDM in any future pregnancy.

II. **The Priscilla White classification system** provides an estimate of the level of microvascular damage present in a patient to assist in effective management during the pregnancy. The White classification system is shown in Table 13-2.

III. **Pregnancy physiology.** Maternal metabolism changes during pregnancy to provide adequate nutrition for both the mother and the fetus. Glucose is transported to the fetus by means of facilitated diffusion. Active transport is needed for amino acids to gain access to the fetus. In the fasting state, maternal glucose levels are lower in pregnancy than in the nonpregnant state (55–65 mg/dL), whereas the concentrations of free fatty acids, triglycerides, and plasma ketones increase. A state of relative maternal starvation exists in pregnancy during which glucose is spared for fetal consumption while alternative fuels are used by the mother. During the second half of the pregnancy, insulin levels increase in part as a result of diabetogenic hormones, predominantly human placental lactogen. Estrogen, progesterone, cortisol, and prolactin are involved as well. Degradation of insulin is also increased during pregnancy.

IV. **Maternal and fetal morbidity and mortality.** Poor control of maternal glucose levels results in significant risk of increased perinatal morbidity and mortality.

   A. **Fetal abnormalities,** including those of the cardiac, renal, and central nervous systems, can occur during the first trimester of pregnancy. Embryogenesis occurs during the third and eighth gestational weeks. Especially during this period of organogenesis, the fetus is extremely sensitive to the maternal environment (i.e., to glycemic control). It is also during this early part of fetal development that the woman often is not aware of her pregnancy. Thus, it is important for diabetic women of reproductive age to receive preconceptual counseling that reinforces the need for pregnancy planning to achieve good glucose control before conception and to maintain it throughout pregnancy. Poorly controlled diabetes carries a fourfold increased risk of congenital anomalies. Potential congenital fetal anomalies associated with DM include the following:

      1. CNS: spina bifida, anencephaly, holoprosencephaly, hydrocephalus

      2. Cardiac (most common): transposition of the great vessels, ventricular septal defect, atrial septal defect, hypoplastic left heart, cardiac hypertrophy, anomalies of the aorta

      3. GI: tracheoesophageal fistula, anal/rectal atresia

TABLE 13-1. COMPARISON OF TYPE 1 AND TYPE 2 DIABETES MELLITUS (DM)

Type 1	Type 2
Formerly known as juvenile-onset DM.	Formerly known as adult-onset DM.
Pathophysiology is insulinopenia.	Includes maturity-onset DM of the young.
Patients are prone to severe hypoglycemia and diabetic ketoacidosis (DKA)	Pathophysiology is tissue resistance to insulin.
	Patients not at risk for DKA but in rare cases may develop hyperosmolar coma.

    4. Genitourinary: renal agenesis, double ureter, cystic kidneys
    5. Skeletal: caudal regression syndrome (most specific)
    6. Situs inversus
    Glycosylated hemoglobin (HbA1C) measurement is often used to assess risk of fetal anomalies, as its level provides an estimate of the three previous months of maternal serum glucose levels.
  B. **Fetal/neonatal sequelae** include spontaneous abortion and fetal death, which are uncommon but significant outcomes in diabetic pregnancies (not increased in class A1 GDM). Other fetal/neonatal sequelae include fetal macrosomia, fetal shoulder dystocia, fetal septal hypertrophy, respiratory distress syndrome (RDS), hyperbilirubinemia, and polyhydramnios. The presence of maternal microvascular disease increases the risk of intrauterine fetal growth restriction.
  C. **Maternal complications** of PDM (type 1/2) include diabetic ketoacidosis (DKA), coronary artery disease, hypertension, infection (increased rate and severity), nephropathy, polycythemia, and retinopathy.
    Other maternal effects of poorly controlled DM during pregnancy include increased risks of preeclampsia, cesarean section, birth trauma, and postpartum infection.
V. **Diagnosis**
  A. **Gestational diabetes.** Diagnosis of diabetes during the first half of pregnancy indicates undiagnosed PDM; GDM is usually a disorder of late gestation.
    1. The universal **screening** currently recommended by the American College of Obstetricians and Gynecologists is as follows.

TABLE 13-2. WHITE CLASSIFICATION SYSTEM FOR DIABETES MELLITUS

Gestational diabetes mellitus (GDM)

Class A	Gestational diabetes
Class A1	Diet-controlled GDM
Class A2	GDM requiring insulin

Pregestational diabetes mellitus

Class B	Diabetes onset at older than 20 yrs of age, or of less than 10 yrs' duration
Class C	Diabetes onset between ages 10 and 19, or of 10–19 yrs' duration
Class D	Diabetes onset at younger than 10 yrs of age, or of 20 yrs' duration or longer
Class F	Diabetes with nephropathy
Class R	Diabetes with proliferative retinopathy
Class H	Diabetes with heart disease
Class T	Diabetes requiring renal transplant

a. During gestational weeks 24–28, a 50-g oral glucose load is administered, followed by measurement of serum glucose level at 1 hour.

b. Accuracy of the screening test is increased if the patient is in a fasting state. However, no dietary preparation is specified for the screen.

2. **Screening thresholds** are as follows:

a. Threshold of greater than or equal to 140 mg/dL diagnoses 90% of GDM; 17% of screened population requires further diagnostic testing.

b. Threshold of greater than or equal to 135 mg/dL diagnoses more than 95% of GDM; 25% of screened population requires further diagnostic testing.

c. If the level is above 190 mg/dL, there are two approaches: consider the patient to have GDM or perform fasting blood glucose testing.
   * If the level is 126 mg/dL or higher, the patient has GDM.
   * If the level is below 126 mg/dL, proceed with the 3-hour glucose tolerance test (GTT).

3. **Interpretation of results.** If the patient's glucose level is equal to or greater than the threshold value chosen, then the 3-hour GTT should be administered.

a. The GTT is performed by administering 100 g of glucose orally in at least 400 mL of water after an overnight fast (for a patient who has been consuming an adequate carbohydrate diet).

b. To date, there is no consensus on which scale (modified O'Sullivan or Carpenter and Coustan) to use in identifying GDM. In 1998, the American Diabetes Association recommended the use of Carpenter and Coustan values. Both sets of recommended glucose values are shown in Table 13-3.

c. If any two or more of the diagnostic values are met or exceeded, then the diagnosis of GDM is made. In patients with significant risk factors and a normal GTT, a follow-up GTT may be performed at 32–34 weeks to diagnose late-onset GDM.

B. **Pregestational diabetes**

1. The **diagnosis** of PDM (types 1 and 2) is made before conception. This evaluation is made according to standard criteria for diagnosing diabetes in adults. A fasting glucose level of 126 mg/dL or higher confirms the diagnosis.

2. **Signs and symptoms** include polydipsia, polyuria, weight loss, obesity; hyperglycemia, persistent glucosuria, ketoacidosis; family history of DM, history of macrosomic infant, and unexplained fetal death—all of which would direct a physician toward further testing and treatment.

VI. **Management of gestational diabetes**

A. **General.** The patient with GDM is at higher risk of developing glucose intolerance later in life. Approximately 40% of women with GDM develop

TABLE 13-3. CRITERION VALUES FOR DIAGNOSIS OF GESTATIONAL DIABETES MELLITUS FROM RESULTS OF ORAL GLUCOSE TOLERANCE TEST

Time since 100-g glucose load	Modified O'Sullivan scale	Carpenter & Coustan scale (1982)
Fasting	≥ 105	95
1 hr	≥ 190	180
2 hrs	≥ 165	155
3 hrs	≥ 145	140

Values are plasma glucose levels in milligrams per deciliter.

DM within 15 years. GDM may be an early manifestation of DM type 2 that is temporarily unmasked by the diabetogenic hormones of pregnancy. Women with GDM are commonly treated on an outpatient basis. The primary focus for women with GDM is dietary control of glucose intake and adequate monitoring of glucose values.

GDM is divided into two categories: A1 (glucose control by diet alone) and A2 (glucose control with diet and insulin). If glucose levels cannot be controlled with diet alone, then insulin therapy should be started.

B. **Diet.** Women with newly diagnosed GDM should be started on an American Diabetic Association diet (see sec. **VII.D**) with a daily intake of 1800–2400 kilocalories.

C. **Glucose monitoring**
   1. The patient should record fasting and 1-hour (or 2-hour) postprandial glucose values (known as paneling) after each meal to determine the adequacy of management.
   2. The threshold values for starting insulin treatment are the following:

Fasting glucose level:	100–105 mg/dL or higher
1-hour postprandial level:	140 mg/dL or higher
2-hour postprandial level:	120 mg/dL or higher

   If the threshold values are consistently exceeded, then insulin therapy should be initiated.
   3. Depending on the recorded glucose levels from paneling, the insulin dosage should be initiated as follows.
      a. Calculate 1.1 U/kg (ideal) body weight.
      b. Usually do not start at more than 60 U insulin/day.
      c. Total daily dose should be divided in half, given every morning and evening.
      d. Morning dose (before breakfast): two-thirds of dose given as neutral protamine Hagedorn (NPH) insulin (peak activity of 5–12 hours), one-third of dose given as regular insulin (peak activity of 2–4 hours).
      e. Evening dose (before dinner): one-half of dose given as NPH, one-half of dose given as regular insulin.
      f. Occasionally, obese patients may require one dose of NPH insulin only, given before bedtime, for adequate control of blood glucose.
   4. The patient should continue paneling, recording fasting and 1-hour postprandial glucose levels after breakfast, lunch, and dinner.
   5. Good control of glucose levels during pregnancy helps reduce the risk of fetal macrosomia, fetal death, and neonatal complications.

D. Regular **exercise** is important in maintaining good glucose control. The patient should be encouraged to maintain a healthy, consistent level of activity throughout her pregnancy, provided there are no complicating factors (i.e., preterm labor, preeclampsia, etc.).

E. **Fetal monitoring**
   1. With GDM type A1, the patient usually can be managed without fetal antenatal testing. The patient is typically seen at 2-week intervals for ongoing diabetic management. If the patient with GDM type A1 has no concurrent disease or obstetric risk factors (i.e., hypertension, fetal growth restriction, previous stillbirth), she needs no antepartum testing beyond that recommended for a normal pregnancy.
   2. Women with GDM type A2 usually require antenatal testing similar to that recommended for PDM. A 36- to 38-week fetal growth ultrasonographic examination is recommended to assess fetal size.
   3. For all women with GDM (types A1 and A2), delivery by 40 weeks' gestation is recommended.

TABLE 13-4. THRESHOLD VALUES IN POSTPARTUM EVALUATION FOR CARBOHYDRATE INTOLERANCE

Time since 75-g glucose load	No DM	Impaired glucose tolerance	Overt DM
Fasting	<110	110–125	≥126
2 hrs	<140	140–199	≥200

DM, diabetes mellitus.
Values are plasma glucose levels in milligrams per deciliter.

F. **Postpartum evaluation.** In the postpartum period, a woman with GDM (A1 and A2) should have a follow-up GTT at 6–12 weeks postpartum to assess for possible PDM. The recommended test to further evaluate for overt DM is as follows: a fasting blood glucose value is taken, then a 75-g oral glucose load is administered, then a 2-hour glucose level is measured. See Table 13-4 for threshold values. If the threshold values are met or exceeded in follow-up testing, the patient should then be followed and treated for overt DM.

VII. **Management of pregestational diabetes**
   A. **General**
      1. In diabetes and pregnancy, fetal glucose levels are similar to maternal glucose levels. Consequently, if maternal glucose control is poor, the fetus will also have hyperglycemia.
      2. Fetal hyperglycemia has been associated with increased incidence of congenital malformations, fetal cardiac septal hypertrophy, spontaneous abortion, unexplained fetal death, and preterm birth.
      3. Potential maternal sequelae of PDM include those experienced by anyone with poorly controlled PDM (i.e., infection, hypertension, coronary heart disease, retinopathy, nephropathy, neuropathy, ketoacidosis), as well as those effects specific to pregnancy (preeclampsia and polyhydramnios).
   B. **Symptoms** of PDM include diaphoresis, tremors, blurred or double vision, weakness, hunger, confusion, paresthesias of lips and tongue, anxiety, palpitations, nausea, headache, and stupor. All of these symptoms may herald a hypoglycemic event. Patients and family members should be instructed in the treatment of hypoglycemia (i.e., consumption of milk, crackers, bread), including the administration of glucagon.
   C. **Preconceptual and pregnancy workup**
      1. The patient should have a preconceptual history and physical examination, an ophthalmologic examination, and measurement of an ECG. Echocardiography and a cardiologic consultation should also be obtained if there is presence of, or concern for, cardiac disease.
      2. The patient should be advised to maintain tight glucose level control.
      3. Measurement of HbA1C may be helpful in evaluating glucose control and assessing risk of fetal malformations. HbA1C levels of 10% or higher are associated with significant risk of fetal malformations. If the HbA1C level is within the normal range, risk appears to be similar to that of nondiabetic women.
      4. A 24-hour urine measurement of creatinine clearance and protein excretion should also be performed for evaluation of kidney function.
      5. The patient should be started on folate 400 µg/day for spina bifida prophylaxis.
      6. The patient should be encouraged to maintain an appropriate activity level or exercise program.
   D. The recommended **diet** for the pregnant woman consists of 1800–2400 kilocalories made up of 15–20% protein, 50–60% carbohydrates, and up to 20% fat.
      1. The patient should be encouraged to maintain tight glucose control.

   2. A nutritional consultation should also be provided as part of preconceptual and pregnancy counseling.
   3. If obesity is present, a weight loss program may be considered before conception.
E. **Medical treatment**
   1. In patients with type 1 DM, insulin requirements are usually increased 50–100% in pregnancy, whereas in patients with type 2 DM, insulin needs usually more than double.
   2. The American Diabetic Association recommends the use of human insulin for pregnant women with DM and for women with DM considering pregnancy.
      a. Patients taking oral hypoglycemic agents or a regimen of 70/30 mixed (NPH/regular) insulin are switched to human NPH and regular insulin.
      b. Oral hypoglycemic medications are not currently used. However, there is some investigational evidence that the newer hypoglycemic agents will be useful in managing diabetes in pregnancy in the near future.
   3. Insulin requirements increase throughout gestation, from approximately 0.7 U/kg (body weight)/day during weeks 6–18, to 0.8 U/kg/day during weeks 18–26, to 0.9 U/kg/day during weeks 26–36, and to 1.0 U/kg/day during weeks 36–40.
   4. The goals for glucose control for the preconceptual and pregnant patient are the following levels:
      • Fasting: 60–90 mg/dL
      • Premeal: less than 100 mg/dL
      • 1 hour postprandial: less than 140 mg/dL
      • 2 hours postprandial: less than 120 mg/dL
      • Bedtime: less than 120 mg/dL
      • 2–6 am: 60–90 mg/dL
   5. Patients with PDM are usually continued on their normal prepregnancy insulin regimen while initial assessment of diabetic control and paneling (recording of blood glucose levels) are performed. Goal glucose values should be discussed with the patient and adjustments in the insulin dosing made accordingly.
   6. If patients are compliant and are still unable to control glycemia, then a long-acting insulin (i.e., ultralente) may be used before breakfast and dinner, together with a short-acting insulin (regular or humalog) before each meal.
   7. If intermittent insulin dosing does not result in good glucose control, then use of an insulin pump providing continuous subcutaneous infusion may be necessary.
      a. Dosing with the insulin pump must be managed carefully, as the risk of severe hypoglycemia in pregnancy is increased and this, coupled with continuous infusion, may worsen the situation.
      b. Although hyperglycemia can have deleterious effects on the patient and fetus, hypoglycemia, if severe, can cause seizures and even death. Thus, patients in whom an insulin pump is to be used must be carefully selected to avoid serious maternal and fetal sequelae.
   8. Hospitalization is usually necessary during pregnancy when there is severe hypoglycemia, severe hyperglycemia, a concurrent infection, or obstetric indications.
F. **Fetal monitoring and pregestational diabetes**
   1. During the first trimester, minimal fetal monitoring is required (i.e., assessment for heart tones by Doppler ultrasonography at each visit during the latter portion of the first trimester).
   2. During the second trimester, measurement of maternal serum alpha-fetoprotein levels, along with levels of unconjugated estriol and human

chorionic gonadotropin, represents the triple screen, which is typically performed at 16–18 weeks' gestation.

    a. Ultrasonography (usually at 18–20 weeks) helps to date the pregnancy and evaluate the fetus for genetic abnormalities and other congenital anomalies that may be present.

    b. Fetal cardiac anomalies are the most common congenital anomalies with PDM, and so a fetal echocardiogram is recommended at 19–22 weeks' gestation.

3. In the third trimester, the fetus should be monitored as follows.

    a. Regular fetal surveillance should be initiated for all pregnancies in insulin-requiring diabetic women.

    b. Fetal surveillance should be performed frequently in the presence of maternal vascular disease, hypertension, ketoacidosis, pyelonephritis, preeclampsia, and poor patient compliance.

    c. In well-controlled DM without associated complications of hypertension and vascular disease, minimal ongoing evaluation of the fetus may be required.

    d. In poorly controlled or complicated DM, the incidence of fetal compromise and death is much higher, and therefore frequent fetal evaluation is required.

    e. Repeat obstetrical ultrasonographic examinations for fetal growth may be considered at 28–30 weeks and then at 36–38 weeks.

    f. If the patient has evidence of microvascular disease, monthly ultrasonographic examinations starting at 24–26 weeks may be necessary to closely follow fetal growth to assess for intrauterine growth restriction (IUGR).

4. Tests commonly used for fetal assessment are the nonstress test, biophysical profile, and contraction stress test.

5. Timing of fetal testing varies.

    a. In a situation in which the patient has extensive complications of DM (i.e., coronary artery disease, nephropathy), fetal assessment may begin at 28 weeks' gestation.

    b. For those women with good glucose control and minimal to no complications, regular fetal evaluation may begin at 32–34 weeks.

    c. Typically, fetal surveillance such as the nonstress test begins around 32 weeks and occurs twice weekly until delivery.

6. Another method of fetal evaluation is Doppler umbilical artery velocimetry.

    a. In pregnant women at risk for vascular disease, Doppler ultrasonographic studies of the umbilical artery can help in assessing fetal outcome.

    b. Umbilical artery waveforms obtained via Doppler ultrasonography should show a progressive decline in the systolic/diastolic (S/D) ratio from early pregnancy until term.

    c. At 30 weeks, the S/D ratio for the umbilical artery should be below 3.0.

    d. The uterine artery S/D ratio should peak around 14–20 weeks and then remain below 2.6 to 26 weeks' gestation.

    e. An elevated umbilical S/D ratio is associated with fetal growth restriction and preeclampsia. With increased resistance of the placenta, the systolic pressure of the umbilical artery increases, which causes an elevated ratio.

G. **Preterm labor and pregestational diabetes**

1. When the patient with DM develops preterm labor, the choice of tocolytics is limited.

2. Sympathomimetics (i.e., terbutaline sulfate, ritodrine hydrochloride) should be avoided because they are known to exacerbate hyperglycemia and may result in ketoacidosis.

3. Indomethacin may be used as long as maternal renal disease or poorly controlled hypertension is absent. Indomethacin should not be given after 32 weeks' gestation.
4. Magnesium sulfate is the tocolytic agent of choice in the presence of preterm labor.
5. Corticosteroids should be given if there is risk of preterm delivery. Caution should be used, however, because of their hyperglycemic effects.

H. **Labor, delivery, and diabetes**
1. The timing of delivery in an insulin-requiring diabetic patient is important.
2. Factors to be considered in choosing the delivery date are maternal glycemic control, presence or absence of maternal complications, estimated fetal weight, fetal well-being (as indicated by antenatal testing), and amniotic fluid volume.
3. In many patients with well-controlled DM, labor may be induced at 39–40 weeks.
4. Amniocentesis is recommended before elective delivery for patients without accurate gestational dating or for gestations of less than 39 weeks.
5. An elevated lecithin/sphingomyelin (L/S) ratio (ratio at lung maturity is 2.0 or higher) is associated with a low incidence of RDS, even if phosphatidylglycerol (PG) is absent.
6. L/S values are affected by blood and meconium. If these are present in amniotic fluid, L/S would not be a good indicator of fetal lung maturity, in contrast to PG level.
7. PG level is useful if blood, meconium, or other contaminants are present in the amniotic fluid.
8. Amniocentesis may need to be repeated until fetal lung maturity is achieved.
9. If antenatal testing gives nonreassuring results, the decision to deliver the fetus requires determination of the risks to the fetus of remaining in utero compared to the risks of delivery of a premature infant.
10. It is essential that the patient be euglycemic during the intrapartum period (glucose level of 100 mg/dL or less).
    a. Maternal hyperglycemia results in fetal hyperglycemia, which then causes fetal hyperinsulinemia. The neonate is then at increased risk of severe hypoglycemia as it loses the maternal infusion of glucose from the umbilical cord and the hyperinsulinemia persists, which can cause seizures and death.
    b. During labor and delivery, continuous intravenous (IV) infusion of insulin and dextrose is the optimal means of glycemic control.
    c. With elective induction of labor, the patient should receive her normal insulin dose the previous evening. On the morning of her induction, the patient's normal insulin dose should be withheld.
    d. Depending on the glucose level on admission, the patient should be started on IV fluids and should be managed as follows:
       (1) Normal saline should be continued until the patient reaches active labor, or when glucose levels fall below 70 mg/dL.
       (2) During active labor or when glucose level is less than 70 mg/dL, IV administration of 5% dextrose (with lactated Ringer's or normal saline) should be started. The infusion fluid is adjusted based on blood glucose levels (Table 13-5).
    e. Short-acting insulin boluses may be added to bring glucose levels to the target range of 80–100 mg/dL.
    f. Blood glucose values should be checked every 1–2 hours and the insulin and fluids adjusted accordingly.
    g. In type 1 DM, exogenous insulin is essential for tissue use of glucose; a low-dose insulin drip should be maintained and hypoglycemia managed with glucose infusion.

TABLE 13-5. LOW-DOSE CONTINUOUS INSULIN INFUSION FOR LABOR AND DELIVERY

Blood glucose (mg/100 mL)	Insulin dosage (U/hr)	Fluids (125 mL/hr)
<100	0	D5 LR
100–140	1.0[a]	D5 LR
141–180	1.5[a]	Normal saline
181–220	2.0[a]	Normal saline
>220	2.5[a]	Normal saline

D5 LR, 5% dextrose with lactated Ringer's solution.
[a]Increase as needed.

11. **Determination of the route of delivery** in an elective procedure remains controversial.
   a. If fetal macrosomia is suspected, a trial of labor could ensue.
   b. If the estimated fetal weight exceeds 4000 g, the risk of shoulder dystocia and traumatic birth injuries increases.
   c. With a suspected birth weight of 4500 g or greater, a cesarean section is indicated.

12. **Management of elective cesarean section**
   a. The patient should withhold her morning insulin dose.
   b. Glucose levels should be monitored frequently during and immediately after surgery.
   c. After delivery, glucose levels should be checked every 4–6 hours, while administering 5% dextrose with lactated Ringer's or normal saline (at approximately 125 mL/hour).
   d. The requirement of tight glucose control during labor and delivery is relaxed.
   e. During the initial postpartum period, short-acting insulin is used only when glucose levels are higher than 150 mg/dL.
   f. Once the patient is taking a full diabetic diet, insulin can be started at one-third to one-half the antepartum dosage or a dosage comparable to her pregestational dosage.

VIII. **Diabetes-associated maternal complications**
   A. **Diabetic ketoacidosis (DKA)** is a metabolic emergency that can be life threatening to both mother and fetus. In pregnant patients, DKA can occur at lower blood glucose levels (i.e., less than 200 mg/dL) and more rapidly than in nonpregnant diabetic patients. Although maternal death is rare with proper treatment, fetal mortality as high as 50% after a single episode of DKA has been reported. Medical illness, usually in the form of infection, is responsible for 50% of cases of DKA; an additional 20% results from neglect of dietary or insulin therapy, or both. In 30% of cases, no precipitating cause is identified. Antenatal administration of steroids to promote fetal lung maturity can precipitate or exacerbate DKA in pregnant diabetic women.
      1. DKA results from either a relative or an absolute deficiency of insulin and an excess of anti-insulin hormones.
         a. The resulting hyperglycemia and glucosuria lead to an osmotic diuresis, which results in the loss of urinary potassium and sodium, as well as fluid loss.
         b. Insulin deficiency increases lipolysis and therefore hepatic oxidation of fatty acids, which leads to the formation of ketones and the development of metabolic acidosis.

2. **Diagnosis**
   a. Signs and symptoms include abdominal pain, nausea and vomiting, polydipsia, polyuria, hypotension, rapid and deep respirations, and impaired mental status, which can vary from mild drowsiness to profound lethargy.
   b. The diagnosis is made by documenting hyperglycemia, acidosis, ketonemia, and ketonuria.
   c. Ketoacidosis usually is defined as a plasma glucose level of more than 300 mg/dL (although effects have appeared at lower levels during pregnancy), plasma bicarbonate level of less than 15 mEq/L, and arterial pH of less than 7.3.
3. **Management**
   a. Initial treatment consists of vigorous IV hydration. One liter of normal saline should be administered in the first hour, followed by 250 mL/ hour thereafter. Three to 5 L may be required in the first 24 hours.
   b. Initial insulin therapy consists of administration of regular insulin at 0.1 U/kg IV push, then an IV infusion of 5–10 U/hour. If glucose levels do not decrease by 25% in the first 2 hours of treatment, the amount of insulin infused should be doubled. Five percent dextrose in water should be started when glucose levels reach 250 mg/dL. The insulin infusion rate should be decreased to 1–2 U/hour when the serum glucose level is found to be below 150 mg/dL. IV insulin and glucose administration should be continued until urine ketones are cleared.
   c. Potassium replacement (20–40 mEq/L) should be started with the initial insulin therapy unless potassium levels are above 5.5 mEq/L, or if urine output is inadequate.
   d. Sodium bicarbonate may be added for patients with an arterial pH lower than 7.10.
   e. Levels of plasma glucose, electrolytes, and arterial blood gases need to be monitored approximately every 4 hours.
   f. When the patient is able to tolerate oral food, her usual insulin regimen may be restarted.

B. **Hypoglycemia.** The strict glycemic control that is recommended during pregnancies complicated by diabetes places patients at increased risk for hypoglycemic episodes. The presence of hyperemesis in early pregnancy also predisposes these patients to severe hypoglycemia. Up to 45% of pregnant patients with type 1 DM experience episodes of hypoglycemia serious enough to require emergency room care or hospitalization. Severe hypoglycemia may have a teratogenic effect in early gestation. The potential adverse effects on the developing fetus are not yet fully understood.
   1. **Symptoms** include nausea, headache, diaphoresis, tremors, blurred or double vision, weakness, hunger, confusion, paresthesias, and stupor.
   2. When **evaluating blood glucose levels,** one must keep in mind that other factors may be involved in altering blood glucose values.
      a. The **Somogyi phenomenon** is a rebound hyperglycemia after an episode of hypoglycemia and is secondary to a counterregulatory hormone release. It manifests as widely varied blood glucose levels over a short period of time (i.e., 2:00–6:00 am), with or without symptoms. Treatment of this phenomenon involves decreasing insulin for the critical time period (i.e., 2:00–6:00 am). If the Somogyi phenomenon is taking place, hypoglycemia resolves and glucose levels stabilize.
      b. The **dawn phenomenon** is an early morning increase in plasma glucose, possibly as a response to growth hormone. The patient is treated by increasing her insulin dose at bedtime to maintain euglycemia.
      c. Differentiating between these two phenomena requires checking the blood glucose level around 3:00 am. If the patient is hypoglycemic, the Somogyi phenomenon may be in effect, and she should consider decreasing her insulin dose at bedtime. If she is euglycemic, she is

appropriately treated; if she is hyperglycemic, she may have the dawn phenomenon and needs to increase her bedtime dose of insulin.

3. **Diagnosis.** The diagnosis is made if the patient is symptomatic or has a blood glucose level lower than 60 mg/dL, or both.

4. **Treatment.** If the patient is experiencing mild symptoms and is otherwise alert and oriented, oral complex carbohydrates should be given (i.e., milk, bread, crackers). If the patient is compromised or severely symptomatic and at risk of aspiration, an ampule of dextrose 10% should be given by IV push immediately, and IV fluids (5% dextrose with Ringer's solution or normal saline) should be started.

C. **Retinopathy.** Proliferative retinopathy is the most common manifestation of vascular disease in diabetics and is one of the principal causes of blindness in adults in the United States. Diabetic retinopathy is believed to be a direct consequence of hyperglycemia, and it is related to the duration of the disease process. The prevalence of any form of retinopathy has been found to be approximately 2% within 2 years of onset of type 1 DM and 98% among patients who have had diabetes (types 1 and 2) for at least 15 years. Retinopathy is classified as either background simple retinopathy or proliferative diabetic retinopathy. Progression to proliferative disease during pregnancy rarely occurs in patients who have either no retinal disease or only background changes. If proliferative retinopathy is present, however, it may worsen in pregnancy and lead to blindness if untreated. If benign retinopathy is diagnosed early in gestation, ophthalmologic follow-up should be performed in each trimester. The presence of proliferative changes calls for more frequent examinations, or therapy, or both. Photocoagulation for diabetic retinopathy is accomplished safely during pregnancy.

D. **Nephropathy** is a progressive disease characterized by increased glomerular permeability to protein, glomerular scarring, and, eventually, renal failure. Diabetic nephropathy develops slowly, appearing an average of 17 years after the onset of DM, and has an estimated prevalence among diabetic pregnant women of 6%. Diabetic nephropathy is of particular concern in the pregnant patient because of its association with chronic hypertension, preeclampsia, fetal growth retardation, nonreassuring fetal heart tones, preterm delivery, and perinatal death (fetal and neonatal).

1. The **diagnosis** is made in the presence of persistent proteinuria of more than 3 g/day, serum creatinine level higher than 1.5 mg/dL, hematocrit less than 25%, and hypertension with mean arterial pressure higher than 107 mm Hg. Creatinine clearance level is an important prognostic indicator because a clearance of less than 50 mL/minute has been associated with a high incidence of severe preeclampsia and fetal loss.

2. Patients with diabetic nephropathy require intensive maternal and fetal surveillance throughout gestation. With intensive management, a fetal survival rate of over 90% has been reported.

E. **Atherosclerosis** is present in many diabetic patients.

1. A complete **history** and physical examination should be performed to elicit any evidence of ischemic heart disease, heart failure, peripheral vascular disease, or cerebral ischemia.

2. **Evaluation** of a pregnant patient with DM should always include an ECG. A maternal echocardiogram and cardiologic consultation should be obtained if clinically indicated.

3. Maternal mortality is increased among diabetic patients with ischemic heart disease. Therefore, preconceptual counseling is essential. If conception occurs, termination of the pregnancy may be considered to preserve the health of the patient.

F. **Spontaneous abortion**

1. Miscarriage among patients with PDM has been reported to range between 6% and 29% and is associated with poor glucose control during the periconceptual period.

2. No increase in incidence of abortion is found in diabetic women with good periconceptual glucose control.

G. **Polyhydramnios** is a common complication during diabetic pregnancies, with a reported incidence of 3–32%. The incidence of polyhydramnios in diabetic patients is 30 times that in nondiabetic controls. Even though polyhydramnios can be associated with abnormalities of the fetal CNS and GI system, no cause is identified in almost 90% of diabetic patients.

1. The pathogenesis of polyhydramnios is not clear. Proposed mechanisms include increased fetal glycemic loads, decreased fetal swallowing, fetal GI obstructions, and fetal polyuria secondary to hyperglycemia.

2. Higher perinatal morbidity and mortality rates have been associated with polyhydramnios. These higher rates can be attributed, in part, to the increased incidence of congenital anomalies and preterm delivery associated with this condition.

H. **Chronic hypertension and preeclampsia**

1. The incidence of chronic hypertension is increased in pregnant patients with PDM, particularly in those with diabetic nephropathy.

2. Bed rest, sodium restriction, and antihypertensive therapy are the principal management strategies.

3. Affected patients must be monitored carefully throughout pregnancy for the potential development of preeclampsia, fetal growth restriction, and fetal distress.

4. When a workup is done on a patient with hypertension or history of preeclampsia, a complete history must be taken and a physical examination performed initially, and an ECG should also be obtained. A renal consultation may be indicated as well.

   a. If the patient is on antihypertensive medications, she should be changed to those medications better suited for pregnancy (i.e., methyldopa).

   b. The patient's urine should be monitored for protein, weight checked for an acute weight gain, and BP monitored at every visit.

   c. The fetus must be evaluated carefully during the third trimester (and second trimester if indicated), with fetal weight estimated and amniotic fluid status, S/D ratio, and fetal heart reactivity assessed.

I. **Preterm labor and preterm delivery**

1. The incidence of preterm labor may be three to four times higher in patients with DM.

2. An association has been made between poor glycemic control during the second trimester and an increased rate of preterm delivery.

   a. Magnesium sulfate is the tocolytic agent of choice in labor in patients with DM.

   b. Corticosteroids should be given if indicated based on risk of preterm delivery. Careful monitoring of blood glucose levels is important when administering betamethasone to diabetic patients.

   c. Antibiotic prophylaxis should also be started according to the presence of risk factors as defined by the American College of Obstetricians and Gynecologists.

IX. **Fetal and neonatal complications associated with diabetes.** Complications during the neonatal period are increased in infants of mothers with both gestational and pregestational DM. The incidence of complications, however, is much higher among infants of patients with PDM, especially those with poor glycemic control, than among those of mothers with GDM.

A. **Congenital malformations.** Because of reductions in intrauterine deaths, in traumatic deliveries, and in RDS, congenital malformations are now the most common contributor to perinatal mortality in pregnancies of women with PDM. Thirty percent to 50% of perinatal mortality can be attributed to congenital malformations. A two- to fourfold higher incidence of major malformations has been documented among infants of insulin-requiring diabetic patients than among infants in the general population. Even though maternal hyperglycemia is considered to be the principal contributing factor for congenital malformations, hypoglycemia and hyperketonemia have also been implicated.

1. The single defect that is considered most characteristic of diabetic fetopathy is sacral agenesis or caudal regression. This rare malformation is diagnosed 200–400 times more frequently in gestations in diabetic patients.

2. A tenfold increase is also seen in the incidence of CNS malformations, including anencephaly, holoprosencephaly, open spina bifida, microcephaly, encephalocele, and meningomyelocele.

3. The rate of cardiovascular anomalies, the most common malformations, are increased fivefold in fetuses of diabetic patients. Defects include transposition of the great vessels, ventricular and atrial septal defects, hypoplastic left ventricle, situs inversus, and aortic anomalies.

4. Malformations of the genitourinary and GI systems are also found, including absent kidneys (Potter's syndrome), polycystic kidneys, double ureter, tracheoesophageal fistula, bowel atresia, and imperforate anus.

B. **Macrosomia** is defined as an estimated fetal weight greater than the ninetieth percentile, or 4000 g, and occurs much more frequently in pregnancies in diabetic women than in nondiabetic women (25–42% versus 8–14%). Maternal diabetes is the most significant single risk factor for the development of macrosomia.

1. Diabetic macrosomia is characterized specifically by a large fetal abdominal circumference and a decrease in the ratio of head circumference to abdominal circumference. These changes are due to the increased subcutaneous fat deposits caused by fetal hyperinsulinemia.

2. Morbidity and mortality rates are higher for macrosomic fetuses. Macrosomic fetuses are at risk of intrauterine death, hypertrophic cardiomyopathy, vascular thrombosis, neonatal hypoglycemia, and birth trauma. Their mothers are also more likely to undergo a cesarean delivery than mothers of smaller infants.

C. **Neonatal hypoglycemia.** Twenty-five percent to 40% of infants of diabetic mothers develop hypoglycemia during the first few hours of life. Poor maternal glycemic control during pregnancy and elevated maternal glucose levels at the time of delivery increase the risk of neonatal hypoglycemia.

1. The **pathogenesis** of neonatal hypoglycemia involves the stimulation in utero of the fetal pancreas by significant maternal hyperglycemia. This stimulation leads to fetal islet cell hypertrophy and beta-cell hyperplasia. When the transplacental source of glucose is eliminated, the newborn exhibits overproduction of insulin.

2. The **clinical signs** of neonatal hypoglycemia include cyanosis, convulsions, tremor, apathy, sweating, and a weak or high-pitched cry. Severe or prolonged hypoglycemia is associated with neurologic sequelae and death.

3. **Treatment** should be instituted when the infant's glucose level drops below 40 mg/dL.

D. **Neonatal hypocalcemia and hypomagnesemia.** Alterations in mineral metabolism are common in infants of diabetic mothers. These alterations are related to the degree of maternal glycemic control.

E. **Neonatal polycythemia.** Thirty-three percent of infants born to diabetic mothers are polycythemic (hematocrit higher than 65%). Chronic intrauterine hypoxia leads to an increase in erythropoietin production, with a resultant increase in red blood cell production. Alternatively, elevated glucose may lead to early and increased red blood cell destruction, followed by increased erythrocyte production.

F. **Neonatal hyperbilirubinemia and neonatal jaundice** occur more commonly in the infants of diabetic mothers than in infants of nondiabetic patients of comparable gestational age. This is due to a delay in in utero liver maturation among infants of diabetic mothers with poor glycemic control.

G. **Neonatal respiratory distress syndrome**
  1. RDS in infants of diabetic mothers is associated with delayed fetal lung maturation. Fetal hyperinsulinemia is thought to suppress production and secretion of the major component of surfactant required for inflation of the lungs.
  2. The reliability of the L/S ratio as a predictor of lung maturity in pregnancies complicated by DM is the subject of controversy.
      a. For many infants, development of RDS is possible with an L/S ratio of 2.
      b. The presence of PG should always be established, because it is associated with the absence of RDS in both normal and diabetic pregnancies.
      c. Nevertheless, a low incidence of RDS can be expected in infants of patients whose disease is well controlled who have a mature L/S ratio, even in the absence of PG.
H. **Fetal and neonatal cardiomyopathy**
  1. Infants of diabetic mothers are at increased risk of developing cardiac septal hypertrophy and CHF. One study reported that up to 10% of these infants have evidence of hypertrophic changes. A strong correlation between the increased risk of cardiomyopathy and poor maternal glycemic control has been documented.
  2. As an isolated finding, cardiac septal hypertrophy is a benign neonatal condition. However, it increases the risk of neonatal morbidity and mortality in infants with sepsis or congenital structural heart disease.
I. **Birth trauma and perinatal hypoxia**
  1. Macrosomic infants are at increased risk for fractured clavicles, facial paralysis, Erb's palsy, Klumpke's palsy, phrenic nerve injury, and intracranial hemorrhage.
  2. Severe injuries may result in permanent morbidity and even death.
  3. Infants of diabetic mothers are also at increased risk for perinatal hypoxic sequelae.

THYROID DISORDERS

I. **General.** Thyroid disease is commonly found in women of reproductive age. The incidence of thyroiditis, thyrotoxicosis, and hypothyroidism in the general population is approximately 1% each. The incidence of nontoxic goiter overall is approximately 5%. Approximately 0.2% of pregnancies are complicated by thyroid disease. The relationship of thyroid function and pregnancy is complex.
II. **Physiology.** Moderate enlargement of the thyroid occurs from increased vascularity and glandular hyperplasia. In a normal pregnancy, however, there is no thyromegaly or nodularity.
  A. Increased levels of altered thyroxine-binding globulin (TBG) occur, and this reduces triiodothyronine resin uptake (T_3RU) and increases levels of thyroxine (T_4) and triiodothyronine (T_3). The serum level of TBG is inversely proportional to T_3RU.
  B. During the first trimester, total serum levels of T_4 increase to 9–16 μg/dL (levels in nonpregnant women are 5–12 μg/dL).
  C. As levels of human chorionic gonadotropin increase during the early part of the first trimester, levels of thyroid-stimulating hormone (TSH) decrease and levels of FT_4 increase. Throughout the remainder of the pregnancy, however, there is no physiologic hyperthyroid state. Levels of TSH, FT_4, and free T_3 remain within the normal range.
  D. If a patient presents with a thyroid nodule or goiter, it should be considered pathologic and evaluated thoroughly.
      1. Measuring the serum levels of total T_3 or T_4 offers the greatest sensitivity for assessing thyroid function when TBG is elevated.
      2. T_3RU levels may be used as an assessment of TBG, which can allow the free T_4 (FT_4) index to be calculated. The FT_4 index is calculated as follows:

$$FT_4 = \text{total } T_4 \times (\text{patient's } T_3RU/\text{normal } T_3RU)$$

      3. The FT_4, when elevated, predicts hyperthyroidism.

TABLE 13-6. THYROID FUNCTION TEST RESULTS IN NORMAL PREGNANCY AND HYPERTHYROIDISM

Test	Normal pregnancy	Hyperthyroidism
Thyroid-stimulating hormone level	No change	Decreased
Thyroxine (T_4)-binding globulin level	Increased	No change
Total T_4 level	Increased	Increased
Free T_4 index	No change	Increased
Total triiodothyronine (T_3) level	Increased	Increased
Free T_3 level	No change	Increased
T_3 resin uptake	Decreased	Increased
Thyroid radioactive iodine uptake	Increased	Increased

4. Although a decreased FT_4 is consistent with hypothyroidism, measuring the TSH level is a better predictor of primary hypothyroidism.
   a. TSH is not bound to protein, does not cross the placenta, and is not affected by pregnancy.
   b. If TSH values are normal and FT_4 is low, then secondary hypothyroidism is likely due to a central hypothalamus-pituitary defect.

III. **Hyperthyroidism.** Thyrotoxicosis occurs in approximately 1 in 2000 pregnancies. Graves' disease is the primary cause of thyrotoxicosis in pregnancy. An autoimmune disease, Graves' disease results in production of thyroid-stimulating antibody (TSA), which mimics TSH and stimulates thyroid function and size increase. Another cause of hyperthyroidism is destruction-induced thyrotoxicosis. Caused by antimicrosomal antibodies, destruction-induced thyrotoxicosis disrupts the gland, so that stored thyroid hormone is released. Differentiating the two causes is important because the treatment differs. Measuring levels of TSA and antimicrosomal antibody helps differentiate the two disorders. Table 13-6 shows test results for normal pregnancy and hyperthyroidism. With thyrotoxicosis, maintaining metabolic control is especially important for the fetus and the mother.

A. Poorly controlled hyperthyroidism can result in preeclampsia, thyroid storm, or CHF for the mother, and preterm labor and delivery, IUGR, and stillbirth for the fetus.

B. Maternal **signs and symptoms** include tachycardia, exophthalmos, thyromegaly, onycholysis, and failure of the nonobese patient to gain weight. Abnormal laboratory test results include increase in serum T_4 level and increase in the FT_4 index.

C. **Management** includes administration of propylthiouracil (PTU) or methimazole, and beta-blockers. The goal is to use the minimum amount of PTU to achieve metabolic control, as it crosses the placenta and potentially can cause fetal hypothyroidism and goiter.

1. **PTU** is the primary medication used (methimazole has been reported to cause aplasia cutis, a fetal scalp disorder). Dosing is as follows: 300–450 mg daily, with the dosage increased until symptoms are diminished and total serum T_4 levels are decreased to high-normal values. Effects of PTU become apparent 3–4 weeks after starting the medication.

2. **Beta-blockers** are used in the treatment of thyrotoxicosis as they can help reduce maternal symptoms of hyperthyroidism. Propranolol hydrochloride is the most widely used beta-blocker.
   a. Onset of action is much faster than that of PTU, as the effect occurs peripherally in reducing the thyroid hormone response.

    b. The patient must be monitored for adverse effects. Beta-blockers can cause decreased ventricular function resulting in pulmonary edema.

    c. The goal of treatment is to reduce the maternal heart rate to a resting state of less than 100 beats/minute.

  3. **Subtotal thyroidectomy** may be performed at any time during the pregnancy if medical management has failed. Maintaining some form of pharmacologic control before surgery provides the best outcome.

IV. **Thyroid storm and heart failure.** Thyroid storm is rarely seen during pregnancy. Heart failure, due to the long-term effects of T_4, is more likely encountered. Heart failure can be exacerbated by pregnancy-associated conditions such as preeclampsia, anemia, or infection.

  A. **Symptoms**

    1. In these hypermetabolic states, the patient often has fever higher than 103°F, tachycardia, widened pulse pressure, and agitation.

    2. The patient may develop hypotension and cardiovascular collapse.

  B. **Treatment**

    1. These emergency states are treated with PTU 1 g and potassium iodide 1 g, by mouth or nasogastric tube.

    2. With thyroid storm, IV beta-blockers may be used, but these should be used cautiously with heart failure.

    3. Other supportive treatments include IV hydration and temperature control.

    4. Further assessment and treatment of other concomitant disorders (i.e., hypertension, infection, anemia) are also crucial to reducing cardiac workload.

V. **Hypothyroidism.** Pregnancy complicated by hypothyroidism is uncommon, as hypothyroidism is associated with infertility.

  A. **Signs and symptoms** include the following: Before delivery, the patient may be asymptomatic or may present with disproportionate weight gain, lethargy, weakness, cold sensitivity, hair loss, myxedematous changes, and dry skin; TSH level is increased, serum T_4 level is low, the FT_4 index is decreased. Type 1 diabetes is associated with an increased incidence of subclinical hypothyroidism during pregnancy.

  B. **Treatment.** Regardless of whether the patient is symptomatic or simply has abnormal thyroid function test results consistent with hypothyroidism, she must be treated to prevent further sequelae.

    1. Replacement of T_4 should be based on the patient's clinical history and laboratory test values. With appropriate replacement of T_4, the patient's pregnancy and development of the fetus can be within normal limits.

    2. Treatment for hypothyroidism is L-thyroxine, starting at 0.05–0.10 mg daily.

      a. The dosage should be increased over several weeks while thyroid function test results are followed, with the goal of finding the dosage that allows the laboratory values to return to the normal range and resolves the patient's symptoms.

      b. A maximum dosage of 0.2 mg/day of L-thyroxine should not be exceeded.

      c. TSH level alone can be followed to determine optimal dosing; however, it can take a month for the effect to be noted in the serum TSH level.

    3. Complications of pregnancy are similar to those of hyperthyroidism, including preeclampsia, IUGR, abruptio placentae, anemia, postpartum hemorrhage, stillbirth, and cardiac dysfunction.

    4. Infants born to hypothyroid mothers optimally treated usually have no evidence of thyroid dysfunction and generally do well.

VI. **Nodular thyroid disease** should be evaluated whenever detected.

  A. Ultrasonographic evaluation and fine-needle aspiration or tissue biopsy should be performed if a thyroid nodule is found.

B. If thyroid carcinoma is found, surgical excision is the primary treatment and should not be postponed because of pregnancy.

PARATHYROID DISORDERS

I. **Physiology**
   A. **General.** Calcium requirements increase during pregnancy due to the need for proper fetal skeletal development. It is recommended that women ingest 1200 mg/day of calcium throughout pregnancy. At term, the fetus has accumulated 25–30 g of calcium. Fetal uptake of calcium is greatest later in pregnancy.
   B. **Maternal.** Levels of ionized calcium do not significantly change during pregnancy. Beginning in the second or third month of pregnancy, total calcium levels decrease, reaching a nadir during the middle of the third trimester. Decreased albumin (and phosphate) account for much of the lower total blood calcium levels. Increased calcium excretion, due to the increased glomerular filtration rate, along with active placental transfer of calcium, also contribute to the decreased maternal calcium levels. There is controversy regarding maternal levels of parathyroid hormone (PTH). Previously it was believed that PTH levels were elevated during pregnancy, which caused a possible physiologic hyperparathyroidism. Recently, however, it has been shown that PTH levels may in fact be significantly decreased during pregnancy.
   C. **Fetal.** Maternal PTH and calcitonin do not cross the placenta. It appears that 25-hydroxyvitamin D is transported across the placenta. However, 1,25-dihydroxyvitamin D probably does not cross the placenta.

II. **Hyperparathyroidism**
   A. **Pathophysiology.** Hyperparathyroidism is rarely diagnosed during pregnancy. Most commonly, a solitary parathyroid adenoma causes hyperparathyroidism. Pregnancy can exacerbate hyperparathyroidism.
   B. **Diagnosis**
      1. **Signs and symptoms**
         a. Initially, symptoms include fatigue, depression, muscle weakness, nausea and vomiting, constipation, and abdominal and back pain.
         b. With impaired renal functioning, polyuria and polydipsia may develop.
         c. Progressive disease is evidenced by bone pain, fractures, and nephrolithiasis.
      2. **Laboratory findings** include elevated free serum calcium and decreased phosphorus levels. Disproportionately high PTH relative to serum calcium may also be found.
      3. ECG abnormalities, including arrhythmias, may be present.
      4. Ultrasonography is recommended for localizing the diseased tissue. If radiation exposure is necessary to identify local disease, it should be kept to a minimum.
   C. **Treatment**
      1. Surgical excision of the parathyroid adenoma is the preferred treatment, although asymptomatic women may be treated with oral phosphate (1.0–1.5 g daily).
      2. With severe disease, medical treatment is recommended before surgery, although it should not significantly delay the surgery.
   D. **Sequelae**
      1. **Fetal.** Increased rates of spontaneous abortion and intrauterine fetal death are the most commonly occurring sequelae.
      2. **Neonatal.** Usually neonates at 1–2 weeks of age are found to have abnormally low calcium levels, although the nadir is reached by 24–48 hours. Hypocalcemia is often transient and probably results from elevated maternal calcium levels in utero, which suppress fetal parathyroid functioning. Tetany and seizures may occur with severe neonatal hypocalcemia.

III. **Hypoparathyroidism**
   A. **Pathophysiology.** Hypoparathyroidism is rare and most commonly occurs iatrogenically as a result of parathyroid removal with thyroid surgery. Other causes include autoimmune disorders, including Addison's disease, chronic lymphocytic thyroiditis, and premature ovarian failure. Pseudohypoparathyroidism may be present; it is evidenced by refractoriness to PTH produced by normal parathyroid glands.
   B. **Signs and symptoms** include weakness, lethargy, paresthesias, muscle cramps, irritability, bone pain, and tetany. Laboratory evaluation shows low calcium and PTH levels and elevated serum phosphate level.
      1. Pregnancy can cause blood to be alkalotic, with an increase in pH; this can increase calcium binding and thus cause tetany.
      2. Trousseau's sign (carpopedal spasm after BP cuff inflation above systolic pressure for several minutes) or Chvostek's sign (upper lip twitching after tapping of the facial nerve) may be present.
   C. **Treatment** includes simply replacement of calcium (1200 mg/day) and vitamin D (10 µg/day), and consumption of a diet low in phosphates.
   D. **Sequelae**
      1. **Fetal.** Poor maternal control of hypoparathyroidism can result in fetal hypocalcemia and skeletal demineralization.
      2. **Neonatal.** During labor and delivery, maternal repletion with calcium gluconate may prevent neonatal tetany.
         a. Alkalosis from maternal hyperventilation in the presence of hypocalcemia may result in neonatal tetany.
         b. Infants exposed to poorly managed maternal hypoparathyroidism can have bone demineralization, subperiosteal resorption, and osteitis fibrosa cystica.

PITUITARY DISORDERS
   I. **Anterior pituitary disorders**
   A. Patients with **prolactin-producing adenomas** usually present with symptoms of amenorrhea, galactorrhea, anovulatory cycles, and infertility.
      1. During normal gestation the pituitary gland increases in size and function due to estrogen stimulation of the lactotrophic cells found in the anterior pituitary; this causes a subsequent rise in serum levels of prolactin.
      2. When a patient presents with symptoms suggestive of a prolactinoma, a confirmatory diagnosis should be made by measuring serum levels of prolactin and performing CT or MRI of the head.
      3. Patients with **microadenomas** (tumor size less than 1 cm) usually have unremarkable pregnancies. The tumor regresses spontaneously following delivery.
      4. **Macroadenomas** (tumors of 1 cm or larger) often cause symptoms associated with a mass effect, such as visual disturbances, headache, and polyuria (diabetes insipidus).
      5. **Treatment.** The patient should be evaluated by an obstetrician, endocrinologist, and ophthalmologist.
         a. Symptomatic prolactin-secreting tumors should first be treated with bromocriptine mesylate (a dopamine receptor stimulator).
         b. Transsphenoidal adenectomy should be reserved for women whose disease does not respond to medical therapy.
         c. Radiotherapy is recommended if medical and surgical treatments fail.
         d. Radiologic evaluation and determination of serum prolactin levels are necessary follow-up measures for a known pituitary micro- or macroadenoma.
   B. **Acromegaly** is the result of an increased level of growth hormone secondary to a pituitary-secreting adenoma.

1. Pregnancy is possible but rare in patients with acromegaly.
2. If a patient with acromegaly becomes pregnant, there appear to be no deleterious or teratogenic effects of the disease on the pregnancy or the fetus.
3. Growth hormone–producing adenomas can be diagnosed by observing increased levels of growth hormone after an oral GTT, and by CT or MRI of the head.
4. For symptomatic growth hormone–secreting adenomas, bromocriptine is the first line of therapy.

II. **Posterior pituitary disorders**

A. The primary disorder associated with the posterior pituitary is diabetes insipidus, which can occur postpartum following pituitary insufficiency.

B. The inciting processes causing diabetes insipidus are Sheehan syndrome (which can occur after an intrapartum or postpartum hemorrhage) and lymphocytic hypophysitis. Acute Sheehan syndrome is characterized by tachycardia, hypotension, hypoglycemia, and failure to lactate. Although the average time before onset of symptoms is approximately 5 years, patients can be symptomatic in the postpartum period.

C. Lymphocytic hypophysitis is due to an autoimmune pituitary process that causes a massive influx of lymphocytes and plasma cells, which destroy the pituitary parenchyma. Up to 25% of cases are associated with other autoimmune diseases. Patients present with headache, visual changes, and other hypopituitary symptoms.

D. Diabetes insipidus is rare. It is associated with decreased or absent vasopressin.

1. Diagnosis is based on the presence of severe polyuria and urinary hypoosmolarity (specific gravity less than 1.005) while the patient is on water restriction.
2. The primary treatment of diabetes insipidus is administration of synthetic vasopressin (L-deamino-I-D-arginine vasopressin) 0.1 mg intranasally three times a day.
3. Oxytocin secretion does not appear to be connected with vasopressin release.

ADRENAL DISORDERS

I. **Pathophysiology.** The adrenal gland is profoundly affected by pregnancy. After an initial decrease in serum corticotropin, levels markedly increase along with levels of plasma renin (and, secondarily, angiotensin and aldosterone levels increase) as pregnancy progresses. Adrenal disorders are not pregnancy induced, but coexisting adrenal disorders do occur in pregnancy.

II. **Cushing syndrome.** Normal pregnancy results in increased serum cortisol levels. Cushing syndrome occurs from long-term exposure to glucocorticoids, either from exogenous steroid use (as in treatment of lupus erythematosus, asthma, sarcoid) or from increased endogenous levels of adrenal corticoid (i.e., increased pituitary adrenocorticotropic hormone production, adrenal hyperplasia, or adrenal neoplasia).

A. Many of the **symptoms** specific to Cushing syndrome are often found in normal pregnancies.

1. Whether the cause is iatrogenic or endogenous, the classic phenotypic presentation is truncal obesity, moon facies, and a buffalo hump.
2. During pregnancy the patient may also present with hypertension, weakness, edema, striae, easy bruising, or evidence of heart failure or GDM.
3. Patients with this disorder are at an increased risk of preterm delivery and perinatal mortality.

B. **Diagnosis** of Cushing syndrome is by observation of increased levels of serum cortisol (with no diurnal variation), together with failure to obtain normal results on dexamethasone suppression testing. Head or abdominal CT or MRI or both are recommended to help localize the causative process.

C. Effective **treatment** of Cushing syndrome is difficult during pregnancy.
   1. Treating hypertension is important.
   2. If pituitary disease is confirmed, surgical excision may be necessary.
   3. With primary adrenal hyperplasia, metyrapone has been used to block cortisol secretion. Metyrapone crosses the placenta and may affect fetal adrenal steroid synthesis.
   4. Surgical removal of an adrenal adenoma is recommended, as the incidence of maternal morbidity may be higher with adrenal adenomas than with hyperplasia.

III. **Adrenal insufficiency** can be due to a primary autoimmune process (Addison's disease), to a secondary pituitary failure, or to adrenal suppression caused by exogenous steroids. Primary adrenal failure results in depletion of all steroid hormones, whereas secondary failure results in significant losses of glucocorticoids only. Adrenal insufficiency is not associated with fetal or neonatal adverse effects.

A. **Addison's disease** presents as generalized, vague symptoms of hypotension, fatigue, anorexia, nausea, and darkening of the skin. Hypoglycemia is often present. Pregnancy can exacerbate adrenal insufficiency.

B. **Diagnosis** is based on low plasma cortisol levels. Adrenocorticotropic hormone stimulation of the adrenal gland with Cortrosyn (0.25 mg IV) results in less than a twofold increase in plasma cortisol levels.

C. **Treatment** of Addison's disease includes maintenance replacement of corticosteroids with hydrocortisone (20 mg each morning and 10 mg each evening), or prednisone (5 mg each morning and 2.5 mg each evening).
   1. For mineralocorticoid replacement, fludrocortisone acetate (0.5–0.1 mg/day) can be used, with close observation if fluid overload is present.
   2. Stress-dose steroids should be given during labor and delivery, and during other times of stress, such as with severe infection.

IV. **Pheochromocytoma** is a rare tumor that may be associated with medullary thyroid carcinoma and hyperparathyroidism (multiple endocrine neoplasia type 2 syndromes), neurofibromatosis, and von Hippel-Lindau disease. In more than 90% of cases, the tumor is found in the adrenal medulla; 10% of tumors are located in sympathetic ganglia. In 10% of cases tumors are bilateral, 10% of tumors are malignant, and 10% are extra-adrenal.

A. When the tumor is diagnosed during pregnancy, maternal mortality is approximately 11% and fetal mortality is 46%. Maternal mortality increases to 55% if the diagnosis is not made until the postpartum period.

B. The tumor secretes catecholamines.
   1. Catecholamines do not cross the placenta and thus do not directly affect the fetus.
   2. Disturbances in the maternal environment can affect the fetus, resulting in fetal growth restriction, fetal stress, and fetal death.
   3. The neonate does not carry additional risks after delivery.

C. The **signs and symptoms** associated with pheochromocytoma can mimic those found in chronic hypertension. They include the following:
   1. Paroxysmal or sustained hypertension, headaches, visual changes, palpitations, diaphoresis, abdominal pain, and anxiety.
   2. Hypoglycemia and postural hypotension can also be found.

D. **Diagnosis** is made by noting increased urine levels of unconjugated norepinephrine, epinephrine, and their metabolites; metanephrine (the most sensitive and specific substrate); and vanillylmandelic acid in a 24-hour urine collection. Abdominal CT or MRI is recommended for localization of the neoplasm.

E. **Treatment** recommendations include surgical intervention regardless of gestational age, and careful pharmacologic control of hypertension.

1. Phenoxybenzamine hydrochloride (alpha-adrenergic long-acting blocker) (10–30 mg two to four times daily) or phentolamine mesylate (short-acting alpha-adrenergic blocker), given intravenously, is recommended as initial treatment.
2. If tachycardia or arrhythmias persist after alpha-adrenergic blockade, then beta-blockers (i.e., propranolol 20–80 mg four times daily) can be given with close monitoring.

F. **Cesarean delivery** is recommended to avoid the catecholamine surges of labor and delivery.

14. HYPERTENSIVE DISORDERS OF PREGNANCY

Lisa Soule and Frank Witter

I. **Classification and definitions**
   A. **Chronic hypertension**
      1. Hypertension is defined as elevation either of systolic BP to 140 mm Hg or higher or of diastolic BP to 90 mm Hg or higher.
      2. Chronic hypertension is defined as hypertension diagnosed before pregnancy or before 20 weeks' gestation, or elevated BP that is first diagnosed during pregnancy and persists after 42 days postpartum.
   B. **Preeclampsia and eclampsia**
      1. **Preeclampsia** is defined as elevated BP and proteinuria after 20 weeks' gestation (except in the presence of trophoblastic disease or multiple gestation, in which cases preeclampsia may appear before 20 weeks' gestation).
         a. **Mild preeclampsia.** The following criteria must be met to confirm the diagnosis of mild preeclampsia:
            (1) **BP** of 140/90 mm Hg or higher after 20 weeks' gestation, measured on two occasions at least 6 hours apart.
            (2) **Proteinuria** greater than 300 mg in a 24-hour urine collection or a score of 1+ on a random urine dipstick test.
            (3) **Edema** frequently accompanies preeclampsia but is not required for diagnosis.
               (a) Edema must be generalized for association with preeclampsia; dependent edema (e.g., low back, legs) is not sufficient.
               (b) Fluid retention is evidenced by rapid weight gain (more than 5 lb in 1 week).
         b. **Severe preeclampsia.** The following criteria are used to confirm the diagnosis of severe preeclampsia:
            (1) **BP** during bed rest of 160 mm Hg systolic or 110 mm Hg diastolic, measured on two occasions at least 6 hours apart
            (2) **Proteinuria** greater than 5 g in a 24-hour collection or a score of 3+ to 4+ on random urine dipstick test
            (3) **Oliguria,** indicated by a 24-hour urine output of less than 400 mL or serum creatinine level higher than 1.2 mg/dL (unless known to be higher previously)
            (4) **Cerebral or visual disturbances,** including altered consciousness, headache, scotomata, blurred vision, or some combination of these
            (5) **Pulmonary edema or cyanosis**
            (6) **Epigastric or right upper quadrant pain**
            (7) **Impaired liver function** without a known cause, indicated by elevated AST level of 70 U/L or higher
            (8) **Thrombocytopenia,** indicated by a platelet count lower than 100,000/mm^3, or evidence of microangiopathic hemolytic anemia, such as abnormal findings on peripheral smear, increased bilirubin level (1.2 mg/dL or higher), or elevated lactate dehydrogenase (LDH) level (600 U/L or higher)
      2. **Eclampsia is preeclampsia accompanied by seizures.**
      3. **HELLP syndrome,** which consists of hemolysis, elevated liver enzymes, and low platelet count, is a form of severe preeclampsia.
         a. **Definition**
            (1) **Thrombocytopenia.** A platelet count of less than 100,000/mm^3 is the most consistent finding in HELLP syndrome.

(2) **Hemolysis** is defined as the presence of abnormal peripheral smear results with burr cells and schistocytes, bilirubin level of 1.2 mg/dL or higher, or LDH level higher than 600 U/L.

(3) **Elevated liver function test results.** AST level is 70 U/L or higher.

b. **Presentation.** Typically, HELLP syndrome occurs in a white multiparous patient older than 25 years, but it is not limited to such patients. It may develop antepartum or postpartum. The majority of cases appear to develop antepartum. The patient frequently is remote from term and complains of epigastric or right upper quadrant pain (90%), nausea and vomiting (50%), and sometimes a nonspecific virus-like syndrome. Ninety percent of patients give a history of malaise of several days' duration before presentation. Patients may present with hematuria or GI bleeding. Hypertension may be absent (20%), mild (30%), or severe (50%).

c. **Physical examination** may reveal right upper quadrant tenderness (80%) and significant weight gain with edema (60%).

d. **Differential diagnoses** include benign thrombocytopenia of pregnancy, idiopathic thrombocytopenic purpura, thrombotic thrombocytopenic purpura, hemolytic uremic syndrome, gallbladder disease, viral hepatitis, pyelonephritis, acute fatty liver of pregnancy, kidney stones, glomerulonephritis, and gastroenteritis.

C. **Chronic hypertension with superimposed preeclampsia** is defined as preeclampsia that occurs in a patient with preexisting chronic hypertension. It is often difficult to differentiate chronic hypertension with superimposed preeclampsia from an exacerbation of chronic hypertension.

D. **Transient hypertension**

1. Transient hypertension, also known as **pregnancy-induced hypertension**, is defined as elevated BP during pregnancy or the first 24 hours postpartum without other signs of preeclampsia or chronic hypertension.

2. Transient hypertension must be differentiated from preeclampsia because transient hypertension is associated with an increased risk of chronic hypertension, whereas preeclampsia or eclampsia is not associated with such a risk.

II. **Preeclampsia**

A. **Epidemiology**

1. **Incidence.** Preeclampsia is reported to occur in 7–10% of all pregnancies extending beyond 20 weeks. It is the third leading cause of maternal mortality, responsible for over 17% of maternal deaths. It is also a major cause of neonatal morbidity and mortality, both directly, via intrauterine growth restriction, and indirectly, through its association with abruptio placentae and the need for preterm delivery. Preeclampsia has been implicated in 10% of perinatal deaths, 20% of labor inductions, 15% of cesarian sections, and 10% of medically indicated preterm deliveries.

2. **Risk factors** for preeclampsia and eclampsia include age younger than 20 years or older than 40 years; nulliparous status; presence of chronic hypertension, lupus erythematosus, diabetes, or renal disease; history of previous eclampsia as primigravida, previous preeclampsia as multipara, or previous superimposed preeclampsia; and positive family history of preeclampsia or eclampsia, multiple gestation, hydatidiform moles, and fetal hydrops.

B. **Pathophysiology**

1. The development of preeclampsia requires the presence of trophoblastic tissue but not necessarily a fetus.

2. There are a number of prominent **pathologic features** of preeclampsia. Derangements are noticed in vascular reactivity, volume homeostasis, thrombogenesis, and regulation of a number of synthetic processes.

3. The temporal sequence of these alterations, and which are causal and which consequences of the disorder, are as yet undetermined.

C. **Diagnosis**

1. **BP values** should be recorded with the woman sitting or in a semirereclining position. Her right arm should be held consistently, roughly horizontally at heart level. Early measurement of the baseline BP is important because BP normally declines in the second trimester.

2. **Symptoms** of preeclampsia or eclampsia may include the following:
   a. Headache
   b. Visual symptoms: blurred vision, scotomata, and blindness (retinal detachment)
   c. Epigastric or right upper quadrant pain
   d. Nausea and vomiting
   e. Dyspnea (from pulmonary edema)
   f. Decreased urine output, hematuria, or rapid weight gain (greater than 5 lb in 1 week)
   g. Constant abdominal pain (resulting from abruptio placentae)
   h. Absence of fetal movement (resulting from fetal compromise)
   i. Premature labor

3. **Physical findings** may include the following:
   a. Elevated BP
   b. Proteinuria
   c. Retinal vascular spasm on funduscopic examination
   d. Bibasilar rales on cardiovascular examination
   e. Right upper quadrant tenderness (secondary to hepatic edema causing stretching of the liver capsule)
   f. Uterine tenderness, or uterine tetany secondary to abruptio placentae on abdominal examination
   g. Nondependent edema (face and hands)

4. **Laboratory findings** *may* include the following:
   a. Increase in hematocrit (resulting from decreased intravascular volume)
   b. Proteinuria greater than 300 mg/dL in a 24-hour collection (or score of 1+ or higher on dipstick test)
   c. Uric acid level higher than 5 mg/dL, which is abnormal in pregnancy but is not used to diagnose preeclampsia
   d. Creatinine level of 0.9 mg/dL or higher, which is abnormal in pregnancy (see sec. **I.B.1.b.(3)**)
   e. Elevated liver enzyme levels, indicated by AST level higher than 70 U/L
   f. Platelet count lower than 100,000/mm^3
   g. Prolonged prothrombin and partial thromboplastin times, which may be a result of primary coagulopathy or abruptio placentae
   h. Decreased fibrinogen, fibrin degradation products, or both as a result of coagulopathy or abruptio placentae

D. **Prevention**

1. **Calcium supplementation.** Ingestion of 2 g of elemental calcium per day has not been shown to be beneficial in the general population; however, in populations at risk with low calcium intake, supplementation may lower the risk of preeclampsia.

2. **Aspirin.** Multicenter randomized clinical trials with aggregate enrollment of more than 27,000 women have demonstrated minimal to no benefit to low-dose aspirin therapy in preventing preeclampsia; therefore, it is not recommended at this time.

3. **Diuretics and salt restriction** have no role in the prevention of preeclampsia.

E. **Management. Definitive treatment for preeclampsia or eclampsia and transient hypertension is delivery.** For patients presenting at more than 34 weeks' gestation with these conditions, delivery should be considered. The urgency of delivery depends on severity.

1. **Mild preeclampsia.** If the gestation is remote from term when mild preeclampsia is discovered, the patient may be managed expectantly. Salt restriction, use of sedatives, and antihypertensive therapy do not improve fetal outcome.
   a. **Outpatient** management. Some compliant patients with mild preeclampsia may be managed at home with home BP monitoring and twice-weekly fetal testing.
   b. **Inpatient** management consists of the following measures:
      (1) Bed rest
      (2) Regular diet (no salt restriction)
      (3) BP measurement every 4 hours while awake
      (4) Daily review of weight, urine output, and symptoms, with examination for edema, deep tendon reflex check, and fetal movement count
      (5) Every-other-day 24-hour urine protein measurement
      (6) Twice weekly hematocrit measurement, platelet count, and measurement of AST level
      (7) Fetal growth sonogram no more frequently than every 2 weeks
      (8) Fetal surveillance with weekly or semiweekly nonstress test (NST) or biophysical profiles
2. **Severe preeclampsia**
   a. The mother's safety must be considered above all. The first priority is to assess and stabilize maternal condition, particularly coagulation abnormalities.
   b. **At 34 weeks' gestation or later,** delivery is the optimal treatment. Immediate delivery by cesarean section is not indicated in every case. Patients in labor, or with a cervical condition favorable to the initiation of labor with oxytocin, can deliver vaginally. Both maternal and fetal conditions must be monitored continuously, however, with hourly assessments and careful attention to intake and output.
   c. **Before 34 weeks' gestation,** patients may be managed expectantly if their BP can be controlled adequately without antihypertensives and if bed rest reduces their symptoms and produces diuresis.
      (1) Between 24 and 34 weeks' gestation, patients who are candidates for expectant management should receive a course of antenatal steroid therapy to induce fetal lung maturity.
      (2) At 24 weeks' gestation and earlier, the prognosis for perinatal survival is extremely poor, and termination of the pregnancy should be considered for maternal welfare.
      (3) Between 25 and 27 weeks' gestation, in selected cases, aggressive in utero therapy at a tertiary care center in consultation with a maternal-fetal medicine specialist may give the fetus a better chance for perinatal survival than immediate delivery. If the patient has none of the factors that necessitate delivery, aggressive antihypertensive therapy (see sec. **II.E.6**) may be used to keep the diastolic BP below 105 until hypertension can no longer be controlled or fetal testing (which may need to be done twice a day) shows increased fetal compromise.
   d. **Inpatient management** of severe preeclampsia. Patients who are eligible to be followed expectantly should receive the following:
      (1) Bed rest
      (2) Seizure prophylaxis for the first 24 hours of hospitalization (see sec. **II.E.4**)
      (3) BP measurement every 4 hours
      (4) Daily examination to assess weight, review systems, check for edema, and check deep tendon reflexes; evaluation of 24-hour urine specimen for volume and protein level measurement; CBC

with platelet count; and measurement of AST, LDH, and bilirubin levels

(5) Daily fetal surveillance including fetal movement counts and NST or biophysical profile

3. **HELLP syndrome.** Management is the same as for severe preeclampsia—delivery. The average time for resolution of symptoms is 4 days. If, however, the only presenting symptom is thrombocytopenia, without elevated levels on liver function tests, antepartum treatment with steroids may be used in cases of gestation shorter than 28 weeks. Dosage is 10 mg intramuscular/intravenous (IV) dexamethasone every 12 hours until platelets exceed 100,000/mm³. If no response is seen by 24–48 hours or the patient's condition worsens, the patient should be delivered. Postpartum patients with thrombocytopenia may be similarly treated with dexamethasone. Quicker postpartum resolution of signs and symptoms may be achieved by removing all trophoblastic tissue through uterine curettage.

4. **Seizure prophylaxis** during labor and for 24 hours postpartum is necessary for all patients with preeclampsia. Some patients with severe preeclampsia need seizure prophylaxis for longer periods before and after delivery than do patients with less severe preeclampsia.

   a. **Magnesium sulfate ($MgSO_4$)**
   (1) Loading dose is 6 g IV administered over 15–20 minutes.
   (2) Maintenance dosage is 2 g/hour IV and may be titrated to higher doses.
   (3) The therapeutic magnesium level is 4–6 mEq/L.
   (4) Magnesium level should be checked 4 hours after administering the loading dose, then every 6 hours as needed.
   (5) $MgSO_4$ (50% solution) may also be given intramuscularly into the upper quadrant of the buttocks. Loading dose is 5 g in both buttocks. Maintenance dose is 3 g in alternating buttocks every 4 hours. Therapeutic range and monitoring are the same as with IV administration.

   b. **Phenytoin (Dilantin)**
   (1) Loading dose is based on maternal weight (Table 14-1).
   (2) The first 750 mg of the loading dose should be given at 25 mg/minute and the remainder at 12.5 mg/minute. If the patient shows a normal cardiac rhythm and has no history of heart disease before initiation of therapy, ECG monitoring is not necessary at this rate of infusion.
   (3) Thirty to 60 minutes after infusion, a serum phenytoin level should be obtained. The therapeutic level is higher than 12 μg/mL. If the findings show levels lower than 10 μg/mL, reloading with 500 mg should be performed and the level rechecked in 30–60 minutes. If levels of 10–12 μg/mL are found, a reloading dose of 250 mg should be administered and the level rechecked in 30–60 minutes.

TABLE 14-1. LOADING DOSE FOR PHENYTOIN (DILANTIN)

Maternal weight (kg)	Dose (mg)
<50	1000
50–70	1250
>70	1500

      (4) If the serum phenytoin level is therapeutic at 30–60 minutes, the level should be rechecked in 12 hours.

      (5) Phenytoin has no tocolytic effect.

  c. **Comparative efficacy.** $MgSO_4$ was shown to be superior to phenytoin in preventing seizures in a recent trial. However, individualization of phenytoin dosage, as recommended here, was not followed in that trial.

5. Conditions that necessitate delivery irrespective of gestational age include the following:

  a. Eclampsia

  b. Thrombocytopenia with a platelet level of less than $100,000/mm^3$

  c. Hemolysis (seen on peripheral blood smear)

  d. Elevated liver enzyme levels

  e. Pulmonary edema

  f. Oliguria

  g. Persistent need for antihypertensive medication, except in selected cases between 25 and 27 weeks' gestation [see sec. **II.E.2.c.(3)**]

6. Antihypertensive therapy is indicated for antepartum, intrapartum, and postpartum patients with a diastolic BP of 105 mm Hg or higher. Acute treatment for severe hypertension in pregnancy involves reducing BP in a controlled manner without reducing uteroplacental perfusion. The goal is not to make the patient normotensive but rather to reduce the patient's diastolic BP to 90–100 mm Hg. A rapid or significant drop in BP interferes with uteroplacental perfusion and results in fetal heart rate decelerations.

  a. **Hydralazine hydrochloride,** administered IV, is the drug of choice for acute BP control.

    (1) The onset of action is 10–20 minutes, with a peak effect in 60 minutes and a duration of effect of 4–6 hours.

    (2) Intermittent bolus infusion should be used rather than continuous infusion.

    (3) Hydralazine decreases BP without sacrificing uteroplacental blood flow.

    (4) Dosing should begin with a 5-mg bolus, and if BP is not in the range of 150–140 mm Hg systolic and 100–90 mm Hg diastolic at 20 minutes, the bolus should be repeated at a dose of 5–10 mg. Boluses may be repeated every 20 minutes, and doses may be increased to a maximum of 20 mg if no response occurs.

    (5) A decrease in urine output may occur 2–3 hours after a bolus when diastolic BP is below 90 mm Hg.

  b. **Labetalol hydrochloride,** administered IV, is an alternative therapy to IV hydralazine for women who cannot be given or have not responded to hydralazine.

    (1) Labetalol has a more rapid onset than hydralazine and, like hydralazine, maintains uteroplacental perfusion.

    (2) Labetalol is contraindicated if maternal heart block of greater than first degree is present.

    (3) Labetalol is given as escalating boluses or a continuous infusion. The escalating bolus protocol begins with boluses every 10 minutes of 20, 40, 80, 80, and 80 mg, to a maximum dose of 300 mg. The continuous-infusion protocol starts at 0.5 mg/kg/hour and increases every 30 minutes by 0.5 mg/kg/hour to a maximum dose of 3 mg/kg/hour.

    (4) Conversion from intermittent boluses to infusion may be accomplished by beginning the continuous infusion after the BP has started to rise but not immediately after the last bolus. Infusion should be started at the lowest rate and titrated to the final infusion rate to avoid overdosing the patient.

c. **Intravenous trimethaphan (Arfonad)**
   (1) Trimethaphan can be used to treat sudden-onset extreme hypertension requiring minute-to-minute titration.
   (2) Trimethaphan is a ganglionic blocker and an extremely potent agent, and it is best used for hypertensive emergencies that occur intraoperatively at the time of delivery. The dosage is 5–30 µg/kg/minute. It is most often administered by an anesthesiologist.

7. **Fluid management.** Patients with preeclampsia frequently are hypovolemic because of loss of fluid into the interstitial spaces due to low serum oncotic pressure and because of increased capillary permeability. These same abnormalities, however, also put these patients at increased risk for pulmonary edema. IV fluids should be restricted to 84–125 mL/hour.

   a. **Oliguria** is defined as urine output of less than 100 mL in 4 hours; it is treated with a 500-mL bolus of crystalloid fluid if the lungs are clear. If no response to this treatment occurs, then another 500-mL bolus can be given. If there is still no response after a total of 1 L has been administered, central hemodynamic monitoring should guide further management.

   b. **Pulmonary edema.** Pulmonary artery catheterization is required to guide therapy for pulmonary edema.

   c. Central venous pressure monitoring does not correlate with pulmonary capillary wedge pressure in all situations; therefore, use of a Swan-Ganz catheter may be required.

   d. Patients usually enter a diuresis phase 12–24 hours after delivery. In cases of severe renal compromise, it may take 72 hours or more for diuresis to appear.

F. **Complications of severe preeclampsia** include renal failure (acute tubular necrosis), acute cortical necrosis, cardiac failure, pulmonary edema, thrombocytopenia, disseminated intravascular coagulopathy, and cerebrovascular accidents.

G. **Perinatal outcome.** Complication of pregnancy by severe preeclampsia is associated with high perinatal mortality and morbidity rates. These high rates are attributable to extreme prematurity, intrauterine growth retardation (IUGR), abruptio placentae, and perinatal asphyxia. Patients whose onset of severe preeclampsia occurs in the second trimester and those with HELLP syndrome and pulmonary edema are at significant risk of maternal morbidity. HELLP syndrome is associated with particularly poor maternal and perinatal outcomes. The reported perinatal fetal mortality rate ranges from 7.7% to 60.0%, and the reported maternal mortality ranges from 0% to 24%. Maternal morbidity is common. Many patients with HELLP syndrome require transfusions of blood and blood products and are at increased risk of acute renal failure, pulmonary edema, ascites, cerebral edema, and hepatic rupture. HELLP syndrome also is associated with high incidences of abruptio placentae and disseminated intravascular coagulopathy.

III. **Eclampsia** is defined as the development of convulsions, coma, or both in a patient with preeclampsia. Eclampsia occurs in 1% of patients with preeclampsia. Although many other conditions can result in seizures during pregnancy, obstetric patients with seizures should be considered eclamptic until proven otherwise. Perinatal mortality in one U.S. series was 12%, attributable to extreme prematurity, abruptio placentae, and IUGR.

A. **Clinical presentation.** Maternal complications may include pulmonary edema, aspiration pneumonitis, abruptio placentae with hemorrhage, cardiac failure, intracranial hemorrhage, and transient blindness.

B. **Pathophysiology.** The etiology of eclamptic seizures is unknown. It is thought that eclampsia occurs when the patient's mean arterial pressure exceeds the upper limit of cerebral autoregulation. The arterioles then fail to protect the cerebral capillaries from the systemic hypertension. Increased cerebral edema, increased intracranial pressure, or both may play a role.

C. **Management.** Eclampsia is an obstetric emergency requiring immediate treatment.
   1. Goals of therapy include the following:
      a. Control of seizures
      b. Correction of hypoxia and acidosis
      c. Control of severe hypertension
      d. Delivery
   2. **Methods of therapy**
      a. **Control of seizures. Magnesium sulfate,** administered parenterally, is the treatment of choice for eclamptic seizures in the United States. The alternative treatment is phenytoin. Treatment protocols for both agents are the same as the protocols for seizure prophylaxis (see sec. **II.E.4**).
         (1) The magnesium maintenance dosage should be decreased as indicated by clinical factors (absent deep tendon reflexes, decreased respiratory rate, oliguria, or renal insufficiency) or plasma magnesium levels.
         (2) Duration of therapy is 24 hours postdelivery or 24 hours after a postpartum seizure.
         (3) Magnesium toxicity may occur when therapeutic levels are exceeded. Loss of patellar reflexes occurs at 8–10 mEq/L, respiratory depression or arrest occurs at 12 mEq/L, and mental status changes may occur at levels higher than 12 mEq/L. To treat magnesium toxicity, magnesium administration should be discontinued and plasma magnesium level determined. Therapy should begin, however, based on a clinical diagnosis. Airway and oxygenation should be maintained; mechanical ventilation may be necessary. Ventilation and oxygenation should be monitored by pulse oximetry. Calcium gluconate should be administered in a dose of 1 g IV over at least 3 minutes. ECG changes and arrhythmias may occur if toxicity is severe. Diuretic agents (furosemide, mannitol) may be administered.
         (4) The loading dose of $MgSO_4$ is 6 g over 15–20 minutes IV. If the patient has a seizure after administration of the loading dose, another bolus of 2 g of $MgSO_4$ can be administered over 3–5 minutes.
         (5) If seizures occur while the patient is receiving magnesium prophylaxis, the magnesium level should be checked. If the level is subtherapeutic (therapeutic range is 4–6 mEq/L), an additional 2-g bolus of $MgSO_4$ should be administered slowly, at a rate not to exceed 1 g/minute. Plasma magnesium level should be measured immediately. If the level is therapeutic, IV phenytoin is used to treat seizures refractory to $MgSO_4$. The treatment protocol for phenytoin is same as the prophylaxis protocol (see sec. **II.E.4**).
         (6) Status epilepticus is treated with diazepam, administered IV at a rate of 1 mg/minute, or up to 250 mg of sodium amobarbital, slowly administered IV.
      b. **Protection of the patient from harm during seizures.** The patient must never be left unattended. Bedside rails should be elevated, and a padded tongue depressor should be available to prevent oral lacerations.
      c. **Control of the airway and ventilation.** Pulse oximetry should be performed or arterial blood gas levels obtained. The patient may require oxygen administration by mask or endotracheal tube. Difficulty in oxygenating patients with repetitive seizures warrants a chest radiographic examination to rule out aspiration pneumonia.
      d. **Treatment of hypertension.** Treatment of hypertension in eclampsia is the same as treatment in preeclampsia (see sec. **II.E.6**).

TABLE 14-2. GRADES OF CHRONIC HYPERTENSION

Grade	Diastolic BP (mm Hg)
Mild	90–104
Moderate	105–114
Severe	≥115

    e. **Delivery of the fetus.** Induction of labor may begin, or a cesarean section may be performed, after the patient is stabilized. Although prompt delivery is desirable, vaginal delivery may be attempted in the absence of other maternal or fetal complications. During the acute eclamptic episode, fetal bradycardia is common and usually resolves spontaneously in 3–5 minutes. Immediate delivery for fetal bradycardia is unnecessary. Allowing the fetus to recover in utero from the maternal seizure, hypoxia, and hypercarbia before delivery is advantageous. If the fetal bradycardia persists beyond 10 minutes, however, abruptio placentae should be suspected. Preparation for emergency cesarean section should always be made in case maternal or fetal condition deteriorates.

    f. **Limitation of fluids except in cases of excessive fluid loss.** Frequent chest auscultation to rule out pulmonary edema and accurate monitoring of urine output using an indwelling Foley catheter are necessary. Pulmonary edema and refractory oliguria are indications for invasive hemodynamic monitoring.

D. **Outcome.** Long-term neurologic sequelae of eclampsia are rare. CNS imaging with CT or MRI should be performed if seizures are of late onset (longer than 48 hours after delivery) or if neurologic deficits are clinically evident. The signs and symptoms of preeclampsia usually resolve within 1–2 weeks postpartum. Approximately 25% of eclamptic patients develop preeclampsia in subsequent pregnancies, with a recurrence of eclampsia in 2% of cases.

IV. **Chronic hypertension** is defined and graded by diastolic pressure and carries increased risks of preterm delivery, superimposed preeclampsia, abruptio placentae, and IUGR.

A. **Grades of chronic hypertension** are listed in Table 14-2.

B. **Baseline information,** including the following data, should be gathered to aid management.
1. History of the duration of hypertension
2. History of current and previous treatments
3. Other cardiovascular risk factors (smoking, increased plasma lipid levels, obesity, diabetes mellitus)
4. Other complicating medical factors (e.g., headaches, myocardial infarction or chest pain, prior stroke, renal disease)
5. Medication with vasoactive drugs (e.g., sympathomimetic amines, nasal decongestants, diet pills)
6. Baseline blood values, including CBC, serum creatinine, serum urea nitrogen, uric acid, and serum calcium
7. Urinalysis findings
8. Twenty-four-hour urine test results for creatinine clearance and protein
9. ECG, if the patient has not had one in the past 6 months
10. Twenty-four-hour urine calcium measurement

C. **Differential diagnosis**
1. Essential hypertension is the cause in 90% of chronic hypertension cases. Other conditions should be ruled out, however, including renal disease; endocrine disorders such as adrenal disease (primary aldosteronism, con-

genital adrenal hyperplasia, Cushing disease, pheochromocytoma), diabetes mellitus, and hyperthyroidism; new onset of a collagen vascular disease such as systemic lupus erythematosus; and cocaine abuse.

2. Worsening chronic hypertension is difficult to distinguish from superimposed preeclampsia. If seizures, thrombocytopenia, pulmonary edema, unexplained hemolysis, or unexplained elevations in liver enzyme levels develop, superimposed preeclampsia should be presumed and the fetus delivered. If these findings are not present, a 24-hour urine calcium measurement may be useful. Patients with preeclampsia have significantly lower 24-hour urinary calcium findings (42 ± 29 mg/24 hours) than pregnant patients with chronic hypertension (223 ± 41 mg/24 hours).

D. **Treatment**

1. Patients with mild hypertension, and some with moderate hypertension, may be managed initially without drug therapy, using the following measures:

   a. Dietary sodium restriction to 4 g
   b. Cessation of smoking and alcohol use
   c. Decrease in activity
   d. Sonography at 18 weeks' gestation, then every 4–6 weeks to follow fetal growth; sonograms may be taken more frequently if indicated, but no more frequently than every 3 weeks
   e. Antepartum testing, to begin at 32 weeks' gestation (or earlier if hypertension is severe or IUGR is suspected)
   f. NST or biophysical profile assessment weekly or biweekly depending on the severity of the hypertension

2. **Angiotensin-converting enzyme (ACE) inhibitors and diuretics should be avoided in pregnancy.** If, however, a diuretic is an essential component in maintaining control for a patient with severe hypertension, it may be continued.

3. **Drug therapy initiated during pregnancy.** Choices for single-agent drug therapy for diastolic BP greater than 105 mm Hg include the following:

   a. **Methyldopa** (Aldomet), 250 mg three times daily, up to 2 g/day, in four doses. Methyldopa is a centrally acting adrenergic inhibitor that decreases systemic vascular resistance and has been shown to be safe in pregnancy. It can produce hepatic damage, so liver enzyme levels should be checked at least once a trimester.
   b. **Hydralazine** often is used as a second agent when maximum dosages of methyldopa are reached. Hydralazine should not be used as first-line oral therapy. It is a peripheral direct vasodilator and can be used effectively in combination with methyldopa or a beta-blocker. Hydralazine can produce a lupus-like syndrome, but usually only when used at dosages higher than 200 mg/day for longer than 6 months. It can lead to fluid retention. The dosage starts at 10 mg four times a day initially and may be increased to a maximum of 200 mg/day.
   c. **Labetalol** is safe for use in pregnancy and can be given to patients who cannot take methyldopa or in whom methyldopa is ineffective. Labetalol is a nonspecific beta- and alpha-blocker, and its use is contraindicated in patients who have greater than first-degree heart block. Labetalol may be used as monotherapy but also works well in combination with hydralazine or a diuretic. The beginning dosage is usually 200 mg two to three times daily; the usual therapeutic dosage is 1600 mg/day, and the maximum dosage is 2400 mg/day.

4. **Drug therapy initiated before pregnancy.** If necessary for adequate BP control, most patients can continue to use the antihypertensive agents they used before pregnancy, with the exception of nifedipine and ACE inhibitors.

   a. **Thiazide diuretics** should not be started late in pregnancy.

    b. **Clonidine** withdrawal may produce acute hypertension. Clonidine may be used safely in pregnancy.

    c. **Beta-blockers** may be used safely in pregnancy.

    d. **Nifedipine** is a calcium channel blocker that is teratogenic in animals but has been used in the third trimester of pregnancy in humans. Nifedipine is potentially hazardous because its use may lead to acute hypotension. It is used as a tocolytic agent and should not be given within 6 hours of $MgSO_4$ administration due to an increased risk of pulmonary edema and hypotension.

    e. **ACE inhibitors** are contraindicated after the first trimester of pregnancy. They are not teratogenic but are associated with fetal death in utero and neonatal renal failure.

5. **Emergency treatment for hypertensive crisis**

    a. IV therapy for patients with hypertensive emergencies in pregnancy is the same as that for patients with preeclampsia (see sec. **II.E.6**).

    b. Sodium nitroprusside may cause fetal thiocyanate and cyanide poisoning and should be used only as a last resort and for no longer than 30 minutes before delivery.

15. CARDIOPULMONARY DISORDERS OF PREGNANCY

Cynthia Holcroft and Ernest Graham

CARDIAC DISORDERS

Cardiovascular disorders complicate 1% of all pregnancies and include preexisting disease as well as conditions that develop during pregnancy or in the postpartum period.

I. **Hemodynamic changes during pregnancy.** The enormous changes in the cardiovascular system during pregnancy carry many implications for the management of cardiac disease in the pregnant patient. These changes influence labor management and appropriate care during the antepartum and postpartum periods.

   A. **Blood volume.** By 32 weeks' gestation, total blood volume expands by 40%, with an increase in the total plasma volume up to 50%. Nonetheless, because the red cell mass only increases by 20%, dilutional anemia results.

   B. **Cardiac output.** Increased stroke volume causes cardiac output to increase 30–50% by 20–24 weeks' gestational age. A marked decrease in cardiac output can occur, however, when a pregnant woman is in the supine position because of caval compression.

   C. **Systemic vascular resistance** decreases during pregnancy. It reaches its nadir during the second trimester and then slowly returns to prepregnancy levels by term.

   D. **Redistribution of blood flow.** During pregnancy, blood flow to the kidneys, skin, and uterus increases. Uterine blood flow reaches as high as 500 mL/minute at term.

   E. **Hemodynamic changes during labor.** Venous pressure increases during labor because uterine contractions cause an increase of venous return from the uterine veins. In turn, this results in higher cardiac output, increased right ventricular pressure, and increased mean arterial pressure.

   F. **Postpartum hemodynamic changes.** In the postpartum period, caval compression decreases, which results in an increase of the circulating blood volume. Higher cardiac output ensues, and a reflex bradycardia may occur. Because of increased blood loss, these hemodynamic changes become less pronounced in patients undergoing cesarean section.

II. **Cardiac diseases in pregnancy**

   A. **Diagnosis and evaluation**

   1. **Signs and symptoms** of cardiac disease overlap common symptoms and findings in pregnancy and include fatigue, shortness of breath, orthopnea, palpitations, edema, systolic flow murmur, and a third heart sound.

   2. **Warning signs.** Because of the difficulty of distinguishing cardiac disease from the changes of normal pregnancy, particular attention must be paid to warning signs, including the following:
      a. Worsening dyspnea on exertion, or dyspnea at rest
      b. Chest pain with exercise or activity
      c. Syncope preceded by palpitations or exertion
      d. Loud systolic murmurs or diastolic murmurs
      e. Cyanosis or clubbing
      f. Jugular venous distention
      g. Cardiomegaly or a ventricular heave

   3. **Evaluation** of cardiac disease includes a thorough history taking and physical examination. Tests include chest radiography to assess cardiomegaly and pulmonary vascular prominence; ECG to assess ischemic, acute, or chronic changes in cardiac function; and echocardiogram to assess ventricular function and structural abnormalities.

B. **Management of patients with known cardiac disease**
   1. Ideally, patients receive preconception evaluation and counseling. If they are already pregnant, however, patients require cardiac assessment as early as possible.
   2. Patients need close **monitoring** throughout pregnancy and preferably are followed by both an obstetrician and a cardiologist. Clinicians must pay close attention to signs or symptoms of worsening CHF. Each visit should include the following:
      a. Cardiac examination and cardiac review of systems
      b. Documentation of weight, BP, and pulse
      c. Evaluation of peripheral edema
   3. If a patient's symptoms worsen, hospitalization, bed rest, diuresis, or correction of an underlying arrhythmia may be required. Sometimes, surgical correction during pregnancy becomes necessary; when possible, procedures should be performed during the early second trimester to avoid the period of fetal organogenesis, but before more significant hemodynamic changes of pregnancy occur.
   4. **Medical management**
      a. **Prophylaxis** for endocarditis. In 1997, the American Heart Association published a consensus statement declaring that the majority of obstetric and gynecologic procedures do not require prophylactic antibiotic treatment for subacute bacterial endocarditis because of the low likelihood of bacteremia (1–5% for a vaginal delivery). Intravenous (IV) antibiotics should be administered on a case-by-case basis if bacteremia is suspected. **For patients at high risk of developing endocarditis (Table 15-1), prophylaxis is optional, both for vaginal hysterectomies and for vaginal deliveries (Table 15-2).** At the same time, many obstetricians still administer prophylaxis for subacute bacterial endocarditis to patients with high-risk lesions due to the relatively low risk of prophylactic antibiotic treatment compared to the complications of endocarditis. Antibiotic prophylaxis consists of 2 g of ampicillin IV or intramuscularly plus 1.5 mg/kg of gentamicin IV or intramuscularly before the procedure, followed by one dose of ampicillin 8 hours postpartum. In the event of penicillin allergy, 1 g of vancomycin IV can be substituted.
      b. Patients with **rheumatic heart disease** require either 1.2 million U of penicillin G every month or daily oral penicillin or erythromycin.
      c. If **anticoagulation** is necessary, heparin sodium remains the drug of choice due to the potential teratogenetic effects of warfarin sodium (Coumadin).
C. **Counseling.** A patient with cardiac disease must be informed about the added risk of pregnancy to herself and her fetus. If the pregnancy poses a serious threat to maternal health, the patient must be offered termination of pregnancy.
III. **Valvar heart disease**
   A. **Mitral valve prolapse** remains the most common congenital heart defect in young women, but it rarely affects maternal or fetal outcome. Signs and symptoms may include a midsystolic click or palpitations.
   B. **Mitral stenosis** is the most common rheumatic heart disease in pregnancy. In this disorder, mitral insufficiency gradually progresses to mitral stenosis. Up to 10 years may elapse before the patient experiences symptoms arising from decreased cardiac output. Eventually, left atrial outflow obstruction develops, which leads to increased atrial pressure and increased pulmonary capillary wedge pressure. Pulmonary congestion later results in pulmonary hypertension and right heart failure. The increased plasma volume of pregnancy imposes great stress on the cardiovascular system of a woman with mitral stenosis because of the fixed cardiac output. Up to 20% of pregnant patients with mitral stenosis

TABLE 15-1. PROPHYLAXIS RECOMMENDATIONS FOR CARDIAC CONDITIONS ASSOCIATED WITH ENDOCARDITIS

Endocarditis prophylaxis recommended	Endocarditis prophylaxis not recommended
High-risk category	Negligible-risk category
Prosthetic cardiac valves	Isolated secundum atrial septal defect
Previous bacterial endocarditis	Surgical repair of atrial septal defect, ventricular septal defect, or patent ductus arteriosus (without residua beyond 6 mos)
Complex cyanotic congenital heart disease	
Surgically constructed systemic pulmonary shunts or conduits	Previous coronary artery bypass graft surgery
	Mitral valve prolapse without valvar regurgitation
Moderate-risk category	Physiologic functional or innocent heart murmurs
Most other congenital cardiac malformations (other than those listed)	Previous Kawasaki disease without valvar dysfunction
Acquired valvar dysfunction (e.g., rheumatic heart disease)	Previous rheumatic fever without valvar dysfunction
Hypertrophic cardiomyopathy	Cardiac pacemakers and implanted defibrillators
Mitral valve prolapse with valvar regurgitation or thickened leaflets, or both	

Adapted from Dajani AS, Taubert KA, Wilson W, et al. Prevention of bacterial endocarditis. Recommendations by the American Heart Association. *JAMA* 1997;277:1794–1801, with permission.

TABLE 15-2. ENDOCARDITIS PROPHYLAXIS RECOMMENDATIONS FOR VARIOUS GENITOURINARY TRACT PROCEDURES

Endocarditis prophylaxis recommended	Endocarditis prophylaxis not recommended
Genitourinary tract	Genitourinary tract
Cystoscopy	Vaginal hysterectomy
Urethral dilation	Vaginal delivery[a]
	Cesarean section[a]
	In uninfected tissue:
	Urethral catheterization
	Uterine dilatation and curettage
	Therapeutic abortion
	Sterilization procedures
	Insertion or removal of intrauterine devices

[a]Prophylaxis optional for high-risk patients.
Adapted from Dajani AS, Taubert KA, Wilson W, et al. Prevention of bacterial endocarditis. Recommendations by the American Heart Association. *JAMA* 1997;277:1794–1801, with permission.

become symptomatic by 20 weeks' gestation, when cardiac output is at its maximum.

1. **Management.** During pregnancy, affected patients should limit their physical activity. If volume overload is present, they should receive careful diuresis. Arrhythmias, especially atrial fibrillation, should be controlled to avoid decreased diastolic filling time. If medical management fails, the patient may require a valve replacement or commissurotomy.

2. **Considerations during labor.** Cesarean section should be performed for obstetric indications only. If significant heart disease exists, especially with pulmonary hypertension, invasive cardiac monitoring with a Swan-Ganz catheter should be considered during labor. The patient should undergo labor in the left lateral position and receive supplemental oxygen.

   a. **Tachycardia** should be prevented because it may lead to decreased cardiac output caused by a decreased diastolic filling time. Verapamil hydrochloride or digoxin may be used to slow the ventricular contraction rate if an atrial arrhythmia is present. Anesthetics may be useful in slowing sinus tachycardia. If an epidural anesthetic is used, care must be taken to prevent hypotension. If necessary, alpha-adrenergic agonists may be used to maintain systemic vascular resistance.

   b. The second stage of labor may be shortened by performing a **forceps delivery or vacuum extraction delivery.**

C. **Mitral regurgitation** may occur in patients with a history of rheumatic fever or endocarditis, idiopathic hypertrophic subaortic stenosis, or, most commonly, mitral valve prolapse. Typically a decrescendo murmur is detected. This murmur, however, is often diminished during pregnancy. In most cases, mitral regurgitation is tolerated well during pregnancy.

   1. In severe cases, the onset of symptoms usually occurs later than in cases of mitral stenosis. Atrial enlargement and fibrillation, as well as ventricular enlargement and dysfunction, may develop. Administration of inotropic agents may be necessary if left ventricular dilatation and dysfunction are present.

   2. During labor, patients with advanced disease may require central monitoring. The pain of labor may lead to an increase in BP and afterload, which cause pulmonary vascular congestion. Therefore, epidural anesthesia is recommended.

D. **Aortic stenosis** is rarely seen in pregnancy. It is a late complication of rheumatic fever that develops over several decades. Patients are usually not symptomatic until the fifth or sixth decade of life. Symptoms, including angina and syncope on exertion, arise from obstruction of the left ventricular outflow tract, which leads to compromised cardiac output. Sudden death from hypotension may occur. After symptoms appear, decompensation is usually rapid, with a 50% mortality in 5 years.

   1. During pregnancy, mortality for patients with aortic stenosis may be as high as 17%.

   2. Because this disorder is characterized by a fixed afterload, adequate end-diastolic volume, and therefore adequate filling pressure, is necessary to maintain cardiac output. Consequently, great care must be taken to prevent hypotension and tachycardia caused by blood loss, regional anesthesia, or other medications. Patients should be hydrated adequately and placed in the left lateral position to maximize venous return. Central monitoring with a Swan-Ganz catheter is recommended in severe cases. Affected patients should receive antibiotic prophylaxis.

E. **Aortic regurgitation** is often a late complication of rheumatic fever that appears 10 years after the acute disease episode. Aortic regurgitation also may be seen with congenital bifid aortic valves or with dilatation of the aortic root, such as occurs in Marfan syndrome. Symptoms usually develop in the fourth or fifth decade of life. Typically, the patient has a high-pitched, blowing murmur. Because of decreased systemic vascular resistance during pregnancy, regurgitation often decreases, and the condition is usually well tolerated.

1. If a patient shows evidence of left heart failure and requires valve replacement, pregnancy should be delayed until after the repair has been completed. If a patient is not yet symptomatic, she should be encouraged to complete her childbearing early, before the onset of symptoms.

2. During labor, afterload reduction by epidural anesthesia is recommended. Bradycardia is poorly tolerated because the increased time of diastole allows more time for regurgitation. A heart rate of 80–100 beats/minute should be maintained.

IV. **Congenital lesions**

A. **Left-to-right shunts** generally are corrected during childhood. If the defect has been corrected, the outcome of pregnancy is usually good. If the defect has not been corrected, pregnancy causes only a slight increase in the degree of shunting. If pulmonary hypertension has caused reversal of the shunt, however, the outcome of pregnancy is dismal, with a high rate of maternal mortality.

1. **Atrial septal defects** are the most common congenital heart lesions in adults. Affected patients usually exhibit a pulmonary ejection murmur and a second heart sound that is split in both the inspiratory and expiratory phases. The defects are usually very well tolerated unless they are associated with pulmonary hypertension. Complications such as atrial arrhythmias, pulmonary hypertension, and heart failure usually do not arise until the fifth decade of life and are therefore uncommon in pregnancy.

   a. For patients without complications, no special therapy or management is necessary during labor.

   b. If the patient has advanced disease, the patient should be observed for the development of atrial dilatation, supraventricular arrhythmias, pulmonary hypertension, and heart failure. During labor, invasive cardiac monitoring should be considered, and arrhythmias and tachycardia should be promptly treated.

2. **Ventricular septal defects (VSDs)** often close spontaneously. Large lesions are generally corrected surgically in childhood, so significant VSDs are rarely seen in pregnancy. Rarely, uncorrected lesions lead to significant left-to-right shunts with pulmonary hypertension, right ventricular failure, and reversal of the shunt.

   a. Because of the increased systemic vascular resistance during labor, epidural anesthesia is recommended. If the patient has pulmonary hypertension or right-to-left shunt, however, this decrease in systemic vascular resistance is poorly tolerated because of decreased perfusion of the lungs. The patient should undergo invasive cardiac monitoring via Swan-Ganz catheter and must be observed carefully for cyanosis in the presence of adequate cardiac output, which signals worsening of the right-to-left shunt.

   b. Fetal echocardiography is recommended. The incidence of VSD in the offspring of affected parents is 4%; however, small VSDs are often difficult to detect antenatally.

3. **Patent ductus arteriosus** is usually tolerated well during pregnancy unless pulmonary hypertension has developed. Because of increased volume, left heart failure and pulmonary hypertension usually worsen during pregnancy. Therefore, pregnancy is not recommended for patients with large patent ductus arteriosus and associated complications.

B. **Right-to-left shunts**

1. **Tetralogy of Fallot** is characterized by right ventricular outflow tract obstruction, ventricular septal defect, right ventricular hypertrophy, and overriding aorta. These conditions cause a right-to-left shunt and cyanosis. If the defect goes uncorrected, the affected patient rarely lives

beyond childhood. If pregnancy does occur, however, the incidence of heart failure is 40%. Affected patients should be observed carefully for evidence of left heart failure. The increased cardiac output associated with labor can lead to a worsening of the right-to-left shunt. The shunt can also worsen during the immediate postpartum period because of the decreases in systemic vascular resistance and blood volume.

   a. During pregnancy, the fetus should be monitored for intrauterine growth retardation. In addition, the patient should be counseled that maternal cyanosis is associated with spontaneous abortion and preterm birth.

   b. Invasive cardiac monitoring is appropriate during labor. Adequate venous return must be maintained; therefore, extreme caution must be exercised if an epidural or spinal anesthetic is used due to the risk of hypotension.

  2. **Coarctation of the aorta.** Severe cases of coarctation of the aorta are usually corrected in infancy. Surgical correction during pregnancy is recommended only if dissection occurs. Coarctation of the aorta is associated with other cardiac lesions as well as berry aneurysms.

   a. Coarctation of the aorta is characterized by a fixed cardiac output. Therefore, the patient's heart cannot meet the increased cardiac demands of pregnancy by increasing its beating rate, and extreme care must be taken to prevent hypotension.

   b. Two percent of infants of mothers with coarctation of the aorta may themselves exhibit cardiac lesions.

  3. **Eisenmenger's syndrome** occurs when an initial left-to-right shunt results in pulmonary arterial obliteration and pulmonary hypertension, which eventually causes a right-to-left shunt. This serious condition carries a maternal mortality rate of 50% during pregnancy and a fetal mortality rate of more than 50% if cyanosis is present. In addition, 30% of fetuses exhibit intrauterine growth retardation. Because of increased maternal mortality, termination of the pregnancy is advised. If the pregnancy is continued, special precautions must be taken during the peripartum period. The patient should be monitored with a Swan-Ganz catheter and care should be taken to avoid hypovolemia. Postpartum death most often occurs within 1 week after delivery; however, delayed deaths up to 4–6 weeks after delivery have been reported.

C. **Marfan syndrome** is an autosomal dominant disorder of the fibrillin gene characterized by weakness of the connective tissues. Cardiovascular manifestations may include aortic root dilatation, mitral valve prolapse, and aneurysms. Genetic counseling is recommended.

  1. Because great variability exists in the clinical expression of Marfan syndrome, individual evaluations concerning the safety and management of the pregnancy must be made. If a patient's cardiovascular involvement is minor and her aortic root diameter is smaller than 40 mm, the risks related to pregnancy are similar to those of the general population. If cardiovascular involvement is more extensive or the aortic root is larger than 40 mm, the risks of complications during pregnancy and aortic dissection are significantly increased.

  2. Hypertension should be avoided and managed with beta-blockers. Beta-blocker therapy should be considered for patients with Marfan syndrome from the second trimester until delivery, particularly if the aortic root is dilated. Regional anesthesia during labor is considered safe.

D. **Idiopathic hypertrophic subaortic stenosis** is an autosomal dominant disorder and manifests as left ventricular outflow tract obstruction secondary to a hypertrophic interventricular septum. Genetic counseling is advised for affected patients.

  1. Patients' conditions improve when left ventricular end-diastolic volume is maximized. Pregnant patients often fare quite well initially because

of an increase in circulating blood volume. Later in pregnancy, however, decreased systemic vascular resistance and decreased venous return caused by caval compression may worsen the obstruction. This may cause left ventricular failure as well as supraventricular arrhythmias from left atrial distention.

2. The following management points should be kept in mind during labor:
   a. Inotropic agents may exacerbate obstruction.
   b. The patient should undergo labor in the left lateral decubitus position.
   c. Medications that decrease systemic vascular resistance should be avoided or limited.
   d. Cardiac rhythm should be monitored and tachycardia treated promptly.
   e. The second stage of labor should be curtailed by operative delivery.

E. **Ebstein's anomaly** is a congenital malformation of the tricuspid valve in which the right ventricle must act as both an atrium and a ventricle. Ideally, if surgical correction is necessary, it should be performed before pregnancy.

F. **Congenital atrioventricular block.** Although affected patients may need a pacemaker, they usually fare well and do not require special treatment during pregnancy.

V. **Cardiomyopathy**

A. **Idiopathic** dilated cardiomyopathy may be caused by an autoimmune response. The heart becomes uniformly dilated, filling pressures increase, and cardiac output decreases. Eventually, heart failure develops and is often refractory to treatment. The 5-year survival rate is approximately 50%; therefore, careful preconceptional counseling is important, even if heart failure is absent.

B. **Peripartum** cardiomyopathy is a dilated cardiomyopathy of unknown cause that develops in the third trimester of pregnancy or the first 6 months postpartum. Of the patients who survive, approximately 50% recover normal left heart function, but the others retain permanent cardiomyopathy. The condition carries a mortality rate of 11–14% if cardiac size returns to normal within 6–12 months, and a mortality rate of 40–80% with persistent cardiomegaly. Due to the high maternal mortality, subsequent pregnancy in both groups is discouraged.

1. Risk factors include multiparity, increased maternal age, multiple gestations, and preeclampsia or eclampsia. Management of peripartum cardiomyopathy includes bed rest; sodium restriction; medical therapy with afterload reducers, diuretics, inotropics, anticoagulants, or some combination of these; and, in cases of advanced disease, transplantation.

2. Invasive cardiac monitoring should be considered during labor until at least 24 hours postpartum. Hydralazine hydrochloride, furosemide, or digoxin, or some combination of these, may be administered, as well as dopamine or dobutamine hydrochloride if necessary. The patient should be given supplemental oxygen and an epidural anesthetic for pain control, and the second stage of labor should be curtailed by operative delivery. Cesarean section is reserved for obstetric indications.

VI. **Arrhythmias.** Nonsustained arrhythmias in the absence of organic cardiac disease are best left untreated. Serious, life-threatening arrhythmias associated with an aberrant reentrant pathway should be treated before pregnancy by ablation. If medical therapy is necessary during pregnancy, established drugs—rather than new or experimental ones—should be used. Artificial pacing should have no effect on the fetus, nor should electrical defibrillation or cardioversion of the maternal heart.

VII. **Ischemic heart disease** is uncommon in pregnancy; however, the incidence has increased because of larger numbers of gravidas who are older or are smokers. Myocardial infarction during pregnancy is rare; the greatest risk factor is age over 35. Usually ischemic heart disease is caused by atherosclerosis, but emboli and coronary vasospasm also occur.

A. Approximately 67% of myocardial ischemia during pregnancy occurs during the third trimester. If myocardial infarction occurs before 24 weeks' gestation, termination of the pregnancy is recommended. If delivery takes place within 2 weeks of the acute event, the mortality rate reaches 50%; survival is much improved, however, if delivery takes place longer than 2 weeks after the acute event.

B. Management of myocardial infarction in a pregnant patient is the same as that in a nonpregnant patient.

C. Cesarean section should be reserved for the usual obstetric indications. If another pregnancy is desired, the patient should receive thorough preconception counseling and evaluation.

PULMONARY DISORDERS

I. **Physiologic changes during pregnancy.** Because of the remarkable amount of pulmonary reserve (during exercise, minute ventilation can increase by 1000%, but cardiac output only increases by 300%), patients with pulmonary disease are less likely to experience deterioration in their conditions during pregnancy.

A. **Structural alterations.** The mucosa of the upper respiratory tract becomes edematous and mucus production increases, which leads to a sensation of stuffiness and chronic cold symptoms. An increase in the subcostal angle occurs in pregnancy even before the uterus increases significantly in size. The transverse diameter and chest circumference also increase early in pregnancy. Later in pregnancy, the diaphragm is elevated, but diaphragmatic excursion with each breath increases.

B. **Oxygen consumption**

1. **Partial pressure of oxygen (PO_2).** Although minute ventilation increases by 30–40% during pregnancy, oxygen consumption increases by only 15–20%. Consequently, PO_2 levels increase to an average of 104–108 mm Hg. The increase in oxygen consumption is attributable to fetal and placental oxygen consumption, increased maternal cardiac output, increased glomerular filtration rate, and increased tissue mass of the breasts and uterus.

2. **Partial pressure of carbon dioxide (PCO_2).** Although carbon dioxide production increases during pregnancy, PCO_2 levels decrease to an average of 27–32 mm Hg because of the increased minute ventilation. This decrease facilitates carbon dioxide exchange between the mother and the fetus. Arterial pH increases only slightly because the decrease in PCO_2 levels is offset by a decrease in serum bicarbonate levels to an average of 18–31 mEq/L as a result of an increased rate of renal excretion.

C. **Tidal volume** increases by 30–40% in pregnancy. Progesterone lowers the carbon dioxide threshold in the respiratory center. The expiratory reserve volume and functional residual capacity decrease in pregnancy, but the respiratory rate and vital capacity remain the same.

D. **Resistance.** Forced expiratory volume and peak expiratory flow rate remain unchanged in pregnancy.

II. **Asthma.** Approximately 1% of pregnancies are complicated by asthma.

A. **Effect of pregnancy**

1. **Maternal effects.** The course of asthma in pregnancy varies, and a patient may be affected differently in one pregnancy than in another. There is no change in the severity of preexisting asthma in 22–49% of pregnancies. The asthma worsens in 9–23% of pregnancies and improves in 29–69% of pregnancies. (These percentages may be easier to remember as a rule of thirds: one-third of patients gets better, one-third gets worse, and one-third remains the same.)

2. **Fetal effects.** An increased risk of growth retardation has been demonstrated, especially if the mother receives long-term steroid therapy.

B. **Surveillance.** At each visit, a pulmonary examination, peak flow measurement, and review of symptoms should be undertaken. In addition, patients may monitor their peak flows at home and begin treatment before they become dangerously symptomatic. Influenza vaccination is recommended for patients with asthma, as well as for any pregnant patient.

C. **Management.** As asthma exacerbations can be severe, they should be treated aggressively in pregnancy.

1. **Medications**

   a. **Beta-sympathomimetic** drugs help control asthma by increasing cyclic adenosine monophosphate release, which causes relaxation of the bronchi. Preparations may be oral (e.g., terbutaline sulfate) or aerosolized (e.g., albuterol or metaproterenol sulfate). Aerosolized preparations cause fewer systemic side effects, such as tachycardia and hyperglycemia.

   b. **Anticholinergics** such as aerosolized ipratropium bromide or glycopyrrolate can also be used to treat severe asthma. Side effects include tachycardia.

   c. **Theophylline** inhibits phosphodiesterase and thereby increases circulating levels of cyclic adenosine monophosphate. Clearance of theophylline increases in the third trimester; therefore, theophylline levels need to be rechecked during this period.

   d. **Steroids.** Aerosolized steroids such as triamcinolone or beclomethasone dipropionate remain active locally with little systemic activity. Systemic steroids are indicated when patients do not respond adequately to other measures. In acute settings, hydrocortisone, 100 mg IV every 8 hours, or methylprednisolone, 125 mg IV every 6 hours, may be used, followed by a tapered dose of oral prednisone. **Upper respiratory infections** may cause acute asthma exacerbations and should therefore be treated aggressively. Patients should be instructed to present at the first sign of infection and should be treated with antibiotics if a bacterial cause is suspected.

2. **Asthma attacks during labor** are rare, possibly because of an increase in endogenous cortisol production. Patients who were given long-term systemic steroids during their pregnancies should receive stress-dose steroids during labor and delivery. Hydrocortisone, 100 mg every 8 hours, or methylprednisolone, 125 mg IV every 6 hours, may be administered. General endotracheal anesthesia should be avoided if possible because of the increased incidence of bronchospasm and atelectasis. Prostaglandin $F_{2\alpha}$ should be avoided for use in postpartum hemorrhage.

3. During **acute exacerbations** requiring hospital observation or admission, patients should be given 30–40% humidified oxygen. The β-mimetics remain the first line of treatment; however, anticholinergics, theophylline, and systemic steroids should also be administered as appropriate. Pulse oximetry should be instituted, and the clinician should have a low threshold for obtaining arterial blood gas measurements. Intubation should be considered if the P_{O_2} begins to fall with a rise in P_{CO_2}. Note that normal P_{CO_2} in pregnancy is 31 mm Hg. Asthmatic patients whose P_{CO_2} level rises above 40 mm Hg are candidates for intubation.

III. **Cystic fibrosis**

A. **Incidence, natural course.** Cystic fibrosis occurs in approximately 1 in 2500 live births. Because of improved treatment of this disease, more and more affected women are reaching childbearing age.

B. **Effect of pregnancy.** Although the rate of maternal mortality is significantly higher in patients with cystic fibrosis than in the general population, this mortality rate is no higher than that of nonpregnant patients with cystic fibrosis. The rate of spontaneous abortions is the same as that of the general population.

C. **Prenatal diagnosis and genetic counseling.** As multiple mutations can cause this disorder, prenatal diagnosis remains problematic. The defective gene can be identified, however, in two-thirds of couples seeking prenatal diagnosis.

   D. **Poor prognostic factors** include a vital capacity of less than 50% of predicted value, cor pulmonale, and pulmonary hypertension.

   E. **Other systemic manifestations.** Affected patients may exhibit pancreatic insufficiency and cirrhosis of the liver.

   F. **Management**

      1. **During labor, fluid and electrolyte balance** should be followed closely. Because of the increased sodium content of sweat in affected patients, they are prone to hypovolemia during labor.

      2. **Breast feeding.** Breast milk should be evaluated for sodium content before the infant is allowed to breast feed, because the sodium content may be elevated significantly. In such cases, breast feeding is contraindicated.

IV. **Infections**

   A. **Tuberculosis (TB).** The incidence of TB is rising in urban areas.

      1. **Diagnosis.** Screening involves subcutaneous placement of purified protein derivative (PPD). Only 80% of results are positive in the setting of reactivation of disease, however, and if a patient previously received the bacille Calmette-Guérin vaccine, the PPD results may remain positive for life. If the PPD test is positive or TB is suspected, chest radiography with abdominal shielding should be performed, preferably after 20 weeks' gestation. A definitive diagnosis of TB can be made with positive culture for *Mycobacterium tuberculosis* or positive finding on acid-fast sputum stain. Sputum samples may be induced using aerosolized saline, and the first morning sputum should be collected for 3 consecutive days.

      2. **Medical treatment.** If a sputum stain finding is positive for acid-fast bacilli, antibiotic therapy should be initiated while final culture and sensitivity results are awaited (which may take up to 6 weeks). Standard treatment consists of isoniazid (INH), 300 mg/day; plus ethambutol, 15 mg/kg/day; plus pyridoxine hydrochloride, 20–50 mg/day. Streptomycin sulfate should be avoided because of the risk of fetal cranial nerve VIII damage. Rifampin should also be avoided during pregnancy unless INH and ethambutol cannot be used.

      3. **INH prophylaxis** for 6–9 months is recommended for asymptomatic patients under 35 years old with positive PPD results and negative findings on chest radiograph. If the patient has converted to positive PPD results within the last 2 years, INH therapy should be initiated during the pregnancy after the first trimester. If the time since conversion is unknown or longer than 2 years, INH therapy should be initiated during the postpartum period. INH prophylaxis is not recommended for patients over the age of 35 due to its hepatotoxicity.

      4. **Effect of pregnancy.** If treated, tuberculosis should not affect the pregnancy, and pregnancy should not alter the course of the disease.

   B. **Pneumonia**

      1. **Signs and symptoms.** Bacterial pneumonia is usually caused by Gram-positive diplococci, namely *Streptococcus pneumoniae*. Symptoms include sudden onset of productive cough, sputum production, fever, chills, and tachypnea. Atypical pneumonias such as that caused by *Mycoplasma pneumoniae* usually present gradually with a nonproductive cough and diffuse, patchy infiltrates on chest radiography.

      2. **Diagnosis** is confirmed by findings on chest radiography and sputum culture testing with Gram's stain.

      3. **Management.** Bacterial pneumonia may be treated with a third-generation cephalosporin until fever abates, followed by antibiotics for a 10- to 14-day total course. *Mycoplasma* pneumonia may be treated with erythromycin or azithromycin dihydrate.

      4. **Medical complications** include bacteremia, empyema, arrhythmias, and respiratory failure.

      5. **Pregnancy complications** include preterm labor, which occurs in 44% of cases, and preterm delivery, which occurs in 36% of cases.

16. RENAL, HEPATIC, AND GASTROINTESTINAL DISORDERS AND SYSTEMIC LUPUS ERYTHEMATOSUS IN PREGNANCY

Kerry L. Swenson and Christian Chisholm

RENAL DISEASE

I. **Renal physiology in pregnancy**
   A. **Structural changes.** During pregnancy, the kidneys increase approximately 1 cm in length and 30% in volume, and the collecting system increases in size by more than 80%, with a greater degree of dilation on the right. This physiologic hydronephrosis and hydroureter is thought to be caused by the enlarged uterus and engorged ovarian vessels. Progesterone may also play a role by relaxing the smooth muscle of the ureters. Renal volume usually returns to normal within the first week postpartum, whereas hydronephrosis and hydroureter may not return to prepregnancy state until 3–4 months after delivery.
   B. **Renal function.** Pregnant women undergo a net accumulation of 500–900 mEq of sodium and 6–8 L of water. With this additional fluid volume, renal plasma flow (RPF) increases by 60–80% by the middle of the second trimester then plateaus later in the third trimester to an increase of 50% over prepregnancy values. Glomerular filtration rate (GFR) begins to increase as early as the sixth week of pregnancy and reaches a peak of 50% more than nonpregnancy values by the end of the first trimester. Because the increase in RPF initially exceeds the increase in GFR, the filtration fraction (GFR/RPF) first decreases. The filtration fraction later increases to prepregnancy values in the third trimester when RPF plateaus and both RPF and GFR are increased equally. Expansion of plasma volume and increase in GFR result in lower mean values for BUN and serum creatinine (8.5 mg/dL and 0.46 mg/dL, respectively). Concentrations of BUN and serum creatinine exceeding 13 mg/dL and 0.8 mg/dL may suggest renal impairment. The changes in RPF and GFR are reflected in an increase in creatinine clearance (110–150 mL/minute), which must be considered when assessing a patient's renal function. Creatinine clearance during pregnancy must be calculated based on a 24-hour urine collection, rather than by formulas based on age, height, and weight, as these parameters do not estimate kidney size in gravid patients.
   C. **Tubular function.** Decreased tubular resorption in pregnancy causes an increased excretion of glucose, amino acids, and protein. Net absorption of most electrolytes occurs. Sodium excretion increases to 20,000–30,000 mEq/day. Due to an increased production of aldosterone, estrogen, and deoxycortisone, however, there is an overall net resorption of 950 mg of sodium per day. A net retention of 300–350 mEq/day of potassium also occurs despite increased aldosterone levels, related to increased reabsorption in the proximal tubules. Increased renal clearance of calcium is balanced by an increase in GI absorption. Ionized calcium remains stable, whereas total calcium levels decrease secondary to a decrease in serum albumin concentration.
   Urinary excretion of glucose increases 10- to 100-fold. The proximal tubule increases its ability to resorb the increased glucose load. Glucose that escapes the proximal tubules is not resorbed secondary to impaired distal reabsorption. Therefore, glucosuria occurs and is routinely observed in a normal pregnancy. Increased urinary glucose increases the susceptibility of pregnant women to bacteriuria and urinary tract infections.
   D. **Routine assessment of renal function.** Proteinuria should be assessed by the use of a urine dipstick test at each prenatal visit. A value of +1 should prompt further evaluation by collection of a clean-catch urine sample for culture as well as microscopic examination. If proteinuria persists with negative

results on urine culture, a 24-hour urine collection should be obtained. These patients should also be evaluated for preeclampsia after 20 weeks' gestation.

II. **Renal disease in pregnancy.** Urinary tract infections are more common in pregnancy. Stasis associated with hydroureter and hydronephrosis, increased urinary nutrients, and increased presence of pathogens are thought to play a role. For patients with a history of multiple urinary tract infections or pyelonephritis, suppressive therapy may be initiated as soon as pregnancy is confirmed.

A. **Asymptomatic bacteriuria (ASB)** is defined as the presence of actively multiplying bacteria within the urinary tract, excluding the distal urethra, without symptoms of infection. ASB is associated with low birth weight and preterm delivery. The prevalence of ASB during pregnancy ranges from 2% to 7%. If left untreated, ASB may progress to acute pyelonephritis in 20% to 30% of pregnant women. Treatment of ASB with the appropriate antibiotics reduces this rate to 3%. All women should undergo screening for bacteriuria at their first prenatal visit. Women with sickle cell trait have a twofold increased risk and should undergo screening for bacteriuria every trimester.

1. **Diagnosis and treatment** is based on the finding of a colony count greater than 10^5 organisms/mL in a clean-catch urine specimen. *Escherichia coli* accounts for 75–90% of infections, whereas *Klebsiella* species, *Proteus* species, *Pseudomonas* species, coagulase-negative *Staphylococcus* organisms, and *Enterobacter* species account for the remainder. Initial therapy (7–10 days) is usually empiric, and a variety of agents, including sulfonamides, nitrofurantoin, ampicillin and the cephalosporins, have been shown to be both safe and effective. Test-of-cure urine cultures should be obtained 1–2 weeks after treatment and again each trimester for the remainder of the pregnancy.

2. **Treatment failures.** Twenty-five percent of women have a recurrence of ASB or urinary tract infection. Treatment should be repeated according to antibiotic sensitivities, and the appropriate antimicrobial should be administered for 1 week. After the second course of treatment, patients should receive prophylactic therapy for the remainder of their pregnancies. Nitrofurantoin 100 mg qd, ampicillin (250 mg qd), and trimethoprim plus sulfamethoxazole (160 mg/800 mg tablet qd) are effective chronic suppressive agents.

B. **Acute cystitis** occurs in approximately 1% of pregnant women. The diagnosis is based on symptoms of urinary frequency, urgency, dysuria, hematuria, and suprapubic discomfort. The bacteriology of acute cystitis is the same as that of ASB, and similar treatment is recommended.

C. **Acute pyelonephritis** occurs in approximately 2% of all pregnancies. Major symptoms include high fever, flank pain, nausea, and vomiting. Frequency, urgency, and dysuria are variably present. Pyelonephritis may increase the incidence of preterm labor and preterm rupture of membranes. Complications, including bacteremia, sepsis, adult respiratory distress syndrome, and hemolytic anemia, are seen more frequently in the gravid patient, possibly due to an increased susceptibility to bacterial endotoxin. Prompt diagnosis and treatment of pyelonephritis in pregnancy is crucial.

1. **Treatment** consists of immediate hospitalization, aggressive intravenous (IV) hydration, use of antipyretics, and administration of broad-spectrum IV antibiotics. Cefazolin sodium and ampicillin plus gentamicin (or clindamycin plus gentamycin for penicillin-allergic women) are most commonly used and should be continued until the patient has been afebrile for at least 48 hours. Dosing of gentamicin every 8 hours is currently preferred over daily dosing in the pregnant patient given pregnancy-related changes in renal function. Gentamicin trough levels should then be followed. Antibiotic therapy should be tailored as necessary based on urine culture sensitivity results.

2. **Treatment failures.** If symptoms do not respond to appropriate antibiotic treatment after 72 hours, antibiotic sensitivity results and dosing

regimens should be reviewed and renal ultrasonography should be performed to evaluate for the presence of anatomic anomalies. After resolution of acute pyelonephritis, the patient should continue antibiotic therapy for a total of 2 weeks followed by suppressive therapy for the remainder of the pregnancy. Recurrence rate is approximately 20%.

D. **Hematuria.** Urolithiasis should be considered in pregnant patients suspected to have a urinary tract infection but with negative urine culture results. Patients with a history of urolithiasis should be advised to keep themselves well hydrated.

1. **Treatment** depends on the patient's symptoms and the gestational age. Initially, IV hydration and analgesics should be administered. Associated infections are treated aggressively. In over one-half of cases, the stone passes spontaneously. Ultrasonography can be used to assess for obstruction, but the usefulness of this modality is hampered by the gravid uterus and the presence of baseline ureteral dilatation during pregnancy. An IVP should be considered for patients with urinary infection that does not respond to 48 hours of antibiotic therapy, declining renal function, severe hydronephrosis on renal ultrasonography, or pain and dehydration from vomiting.

2. **Indications for intervention** include calculus pyelonephritis, persistent severe hydronephrosis with impairment of renal function, and protracted pain or sepsis. Approximately one-third of pregnant women with symptomatic stones require surgical intervention for stone extraction. Extracorporeal shock-wave lithotripsy is contraindicated in pregnancy.

E. **Chronic renal disease** can be categorized as mild, with a serum creatinine level of less than 1.4 mg/100 mL; moderate, with serum creatinine level higher than 1.4 but less than 2.5 mg/100 mL; or severe, with serum creatinine level higher than 2.5 mg/100 mL. In general, as renal disease progresses and function declines, the ability to conceive and to sustain a viable pregnancy decreases. Normal pregnancy is rare when renal function declines to the point at which preconception serum creatinine and BUN levels exceed 3 mg/dL and 30 mg/dL, respectively. Pregnant women with preexisting renal disease are at risk for deterioration of renal function, even to the point of renal failure, and superimposed preeclampsia. In general, patients with mild renal dysfunction experience little or no disease progression during pregnancy, whereas patients with moderate to severe renal insufficiency are at greatest risk for potentially irreversible deterioration of their renal function. Furthermore, chronic renal disease complicated by hypertension imposes a substantially increased risk to both patient and fetus.

1. **Pregnancy outcome.** Chronic renal disease is associated with increased perinatal mortality, preterm birth, and intrauterine growth restriction (IUGR). Outcomes depend on the degree of associated hypertension and renal insufficiency in each case. Patients with glomerulonephritis or nephrosclerosis appear to be at greatest risk for poor pregnancy outcomes.

2. **Antepartum management** should include the following:
   a. Early pregnancy diagnosis and accurate dating
   b. Baseline laboratory studies, preferably performed preconception, including BP, serum creatinine level, serum electrolyte levels, BUN level, 24-hour urine collection for protein excretion and creatinine clearance testing, urinalysis, and urine culture
   c. Biweekly antenatal visits until 28–32 weeks' gestation, then weekly visits until delivery
   d. Laboratory studies repeated each trimester and when clinically indicated
   e. Serial ultrasonographic examinations for assessment of fetal growth
   f. Antepartum tests of fetal well-being should begin at 28 weeks' gestation for patients with severe disease and as late as 34 weeks' gestation for patients with mild disease.

3. **Pregnancy and dialysis.** Pregnancy occurs in only 1 in 200 women on long-term dialysis. Control of BP is important, especially during dialysis, when BP can fluctuate widely. Volume shifts during dialysis should be avoided, and particular attention must be paid to electrolyte balance. Later in pregnancy, the fetal heart rate should be continuously monitored during dialysis. Patients should receive longer and more frequent dialysis sessions to maintain a BUN level of less than 50 mg/dL. Chronic anemia is common. Hematocrit should be maintained above 25% with transfusions or erythropoietin therapy or both. Successful pregnancies have been achieved with the use of long-term ambulatory peritoneal dialysis or long-term cycling peritoneal dialysis. High rates of preterm delivery, IUGR, and abruptio placentae are associated with these procedures. Antepartum testing should begin at 28 weeks' gestation.

4. After successful **renal transplantation,** approximately 1 in 50 women becomes pregnant. These women have an increased incidence of infection, preeclampsia, preterm labor, premature rupture of membranes, and low-birth-weight offspring. Women who have undergone renal transplantation should meet the following criteria for the greatest chance of a successful pregnancy outcome:

   a. Serum creatinine level less than 2 mg/dL.
   b. Minimal or well-controlled hypertension.
   c. Minimal or no proteinuria.
   d. Good general health.
   e. Elapsed time from transplant surgery of 18–24 months.
   f. No evidence of pelvicaliceal distension on recent IVP.
   g. Response to immunosuppressive therapy that is stable at 15 mg/day or less of prednisone and 2 mg/kg/day or less of azathioprine. If the patient is on prednisone, screening for gestational diabetes should be undertaken at 20–24 weeks' gestation and repeated at 28–32 weeks' gestation if the results of the initial screen are negative. Antepartum testing should begin by 28 weeks' gestation. If the patient is taking cyclosporine A, levels should be monitored monthly.

HEPATIC DISEASE

I. **Hepatic physiology in pregnancy.** In pregnancy, liver enzymes remain at normal levels and may even decrease related to hemodilution. Levels of lipids, fibrinogen, and alkaline phosphatase increase progressively throughout pregnancy, and albumin levels decrease by 20% early in the first trimester. As the enlarging uterus expands into the upper abdomen, the liver is displaced posteriorly and to the right. This displacement actually decreases estimated size on physical examination. Thus, any palpable liver in pregnancy should be treated as abnormal and appropriate workup should be performed.

II. **Hepatic disorders associated with pregnancy**

   A. **Intrahepatic cholestasis of pregnancy** is the most common liver disorder unique to pregnancy. It is uncommon in the United States and almost nonexistent among African-Americans, but affects up to 2% of pregnancies in Chile and is fairly common in Scandinavian and Mediterranean populations. The bile ducts and hepatocytes of these patients have an increased susceptibility to the elevated concentrations of estrogen and progesterone in pregnancy. Complications of pregnancy include preterm labor, fetal distress, and fetal death. These risks increase progressively to term regardless of progression of symptoms. Some studies, however, have shown a correlation between the level of maternal serum bile acids and risk to the fetus. Antepartum fetal testing is recommended but may not reliably indicate fetal well-being, as death is usually sudden. Therefore, labor should be induced at term. In moderate to severe cases, administration of corticosteroids and amniocentesis to test for fetal lung maturity followed by induction of labor at 36–37 weeks may be considered. A recurrence rate of approximately 70% has been reported, with subsequent pregnancies more severely affected.

B. **Diagnosis.** The presenting symptom is almost always severe pruritus. A mild jaundice may develop in approximately 50% of patients and resolves quickly after delivery. Anorexia, malaise, steatorrhea, and dark urine are also common complaints. Patients should be observed for malnutrition, weight loss, and deficiency of fat-soluble vitamins, especially vitamin K. Prothrombin time should be checked periodically. Differential diagnosis includes viral hepatitis and gallbladder disease. Other causes of these symptoms should be ruled out, especially if fever, abdominal pain, hepatomegaly, or splenomegaly is present. Laboratory studies are remarkable for the following: elevated serum alkaline phosphatase level, five to ten times above normal; elevated total bilirubin level, rarely higher than 5 mg/dL; elevated serum bile acid levels, up to ten times above normal; moderate elevation in serum aminotransferase activity.

Management is aimed at reducing the symptoms. Cholestyramine given in dosages of 8–16 g/day in three to four divided doses has been shown to be effective in reducing pruritus. The prothrombin time should be checked weekly, as cholestyramine decreases intestinal absorption of vitamin K. Vitamin K should be administered at 10 mg daily until the prothrombin time normalizes. Diphenhydramine may provide relief in some patients. Dexamethasone 12 mg/day for 7 days has also been shown to be somewhat effective. In addition, phenobarbital at a dose of 90 mg at bedtime has been used when patients cannot tolerate cholestyramine. Use of ursodeoxycholic acid (UDCA), a hydrophilic bile salt, has exhibited some success. After delivery, symptoms usually abate within 2 days. Oral contraceptives should be prescribed cautiously for these patients, because cholestasis may develop postpartum when oral contraceptives are taken.

III. **Hepatic disorders coincident with pregnancy**
   A. **Acute hepatitis.** See Chap. 11.
   B. **Acute liver failure** in pregnancy is complicated by a high rate of maternal and fetal morbidity and mortality. Poor prognostic indicators include coincident renal impairment, metabolic acidosis, hypotension, hyponatremia, and thrombosis. Assessment for potential liver transplant should be performed as early in the pregnancy as possible. Doppler ultrasonographic examination of the hepatic veins should be performed, and liver function test results should be followed to evaluate severity of disease. Appropriate laboratory evaluations include hepatitis panel, human immunodeficiency virus test, and toxicology screen, including tests for ethanol and acetaminophen. Differential diagnosis includes viral hepatitis, acute fatty liver of pregnancy, preeclampsia, HELLP syndrome (hemolysis, elevated liver enzymes, and low platelet count), thrombotic thrombocytopenia purpura, hemolytic uremic syndrome, Wilson's disease, toxin-induced and alcoholic hepatitis, and Budd-Chiari syndrome.
   C. **Cirrhosis.** Women with cirrhosis have a high rate of infertility. Those who do conceive have an extremely high risk of spontaneous abortion, fetal death, and neonatal death. Portosystemic decompression improves the outcome of these pregnancies; it is best performed before conception but may be performed during pregnancy. The severity of hepatic dysfunction, rather than the cause of the cirrhosis, is predictive of maternal and fetal prognosis. The most common complication of cirrhosis is esophageal varices. Other complications include postpartum hemorrhage, ascites, peritonitis, splenic artery aneurysm, portal vein thrombosis, coma, and death. Maternal mortality is estimated to be 10–18%. Vaginal delivery in these patients is safe and actually is preferred to cesarean delivery due to the high rate of postoperative complications. A prolonged second labor stage should be avoided, and early intervention with forceps is encouraged.
   D. **Budd-Chiari syndrome** is a veno-occlusive disease of the hepatic veins resulting in hepatic congestion and necrosis. The hypercoagulable state of pregnancy is thought to play a role in the disease process, as can use of oral

contraceptive pills. The disease is marked by abdominal pain with an abrupt onset of ascites and hepatomegaly. Diagnosis is made by Doppler ultrasonographic imaging of the liver to determine venous patency as well as direction and amplitude of blood flow. Maternal and fetal prognosis are poor. Abdominal ascites occurs rapidly and is frequently resistant to medical management. The risk of thrombosis remains high, even with therapeutic anticoagulation therapy. A workup for hypercoagulable disorders, paroxysmal nocturnal hemoglobinuria, hemolytic anemia, and thrombotic thrombocytopenic purpura should be performed.

GALLBLADDER DISEASE

I. **Cholelithiasis in pregnancy.** Presenting symptoms of cholelithiasis include right upper quadrant pain, nausea, and vomiting, usually associated with fatty meals. Diagnosis is usually made by ultrasonography, but endoscopic retrograde cholangiopancreatography and percutaneous transhepatic cholecystography may be performed safely with proper shielding of the fetus. Management includes bed rest, bowel rest, IV hydration, and antibiotic therapy. Cholecystectomy and fiberoptic endoscopic cannulation for retrieval of stones may be performed in pregnancy. These invasive procedures are optimally performed in the second trimester when risk of spontaneous abortion is decreased and displacement of the liver and gallbladder by the enlarging uterus is minimal. Dissolution of stones with bile acids and lithotripsy is contraindicated in pregnancy.

II. **Cholecystectomy** is second only to appendectomy as the most common nonobstetric surgery performed in pregnant women. This procedure may be performed laparoscopically in the first half of pregnancy or as an open procedure in the latter half.

GASTROINTESTINAL DISEASE

I. **Gastroenteritis.** Viral enteritis caused by the Norwalk agent is the most common infectious disease of the GI tract during pregnancy. Patients usually present with nausea, cramping, vomiting, diarrhea, headache, and myalgia. Low-grade fever is common. The symptoms last 48–72 hours, and treatment is supportive. In cases of severe dehydration, intravenous hydration is indicated.

II. **Hyperemesis gravidarum.** Nausea and emesis are common in pregnancy. Hyperemesis gravidarum, defined as nausea and vomiting associated with dehydration, weight loss, or electrolyte disturbances, affects 0.5–10.0 of 1000 pregnancies. The peak occurrence is between the eighth and twelfth weeks of pregnancy.

A. The **etiology** of hyperemesis gravidarum is unknown but is believed to involve hormonal, neurologic, metabolic, toxic, and psychosocial factors. Laboratory findings include ketonuria, increased urine specific gravity, elevated hematocrit and BUN level, hyponatremia, hypokalemia, hypochloremia, and metabolic alkalosis. Test for serum human chorionic gonadotropin β-subunit and thyroid function tests usually are performed because molar pregnancy and hyperthyroidism can cause hyperemesis. Some patients with hyperemesis gravidarum have transient hyperthyroidism. Whether or not to treat the transient hyperthyroidism is controversial, because in most cases it resolves spontaneously as pregnancy continues.

B. **Treatment** should be tailored to the severity of symptoms. Therapy usually includes IV hydration and antiemetic therapy. Patients may need to be hospitalized for intractable emesis, correction of any electrolyte abnormalities, and hypovolemia. In severe cases in which prolonged IV hydration is anticipated, parenteral nutrition and vitamin supplementation may be instituted; this should include thiamine supplementation [100 mg qd intramuscularly (IM) or IV] to avoid Wernicke's encephalopathy. Oral feedings should be introduced slowly when tolerated, starting with clear liquids and progressing to a bland solid diet consisting of small, carbohydrate-rich meals. Fatty and spicy foods should be avoided. When pregnant women do not respond to the medical and supportive care of obstetric and nursing professionals, a psychiatric consultation is advisable.

C. The risk-benefit ratio of medication therapy for hyperemesis should be determined on a case-by-case basis. Medicines shown to be effective include the following [the U.S. Food and Drug Administration (FDA) has approved no drugs for treatment of nausea and vomiting in pregnancy]:

1. Pyridoxine (vitamin B_6), 25 mg three times daily (tid) by mouth (PO)
2. Phosphorylated carbohydrate solution (Emetrol), 15–30 mL every 15 minutes for a maximum of five doses
3. Doxylamine succinate (Unisom), 25 mg every night; best results when used with pyridoxine
4. Metoclopramide hydrochloride (Reglan), 5–10 mg tid, PO or IV
5. Promethazine hydrochloride (Phenergan) 12.5–25.0 mg four times daily (qid), PO, IV, IM, or rectally (PR)
6. Prochlorperazine (Compazine), 5–10 mg tid, PO, IV, or PR
7. Chlorpromazine (Thorazine), 10–25 mg qid, PO; 25–50 mg qid, IV or IM; 50–100 mg tid PR
8. Ondansetron hydrochloride (Zofran), 4–8 mg tid
9. Methylprednisolone (Medrol), 48 mg qd, PO for 3 days, followed by a taper

III. **Gastroesophageal reflux disease,** with resultant heartburn, is very common during pregnancy. Heartburn usually is more severe after meals and is aggravated by recumbent position. Treatment of reflux during pregnancy consists primarily of neutralizing or decreasing the acid material that is being regurgitated. Measures that may provide symptomatic relief include elevating the head of the bed, consuming small meals, following a reduced-fat diet, refraining from ingesting meals or liquids other than water within 3 hours of bedtime, stopping smoking, and avoiding chocolate and caffeine. For relatively severe symptoms, treatment with over-the-counter antacids after meals and at bedtime or the use of sucralfate (1 g tid) should be considered. In refractory cases, an H_2 blocker (all FDA category B) should be administered. The most commonly prescribed are cimetidine and ranitidine. There are limited data evaluating the safety of the proton pump inhibitors lansoprazole and omeprazole in pregnancy. Metoclopramide hydrochloride (Reglan) can be helpful in reducing reflux and is FDA category C.

IV. **Peptic ulcer disease (PUD)** during pregnancy is uncommon. Patients who develop PUD before pregnancy frequently experience fewer symptoms during pregnancy and may even become asymptomatic. The **treatment** of PUD during pregnancy consists primarily of taking antacids after meals and at bedtime; avoiding fatty foods, caffeine, alcohol, chocolate, and nicotine, which may trigger gastric retention; avoiding aspirin and other nonsteroidal anti-inflammatory drugs (NSAIDs); and taking an H_2-receptor antagonist such as cimetidine or ranitidine. Indomethacin should be avoided as a tocolytic agent in patients with a history of PUD. For nonpregnant individuals, proton pump inhibitors offer the quickest healing rates. However, the safety of these agents in pregnancy is not well documented. An association has been found between *Helicobacter pylori* infection of the GI tract and peptic ulcer disease. The gold standard method of diagnosis is endoscopy with biopsy. Serum serology and breath analyzer tests are also being used. Nonpregnant patients with positive test results are treated with combination antibiotic regimens along with bismuth and a proton pump inhibitor. Currently, no guidelines exist for treatment of this condition in pregnancy, and the need for multiple therapeutic agents poses additional risks. Symptoms may be adequately treated with acid-reduction therapy. Therefore, diagnosis and treatment of *H. pylori* infection is usually deferred to the postpartum period.

V. **Inflammatory bowel disease (IBD).** The age of peak incidence for ulcerative colitis is 20–35 years, and for Crohn's disease, 15–30 years. These diseases frequently coincide with childbearing. The fertility rate is unaffected in patients with ulcerative colitis. Reduced fertility has been associated with Crohn's disease, possibly because of the chronic pelvic adhesions that may result from the inflammatory process. Studies evaluating fetal risk in pregnancies complicated by IBD have shown no difference from overall risk in the general population. Some concern exists over the effect of pregnancy on the disease process. Most studies, however, have shown an improvement in symptoms. Disease activity during pregnancy appears to reflect the degree of activity at conception.

A. **Treatment.** The medical management of IBD in pregnant patients is similar to that in nonpregnant patients, with a few exceptions. The mainstay of medical therapy for IBD is sulfasalazine and corticosteroids. All of these agents have been shown to be safe in pregnancy. Because sulfasalazine may interfere with the absorption of folate, supplemental folate should be prescribed to pregnant women. Immunosuppressive agents such as azathioprine or 6-mercaptopurine are occasionally used in IBD and have been shown to be safe in pregnancy. Experience is limited, however. If the agent has been effective in keeping the disease in remission, consideration should be given to continuing the therapy in pregnancy. An alternate approach involves discontinuing the agent around conception while continuing or substituting sulfasalazine. Antibiotics, particularly metronidazole hydrochloride, are useful for treating perirectal abscesses and fistulas complicating IBD. Pregnant women treated with metronidazole have not shown an increase in fetal complications.

B. **Surgical intervention** is indicated for severe complications of IBD. Intestinal obstruction, perforation, unremitting GI bleeding, and the development of toxic megacolon may necessitate surgical intervention.

C. The **method of delivery** chosen may be affected by IBD. Vaginal delivery can be undertaken by most women with IBD unless severe perineal disease exists. Crohn's disease may be associated with perineal scarring, which may make vaginal delivery difficult. Active perineal disease or perineal fistula in patients with Crohn's disease may prevent adequate healing of a perineal laceration or episiotomy. Consideration should be given to performing a cesarean section in these patients. Episiotomy is generally not contraindicated in ulcerative colitis. If a patient has been on prolonged corticosteroid therapy, stress-dose IV corticosteroids should be administered during labor. When cesarean section is necessary, difficult intraperitoneal adhesions should be expected and preparations made accordingly.

VI. **Pancreatitis** is an uncommon cause of abdominal pain in pregnancy, with an incidence of 1 in 1000 to 1 in 3800 pregnancies.

A. The **clinical presentation** is similar to that of the nonpregnant patient: midepigastric or left upper quadrant pain with radiation to the back, nausea, vomiting, ileus, and low-grade fever. Whereas gallstones and alcohol abuse are equal contributors to the development of the disease in nonpregnant women, during pregnancy cholelithiasis is the most common cause. Elevated levels of serum amylase, lipase, or both remain the key finding in the diagnosis of acute pancreatitis. Ultrasonographic evaluation is of limited use in the evaluation of acute pancreatitis in pregnant patients because of the enlarged uterus and overlying bowel gas.

B. **Management** is principally conservative and is aimed at resting the GI tract and preventing complications. Most cases of gallstone pancreatitis can be managed successfully with conservative treatment during pregnancy, with elective cholecystectomy delayed until postpartum. Cholecystectomy can be performed safely during pregnancy if necessary. Exploratory laparotomy is indicated in women with unrelenting disease and in those in whom the diagnosis is uncertain. It is important to postpone definitive biliary surgery until the acute inflammation has subsided. Endoscopic retrograde cholangiopancreatography with shielding of the maternal abdomen can be performed under IV sedation during the second trimester.

VII. Acute **appendicitis** is discussed in Chap. 19.

SYSTEMIC LUPUS ERYTHEMATOSUS

I. **Etiology.** Systemic lupus erythematosus (SLE) is a multiorgan disease primarily affecting young women in their reproductive years and is relatively common in pregnancy. African-American women have a risk of SLE five times that of white women. Fertility rate is normal in women with SLE, except in those with severe end-organ disease and those who have had cyclophosphamide therapy. An increased rate of spontaneous abortions is seen, however. The optimal time to conceive is during remission.

II. **Diagnosis** of SLE is based on the history, physical examination, and laboratory tests. SLE should be ruled out in any pregnant woman with a photosensitive rash, polyarthritis, undiagnosed proteinuria, false-positive syphilis test, or multiple spontaneous abortions. Abnormal laboratory test findings include positive antinuclear antibody test results (higher than 1 in 160; patterns common in SLE include homogeneous, nucleolar, and rim only); elevated anti–SSA (anti-Ro) and anti–SSB (anti-La) antibody titers; decreased C3 and C4 complement levels; positive results on lupus anticoagulant test (dilute activated partial thromboplastin time test, kaolin clotting time test, or Russell viper venom time test); and elevated anticardiolipin antibody or anti–double-stranded DNA (dsDNA) antibody titers.

III. **Effect of pregnancy on SLE.** Pregnancy does not appear to alter the long-term prognosis of most SLE patients. Transient lupus flares are more likely during pregnancy than at other times and can occur during any trimester and in the early postpartum period. These flares are usually mild and involve primarily cutaneous and articular symptoms. It is very difficult to differentiate between a lupus flare and other disease states associated with pregnancy such as preeclampsia.

IV. **Effect of SLE on pregnancy.** Patients with SLE have an increased risk of spontaneous abortion, IUGR, premature birth, cesarean delivery, and fetal death. Management of SLE in pregnancy consists of the following.

A. **First trimester.** Initial laboratory studies include CBC, creatinine level, 24-hour urine collection for measurement of protein and creatinine, microscopic urinalysis, and a lupus panel (antinuclear, anti-Ro, and anti-La antibody titers, lupus anticoagulant levels, and anticardiolipin antibody and anti-dsDNA antibody titers). An obstetric ultrasonographic examination should be performed to determine gestational age and viability of the fetus.

B. **Second trimester.** Repeated laboratory studies include CBC, creatinine level, 24-hour urine collection for measurement of protein and creatinine, and microscopic urinalysis. Obstetric ultrasonography should be performed every 4 weeks after 20 weeks' gestation to monitor fetal growth. In women positive for anti-Ro or anti-La antibodies, careful ultrasonography should begin at 16–18 weeks' gestation to assess for possible heart block.

C. **Third trimester.** Fetal testing, with weekly nonstress tests and weekly measurement of biophysical profile, may be initiated as early as 28 weeks based on clinical scenario. Serial growth ultrasonographic studies and fetal echocardiograms should be obtained. In the presence of IUGR, fetal Doppler ultrasonographic studies should be performed. Treatment with dexamethasone or betamethasone should be initiated in patients with poor fetal test results or worsening maternal disease in anticipation of a preterm delivery.

D. **Lupus flare.** Most lupus flares are diagnosed clinically when patients present with fever, malaise, and lymphadenopathy. Laboratory findings include low C3 or C4 complement levels, active sediment on urine microscopic analysis (defined by more than 20 red blood cells or WBCs per high-power field or cellular casts), elevation in anti-dsDNA antibody titer, and hemolytic anemia, thrombocytopenia, and leukopenia. Distinguishing a lupus flare from preeclampsia in pregnant patients can be challenging. Factors that are not helpful include the level of proteinuria and the presence of thrombocytopenia, hypertension, or hyperuricemia. Factors that are useful include complement levels, which are low in lupus flare and usually normal in preeclampsia; serum hepatic transferase levels, which are generally normal in a lupus flare but may be elevated in preeclampsia; the presence of red blood cell casts in the urine, which implies active lupus; and very gradual onset of proteinuria, which is characteristic of lupus flare. In preeclampsia, proteinuria appears abruptly or increases from baseline values rapidly. If differentiation between preeclampsia and a lupus flare becomes crucial to determine further management, renal biopsy may be performed.

V. **Treatment**
  A. **Corticosteroids** can be used during a lupus flare. The usual dosage is 60 mg of prednisone daily for 2–3 weeks, which then is tapered to the lowest dosage that controls symptoms. Patients should be monitored closely for the development of glucose intolerance, hypertension, and preeclampsia, which have been associated with corticosteroid therapy.
  B. Because of the fetal risks associated with **NSAID use,** pregnant women with SLE usually are switched from other NSAIDs to aspirin. In the Hopkins Lupus Pregnancy Center, low-dose, or "baby," aspirin (81 mg) is administered to women with prior fetal loss and antiphospholipid antibodies and to those who have a history of pregnancy-induced hypertension or preeclampsia.
  C. **Immunosuppressive agents** are used only for patients with significant organ involvement.
  D. **Antimalarial drugs.** Hydrochloroquine is currently being used to treat SLE. Controversy exists over whether or not to continue hydrochloroquine throughout pregnancy. Studies have not shown any adverse effects on the fetus and have suggested that continuing the medication may be more beneficial than risking losing control of the disease activity.
  E. **Antihypertensives** are used by many SLE patients before pregnancy or are initiated during pregnancy when hypertension develops. Antihypertensive agents with good safety records in pregnancy include methyldopa, hydralazine hydrochloride, and labetalol hydrochloride (see Chap. 8, sec. **II.E.6**).
  F. In pregnant women, the presence of **antiphospholipid antibodies** (lupus anticoagulant or anticardiolipin) is associated with fetal death, particularly in the second trimester. Studies have shown that treatment with low-dose aspirin and moderate-dose heparin sodium improve fetal outcome. Use of low-dose aspirin and prednisone has improved fetal outcome but with more maternal complications. Therapy with low-dose aspirin, heparin, or warfarin sodium usually is recommended for approximately 3 months after delivery for women with a history of thromboembolic events.

VI. **Neonatal lupus syndrome** consists of a transient rash in the newborn period, complete heart block, or both. Neonatal lupus is a rare syndrome that occurs in a minority of infants delivered only to mothers who have antibodies to the Ro (SSA) or La (SSB) antigens, or both. Among infants at risk, fewer than 25% develop cutaneous manifestations, whereas fewer than 3% develop congenital heart block. In subsequent pregnancies, the risk of recurrence of cutaneous neonatal lupus is approximately 25% and the risk of heart block is between 8% and 16%.

Although no treatment has been proven to be effective in reversing fetal heart block in utero, the administration of dexamethasone to the mother may be beneficial in preventing extension of the fetal myocarditis.

17. HEMATOLOGIC DISORDERS OF PREGNANCY

Suzanne Davey Shipman and Christian Chisholm

I. **Anemia** in pregnancy is defined as a hemoglobin concentration of less than 10.5 g/dL. Microcytic anemia is characterized by a mean corpuscular volume (MCV) of less than 80 fL; the two most common causes of microcytic anemia are iron deficiency and the thalassemias. If the MCV is 80–100 fL, the anemia is normocytic; a relatively common cause of normocytic anemia is sickle cell disease. Macrocytic anemia is present if the MCV is greater than 100 fL; the most common causes of macrocytic anemia are deficiency of vitamin B_{12} and folate deficiency.

   A. **Physiologic anemia of pregnancy.** During pregnancy, plasma volume increases 25–60%, starting at 6 weeks' gestation and continuing through delivery. The red blood cell (RBC) mass increases only 10–20% in pregnancy. The disproportionate increase in plasma volume compared with RBC mass results in hemodilution, and hematocrit falls 3–5%.

   B. **Iron deficiency anemia**
      1. **Diagnosis** is based on the slow onset of symptoms such as fatigue, headache, and malaise. In severe cases, pallor, glossitis, stomatitis, koilonychia (in which the outer surfaces of the nails are concave), pica, splenomegaly, shortness of breath, or high-output heart failure can occur.
      2. **Laboratory findings.** The diagnosis is confirmed by the presence of small, hypochromic erythrocytes of various shapes and sizes, an MCV of less than 80 fL, mean corpuscular hemoglobin concentration of less than 30 g/dL, and serum ferritin level of less than 10 ng/mL.
      3. **Treatment** consists of administration of iron sulfate, 325 mg twice daily. The hemoglobin level should increase within 6–8 weeks. For patients who do not respond to or cannot tolerate oral therapy, intravenous iron dextran is an alternative.

   C. **Thalassemias.** There are two types of thalassemia, α and β, which result from decreased production of structurally normal α- and β-globulin chains, respectively. Both diseases are transmitted as autosomal recessive traits. Table 17-1 shows the various types of α and β thalassemias. In β thalassemia, the reduction in β-globin synthesis leads to redundant α-globin chains. These are insoluble; they precipitate freely as Heinz bodies and damage the developing cell, which leads to intramedullary hemolysis and ineffective erythropoiesis. Conversely, α thalassemia results from a reduction in the synthesis of α-chains, so that insufficient amounts are available for combination with non-α globins and for assembly of hemoglobin. The usual cause of α thalassemia is deletion of α-globin genes.
      1. **Diagnosis.** Thalassemia is generally a microcytic hypochromic anemia, with an MCV of less than 80 fL.
      2. **Laboratory findings.** Quantitative hemoglobin electrophoresis is required for diagnosis. In homozygous β thalassemia, levels of hemoglobin F (HbF) are increased by 20–60% and may be as high as 90%. Homozygotes are severely anemic with hemoglobin levels of less than 5 g/dL in the absence of transfusion. MCV and mean corpuscular hemoglobin level are decreased, and the reticulocyte count is elevated. In heterozygous β thalassemia, the level of hemoglobin A_2 (HbA_2) is increased (4–6%), and a slight increase in HbF level may be present (1–3%). Reticulocyte counts may be elevated (1–3%). Low MCV and elevated HbA_2 level are the criteria for diagnosing carriers. Asymptomatic carriers of α thalassemia often have normal amounts of HbA_2 and HbF, so pedigree studies are often helpful during workup of these patients. Suspicion for

TABLE 17-1. α AND β THALASSEMIAS AND THE DEGREE OF ASSOCIATED ANEMIA

	Number of α chains in α thalassemia			
	0	**1**	**2**	**3**
Diagnosis	Hydrops fetalis	Hemoglobin H disease	Silent carrier	Silent carrier
RBC morphology	Increased nucleated RBC	Microcytic Heinz bodies, targets	Microcytic slight hypochromasia	Normal
Hemoglobin electrophoresis	Increased hemoglobin Bart	Increased hemoglobin H cells	Decreased hemoglobin A_2	Normal
Prognosis	Death	Moderate to severe anemia	Mild anemia	No symptoms

	Number of β chains in β thalassemia	
	0	**>0**
Diagnosis	Cooley's anemia, homozygous	Heterozygous
RBC morphology	Decreased MCV, target cells, hypochromia, nucleated RBCs	Decreased MCV, stippling
Hemoglobin electrophoresis	Increased hemoglobin F	Increased hemoglobin A_2
Prognosis	Death in childhood without transfusion	Mild to moderate anemia

MCV, mean corpuscular volume.

the presence of α thalassemia is raised by the finding of microcytosis and a normal RDW with minimal or no anemia in the absence of iron deficiency or β thalassemia. If a pregnant woman is found to be a carrier of thalassemia, her partner is offered testing. DNA-based prenatal testing using amniocentesis or chorionic villus sampling is available if both members of the couple are found to be carriers.

3. **Treatment** varies depending on the severity of the disease. Asymptomatic α thalassemia carriers and patients with heterozygous β thalassemia require no special care other than counseling and information about the availability of prenatal diagnosis. Iron supplementation should be given when red cell ferritin and plasma ferritin levels indicate the need for it; iron overload with resulting hemochromatosis may be the result of overtreatment with iron. Homozygous β thalassemia patients may need multiple blood transfusions and splenectomy. All homozygous patients should receive supplemental folate to meet the requirements of accelerated erythropoiesis.

4. **Antepartum fetal testing** is essential in anemic patients. Patients with thalassemia should undergo frequent fetal sonography to assess fetal growth as well as nonstress testing to evaluate fetal well-being. Asymptomatic carriers require no special testing.

D. **Sickle cell disease** describes a group of hemoglobinopathies [sickle cell hemoglobin or hemoglobin S (HbS), sickle cell hemoglobin C (HbSC), sickle thalassemia hemoglobin (HbS-Thal)] that may cause severe symptoms during pregnancy or may be quiescent in an unaffected hemoglobin A/hemoglobin S (HbAS) carrier. Homozygosity for HbS (HbSS) is the most common of these phenotypes, affecting 1 in 708 African-Americans. Affected patients may experience hemolytic anemia, recurrent pain crises, infection, and infarction of more than one organ system. In HbS, valine replaces glutamate at the sixth position of both β-chains of hemoglobin. HbS, when deoxygenated, forms insoluble tetramers inside RBCs. The tetramers cause the RBCs to become rigid and, consequently, trapped in the microvasculature, which causes vascular obstruction, ischemia, and infarction. This may lead to a vaso-occlusive crisis, which may be associated with fever as well as skeletal, abdominal, and chest pain. Vaso-occlusive crises may be initiated by an event such as hypoxia, acidosis, dehydration, infection, or psychologic stress. Patients with sickle cell disease are at increased risk for sickling during pregnancy because of increased metabolic requirements, vascular stasis, and relatively hypercoagulable state.

1. **Diagnosis.** Most affected patients are diagnosed in childhood. Some present in pregnancy with previously undiagnosed symptoms such as a pain crisis or infection, splenic sequestration, or acute chest syndrome, which is associated with chest pain, pulmonary infiltrates, leukocytosis, and hypoxia. Jaundice may result from RBC destruction.

2. **Laboratory findings.** The anemia is normocytic, with a hemoglobin concentration of 5–8 g/dL and hematocrit of less than 25%. The reticulocyte count is increased. The peripheral blood smear may show sickle cells and target cells. Diagnosis is confirmed by hemoglobin electrophoresis. All African-American patients should undergo a hemoglobin electrophoresis to assess carrier status. If both the patient and the father of the baby are found to be hemoglobinopathy carriers, genetic counseling is indicated. Amniocentesis or chorionic villus sampling may be performed for prenatal diagnosis.

3. **Treatment.** Folic acid supplements are administered to maintain erythropoiesis. Infections are treated aggressively with antibiotics. Severe anemia (hemoglobin level of less than 5 g/dL, hematocrit of less than 15%, or reticulocyte count of less than 3%) is treated with blood transfusion. Pain crises are managed with oxygen, hydration, and analgesia. Controversy surrounds prophylactic exchange transfusion. The advantages of transfusion are an increase in HbA level, which improves oxygen-carrying capacity, and a decrease in HbS-carrying erythrocytes. Risks of transfusion are hepatitis, human immunodeficiency virus (HIV) infection, transfusion reaction, and alloimmunization. Treatment for acute chest syndrome is the same as for pain crises. Splenic sequestration is treated with blood transfusion.

4. **Pregnancy considerations.** An increase in prematurity, stillbirth, low-birth-weight babies, spontaneous abortion, and intrauterine growth restriction is associated with sickle cell disease. The intensity of fetal surveillance varies according to the clinical severity of the disease. In advanced cases, semiweekly nonstress testing and biophysical profile measurement should begin at 32 weeks' gestation, and serial sonography is used to diagnose fetal growth restriction. After delivery, patients should practice early ambulation and wear pressure stockings to prevent thromboembolism. Use of intrauterine devices and combination oral contraceptives is contraindicated. Progestin-only pills, depot medroxyprogesterone, subcutaneous implants, or barrier devices are recommended for contraception. Use of medroxyprogesterone acetate (Depo-Provera) injections has been found to decrease the number of pain crises.

5. **Heterozygous status (HbAS)** is common (4–14%) in African-Americans. Women with sickle cell trait are at increased risk of renal infection, papillary necrosis, and, rarely, splenic infarction. There is no direct fetal compromise from maternal sickle cell trait. Patients should be screened each trimester for asymptomatic urinary tract infections.

E. **Megaloblastic anemia** is characterized by macrocytosis (MCV of greater than 100 fL).

Macrocytosis results from impaired DNA synthesis. Nuclear maturation is delayed, which affects erythrocytes, leukocytes, and thrombocytic cell lines; this in turn leads to anemia, leukopenia, hypersegmented polymorphonuclear leukocytes, and thrombocytopenia. Altered DNA synthesis stems from nutritional causes in 95% of cases. Megaloblastic anemia usually is slowly progressive. It can manifest as bleeding caused by thrombocytopenia or as an infection resulting from leukopenia.

1. The cause of **folate deficiency** is insufficient dietary intake. Folic acid requirements increase from 50 μg/day in the nonpregnant state to 800–1000 μg/day in pregnancy. Phenytoin, nitrofurantoin, trimethoprim, and alcohol decrease absorption of folic acid. Folic acid deficiency is associated with neural tube defects, abruptio placentae, preeclampsia, prematurity, and intrauterine growth restriction.

2. A less common cause of megaloblastic anemia is **vitamin B_{12} deficiency,** which often is a result of a long-term vegetarian diet or decreased intestinal absorption due to active tropical sprue, regional enteritis, GI resection, or chronic giardiasis. Pernicious anemia, which results from decreased release of gastric intrinsic factor causing malabsorption of vitamin B_{12}, is age related and often accompanied by infertility, and thus it is rarely seen in pregnancy.

3. **Laboratory findings.** In megaloblastic anemia, MCV usually is greater than 100 fL, but the anemia can be normochromic, with normal mean corpuscular hemoglobin and mean corpuscular hemoglobin concentration. The peripheral blood smear shows hypersegmented neutrophils and erythrocyte inclusions. The fasting serum folate level is less than 6 μg/L (normal is 6–12 μg/L). RBC folate is less than 165 μg/L. In severe disease, serum iron concentration and serum lactate dehydrogenase increase. In vitamin B_{12} deficiency, the findings are similar to those in folate deficiency. Serum B_{12} level is less than 190 ng/L (normal is 190–950 ng/L).

4. **Treatment.** Folate deficiency is treated with folic acid 1 mg orally three times daily. Good dietary sources of folate include dark green leafy vegetables, orange juice, strawberries, liver, and legumes. Within 7–10 days, the WBC and platelet counts should return to normal. Hemoglobin gradually increases to normal levels after several weeks of therapy. Vitamin B_{12} therapy entails 6 weekly injections of 1 mg of cyanocobalamin. Affected patients may require monthly injections for life. These women usually require treatment with iron and folate as well. Of note, replacement of folic acid can mask vitamin B_{12} deficiency.

II. **Thrombocytopenia**

A. **Maternal thrombocytopenia** (platelet count of less than 150,000/mL) occurs in 5–7% of all pregnancies. The most common clinical signs are petechiae, easy bruising, epistaxis, gingival bleeding, and hematuria. A patient with a platelet count of more than 20,000/mL is at low risk for bleeding, but the risk increases as the platelet count drops below 20,000/mL. Causes of maternal thrombocytopenia include gestational thrombocytopenia (73.6%), pregnancy-induced hypertension (21%), immunologic causes (3.8%), and rare causes such as disseminated intravascular coagulopathy, thrombotic thrombocytopenic purpura, hemolytic uremic syndrome, HIV infection, and drug effects.

1. **Gestational thrombocytopenia** is a benign condition that occurs in 4–8% of pregnancies.

a. **Diagnosis.** Gestational thrombocytopenia is usually a diagnosis of exclusion, for which the following three cardinal criteria are present: mild thrombocytopenia (70,000–150,000/μL), no prior history of thrombocytopenia, and no bleeding symptoms. The pathophysiology is unknown but may be related to increased physiologic platelet turnover. Gestational thrombocytopenia usually resolves by 6 weeks postpartum and can recur in subsequent pregnancies.

b. **Management.** The first step is taking a careful history to exclude other causes of thrombocytopenia. One should review prior platelet counts both during and before the pregnancy. In gestational thrombocytopenia, *no intervention is necessary.* Approximately 2% of the offspring of mothers with gestational thrombocytopenia have mild thrombocytopenia (higher than 50,000/μL). None have severe thrombocytopenia.

2. **HELLP (hemolysis, elevated liver enzymes, and low platelet) syndrome** is the most common pathologic cause of maternal thrombocytopenia. It occurs in approximately 10% of women who have severe preeclampsia. HELLP syndrome results from increased platelet turnover related to either endothelial damage or consumptive coagulopathy. Symptoms spontaneously resolve by the fifth postpartum day. Around 0.4% of the offspring of mothers with HELLP syndrome have mild thrombocytopenia, mainly as a consequence of prematurity. Preeclampsia may be difficult to distinguish from thrombotic thrombocytopenic purpura, especially when thrombocytopenia, microangiopathic hemolysis, and renal failure are present. Measurement of antithrombin III levels may help make the diagnosis, as antithrombin III activity is decreased in severe preeclampsia but normal in thrombotic thrombocytopenic purpura and hemolytic uremic syndrome.

3. **Idiopathic thrombocytopenic purpura (ITP)** is the most common autoimmune disease in pregnancy, occurring in 1–2 of 1000 pregnancies. The pathophysiology is well understood, even if the cause is not. Lymphocytes produce antiplatelet antibodies directed at platelet surface glycoproteins. The immunoglobulin G (IgG)–coated platelets are cleared by splenic macrophages, which results in thrombocytopenia. The course of ITP is unaffected by pregnancy. Placental transfer of the IgG platelet antibodies can result in fetal or neonatal thrombocytopenia.

a. **Diagnosis.** Isolated maternal thrombocytopenia occurs without splenomegaly or lymphadenopathy. Secondary causes of maternal thrombocytopenia should be excluded (e.g., preeclampsia, HIV infection, systemic lupus erythematosus, drugs). Maternal bone marrow examination reveals normal or increased megakaryocytes. Detection of platelet-associated antibodies is consistent with but not diagnostic of ITP. These antibodies are detected in 30% of patients with nonimmune thrombocytopenia. The absence of platelet-associated IgG makes the diagnosis less likely. Currently, no diagnostic test exists for ITP.

b. **Antenatal management.** Patients with ITP may experience greater morbidity from the therapeutic regimens used to treat the disease than from the disease itself. The goal of therapy is to raise the platelet count to a safe level (more than 20,000–30,000/μL) with the least amount of intervention possible; it is important to remember that a safe platelet count is not necessarily a normal platelet count.

When the maternal platelet count falls below 20,000–30,000/μL, treatment is initiated with prednisone at 1–2 mg/kg/day; dosage is tapered after the platelet count rises to a safe level. Steroids are thought to suppress antibody production, inhibit sequestration of antibody-coated platelets, and interfere with the interaction between platelets and antibody. Within 3 weeks, 70–90% of patients respond to therapy. High doses of intravenous infusion of gamma globulin (IVIG) (400 mg/kg/day for 5 days a week for 3 weeks or 1 g/kg/day for 1 week) are recommended for patients who do not respond to steroids. The proposed mechanism of action of IVIG is prolongation of the clearance time of IgG-coated platelets by the maternal reticuloendothelial system. Eighty percent of patients treated with IVIG respond within days, and remission lasts 3 weeks. The main drawback of IVIG treatment is its cost. **Splenectomy** rarely is indicated during pregnancy. Immunosuppressive therapy is controversial and usually not pursued. Although the efficacy of these treatments in increasing maternal platelet count is well established, they are potentially harmful to the developing fetus.

c. **ITP and fetal or neonatal thrombocytopenia.** Ten percent to 15% of pregnancies complicated by ITP are associated with severe fetal or neonatal thrombocytopenia (platelet count <50,000/μL). It is generally accepted that no correlation exists between fetal and maternal platelet counts. However, no association between the presence or the level of maternal platelet antibodies and fetal platelet count exists either. This lack of association may be explained by the fact that fetal thrombocytopenia is related not only to the level of antiplatelet antibodies but also to the fetal reticuloendothelial system and the fetal capacity to produce platelets.

The neonatal platelet count declines after delivery, reaching a nadir at 48–72 hours of life. As many as 34% of neonates with severe thrombocytopenia experience hemorrhagic sequelae. The incidence of intracranial hemorrhage in one series was 1.5%, with a perinatal mortality of 0.5%. Unlike alloimmune thrombocytopenia, in which 50% of the intracranial hemorrhages occur in utero, no convincing evidence attributes in utero intracranial hemorrhage to maternal ITP. Notification of a pediatrician for close monitoring of the neonatal platelet count is very important in preventing the devastating sequelae of neonatal intracranial hemorrhage.

d. **Intrapartum management.** For years, the assumption that a fetus with a platelet count lower than 50,000/μL is at significant risk for intracranial hemorrhage, coupled with the belief that cesarean delivery is less traumatic than spontaneous vaginal delivery, led to the recommendation of cesarean delivery for severe fetal thrombocytopenia in ITP patients. Fetal platelet counts were determined either by scalp sampling or by cordocentesis. There is currently no recommendation to assess fetal platelet counts to determine route of delivery, however, in light of the evidence that intracranial hemorrhage is a neonatal event, not an intrapartum event. In a retrospective study, the incidence of neonatal intracranial hemorrhage was lower with vaginal delivery than with cesarean (0.5% versus 2.0%). The investigators, however, did not subdivide the cesarean section group into those with elective surgeries and those with surgeries performed after the onset of labor. Other reviews found equal morbidity in thrombocytopenic neonates after cesarean or vaginal delivery. Without evidence that cesarean section provides fetal benefit, we believe spontaneous vaginal delivery without antepartum or intrapartum fetal platelet determination to be the most reasonable method of delivery for women with ITP.

e. **Surgery.** Excessive surgical bleeding is rare when the platelet count is more than 50,000/μL. Platelet transfusions may be used to elevate the platelet count to this level before surgery. Platelet transfusions are available both as platelet concentrates and as platelet-enriched plasma. Each unit of platelets transfused increases the platelet count 5000–10,000/μL. In the presence of clotting abnormalities, use of epidural anesthesia can increase the patient's risk of intraspinal hematoma. When the platelet count is more than 100,000/μL, the patient is a candidate for regional anesthesia. If the platelet count is between 50,000 and 100,000/μL, however, measurement of bleeding time might help to determine whether the patient is at increased risk for intraspinal bleeding. If the bleeding time is prolonged, epidural anesthesia should be avoided.

B. **Fetal or neonatal thrombocytopenia. Alloimmune thrombocytopenia** is the result of a fetal-maternal platelet incompatibility analogous to the incompatibility that causes Rh hemolytic disease. In alloimmune thrombocytopenia, the fetal platelets carry a specific paternal antigen that is not present on maternal platelets. These fetal platelets can traverse the placenta and immunize the mother. The IgG maternal antiplatelet antibodies cross to the fetal circulation and cause fetal thrombocytopenia. Unlike in ITP, the maternal platelet count is normal in alloimmune thrombocytopenia; it is only the fetus who becomes thrombocytopenic.

1. **Incidence and complications.** Unlike with Rh disease, 20–59% of diagnosed cases of neonatal alloimmune thrombocytopenia occur in primiparous women. In approximately 80% of cases, the thrombocytopenia is a benign, self-limited condition of 1–16 weeks' duration postpartum. Twenty percent of affected offspring have intracranial hemorrhage, half of which cases occur in utero. Ninety percent of subsequent pregnancies are likely to be equally or more severely affected. If alloimmune thrombocytopenia has complicated a previous pregnancy, appropriate prenatal management entails determination of fetal platelet genotype so that antenatal treatment can be initiated if the fetus is at risk.

2. **Five major human platelet antigen systems** have been described: PLA I, Bak, Br, Ko, and Pen (also known as HPA 1–5). The platelet antigens are localized on platelet membrane glycoprotein complexes. All are implicated in alloimmune thrombocytopenia. These human antigen systems are biallelic and are inherited as autosomal codominant traits. Parental genotypes determine whether the fetus is potentially at risk. When a father is homozygous for a platelet antigen allele lacking in the mother, all of the offspring are at risk for alloimmune thrombocytopenia. When the father is heterozygous, however, only half of the fetuses are at risk. When the father is heterozygous, amniocentesis can be performed to determine whether the fetus is at risk.

3. **Management.** Optimal management of pregnant patients at risk of alloimmune thrombocytopenia is still evolving. Therapeutic options include maternal administration of steroids alone, maternal administration of IVIG with or without steroids, and fetal platelet transfusions using washed, irradiated maternal platelets. Fetal blood sampling is often performed at 20–22 weeks' gestation, after which therapy is initiated based on the initial fetal platelet count. If a previous offspring was severely affected, therapy is initiated as early as 12 weeks in subsequent pregnancies. More than one fetal blood sampling procedure may be necessary, particularly if failure of maternal therapy necessitates serial fetal platelet transfusions. At the time of labor, fetal blood sampling can be offered to the patient before allowing vaginal delivery. The patient also might choose an elective cesarean near term.

III. **Thromboembolic disease.** The absolute risk of symptomatic venous thrombosis is between 0.5 and 3.0 per 1000 women during pregnancy. The risk of thromboembolic disease is five times greater in pregnancy than in the nonpregnant state. Pregnancy-associated changes in coagulation include increases in levels of clotting factors (I, VII, VIII, IX, X), decreases in levels of protein S, decreases in fibrinolytic activity, increased venous stasis, vascular injury associated with delivery, increased activation of platelets, and resistance to activated protein C. Antepartum deep venous thromboses (DVT) occur in all three trimesters with equal frequency. A significant number of embolic events also occur after delivery. The risk of DVT increases three- to sixteenfold after cesarean delivery. DVT risk also increases with age, multiparity, and prior thromboembolism (Table 17-2). PE is more common postpartum.

A. A **superficial thrombus** is the most common type of thrombosis in pregnancy. These clots rarely travel to the deep venous system. Superficial thromboses are treated with elevation of the affected body part and applica-

TABLE 17-2. RISK FACTORS FOR DEEP VENOUS THROMBOSIS AND THROMBOEMBOLIC DISORDERS

Hereditary thrombophilia	Other
Factor V Leiden mutation (5–9%)	Prior history of deep venous thrombosis
Antithrombin III deficiency (0.02–0.2%)	Mechanical heart valve
Protein C deficiency (0.2–0.5%)	Atrial fibrillation
Protein S deficiency (0.08%)	Trauma, prolonged immobilization, major surgery
Hyperhomocystinemia (1–11%)	Other familial hypercoagulable states
Prothrombin gene mutation (2–4%)	Antiphospholipid syndrome

tion of moist heat. No anti-inflammatory agents or anticoagulants are administered for this benign disease.

B. **Deep venous thrombosis** occurs in the lower extremities or in pelvic veins. Leg edema, calf pain, and Homans sign are not particularly helpful in diagnosis because these effects can all be produced by many other causes, and DVT may be present without any of them.

1. **Diagnosis** by Doppler ultrasonography. In femoral veins, the interpretation of Doppler ultrasonography may be difficult if the patient is in the supine position with uterine compression of the inferior vena cava, especially after 20 weeks' gestation.

   a. **Noninvasive testing**

      (1) **Compression ultrasonography.** Sensitivity is 95% for proximal DVT and 73% for distal DVT, and specificity is 96% for detecting all DVT. This method uses compression from the ultrasonic transducer probe to detect an intraluminal filling defect.

      (2) **Impedance plethysmography.** Sensitivity is 83% for detecting proximal DVT in the symptomatic nonpregnant patient; specificity is 92%.

   b. **Invasive testing**

      (1) **Limited venography** with abdominal shielding (less than 0.05 rad).

      (2) **Full venography:** bilateral venography without shielding (less than 1.0 rad). This method can be used if iliac or pelvic thrombosis is suspected.

   c. The role of MRI is still not well defined for the pregnant patient.

2. **Treatment**

   a. **Intravenous heparin** sodium is the treatment for acute thromboembolism. The appropriate dosage is a 70–100 U/kg IV bolus of heparin, followed by infusion of 15–20 U/kg/hour, with the target of an activated partial thromboplastin time (aPTT) of 1.5–2.5 times control. After initial inpatient treatment, which should be maintained for at least 5–7 days, therapy should be continued with subcutaneous heparin injections every 8–12 hours for at least 3 months after the acute event. Some recommend continuing therapeutic anticoagulation for the remainder of the pregnancy or until 6–12 weeks postpartum.

   b. The major concerns with heparin use during pregnancy are heparin-induced osteopenia and thrombocytopenia. Platelet counts should be checked on day 5 and then periodically for the first 2 weeks of heparin therapy. Heparin does not cross the placenta and therefore does not have the potential to cause fetal bleeding or teratogenicity. Bleeding at the uteroplacental junction is possible.

    c. **Low-molecular-weight heparin (LMWH).** Enoxaparin sodium or dalteparin sodium may be used as either anticoagulation prophylaxis or anticoagulation therapy during pregnancy. Because data are lacking regarding adequate dosing during pregnancy, anti–factor Xa levels may be monitored. According to a study by Casele et al. (*Am J Obstet Gynecol*, 181/1113, 1999) the pharmacokinetics of LMWH (specifically enoxaparin) is different in pregnant patients than in the same patients postpartum; it also changes throughout gestation. These investigators concluded that twice-daily dosing of enoxaparin may be necessary to maintain anti–factor Xa activity above 0.1 IU/mL throughout a 24-hour period. They recommend periodic monitoring of peak anti–factor Xa activity (approximately 3.5 hours after a dose) and predose activity. Patients should be counseled to stop taking their LMWH at the onset of labor. There is concern regarding the safety of epidural anesthesia with the use of twice-daily LMWH, and the American Society of Regional Anesthesia has recommended that epidurals be withheld until 24 hours after the last heparin injection. For patients receiving low-dose, once-daily LMWH, epidural anesthesia should be withheld for 10–12 hours after the last dose (*Chest*, 114(5)/524–530,1998; ACOG Practice Bulletin No. 19, 2000).

    d. **Warfarin sodium** use is contraindicated in pregnancy because it has been found that one-third of fetuses exposed to warfarin late in pregnancy developed CNS injuries, hemorrhage, or ophthalmologic abnormalities. Fetuses exposed to warfarin in the first trimester (between 6 and 12 weeks' gestation) had a high incidence of congenital anomalies (including a skeletal embryopathy resulting in stippled epiphyses and nasal and limb hypoplasia) and miscarriage. Studies of patients on long-term anticoagulation therapy with warfarin showed that, when warfarin was replaced with heparin at 6 weeks' gestation, none of the patients delivered children with warfarin embryopathy.

C. **Pulmonary embolism.** The symptoms of dyspnea, pleuritic chest pain, tachypnea, and tachycardia typically associated with pulmonary embolism are all common in pregnancy for other reasons. Normal arterial blood gas values also are altered in pregnancy, so these findings must be interpreted using pregnancy-adjusted normal values.

    1. **Diagnostic studies.** The chest radiograph is important, because it helps rule out other disease processes and enhances interpretation of the ventilation-perfusion ($\dot{V}/\dot{Q}$) scan. A $\dot{V}/\dot{Q}$ scan is necessary for diagnosing pulmonary embolism. A normal scan finding is accurate in excluding pulmonary embolism. Most fetal exposure to radiation occurs when radioactive tracers are excreted in the maternal bladder. Therefore, fetal radiation exposure can be limited by prompt and frequent voiding after the $\dot{V}/\dot{Q}$ procedure. The total radiation exposure during a $\dot{V}/\dot{Q}$ scan is 0.215 rad, with the perfusion portion (technetium) contributing 0.175 rad, and the ventilation portion (xenon) contributing 0.040 rad. Radiation exposure from a two-view chest radiograph is 0.00007 rad. High-probability results on scans may be accepted as an indication for treatment because the reliability of $\dot{V}/\dot{Q}$ testing is 90%. Intermediate- or low-probability results require arteriography for further evaluation before a commitment to long-term anticoagulation is made. If noninvasive testing reveals a proximal DVT, then anticoagulation therapy should be initiated. Pulmonary angiography poses fewer radiation risks to the fetus than might be expected. Spiral CT of the chest may also be considered for the diagnosis of pulmonary embolism. This modality has not yet been used extensively in pregnancy, but the sensitivity and specificity of spiral CT for diagnosing central pulmonary artery embolus are approximately 94% in the nonpregnant patient.

    2. **Treatment** is the same as that for DVT. As with DVT, the most important time to provide prophylaxis for future pregnancies is during the 6-

week postpartum period. No difference exists between the prophylaxis provided to a patient who experienced a DVT and that provided to a patient who experienced a pulmonary embolism. Prophylactic therapy consists of heparin, 5000 U subcutaneously every 12 hours. See later for other options.

D. **Thromboprophylaxis in pregnancy**
  1. Highest-risk patients should have adjusted-dose heparin prophylaxis (adjusted-dose heparin every 8 hours to maintain an aPTT of at least 1.5 times the control level, or, as an alternative, LMWH twice daily). The patients at highest risk are those who have
      a. Artificial heart valves (some investigators recommend warfarin therapy after the first trimester in certain circumstances)
      b. Antithrombin III deficiency
      c. Antiphospholipid syndrome
      d. History of rheumatic heart disease with current atrial fibrillation
      e. Homozygous factor V Leiden mutation, homozygous prothrombin G20210A mutation
      f. Patients receiving chronic anticoagulation for recurrent thromboembolism
      g. History of a life-threatening thrombosis or recent thrombosis
  2. Other recommendations based primarily on consensus and expert opinion (ACOG Practice Bulletin No. 19, 2000) include the following:
      a. Pregnant patients with a history of isolated venous thrombosis directly related to a transient, highly thrombogenic event such as orthopedic trauma or complicated surgery in whom an underlying thrombophilia has been excluded may be offered heparin prophylaxis or no prophylaxis during the antepartum period. Such patients, however, should be counseled that their risk of thromboembolism is likely to be higher than that of the general population. Prophylactic warfarin should be offered for 6 weeks postpartum.
      b. Pregnant patients with a history of idiopathic thrombosis or thrombosis related to pregnancy or oral contraceptive use, or a history of thrombosis accompanied by an underlying thrombophilia other than homozygosity for the factor V Leiden mutation, heterozygosity for both the factor V Leiden and the prothrombin G20210A mutation, or antithrombin III deficiency should be offered antepartum and postpartum low-dose heparin prophylaxis.
      c. Patients who have no history of thrombosis but who have an underlying thrombophilia and have a strong family history of thrombosis also are candidates for antepartum and postpartum prophylaxis. At the minimum, postpartum prophylaxis should be offered.
      d. It is unclear whether patients with a history of thrombosis associated with protein C or protein S deficiency should receive low-dose or adjusted-dose heparin prophylaxis during pregnancy.
      e. Patients at risk for thrombosis should receive warfarin postpartum for 6 weeks to achieve an international normalized ratio of 2.0–3.0. Heparin should be given immediately postpartum with warfarin for at least 5 days until the international normalized ratio is in the therapeutic range.
  3. Prophylactic heparin regimens in pregnancy
      a. Unfractionated heparin
          (1) Low-dose prophylaxis 5000–7500 U every 12 hours during the first trimester; 7500–10,000 U every 12 hours during the second trimester; 10,000 U every 12 hours during the third trimester unless the aPTT is elevated. The aPTT may be checked near term and the heparin dose reduced if prolonged. Alternately, 5,000–10,000 U every 12 hours may be used throughout pregnancy.

           (2) Adjusted-dose prophylaxis: more than 10,000 U two or three times a day to achieve an aPTT of 1.5–2.5

     b. LMWH

           (1) Low-dose prophylaxis:

               (a) Dalteparin, 5000 U once or twice daily

               (b) Enoxaparin, 40 mg once or twice daily

           (2) Adjusted-dose prophylaxis

               (a) Dalteparin, 5000–10,000 U every 12 hours

               (b) Enoxaparin, 30–80 mg every 12 hours

18. ALLOIMMUNIZATION

Suzanne Davey Shipman and Christian Chisholm

ALLOIMMUNIZATION BY RH ANTIGENS

I. **The Rh blood group system**

A. A high degree of polymorphism characterizes the Rh blood group. Five major antigens are identified with typing sera, and many variant antigens are known to exist.

B. The **Fisher-Race nomenclature** is used most commonly to classify Rh antigens. The nomenclature assumes the presence of three genetic loci, each with two major alleles, C, c, D, d, E, e. No antiserum specific for the hypothetical d antigen has been found. The Rh antigen complex is the final expression of a group of at least these five possible antigens. An individual who expresses the D antigen is termed Rh positive; one who does not express this antigen is termed Rh negative.

C. The **D^u antigen** is one of the most common of approximately 36 antigenic variants. D^u antigen is an incomplete form of D antigen. According to the American Association of Blood Banks, the D^u designation has been changed to "weak D positive" [*American Association of Blood Banks Association Bulletin*, 98(2)/1–6, 1998]. Patients with this designation are considered Rh D positive and should not receive anti–D immune globulin. Rh D antigens are expressed on the surface of erythrocytes in a weaker concentration than in most Rh D–positive individuals. Mothers who are weakly D positive are not at risk for sensitization.

II. **The Rh antigen.** Rh antigens consist of polypeptides embedded in red blood cell (RBC) membranes and appear by 52 days' gestation. At least three different D-antigen epitopes exist.

III. **Rh alloimmunization requirements.** All of the following criteria must be met for alloimmunization to occur:

A. The fetus must have Rh-positive RBCs, and the mother must have Rh-negative RBCs.

B. **Fetomaternal transfusion (FMT).** A sufficient number of fetal RBCs (0.1 mL or more) must gain access to maternal circulation.

C. **Maternal immunocompetence.** The mother must mount an immune response to produce antibody directed against D antigen.

IV. **Incidence.** The highest proportion of Rh-negative individuals is found among the Basque communities of France and Spain, with a prevalence of 25% to 40%. Overall, 15% of white Americans, 7–8% of African-Americans, and 7% of Hispanic Americans are Rh negative. In the white U.S. population, an Rh-negative woman has an 85% chance of mating with an Rh-positive man, and an Rh-positive man has a 70% chance of producing an Rh-positive fetus; thus, a 60% chance of an Rh-incompatible pregnancy exists for any Rh-negative woman. The incidence of alloimmunization is 0.2%.

V. **Pathophysiology**

A. Initial immunoglobulin M response is followed by long-standing immunoglobulin G production. Immunoglobulin G crosses the placenta by receptor-mediated endocytosis via receptors for the Fc portion of immunoglobulin G, and substantial transfer can occur after 20 weeks. Antibody binds to antigen, which causes disruption of red cell membranes and hemolysis. The fetus responds to anemia by increasing erythropoietin production. Both marrow and extramedullary sites of hematopoiesis are stimulated. Control of erythroid maturation is poor, and immature forms are found in peripheral circulation (**erythroblastosis fetalis**).

B. Factors leading to **fetal hydrops**

1. Reduced hepatic protein synthesis

2. Intrahepatic changes causing portal hypertension
3. Increased cardiac output and hydrostatic pressure
4. Increased capillary permeability

VI. **Fetomaternal transfusion** sufficient to cause alloimmunization most commonly occurs at delivery. At most deliveries, less than 0.1 mL is transfused; in only 0.2% to 1.0% is the volume greater than 30 mL. The amount of FMT necessary to cause alloimmunization varies with the immunogenic capacity of the RBCs and the immune responsiveness of the mother. FMT is detected in 6.7% of first trimester pregnancies, 13.9% of second trimester pregnancies, and 29.0% of third trimester pregnancies. FMT also can be detected in 15% to 25% of amniocentesis procedures in the second and third trimesters, even with ultrasonographic guidance. The incidence of FMT is higher in terminated pregnancies than in spontaneous abortions. As many as 30% of Rh-negative individuals are immunologic "nonresponders" and do not appear to be at risk for Rh alloimmunization. ABO incompatibility between the mother and fetus has a protective effect against Rh sensitization, as ABO-incompatible RBCs are cleared more rapidly.

VII. **Administration of Rh D immune globulin.** In the United States, the use of Rh immune globulin at 28 weeks has produced a 100-fold reduction in cases of antepartum sensitization to the Rh D antigen.

A. Anti–D immune globulin is administered intramuscularly to prevent active immunization. Three hundred micrograms is administered within 72 hours of delivery or fetomaternal hemorrhage (FMH). The 72-hour time frame is an artifact of study methodology. Administration of Rh immune globulin as late as 14–28 days postpartum may be effective in preventing alloimmunization.

B. Overall, 16% of Rh-negative women become alloimmunized by their first Rh-incompatible (ABO-compatible) pregnancy if they are not treated with Rh immune globulin. This rate decreases to 1.5% if Rh immune globulin is administered within 72 hours after delivery, and further decreases to 0.1% if antepartum prophylaxis is given at 28 weeks' gestation.

C. Other indications for administration of Rh_0 D immune globulin include the following:

1. First trimester spontaneous or therapeutic abortion. Whether to administer Rh D immune globulin to a patient with threatened abortion and a live embryo or fetus at or before 12 weeks of gestation is controversial, and no evidence-based recommendation can be made.
2. Ectopic pregnancy.
3. Amniocentesis, chorionic villus sampling, and fetal blood sampling.
4. Molar pregnancy.
5. Second or third trimester bleeding.
6. Fetal death from suspected FMH in the second or third trimester.
7. External cephalic version.
8. Abdominal trauma.

D. For FMH, 10 µg/estimated mL of whole fetal blood should be administered. Quantitation of FMH requires a Betke-Kleihauer smear of maternal blood. This test determines the percentage of fetal red blood cells in the maternal blood. The percentage of fetal RBCs is multiplied by maternal blood volume, then by maternal hematocrit; the end product represents the volume of fetal RBCs in the maternal circulation.

E. The half-life of Rh D immune globulin is 24 days, although titers decrease over time. If delivery occurs within 3 weeks of the standard antenatal anti–D immune globulin administration, the postnatal dose may be withheld in the absence of excessive FMH. The same is true when anti–D immune globulin is given for antenatal procedures, such as external cephalic version or amniocentesis, or for third trimester bleeding.

VIII. **Management of pregnancy in unsensitized Rh-negative women**

A. Patients who are Rh negative, D^u negative

1. At less than 20 weeks' gestation, the following tests should be performed: determination of ABO blood group, determination of Rh type, antibody screen.

2. At 28 weeks' gestation, the antibody screen should be repeated. If the results are negative, 300 μg of Rh immune globulin should be administered. If the antibody screen results are positive, management should be as for pregnancy in an Rh-immunized woman.

3. After delivery, if the neonate is Rh negative or D^u positive, the antibody screen should be repeated and a test performed for excessive FMH. If the antibody screen results are negative and estimated FMH is less than 30 mL of whole blood, 300 μg of Rh immune globulin should be administered. If the antibody screen results are negative and the estimated FMH is greater than 30 mL, Rh immune globulin, 300 μg per 30 mL of estimated fetal blood, should be administered if the neonate is Rh positive or D^u positive. If the antibody screen results are positive (titer greater than 1:4), the woman should be managed as Rh immunized in her next pregnancy. Lower titers probably result from passively administered Rh immune globulin, and patients with low titers are candidates for receipt of Rh immune globulin in subsequent pregnancies.

B. Infrequently, an Rh-negative woman is found to have "weak" Rh antibody, detectable only by very sensitive techniques. The majority of these women are not Rh immunized and should be given prophylactic Rh immune globulin according to protocol.

IX. **Management of pregnancy in D^u-positive patients.** D^u-positive mothers should be treated as if they were Rh positive. One should beware when previously typed Rh-negative mothers are found to be D^u positive during pregnancy or postpartum. Such a finding usually results from the presence of a large number of fetal cells in the maternal circulation. A check should be made for FMH, and the patient should be treated with Rh immune globulin.

X. **Management of pregnancy in Rh-alloimmunized women.** The fetus should be assessed. Any patient with an anti–D antibody titer higher than 1:4 should be considered Rh sensitized (Fig. 18-1).

A. **Estimated gestational age.** An accurate estimate of gestational age should be obtained, as this is crucial to timing of amniocentesis, cordocentesis, and delivery.

B. **Paternal status.** The Rh antigen status of the baby's father should be determined. If the father is Rh negative, no further intervention is needed. One should confirm with the mother *in private* that the apparent father is the only possible father. Paternal blood is tested for the phenotype for the specific antigen; typing and screening is not helpful.

1. If the father is negative for the antigen in question, the fetus is not at risk. Maternal antibody titers and fetal growth should be followed.

2. If the father is homozygous for the antigen in question, the fetus is at risk for fetal hemolytic disease. Serial fetal assessment should be begun and tertiary care referral ensured.

3. If the father is heterozygous for the antigen in question, the likelihood is 1:2 that the fetus is at risk. Fetal antigen status should be evaluated by cordocentesis for direct testing of fetal red cell antigen status or by amniocentesis for genetic testing of fetal status by polymerase chain reaction.

C. **Determination of the antibody titer.** In first pregnancies in sensitized women, the antibody titer that determines the need for amniocentesis is called the **critical titer**; this is generally 1:16. After the critical titer is reached and the need for amniocentesis established, determination of titers is not useful in management. Eighty percent of severely affected patients have stable titers.

1. If the antibody titer is less than the critical titer in the first pregnancy of a sensitized woman, titer determination should be repeated every 2–4 weeks, beginning at 16–18 weeks' gestation.

2. If the titer is less than 1:8 and the patient has previously carried an infant with fetal hemolytic disease, titer determination should be repeated every 2–4 weeks and fetal progress should be followed with serial ultrasonographic examinations.

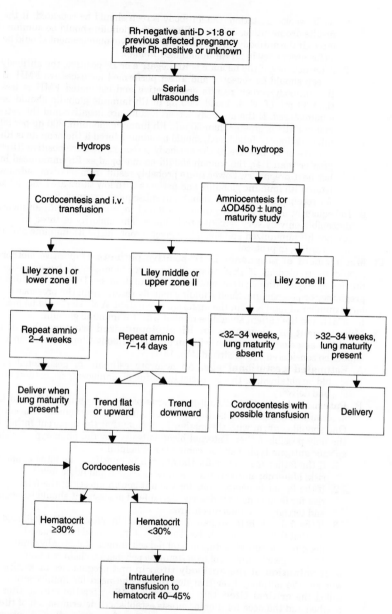

FIG. 18-1. Flow diagram outlining the management of a pregnancy complicated by Rh sensitization. The timing of the first amniocentesis is based on the history, maternal titer, and gestational age. In addition to assessment of amniotic fluid bilirubin or umbilical cord hematocrit, daily monitoring of fetal movements by patients after 26–28 weeks' gestation, nonstress tests one to two times weekly, and ultrasonographic examinations every 1–2 weeks are recommended. ΔOD450, spectrophotometric peak at 450 nm amnio, amniocentesis. (From Gabbe SG, Nieble JK, Simpson JL. *Obstetrics: normal and problem pregnancies,* 3rd ed. New York: Churchill Livingstone, 1996, with permission.)

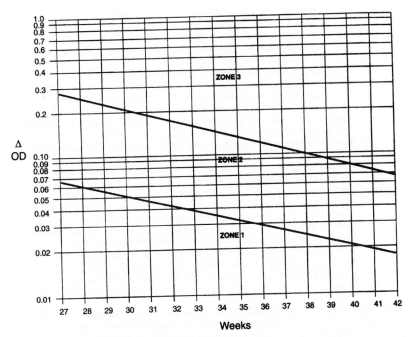

FIG. 18-2. Liley graph depicting degrees of Rh sensitization. ΔOD, optical density at 450 nm. (From Liley AW. Liquor amnii analysis in management of pregnancy complicated by rhesus sensitization. *Am J Obstet Gynecol* 1961;82:1359–1370, with permission.)

   3. If the titer is higher than the critical titer, further evaluation with amniocentesis is necessary beginning at 26 weeks' gestation or earlier.
   D. **Obstetric history.** A history of sensitization in previous pregnancies is useful. Fetal hemolytic disease tends to be as severe or more severe in subsequent pregnancies compared with the first. If a previous fetus was hydropic, an 80% chance exists that the next Rh-positive fetus will be hydropic. Fetal hemolytic disease also tends to develop at the same time or somewhat earlier in subsequent pregnancies. Obstetric history is not significant, however, if the previous pregnancy was the first in which sensitization occurred, because few fetuses in the first pregnancy develop hydrops.
   E. **Analysis of the amniotic fluid.** In 1956, Bevis determined that the bilirubin concentration of amniotic fluid in pregnancies complicated by Rh sensitization correlated with severity of fetal hemolysis. In 1961, Liley showed that the spectrophotometric peak at 450 nm (ΔOD450) was directly proportional to the concentration of bilirubin in amniotic fluid after the second trimester.
      1. Three prognostic zones have been described: zone 3 (upper, severely affected) to zone 1 (lower, unaffected or mildly affected). Zone 2 encompasses a wide range of severity. It is important to establish the ΔOD450 trend. Amniotic fluid bilirubin concentration decreases as normal pregnancy advances, so a horizontal or rising trend is ominous (Fig. 18-2).
      2. Interpretation of amniotic fluid findings
         a. A single ΔOD450 value is often insufficient for accurate analysis; a trend is more reliable.

b. Relying solely on ΔOD450 values may lead to a false impression of severity. Fetal blood sampling is indicated when ΔOD450 values increase or fall into upper zone 2 or zone 3.

c. Controversy exists about the reliability of extrapolating Liley graph values before 26 weeks' gestation.

F. **Analysis of fetal blood.** Ultrasonographically guided vascular puncture techniques were developed to determine fetal blood type, hematocrit, and blood gas values. These techniques also enabled intravascular fetal blood transfusion. Fetal blood analysis is the first step in the care of the fetus at risk for severe hemolytic disease in many centers. There is a 1% or lower fetal loss rate with cordocentesis in experienced hands.

G. **Ultrasonographic and Doppler flow studies.** Ultrasonographic evidence of cardiac failure is a late sign of hydrops (hematocrit less than 15%). Findings suggesting a lesser degree of anemia include increased placental thickness, increased umbilical vein diameter, increased size of the fetal liver, pericardial effusion, bowel wall edema (visualization of both sides of the fetal bowel), polyhydramnios, and abnormalities of pulsed Doppler flow-velocity waveforms, especially in the middle cerebral artery.

H. **Evaluation of the need for intrauterine transfusion.** The need for intrauterine transfusion is based on ΔOD450 values and trends. Severe anemia is suspected when ΔOD450 values rise into the upper third of zone 2 before 30 weeks' gestation or into zone 3 before 32 weeks' gestation. A single ΔOD450 value in zone 3 before 32–34 weeks' gestation also may indicate severe anemia. Sonographic evidence of hydrops implies a hematocrit of less than 15%.

XI. **Intrauterine transfusion in pregnancies complicated by Rh alloimmunization** offers an alternative to preterm delivery in cases of severe fetal hemolytic disease. The goals of intrauterine transfusion are to correct anemia, thus improving oxygenation, and to reduce extramedullary hematopoietic demand, thus decreasing portal venous pressure and improving hepatic function. In 1963 Liley reported the first successful intraperitoneal intrauterine transfusion. Rodecke and colleagues in 1981 performed successful intravascular transfusions using a fetoscopic technique. Ultrasonographically guided transfusion is now performed. The needle is placed into the umbilical vein at its insertion into the placenta or into the intrahepatic portion of the same vessel. Crossmatched, cytomegalovirus-negative, irradiated packed red blood cells are used.

A. Intraperitoneal versus intravascular transfusion

1. Intravascular transfusion (IVT) allows the degree of fetal anemia to be measured, which thus permits precise calculation of the amount of blood required.

2. IVT provides immediate correction of the anemia, reversing fetal hydrops more quickly.

3. Use of IVT alone increases the total number of procedures required, because the volume transfused is smaller than in intraperitoneal transfusion (IPT).

4. The risk of fetal death is 2% per procedure for IPT and 4% per procedure for IVT. Eighty-four percent of fetal IVT procedures have good outcomes, with 94% survival of nonhydropic fetuses and 74% survival of hydropic fetuses.

B. General risks of intrauterine transfusion include rupture of membranes, FMH, and infection.

XII. **Timing of delivery.** In cases of mild fetal hemolysis, delivery should occur around 37 weeks' gestation after fetal lung maturity is confirmed. In cases of severe sensitization, the decision to deliver is individualized, with every attempt made to bring the fetus to at least 32 weeks' gestation using transfusions. Correction of hydrops in utero results in better neonatal outcome, regardless of gestational age.

XIII. **Perinatal outcome.** The earlier a transfusion is required, the poorer the outcome. The presence of fetal hydrops at the time of first transfusion is associated with a poor outcome.

ALLOIMMUNIZATION BY OTHER ANTIGENS

I. **Sensitization caused by minor antigens.** Maternal antibodies to minor antigens are detected as frequently as or more frequently than anti–D antibody. The incidence of sensitization caused by these minor antigens is increased in multiparas and in women who received a blood transfusion in the past.

   A. **Lewis antigens.** Le^a and Le^b are not true RBC antigens but are secreted by other tissues and acquired by RBCs. Fetal RBCs acquire little antigen and react weakly with antibodies (a mnemonic is "Lewis lives").

   B. The most commonly encountered potentially serious antibodies are anti-Kell; anti-E, anti-c, and anti–c+E (part of Rh complex); and anti-Fy^a (Duffy). Mnemonics are "Kell kills," "Duffy dies."

   C. **Anti-Kell sensitization**

      1. **Diagnosis.** The fetal anemia produced by anti-Kell sensitization is qualitatively different from that of Rh disease. The primary cause of the anemia is suppression of fetal erythropoiesis rather than hemolysis; therefore, the Δ OD450 value in cases of anti-Kell anemia may not be as elevated for a given degree of fetal anemia as it is in Rh disease because the test measures fetal bilirubin.

      2. **Management** should include the use of cordocentesis, rather than ΔOD450 value, to determine fetal anemia. It is worth determining paternal antigen status, because 90% of the population is Kell antigen negative, and only 0.2% is homozygous Kell positive.

II. **ABO incompatibility** occurs in 20% to 25% of pregnancies. This condition does not cause fetal hemolysis. It is a pediatric, not an obstetric, problem and manifests as mild to moderate hyperbilirubinemia during the first 24 hours of life.

19. SURGICAL DISEASE AND TRAUMA IN PREGNANCY

Ada Kagumba and Michael Lantz

GENERAL CONSIDERATIONS FOR THE PREGNANT SURGICAL PATIENT

The diagnosis and management of surgical disease during pregnancy is a challenge for the obstetrician and the surgeon, both of whom must strive to maintain the pregnancy and provide definitive therapy as promptly as possible. Surgical disease in pregnancy is complicated by the masking of symptoms by the physiologic changes of pregnancy, specific obstetric pathology, delay in diagnosis or treatment, and potential harm to the fetus of intervention.

I. **Physiologic and anatomic changes in pregnancy**
   A. The enlarging uterus displaces abdominal organs and brings adnexal structures into the abdomen.
   B. Compression of the inferior vena cava by the uterus decreases venous return and may cause supine hypotension syndrome.
   C. Relative leukocytosis may make determination of infection difficult, especially when leukocytosis is a key variable in determining infective etiology.
   D. Increased plasma volume and decreased hematocrit, as well as relatively decreased BPs, make evaluation of acute blood loss difficult.
   E. The ability of the omentum to contain peritonitis is reduced during pregnancy.
   F. The patient's hypoalbuminemic state predisposes to edema.

II. **Complications of nonobstetric surgery** in the pregnant patient include preterm labor, preterm delivery, and fetal loss. Recent abdominal surgery, however, does not complicate vaginal delivery, nor has incisional dehiscence been associated with vaginal delivery.

III. **Diagnostic radiology in the pregnant patient.** Teratogenic and oncogenic risks of ionizing radiation are highest between 8 and 15 weeks' gestation. Exposure of the fetus to less than 10 rad is believed to pose little risk.

IV. **Management of the pregnant surgical patient**
   A. Optimal timing for surgery is during the second trimester. Surgery during the first trimester carries an increased risk of spontaneous abortion because of possible disruption of the corpus luteum. Preterm labor and inadequate operative exposure complicate third trimester surgery.
   B. Intraoperative management should include left lateral uterine displacement, avoidance of uterine manipulation, optimal maternal oxygenation, and external fetal monitoring if gestational age is in the viable range.
   C. **Perioperative care.** Current data do not support the use of tocolytic agents intraoperatively.

ACUTE ABDOMEN IN PREGNANCY

I. **Acute appendicitis** is the most common surgical complication of pregnancy, affecting approximately 1 in 1500 pregnancies. It usually occurs with the same frequency in each trimester and in the puerperium.
   A. **Clinical presentation** includes anorexia, nausea, vomiting, fever, abdominal pain (the location of which depends on gestational age), abdominal tenderness, rebound tenderness, and, less commonly, leukocytosis.
   B. **Diagnostic evaluation.** Clinical suspicion is essential in making the diagnosis. Unfortunately, the classic signs of appendicitis, including right lower quadrant pain preceded by periumbilical pain, rebound tenderness, and obturator, psoas, or Rovsing's signs, are often absent in the pregnant patient. The leukocyte count may or may not be elevated, although a shift to the left is a significant finding. Ultrasonography may be useful in ruling out other diagnoses.

C. **Therapy**
1. **Laparoscopy** may be useful if the diagnosis is uncertain (e.g., in the presence of a history of pelvic inflammatory disease). After 12–14 weeks' gestation, however, laparoscopy carries an increased risk of uterine perforation, so open laparoscopy is advisable. Due to risk of perforation and poor exposure, laparoscopy is contraindicated during the third trimester.
2. **Laparotomy** is indicated if clinical suspicion of appendicitis is high, regardless of the stage of gestation. The location of the incision depends on gestational age. The acceptable rate of laparotomy with negative findings is 20% to 35%.
3. **Antibiotics** should be administered postoperatively in cases of perforation, peritonitis, or periappendiceal abscess.
4. The role of tocolytic agents pre- or postoperatively is not known.

D. **Obstetric complications** of appendicitis include preterm labor (10–15%), spontaneous abortion (3–5%), and maternal mortality. If the delay in diagnosis is longer than 24 hours, morbidity is increased, with significant rates of perforation and fetal loss. Maternal mortality may approach 5%, largely because of surgical delay.

E. **Differential diagnosis** includes ectopic pregnancy, pyelonephritis, acute cholecystitis, pelvic inflammatory disease, preterm labor, abruptio placentae, degenerating myoma, round ligament pain, adnexal torsion, and chorioamnionitis. Pyelonephritis is the most common misdiagnosis.

II. **Acute cholecystitis** is the second most common surgical complication of pregnancy, with an incidence of 1 in 4000. Pregnant patients are predisposed to cholelithiasis because of their increased gallbladder volume, decreased intestinal motility, and delayed emptying of the gallbladder. Progesterone causes decreased contraction of the gallbladder; therefore, preexisting gallstones rarely cause acute cholecystitis.

A. **Clinical presentation** is similar to that for nonpregnant patients. Symptoms may be localized to the flank, right scapula, or shoulder.

B. **Diagnostic evaluation** should consist of blood work, including leukocyte count, serum amylase level, and total bilirubin level, and ultrasonography of the right upper quadrant to visualize calculi, wall thickness, presence or absence of pericholecystic fluid, and common duct dilatation. Experience with endoscopic retrograde cholangiopancreatography (ERCP) during pregnancy is limited, but the procedure may be considered if common bile duct stones are present. If ERCP is warranted, the amount of fluoroscopy may be kept to a minimum.

C. **Differential diagnosis** includes acute fatty liver, abruptio placentae, pancreatitis, acute appendicitis, HELLP syndrome (hemolysis, elevated liver enzymes, and low platelets), and pneumonia.

D. **Therapy**
1. Nonoperative management may be sufficient and includes bowel rest, intravenous hydration, nasogastric suction, antibiotic therapy, analgesic administration, and fetal monitoring.
2. Successful use of ERCP with sphincterotomy and percutaneous cholecystostomy has been reported. Cholecystectomy can be performed safely postpartum. Surgical management is required in approximately 25% of cases and is indicated in cases of failure of conservative therapy, recurrence in the same trimester, suspected perforation, sepsis, or peritonitis. Surgery is safest during the second trimester. The physician should consider delaying first trimester cases until the second trimester, and delaying third trimester cases until postpartum. Once again, open laparoscopy may be preferable in early pregnancy. Intraoperative cholangiography should be avoided unless gallstone pancreatitis is suspected.

III. **Ovarian torsion and ruptured corpus luteum.** Adnexal torsion is an uncommon complication of pregnancy and occurs when an enlarged ovary twists on its pedicle. The common causes of adnexal torsion are corpus luteum cysts, dermoids and other neoplasms, and ovulation induction.

A. **Clinical presentation** is characterized by mild to severe distress associated with acute, usually unilateral, pain, with or without diaphoresis; nausea; and vomiting. An adnexal mass may be palpable.

B. **Diagnostic evaluation** includes ultrasonography with Doppler flow studies to visualize cysts, rule out ectopic pregnancy, and evaluate blood flow to the ovaries.

C. **Differential diagnosis** includes acute appendicitis, ectopic pregnancy, diverticulitis, small bowel obstruction, pelvic inflammatory disease, and pancreatitis.

D. **Complications** of torsion include adnexal infarction, chemical peritonitis, and preterm labor.

E. **Therapy**

1. **Conservative management,** once an intrauterine pregnancy has been confirmed by ultrasonography, is indicated for ruptured corpus luteum cysts, which usually regress by 16 weeks' gestation.

2. **Operative management** is indicated for an acute abdomen and cases of suspected torsion or infarction. Whether the ovary should be removed or untwisted depends on the assessment of viability of the ovary that has undergone torsion. Persistent cysts, cysts larger than 6 cm, or cysts with solid elements may also require surgery. Depending on gestational age, laparoscopy may be considered when the diagnosis is uncertain.

3. **Progestins** should be administered postoperatively to prevent spontaneous abortion during the first 10 weeks of pregnancy, especially when the ovary containing the corpus luteum of pregnancy is involved.

TRAUMA IN PREGNANCY

I. **Incidence and etiology.** One in twelve pregnancies is complicated by trauma. Motor vehicle collisions are the most common cause, followed by falls and domestic abuse and assaults. Maternal outcome is similar to that in trauma to nonpregnant women.

II. **Assessment of the pregnant trauma patient**

A. **The mother should first be stabilized.**

B. **A primary survey should be conducted.**

1. An airway should be established and maintained as for nonpregnant patients.

2. Breathing. Oxygen should be administered by nasal cannula, face mask, or endotracheal tube to maintain saturation at 95% or greater. Intubation should be performed early. Maternal oxygen saturation of 91% correlates with a fetal partial oxygen pressure of approximately 60 mm Hg.

3. Circulation

a. The patient should be placed in the left lateral decubitus position, or the uterus should be manually deflected to the left with a wedge under the right hip, if gestational age is greater than 20 weeks.

b. Two large-bore intravenous catheters should be placed.

c. Crystalloid in the form of lactated Ringer's solution or normal saline should be administered in a 3:1 ratio to the estimated blood loss.

d. Transfusion is indicated if the estimated blood loss is greater than 1 L. Because of increased blood volume during pregnancy, patients may lose up to 1500 mL of blood before clinical instability becomes apparent.

e. Vasopressors should be avoided if possible because they depress uteroplacental perfusion, but vasopressors should not be withheld if they are indicated, such as in cases of cardiogenic or neurogenic shock.

C. **A secondary survey should be conducted.**

1. The entire body should be examined, particularly the abdomen and uterus, after the patient has been stabilized.

2. Fetal surveillance is performed to assess well-being and estimate gestational age.

D. **Diagnostic tests should be performed.**

1. Diagnostic peritoneal lavage is more risky in pregnant than in nonpregnant patients but still has a morbidity rate of less than 1%. It may be

indicated in cases of blunt trauma or stab wounds if the patient has altered sensorium, unexplained shock, major thoracic injury, or multiple orthopedic injuries.

2. CT scan should be performed if the patient is stable.
3. Ultrasonography is less useful for assessing injury than other modalities; it may be used, however, for screening or for obstetric indications—for assessment of fetal age, viability, and well-being.
4. Laboratory studies include test for Rh status, determination of blood type and crossmatch for anticipated needs, CBC, Kleihauer-Betke test, measurement of coagulation profile, and toxicology screen including blood alcohol levels.

E. **Cesarean section** for fetal distress, abruptio placentae, uterine rupture, or unstable pelvic or lumbosacral fracture in labor may be considered if the mother is in stable condition, depending on gestational age, condition of fetus, and extent of injury to the uterus.

F. The **use of tocolytic agents** in cases of trauma is controversial but not contraindicated. Standard tocolytic agents produce symptoms such as tachycardia, hypotension, and altered sensorium that may complicate management of the trauma patient in preterm labor.

III. **Blunt trauma** most commonly is caused by motor vehicle collisions. Pregnant women should be instructed to wear seat belts with three-point restraints and with the lap belt secured over the bony pelvis and not across the fundus.

A. **Complications** include retroperitoneal hemorrhage (which is more common in the pregnant than in the nonpregnant patient due to marked engorgement of pelvic vessels from increased intravascular volume), abruptio placentae, preterm labor, placental laceration, uterine rupture, and direct fetal injury. These complications are more likely in the presence of pelvic fractures. Splenic rupture is the most common cause of intraperitoneal hemorrhage. Bowel injuries, in contrast, are less common during pregnancy than at other times. Fetal death is caused most commonly by maternal death and correlates with severe injuries, expulsion from the vehicle, and maternal head injury.

B. **Evaluation**
1. Laboratory tests, as listed in sec. **II.D.4**, should be performed, including hematocrit, blood type and screen, and Kleihauer-Betke test.
2. Nitrazine and fern tests of vaginal secretions should be performed to rule out rupture of membranes.
3. Radiographic studies with abdominal shielding should be performed as indicated.

C. **Abruptio placentae** in the trauma patient occurs in up to 38% of cases of blunt trauma with major maternal injury and in up to 2.4% of cases of blunt trauma with minor maternal injury. See Chap. 10 for a complete discussion of evaluation and management.

IV. **Penetrating trauma.** Management of pregnant patients with penetrating trauma is the same as that of nonpregnant women. Tetanus toxoid should be administered if indicated.

A. **Gunshot wounds.** The incidence of fetal mortality from gunshot wounds is 40% to 70%, whereas maternal mortality occurs in 5% of patients. As with blunt injuries, the incidence of bowel injuries is decreased in pregnant patients.
1. Evaluation includes thorough examination of all entrance and exit wounds. Radiographs may help localize the bullet, and CT may also be helpful.
2. Management. Surgical exploration is mandatory in gunshot wounds to the abdomen or flank.

B. **Stab wounds** carry a more favorable prognosis than gunshot wounds. Evaluation consists of local exploration of the wound. Diagnostic peritoneal lavage may be considered if the fascia has been penetrated. CT may be helpful in assessing the extent of the injury. Laparotomy is indicated if intraperitoneal bleeding is suspected.

V. **Burns.** Less than 4% of those suffering burn injuries are pregnant. The pregnancy itself does not appear to influence maternal outcome. Fetal outlook is dependent on severity of the burn. If more than 30% of the total body surface area is affected, delivery should be expedited if there is a good probability of fetal survival.

VI. **Abuse and domestic violence.** Twenty-two percent to 35% of women presenting with any complaint in the emergency department have injuries related to physical abuse. Injuries are more likely to be proximal and midline injuries, especially to the neck and face. It is important to help identify probable victims and to work to obtain appropriate support and intervention. In some states, domestic violence is the leading cause of maternal mortality (see Chap. 29).

VII. **Cardiopulmonary resuscitation in pregnancy.** Because cardiac arrest in a pregnant patient is usually the result of an acute insult rather than a chronic illness, maternal survival is more common than in the general population. The chance of fetal survival is also improved by the generally healthy state of the pregnant patients who experience cardiac arrest.

    A. **Causes** of cardiac arrest in the pregnant patient other than trauma include pulmonary embolism, amniotic fluid embolism, stroke, maternal cardiac disease, and complications of tocolytic therapy such as pulmonary edema (seen with beta-adrenergic agonists).

    B. **Standard resuscitative protocols** should be followed without modification. Compression of abdominal and pelvic vessels by the gravid uterus can be minimized by manually deflecting the uterus to the left during chest compression.

    C. **Pharmacologic agents** should be administered as indicated; pressors, however, should be avoided if possible, because they decrease uteroplacental perfusion.

VIII. **Postmortem cesarean section or emergency cesarean section** to save the fetus may be considered after severe maternal injury if the fetus is considered to be viable and neonatal support is available. Cesarean section is contraindicated in unstable patients because blood loss from surgery can precipitate death.

    A. **Technique.** A sterile field is unnecessary and time-consuming to establish. The procedure should be performed immediately at bedside. Cardiopulmonary resuscitation should be continued. If it is believed that maternal survival is possible, broad-spectrum antibiotic prophylaxis should be administered. Careful documentation of the indications for and circumstances surrounding the procedure is essential, because legal issues often arise in the aftermath of maternal death.

    B. **Timing** of postmortem cesarean section is critical to its success. The decision to perform the procedure should be made within 4 minutes of cardiac arrest, with delivery within 5 minutes. Chances of fetal survival are excellent if delivery occurs within 5 minutes and poor if delivery occurs after 15 minutes. Nevertheless, infant survival after cesarian delivery more than 20 minutes postarrest has been reported; therefore, if any signs of fetal life are present at any time after maternal death, an attempt at delivery should be made. In cases of maternal brain death, however, delivery is not emergent if the fetus is mature, a normal fetal heart rate is present, and signs of fetal distress are absent; in such cases, the patient's family should be consulted before surgery is performed.

20. POSTPARTUM CARE AND BREAST FEEDING

Julia Cron, Rita Driggers, and David Nagey

POSTPARTUM CARE

I. **In-hospital postpartum care.** Immediate postpartum care involves monitoring of vital signs, pain management, and surveillance for complications such as postpartum hemorrhage. Particular attention should be paid to cesarean section, with recognition that they are postsurgical and should receive appropriate additional monitoring. As concern for postpartum complications eases, increasing attention should be turned to parental education. Important issues to cover during this time include maternal self-care, appropriate sexual and physical activity, and infant nutrition.

   A. **Common postpartum complications**

      1. **Postpartum hemorrhage** has been defined as either a 10% change in hematocrit between admission and the postpartum period or a need for erythrocyte transfusion. The differential diagnosis of postpartum hemorrhage should include uterine atony; vaginal, cervical, or perineal laceration; and retained products of conception. Less commonly, uterine rupture, uterine inversion, and hereditary or acquired coagulopathies should be considered. Vaginal bleeding after a normal vaginal delivery is prevented by uterine contraction. Uterine atony is defined as insufficient postpartum uterine contractions to provide hemostasis. Risk factors for developing uterine atony include multiple gestation, grand multiparity (parity greater than 6), prolonged labor or oxytocin induction or both, multiple gestation, and advanced age. Initial management of uterine atony is careful inspection for lacerations followed by bimanual uterine massage, which permits stimulation of uterine contractions as well as verification that the uterus is intact and free of retained products. After bimanual massage and verification that the uterus is empty and intact, uterotonic agents can be administered while continuing with uterine massage (Table 20-1).

      If the initial response to therapy is not successful, consideration must be given to exploratory laparotomy. Coagulation studies should also be performed to rule out hereditary coagulopathies or coagulopathies acquired as a result of excessive blood loss or significant infection. Observation of the patient's blood in an undisturbed glass tube with no additives can be reassuring if it clots within a few minutes and lyses several minutes later.

      2. **Postpartum febrile morbidity** is defined as a temperature higher than 38.0°C on at least two occasions, at least 4 hours apart, after the first 24 hours postpartum. The differential diagnosis should include breast engorgement, atelectasis, urinary tract infection, and endomyometritis. Endomyometritis is a complication of 1–3% of vaginal deliveries and 10–50% of cesarean deliveries. The primary pathogen involved differs depending on the postpartum day (postpartum days 1–2: group A Streptococcus; postpartum days 3–4: enteric organisms; postpartum day 7 or greater: Chlamydia trachomatis). Endomyometritis should be treated with intravenous (IV) antibiotics until the patient is afebrile for 24 hours. The American College of Obstetricians and Gynecologists (ACOG) recommends initial treatment with gentamycin (1.5 mg/kg every 8 hours) and clindamycin (900 mg every 8 hours), with the addition of ampicillin (2 g every 6 hours) if Enterococcus is suspected or if fever persists after initial treatment. Some practitioners begin initial therapy with the triple antibiotic regimen.

TABLE 20-1. UTEROTONIC AGENTS

Agent	Dosage	Comments/relative contraindications
Oxytocin	10–40 U/L IV infusion; 10–40 U IM	Do not give IV push
Methylergonovine maleate	0.2 mg IM or PO every 2–4 hrs	Preeclampsia or hypertension
15S-methyl prostaglandin $F_{2\alpha}$	0.25 mg IM every 15 mins to a maximum of 8 doses	Asthma; significant renal, hepatic, or cardiac disease

Adapted from the American College of Obstetricians and Gynecologists (ACOG) Bulletin on Postpartum Hemorrhage, 1998.

Outpatient oral antibiotic therapy has been shown to be unnecessary. Patients who have persistent temperature elevation despite antibiotic treatment should be assessed for other complications such as retained products of conception (especially if their bleeding is heavier than usual), pelvic abscess, wound infection, ovarian vein thrombosis, and septic pelvic thrombophlebitis. All maternal fevers should be reported to the newborn nursery.

3. **Hypertension** is defined as BP of 140/90 or higher taken with the patient in a seated position on two or more occasions 4 or more hours apart. Because some women may develop preeclampsia or eclampsia postpartum, even in the absence of antenatal complications, particular attention should be paid to maternal BP postpartum. Any pressure reading of 140/90 or higher should be evaluated by repeating BP measurements, checking urine protein, and eliciting symptoms of preeclampsia. In those women who had antenatal preeclampsia, effective postpartum diuresis as well as normalization of BP should be documented. It is normal, however, for hypertension resulting from preeclampsia to persist for up to 6 weeks.

B. **Immunizations**
1. **Rh immunoglobulin.** An unsensitized Rh-negative woman who delivers an Rh-positive infant should receive 300 µg of Rh immunoglobulin within 72 hours of delivery even if Rh immunoglobulin was given in the antepartum period. Additional doses may be necessary if there had been antepartum fetal-maternal hemorrhage. The blood bank providing the Rh immunoglobulin should perform testing to assess the potential need for additional doses.
2. **Rubella vaccine.** Mothers who are not immune to rubella virus should receive MMR (measles-mumps-rubella) vaccine just before discharge (it is a live virus, and therefore exposure to pregnant women should be avoided). Use of monovalent rubella vaccine (e.g., Rubivax) is no longer considered appropriate because MMR is more cost effective and because many of the women without immunity to rubella also lack immunity to rubeola (measles). Breast feeding is not a contraindication to MMR vaccination. The peripartum period is an appropriate time to offer hepatitis A or hepatitis B vaccination, or both, to women at risk for these diseases.

II. **Discharge.** When there are no complications, mothers may be discharged 24–48 hours after vaginal delivery and 24–96 hours after cesarean delivery. The following criteria should be met.
A. Vital signs are stable and within normal limits.

B. Uterine fundus is firm and decreasing in size (within 24 hours postpartum, a uterus without fibroids should decrease to 20 weeks' size).

C. The amount and color of lochia is appropriate—red, less than a heavy period, and decreasing.

D. Urine output is adequate.

E. Any surgical incisions or vaginal repair sites are healing well without signs of infection.

F. The mother is able to eat, drink, ambulate, and void without difficulty.

G. No medical or psychosocial issues are identified that preclude discharge.

H. The mother has demonstrated knowledge of appropriate self-care and care of her infant.

I. The issue of contraception has been addressed.

J. Appropriate immunizations and Rh immunoglobulin, if appropriate, have been administered.

K. Follow-up care has been arranged for mother and infant.

L. Infant nutritional needs have been addressed.

III. **Outpatient postpartum care**

A. **Timing.** Women should be seen 4–6 weeks postpartum unless a problem identified in the early puerperium requires closer follow-up. For example, women with hypertensive complications should have a BP check within 1 week of discharge.

B. **The postpartum visit** should address the following.

1. **Physical examination** including BP, breast examination, abdominal examination, and pelvic examination
   a. Vaginal repairs should be healing.
   b. At 2 weeks postpartum, the nonmyomatous uterus is usually not palpable abdominally.
   c. By 6 weeks postpartum, the nonmyomatous uterus should return to 1.5–2.0 times its nonpregnant size.

2. **Quantity and quality of lochia**
   a. By 6 weeks postpartum, lochia should be essentially gone.
   b. If lochia is persistent, it should be reevaluated at 10–12 weeks. At that time, if bleeding continues, a full evaluation is warranted, including measurement of serum human chorionic gonadotropin.

3. **Pain control**
   a. Perineal discomfort can be treated with sitz baths, ice packs, and analgesics.
   b. Women with significant pain deserve further evaluation for perivaginal hematomas or other complications.

4. **Birth control.** See Chap. 28, Fertility Control.

5. **Sexual activity**
   a. When the perineum is healed and bleeding is decreased, sexual activity may be safely resumed.
   b. If the patient reports significant dyspareunia, further evaluation is necessary.

6. **Feeding method** with attention to any difficulties with breast feeding

7. **Depression screening** and assessment of general psychosocial well-being
   a. If there is evidence of depression, antidepressant medication should be considered, and the patient should be referred for mental health care.
   b. Thyroid-stimulating hormone level should be determined to rule out postpartum hypothyroidism.

8. **MMR and other immunizations** if not addressed before discharge

9. **Antenatal complications** should be addressed.
   a. Women with preeclampsia should be followed to rule out chronic hypertension or nephrotic syndrome.
   b. Women with gestational diabetes should be screened for diabetes (Table 20-2).

TABLE 20-2. DIABETIC SCREENING IN THE NONPREGNANT PATIENT

	Fasting glucose level (mg/dL)	Glucose level 2 hrs after 75-g load (mg/dL)	Management
Normal	<110	<140	Annual screening
Carbohydrate intolerant	110–125	140–199	Diet and exercise modification Annual screening
Diabetic	≥126	≥200 Random glucose level ≥200 with symptoms	Treatment as indicated

The fasting plasma glucose test is the preferred test for diagnosis of diabetes. An initial abnormal value must be confirmed, on a subsequent day, by measurement of fasting plasma glucose level, plasma glucose level after glucose load, or random plasma glucose level if symptoms are present.
Adapted from the American Diabetes Association Clinical Practice Recommendations 2001.

BREAST FEEDING

I. **Recommendations.** The American Academy of Pediatrics recommends exclusively breast feeding for the first 4–6 months of life and breast feeding with solids for at least 1 year. Breast feeding should be encouraged as soon after delivery as possible. Infants and mothers who initiate breast feeding within the first hour after delivery have a higher success rate than those who delay breast feeding. Newborns should be fed every 2–3 hours until satiety. Feeding for at least 5 minutes at each breast at each feeding on postpartum day 1 and gradually increasing feeding time over the next few days will allow optimal milk letdown without resulting in sore nipples. There is no need to limit feeding time. Frequent breast feeding helps establish maternal milk supply, prevents excessive engorgement, and minimizes neonatal jaundice.

Breast feeding may be associated with initial minor discomfort, but painful breasts should be assessed and positioning should be reevaluated. Nipple tenderness can be treated with lanolin cream. In addition, women should begin nursing on the less sore breast, should change nursing position to rotate stress points on nipples, and should be instructed to break suction before removing the infant from the breast.

Women who are breast feeding require 500–1000 kcal per day more than nonlactating women. Breast-feeding women are at increased risk of deficiencies in magnesium, vitamin B_6, folate, calcium, and zinc. Human milk may not provide adequate iron for premature newborns or infants who are older than 6 months. Supplemental iron should be given to these infants and to infants whose mothers are iron deficient.

II. **Statistics on breast feeding**
A. In 1971, 24.7% of mothers left the hospital breast feeding.
B. In 1998, 64.3% of mothers left the hospital breast feeding (44.9% of African-American mothers).
C. In 1998, 28.6% of mothers were breast feeding at 6 months.
D. Women with the highest breast-feeding rate are college educated, are older than 30 years, are residents of the Mountain or Pacific census regions, and are not enrolled in the Women, Infants, Children (WIC) program.
E. Women with the lowest breast-feeding rate are African-American, did not complete high school, are younger than 20 years, are residents in the East South Central census region, and are enrolled in the WIC program.

   F. Women enrolled in the WIC program have the most rapid rate of increase in breast feeding.

   G. Healthy People 2010 goals are 75% breast feeding in early postpartum period, 50% at 6 months, and 25% at 12 months.

III. **Benefits for newborns.** Breast feeding provides the baby excellent nutrition with changing nutritional content to match nutritional needs. For example, breast milk includes increased protein and minerals shortly after delivery and increased water, fat, and lactose later. Breast milk nutritional content changes during pregnancy as well, so that a baby born prematurely will receive nutrition more appropriate to his or her needs at the time.

     Breast feeding also provides protection against infection. Secretory immunoglobulin A is present in high quantities in colostrum and thus provides the baby with passive immunity to the infections to which the mother has immunity. Breast milk promotes phagocytosis by macrophages and leukocytes, thus boosting cellular immunity. Bifidus factor is present in breast milk and promotes proliferation of *Lactobacillus bifidus,* which decreases colonization by pathogens that cause diarrhea.

     Based on research in developed countries among middle-class populations, breast feeding decreases rates or severity, or both, of lower respiratory tract infections, otitis media, bacteremia, bacterial meningitis, urinary tract infections, botulism, diarrhea, and necrotizing enterocolitis.

     Because the protein in breast milk is species (human) specific, the delayed introduction of foreign protein also delays and reduces the development of allergies to some environmental allergens. Breast feeding has been shown to decrease the incidence and severity of eczema.

IV. **Benefits for mothers.** Oxytocin release during milk letdown causes increased uterine contractions, hastens uterine involution, and thus decreases postpartum blood loss. Women who breast feed experience a decreased risk of ovarian and premenopausal breast cancer that is proportional to the time spent breast feeding. Breast-feeding mothers also experience a decreased incidence of osteoporosis and postmenopausal hip fracture, and a decreased incidence of pregnancy-induced long-term obesity. Breast feeding supports bonding between mother and child and clearly results in decreased costs compared to formula feeding.

     Breast feeding delays postpartum ovulation and facilitates birth spacing (see sec.**VIII.A**).

V. **Contraindications.** Although not contraindications, some structural problems make breast feeding difficult and sometimes impossible. These include tubular breasts, hypoplastic breast tissue, true inverted nipples (which are very rare!), and surgical alterations that sever the milk ducts.

   The following are strict contraindications to breast feeding:

   A. Maternal use of illegal substances or excessive alcohol.

   B. Infant with galactosemia (infants with phenylketonuria may consume only up to 20 oz of breast milk per day).

   C. Maternal human immunodeficiency virus infection.

   D. Maternal active, untreated tuberculosis. Women can give their infant expressed breast milk and can breast feed once their treatment regimen is well established.

   E. Maternal active, untreated varicella. Once the infant has been given varicella zoster immunoglobulin, the infant can receive expressed breast milk if there are no lesions on the breast. Within 5 days of the appearance of the rash, maternal antibodies are produced, and thus breast feeding would be beneficial in providing passive immunity.

   F. Active herpes lesions on the breast.

VI. **Noncontraindications**

   A. Congenital or acquired cytomegalovirus infection in otherwise healthy, term infants. Such infants actually do better if they are breast fed because maternal antibodies (and virus) are in breast milk.

TABLE 20-3. MEDICATIONS CONTRAINDICATED DURING BREAST FEEDING

Medication	Reason for discontinuation
Bromocriptine mesylate	Lactation suppression
Cocaine	Cocaine intoxication of the newborn
Ergotamine tartrate	Vomiting, diarrhea, convulsions in the newborn
Lithium	One-third to one-half of maternal drug levels found in the newborn
Phencyclidine	Potent hallucinogen
Radioactive elements	Enter newborn bloodstream
Cyclophosphamide	Possible neutropenia and immune suppression in the newborn, unknown effect on growth or association with carcinogenesis
Cyclosporine	Same as for cyclophosphamide
Doxorubicin hydrochloride	Same as for cyclophosphamide
Methotrexate sodium	Same as for cyclophosphamide

Adapted from the American Academy of Pediatrics, Committee on Medications, 1994.

B. Maternal chronic hepatitis B if the infant has received hepatitis B immunoglobulin and the hepatitis B vaccine. (Women who have had acute hepatitis B infection during pregnancy should not breast feed.)
C. Maternal acute hepatitis A if the infant has received hepatitis A immunoglobulin and hepatitis A vaccine.
D. It is controversial whether women with hepatitis C should breast feed or not. Although there is no strong evidence that there is increased transmission with breast feeding, some providers discourage breast feeding in women with hepatitis C.

VII. **Breast feeding and maternal medications.** Use of nearly all antineoplastic, thyrotoxic, and immunosuppressive medications is contraindicated during breast feeding (Table 20-3). In general, breast feeding may be continued during maternal antibiotic therapy. Although all major anticonvulsants are secreted in breast milk, they need not be discontinued unless the infant shows signs of excessive sedation. The website of the American Academy of Pediatrics contains updated information on medication use in breast feeding (see Appendix D).

VIII. **Contraception during lactation.** In the non–breast-feeding woman, the average time to first ovulation is 45 days (range, 25–72 days). The mean time to ovulation is 190 days in women who are breast feeding.
A. **The lactational amenorrhea method** has been shown to provide 95–99% protection in the first 6 months postpartum if strict criteria are followed. Feedings need to be every 4 hours during the day and every 6 hours at night. Supplemental feedings should not exceed 5–10% of the total.
B. **Nonhormonal methods** (condom, intrauterine device, sterilization) are the preferred methods of contraception in lactating women.
C. **Progestin contraceptives** (progestin-only minipills, progestin injectables, progestin implants) do not affect the quality of breast milk and may actually increase the volume of milk; thus, these are the preferred method of hormonal contraception for breast-feeding women. The progestin from pills, injectables, and implants has been shown to be present in breast milk. Despite the lack of evidence suggesting adverse effects on infants, there is a theoretical risk of harmful consequences from exogenous steroids. Therefore, there is some question as to when to initiate progestin contraception.

The ACOG recommends initiating progestin pill use 2–3 weeks postpartum, administering injectables at 6 weeks postpartum, and inserting implants at 6 weeks postpartum. Starting progestin contraceptives earlier may be acceptable for those patients who are unwilling or unable to use nonhormonal contraceptives and who are not willing to risk a repeat pregnancy. It is important to note the decreased efficacy of progestin-only pills and the need to take them at the same time every day (see Chap. 28, Fertility Control).

D. **Combination estrogen-progestin contraceptives.** Estrogen-containing oral contraceptive pills (OCPs) have been shown to reduce the quantity and quality of breast milk. The World Health Organization recommends waiting at least 6 months before initiating combination OCPs. U.S. Food and Drug Administration labeling recommends not using combination OCPs until the child is completely weaned. The ACOG recommends that, if combination OCPs are preferred, they should not be started before 6 weeks postpartum, and they should only be started after lactation is well established and the infant's nutritional status is well monitored. As with progestin-only contraceptives, some providers may initiate the use of combination OCPs earlier if lactation is well established, the patient declines other forms of contraception, and the risk of repeat pregnancy is significant.

IX. **Mastitis** is a breast infection that occurs in 1–2% of breast-feeding women, usually between the first and fifth weeks postpartum. It is characterized by a localized sore, reddened, indurated area on the breast that is often accompanied by fever, chills, and malaise.

A. **Etiology and treatment.** Forty percent of cases are due to *Staphylococcus aureus* infection. Treatment is dicloxacillin, 500 mg four times daily for 10 days. Women should continue to express milk, starting on the affected side to encourage more complete emptying.

B. **Differential diagnosis** includes the following:

1. Clogged milk ducts: a tender lump in the breast not accompanied by systemic symptoms; resolves after application of warm compresses and massage.

2. Breast engorgement: bilateral, generalized tenderness of breasts, often occurring 2–4 days postpartum and associated with low-grade fevers. May be treated with application of warm compresses followed by hand or pump expression of milk and continued breast feeding.

3. Inflammatory breast cancer: a rare form of breast cancer that presents with breast tenderness and breast skin changes.

4. Breast abscess: a firm, tender, usually well-circumscribed mass. Breast sonography may be required for diagnosis, and incision and drainage are necessary for treatment.

X. **Decreased milk supply.** The normal amount of milk produced by the end of the first postpartum week is 550 mL per day. By 2–3 weeks, milk production is increased to approximately 800 mL per day. Milk production peaks at 1.5–2.0 L per day. Before gaining weight, newborns who are breast fed may be expected to lose 5–7% of birth weight in the first week. If the loss is greater than 5–7% or if the weight loss is rapid, adequacy of breast feeding should be assessed. Glycogen stores in full-term infants generally provide sufficient initial nutrition. Therefore, supplemental feeding should be avoided unless medically indicated. Frequent breast feeding helps to maintain milk stores.

Poor nourishment and psychologic stress can decrease milk supply. Sheehan syndrome (postpartum pituitary necrosis) can result in lack of milk production.

21. OBSTETRIC ANALGESIA AND ANESTHESIA

Betty Chou and Andrew P. Harris

I. **Introduction.** Although the use of anesthesia or analgesia during labor and delivery must be individualized to each patient, the common goal is to maximize outcomes for both the mother and the neonate. Some laboring patients may not want or need anesthesia; however, others may desire a higher level of pain control or the mode of delivery may necessitate anesthetic intervention.

   A. **Definitions. Analgesia** is defined as relief of pain without the loss of consciousness or motor function. **Anesthesia** is defined as the loss of feeling or sensation and can include the loss of consciousness, motor power, and autonomic reflex activity.

   B. **Types of analgesia or anesthesia.** The spectrum of anesthetic techniques useful in obstetrics includes the following: systemic, local infiltration, peripheral nerve block, major regional analgesia and anesthesia (spinal and epidural blocks), and general anesthesia. Each technique entails varying levels of pain control, alterations to the progression of labor, and effects on the parturient and fetus.

      1. **Analgesia for labor.** The goal is to achieve adequate pain control without depressing the parturient or fetus or affecting the progress of labor. Nonpharmacologic approaches to pain control (e.g., Lamaze method and attendance of a doula) may be desired by the patient. However, systemic analgesia, epidural anesthesia, and combined spinal-epidural techniques are more often used.

      2. **Analgesia and anesthesia for vaginal delivery.** For an anticipated vaginal birth, the caregiver must consider various factors when selecting an analgesic or anesthetic, including effectiveness of analgesia, maternal safety, fetal safety, alterations to maternal pushing efforts, and alterations to the musculature of the birthing canal. Major regional anesthesia (epidural or spinal block) is the technique of choice; local infiltration of the perineum and paracervical and pudendal blocks are used less frequently. Rarely, general anesthesia can be used for emergency forceps delivery, shoulder dystocia, or difficult vaginal breech delivery.

      3. **Analgesia and anesthesia for cesarean section.** The anticipated length of surgery, medical conditions of the mother, maternal and fetal safety, and urgency of the delivery should dictate the type of anesthetic administered. Major regional anesthesia and, less often, general anesthesia are used. Rarely, local infiltration can be used in cases of emergency cesarean section in which rapid general anesthesia is not possible.

      4. **Analgesia for postoperative pain.** Systemic and regional pain control methods have been found to be quite effective. In particular, patient-controlled intravenous (IV) and epidural anesthesia are often used until the patient can tolerate oral analgesics.

II. **Nonpharmacologic techniques.** Some patients may prefer to use nonpharmacologic methods to help prepare for and manage the pains of labor and vaginal delivery. Lamaze or Bradley childbirth education are favored by some. Others may desire a doula, a trained layperson, to provide continuous support throughout the labor. The goal is to minimize the amount of pharmacologic intervention, as tolerated.

III. **Systemic analgesia**

   A. **Indications.** Systemic medications can be given in the latent or active phase of labor for effective pain relief. They can also be used for postoperative pain control.

TABLE 21-1. NARCOTIC PAIN CONTROL

Medication	Dose	Peak effect	Duration
Meperidine hydrochloride (Demerol)	25–50 mg IV	7–8 mins	1.5–3.0 hrs
	50–75 mg IM	45 mins	3–4 hrs
Fentanyl	25–50 μg IV	3–5 mins	30–60 mins
	50–100 μg IM	30 mins	1–2 hrs
Morphine sulfate	2–3 mg IV	20 mins	4–6 hrs
	5–10 mg IM	1–2 hrs	4–6 hrs
Butorphanol tartrate (Stadol)	1–2 mg IV	4–5 mins	3–4 hrs
	1–2 mg IM	30–60 mins	3–4 hrs
Nalbuphine hydrochloride (Nubain)	5–10 mg IV or IM	30–45 mins	3–6 hrs

1. **Narcotics** are the most effective systemic medication for pain control (Table 21-1).
2. **Sedatives and tranquilizers.** A wide variety of these medications, such as phenothiazine, promethazine hydrochloride, and hydroxyzine hydrochloride, are used to supplement narcotic analgesia. Although these medications have the added benefit of an antiemetic effect and reduced narcotic demand, they do cause increased sedation.

B. **Advantages.** The advantage of this mode of analgesia is the ease of administration (orally, intramuscularly, subcutaneously, intravenously) and relatively low risk to mother and fetus.

C. **Limitations.** Narcotics may provide inadequate pain relief for many patients.

D. **Risks.** The parturient can experience respiratory depression, orthostatic hypotension, nausea, vomiting, and delayed gastric emptying with increased risk of aspiration. The neonate can experience respiratory depression, lower Apgar scores, and neurobehavioral abnormalities. Narcotic administration should be minimized just before delivery to prevent delivery of a depressed neonate. Naloxone hydrochloride can be administered to antagonize the respiratory depression caused by narcotics. The usual dosage of naloxone is 0.1–0.4 mg IV for adults and 0.1 mg/kg IV for neonates.

IV. **Local infiltration (field block)**

A. **Indications**

1. **Vaginal delivery.** Local infiltration of an anesthetic agent may be required to perform an episiotomy or repair any lacerations or episiotomies after vaginal delivery. Perineal infiltration with 5–15 mL of 1% lidocaine (or 0.25–0.5% bupivacaine hydrochloride, 2% chloroprocaine hydrochloride, or 1% mepivacaine hydrochloride) can provide sufficient analgesia for an episiotomy or repair and occasionally for an outlet operative delivery. The medication, which should not be mixed with epinephrine, must not be directly injected into a blood vessel. Extravascular placement can be verified by withdrawing on the syringe before injecting any anesthetic agent.

2. **Cesarean section.** Occasionally, cesarean sections must be performed under local anesthesia in an emergency situation when alternate anesthesia is not immediately available or possible. Dilute concentrations of an agent such as lidocaine (0.5–1.0% to a maximum of 7 mg/kg) or chloroprocaine (1–2%) is used to infiltrate the skin and abdominal wall and bathe the parietal and visceral peritoneum. Local anesthesia alone is usually inadequate pain relief and is used only in rare emergency cases.

B. **Advantages.** The advantages of local infiltration are its ease of administration and minimal negative effects on the parturient and fetus.

C. **Limitations.** Field block offers no relief from the pains of uterine contractions. In addition, if the caregiver is concerned about a difficult vaginal delivery or a possible cesarean section, the patient should be advised that major regional anesthesia is highly recommended if timing permits.

V. **Peripheral nerve block.** This form of analgesia involves injection of a local anesthetic agent in the vicinity of discrete peripheral nerves in the pelvis (paracervical or pudendal areas) to achieve pain control.

A. **Paracervical block**

1. **Indications.** The paracervical block is a rarely used method of analgesia that can provide relief from uterine contractions. This block involves the transvaginal injection of a total of 10–20 mL of 1% lidocaine (or 2% chloroprocaine) just lateral to the cervix bilaterally at the 4 and 8 o'clock positions). This technique blocks the sensory nerves from uterus, cervix, and upper vagina.

2. **Limitations.** The sensory fibers from the perineum are not affected. Therefore, the paracervical block has no benefit outside of the first stage of labor. In addition, it is difficult to administer late in the first stage.

3. **Risks.** Although it is easy to perform and does not cause maternal hypotension, paracervical anesthesia can cause local vasoconstriction, increased uterine tone, and decreased perfusion to the uterus. There is an increased risk for fetal depression and transient fetal bradycardia.

B. **Pudendal block**

1. **Indications.** This method is used to achieve perineal analgesia and help the patient tolerate the pain of the second stage of labor and any postdelivery repairs. It is administered by transvaginally injecting a total of 10–20 mL of 1% lidocaine (or 2% chloroprocaine) just posterior to the ischial spines bilaterally. This method blocks the pudendal nerve, which provides afferent fibers to the genitalia and perineum.

2. **Limitations.** Complete analgesia may require infiltration of the perineum with a local anesthetic. In addition, if a complicated vaginal delivery or possible cesarean section is predicted, major regional anesthesia should be recommended.

3. **Risks.** The pudendal block carries little risk to the fetus. Its rare complications to the mother include accidental sciatic nerve block, formation of a hematoma, or puncture of the rectum.

VI. **Major regional anesthesia and analgesia.** This is the most commonly used form of anesthesia today. It involves the injection of anesthetic/analgesic agents into the epidural or subarachnoid (spinal) space to achieve adequate analgesia for vaginal delivery or anesthesia for cesarean section while allowing the parturient to maintain full consciousness.

A. **Epidural anesthesia**

1. **Indications.** An epidural block can be used for establishing analgesia during labor, analgesia and anesthesia for nonoperative and operative vaginal delivery, and anesthesia for cesarean section. After a cesarean section, postoperative pain can be managed with epidural patient-controlled anesthesia quite successfully.

2. **Application.** A 19- or 20-gauge plastic indwelling catheter is placed into the epidural space at the level of L2–L5. Verification of placement into the epidural space includes the inability to aspirate blood or cerebrospinal fluid and the administration of a test dose that does not indicate IV or subarachnoid placement. Repeated epidural injections, patient-controlled pumps, and continuous infusion of a mixture of local anesthetic plus narcotic analgesic (e.g., bupivacaine and fentanyl) has allowed lower concentration of medications to be used for effective pain control with minimal risk to patient and fetus.

3. **Advantages.** There is often less fetal depression and respiratory compromise to the mother than with general anesthesia or systemic narcot-

ics. The epidural anesthetic can be titrated to fulfill the pain control needs of the parturient, maintain her full consciousness, and allow her to push in a vaginal delivery. In addition, it is the only mode of anesthesia that can be used throughout all stages of labor and vaginal delivery as well as be dosed for proper anesthesia for a cesarean section.

4. **Limitations.** An epidermal block takes longer to initiate than spinal or general anesthesia. Therefore, it is not indicated for expected imminent vaginal delivery or an emergent cesarean section.

5. **Contraindications.** Possible contraindications include neurologic problems (e.g., sciatica), spine abnormalities, infection at the site, acute maternal hemorrhage, or bleeding disorders.

6. **Risks**
   a. **Maternal hypotension.** The most common complication of an epidural block is maternal hypotension, which can cause uteroplacental insufficiency and can lead to fetal distress. Prophylactic intravascular volume expansion with 500–1000 mL of lactated Ringer's solution is usually administered before placing an epidural catheter. If hypotension still occurs, additional IV fluids, ephedrine (10.0 mg IV), or both may be needed. Left uterine displacement (placement of the patient in left lateral tilt position) can be helpful.
   b. **Accidental dural puncture ("wet tap").** Complications after a wet tap include spinal headache. Treatment includes administration of abdominal binders, administration of caffeine, and increased fluid intake. Severe cases may require injection of autologous blood in the epidural space near the dural puncture (i.e., "blood patch").
   c. **Accidental intravascular injection.** CNS toxicity from intravascular injection of an anesthetic includes dizziness, slurred speech, metallic taste, tinnitus, convulsions, and in rare cases cardiac arrest. Treatment is supportive and may involve establishing an airway to provide assisted ventilation and administering short-acting benzodiazepines or barbiturates for seizure control.
   d. **Accidental subarachnoid injection.** If accidental subarachnoid placement of the catheter is not detected by a test dose, a usual epidural dose may result in high or total spinal anesthesia, leading to apnea and hypotension that must be rapidly treated with supportive care.
   e. **Effect on progress of labor.** If an epidural block is too dense or administered too early in labor, the musculature of the pelvic floor can become too relaxed, which potentially results in malrotation of the fetal head during descent. In addition, the parturient may lose the urge or ability to push effectively because of lack of sensation. As a result, the duration of the second stage of labor may be prolonged.

B. **Spinal anesthesia and analgesia**
   1. **Indications.** Spinal analgesia may be administered for labor and vaginal delivery. Spinal anesthesia can be used for cesarean sections.
   2. **Application.** For cesarean section, a local anesthetic (tetracaine hydrochloride, bupivacaine, or lidocaine) is injected into the subarachnoid space through a needle placed at the level of L2–L5. A sensory level of T5 is preferable for adequate anesthesia for a cesarean section. For labor and vaginal delivery, small amounts of narcotic (fentanyl, sufentanil citrate, or morphine sulfate) or local anesthetic or both can be used for analgesia. T10–L1 block is needed to minimize the pain of uterine contractions and S2–S4 block is needed for perineal analgesia.
   3. **Advantages.** The advantages of the spinal block are its rapid onset of effect and ease of administration (relative to an epidural).
   4. **Limitations.** The analgesia of a spinal block lasts only for a limited time period. Therefore, this type of anesthesia is not indicated to relieve the pain of a lengthy labor. Likewise, if concern exists about a very com-

plicated, prolonged cesarean section, epidural or general anesthesia is preferred. Spinal anesthesia is not appropriate for an extremely emergent cesarean section.

5. **Contraindications.** These are the same as those listed for epidural anesthesia (see sec. **VI.A.5**).

6. **Risks.** As with the epidural block, the spinal block can have complications associated with induced maternal hypotension, spinal headache, and high block (see risks of epidural anesthesia, sec. **VI.A.6**). Spinal headache can be less likely if a smaller-caliber needle (e.g., 26 or 27 gauge) is used. Respiratory depression and pruritus may occur after spinal analgesia with narcotics [treatment is with naloxone hydrochloride (Narcan)].

C. **Combined spinal-epidural anesthesia (CSE)**

1. **Indications.** This type of anesthesia is useful for providing analgesia or anesthesia or both for labor, vaginal deliveries, or cesarean sections.

2. **Application.** The most frequently used technique is the needle-through-needle method. The epidural space is identified, a spinal needle is then passed through the epidural needle and advanced beyond its tip to puncture the dura, and spinal anesthesia is administered. The spinal needle is then removed, and an epidural catheter is placed through the remaining needle.

3. **Advantages.** The CSE combines the rapidity, density, and reliability of the spinal block with the facility to modify or prolong the anesthesia with use of the epidural catheter.

4. **Contraindications.** These are the same as those listed for epidural anesthesia (see sec. **VI.A.5**).

5. **Risks.** In addition to the risks of spinal and epidural anesthesia, there may be difficulty interpreting the epidural test dose after a spinal block has been administered.

VII. **General anesthesia.** This form of anesthesia is used far less than regional anesthesia. It requires endotracheal intubation to protect the parturient's airway and minimize the risk of aspiration.

A. **Indications.** Because of its rapid induction, general anesthesia is usually used for extremely emergent cesarean sections and less often for emergent vaginal deliveries (forceps delivery, severe shoulder dystocia, difficult breech delivery). It may also be used when a patient is hypovolemic or has a contraindication to use of regional anesthesia.

B. **Application.** The most popular regimen is to use sodium thiopental (3–4 mg/kg) or ketamine hydrochloride (1–2 mg/kg) as the induction agent, followed by succinylcholine chloride (1 mg/kg) for muscle relaxation to facilitate intubation. Preoxygenation with 100% oxygen increases the oxygen stores in the maternal lungs. Additional inhalation agents (halothane, isoflurane, nitrous oxide) are commonly used.

C. **Advantages.** General anesthesia has the advantages of providing rapid induction and producing less hypotension.

D. **Limitations.** Because of its increased risks to the mother and fetus, general anesthesia is usually reserved for situations when all other forms of anesthesia are contraindicated or inadequate.

E. **Risks.** Data suggest that the rate of maternal death contributable to general anesthesia may be at least double the rate due to regional anesthesia. The primary cause of death associated with general anesthesia is difficulty with airway management.

1. **Failed intubation or aspiration.** A careful preoperative evaluation should be performed to identify any potential challenges to intubation. Awake intubation may be necessary. Preoxygenating with 100% oxygen decreases the risk of hypoxia. To reduce the risk of aspiration, cricoid pressure is applied until the endotracheal tube is inserted and the cuff is inflated. Ideally, the patient should have an empty stomach. An ant-

acid is also administered before general anesthesia to increase the pH of the stomach contents.

2. **Increased uterine bleeding.** Because halogenated anesthetic agents (halothane, isoflurane) cause uterine relaxation, their prolonged use may increase blood loss, although several studies have shown no increased blood loss when these agents are used appropriately.

3. **Fetal depression.** General anesthetics have the potential for causing neonatal depression. In addition, induction of general anesthesia is associated with a significant decrease in uterine blood flow.

Section Three. GYNECOLOGY

22. ANATOMY OF THE FEMALE PELVIS

Alice W. Ko and Geoffrey W. Cundiff

I. **Abdominal wall.** The abdominal wall is outlined cephalad by the lower edge of the rib cage; caudally by the iliac crests, inguinal ligaments, and pubic bones; and dorsolaterally by the lumbar spine and its adjacent muscles.

   A. **Layers of the anterior abdominal wall.** The layers are shown in transverse section in Figs. 22-1 and 22-2.

   1. **Skin**

   2. **Subcutaneous layer (subcutaneum).** This layer consists of fat globules in a meshwork of fibrous septa.

      a. **Camper's fascia** is the more superficial aspect of the subcutaneum, which contains more fat than fibrous tissue and has a less organized texture than Scarpa's fascia.

      b. **Scarpa's fascia** is the deeper portion of the subcutaneum and contains more fibrous tissue with a more organized consistency than Camper's fascia.

      Camper's and Scarpa's fasciae are not clearly delineated layers seen during surgery but represent regions of the subcutaneous layer.

   3. **Musculoaponeurotic layer.** Located immediately below the subcutaneum, it consists of layers of fibrous tissue (called the **rectus sheath**) and muscle that hold the abdominal viscera in place. This layer is anatomically different above and below the **arcuate line.** The rectus sheath surrounds the abdominal muscles and provides support for the muscles anteriorly and posteriorly except for the posterior aspect below the arcuate line.

      a. **Muscles of the anterior abdominal wall**

         (1) **Vertical muscles**

            (a) The **rectus abdominis muscle** is a paired muscle, found on either side of the midline, that originates from the sternum and cartilages of ribs 5–7 and inserts into the anterior surface of the pubic bone.

            (b) The **pyramidalis muscle,** also a paired muscle, sits ventral to the rectus abdominis muscle and arises from the pubic bones to insert into the linea alba several centimeters caudal to the symphysis. Their development varies among individuals and their strong attachment to the midline (linea alba) makes separation of their attachment difficult by blunt dissection. Also, the pyramidalis fibers point toward the midline, which assists in locating the midline during a midline incision.

         (2) **Oblique flank muscles** lie lateral to the rectus abdominis muscles. Most superficial is the external oblique, then the internal oblique, and then the transversus abdominis. Despite the fact that these muscles do not generally run parallel to one another, their orientation is primarily transverse. Thus, vertical skin incisions are under more tension, which results in an increased incidence of wound dehiscence than with transverse incisions.

            (a) The **external oblique muscle** originates from the lower eight ribs and iliac crest and runs obliquely anteriorly and inferiorly.

            (b) The **internal oblique muscle** originates from the anterior two-thirds of the iliac crest, the lateral part of the inguinal ligament, and the thoracolumbar fascia in the lower posterior

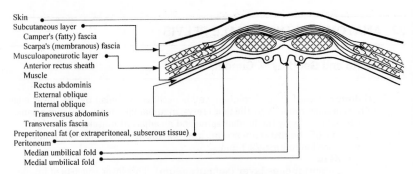

FIG. 22-1. Layers of the anterior abdominal wall caudal to the arcuate line.

flank. These muscles predominantly run perpendicular to the external oblique, but, toward the lower abdomen, their fibers progressively angle more like those of the external oblique.

(c) The **transversus abdominis muscle** is the innermost of the three layers mentioned earlier, and its fibers run transversely. They originate from the lower six costal cartilages, the thoracolumbar fascia, the anterior three-fourths of the iliac crest, and the lateral inguinal ligament. The nerves and vasculature of the flank are found between the internal oblique and transversus abdominis muscles, and injury to these structures can occur here.

b. The **rectus sheath (conjoined tendon)** is comprised of the aponeuroses of the external oblique, internal oblique, and transversus abdominis muscles. Anterior to the rectus abdominis muscles, the rectus sheath is called the **anterior rectus sheath,** and posterior to the rectus abdominis muscles, the rectus sheath is called the **posterior rectus sheath.**

(1) The **arcuate line (linea semicircularis, semilunar fold of Douglas),** semicircular in shape, is located midway between the umbilicus and symphysis pubis but has also been described as delineating the lower one-fourth of the abdominal wall from the upper three-fourths. The arcuate line marks the lower edge of the posterior rectus sheath and thus the point below which the fibers

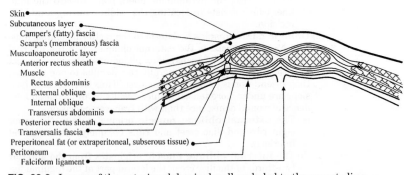

FIG. 22-2. Layers of the anterior abdominal wall cephalad to the arcuate line.

of the posterior rectus sheath run anterior to the rectus abdominis muscles and thereby become part of the anterior rectus sheath.

(2) The **anterior rectus sheath below the arcuate line** is comprised of the conjoined aponeuroses of the external oblique, internal oblique, and transversus abdominis muscles.

(3) The **anterior rectus sheath above the arcuate line** is comprised of the conjoined aponeuroses of the external oblique and the ventral half of the internal oblique muscle.

(4) The **posterior rectus sheath** is located only above the arcuate line. In fact, it is its lower margin that delineates the arcuate line. The posterior sheath is comprised of the conjoined aponeuroses of the dorsal half of the internal oblique and the transversalis muscle. This layer is usually encountered in vertical incisions at the most cephalad aspect and not in Pfannenstiel or low transverse incisions.

(5) The **linea alba** is the midline ridge of the rectus abdominis muscles. Cephalad to the arcuate line, the linea alba marks the fusion of the anterior and posterior rectus sheaths.

(6) The **semilunar line of the rectus sheath** marks the lateral border of the rectus muscle.

(7) The **transversalis fascia** is located just underneath the rectus abdominis muscles suprapubically and is separated from the peritoneum below by a variable layer of adipose tissue. This is the region that is taken down in layers just above the bladder.

4. **Peritoneum.** A single layer of serosa, the peritoneum has five vertical folds on the posterior aspect of the anterior abdominal wall, which converge toward the umbilicus. The peritoneum is believed to reepithelialize in 24 hours; thus, sterile wound dressings should remain in place for 24 hours postoperatively.

a. The **median umbilical fold** is a single fold caused by the presence of the **median umbilical ligament (obliterated urachus).**

b. The **medial umbilical folds** are paired folds located lateral to the median umbilical fold. These are caused by the presence of the **obliterated umbilical arteries** that once connected the internal iliac vessels to the umbilical cord.

c. The **lateral umbilical folds** are raised by the inferior epigastric arteries and veins. They are significantly less prominent than the middle umbilical folds and frequently cannot be distinguished.

5. **Bladder reflection.** The apex of the bladder blends into the median umbilical ligament and is highest in the midline. Therefore, incising the peritoneum lateral to the midline is helpful to avoid bladder injury.

B. **Vasculature of the anterior abdominal wall.** The vasculature of the abdominal wall can be separated into those vessels that predominantly supply the subcutaneum and those that predominantly supply the musculofascial layer (Fig. 22-3).

1. **Subcutaneous supply**

a. The **superficial epigastric arteries** supply the skin and subcutaneous tissues. These are the only *epigastric* vessels located in the subcutaneous tissue and should *not* be confused with the superior and inferior epigastric arteries that are located in the musculofascial layers. The superficial epigastric vessels stem from the femoral vessels after the femoral vessels descend through the femoral canal. The vessels can be found 5.5 cm from the midline just above the pubis and 4.5 cm from the midline at the level of the umbilicus.

b. The **superficial external pudendal arteries** run from the femoral artery toward the mons pubis. As these arteries contain many branches, bleeding in this area can be heavier than in any other area in the subcutaneum.

c. The **superficial circumflex iliac arteries** run laterally from the femoral artery to the flank.

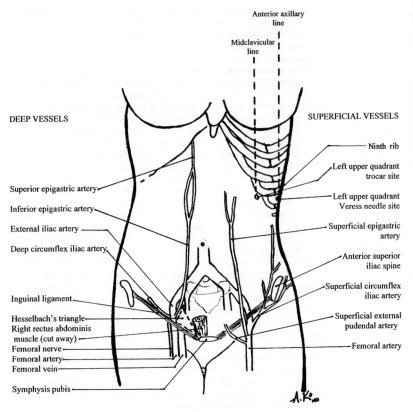

FIG. 22-3. Vasculature and laparoscopic landmarks of the anterior abdominal wall.

2. **Musculofascial supply.** The blood supply to the musculofascial layer of the lower abdominal wall parallels the subcutaneous supply.
    a. The **superior epigastric artery** stems from the internal thoracic artery (which stems from the subclavian artery) and runs caudally to form anastomoses with the inferior epigastric artery.
    b. The **inferior epigastric artery** has *two* associated veins and branches from the external iliac artery just proximal to the inguinal ligament. It runs toward the umbilicus, creating the lateral umbilical fold. The artery intersects the rectus abdominis muscle's lateral border midway between the pubis and umbilicus. Caudal to this site of intersection, the artery runs deep to the transversalis fascia and lateral to the rectus. Cephalad to that site, it crosses the transversalis fascia and runs between the dorsal aspect of the rectus and the posterior rectus sheath. Once it enters the posterior rectus sheath, the vessel has numerous branches that supply the musculofascial layer, the subcutaneum, and the skin, and anastomoses with branches of the superficial and superior epigastric arteries.

       Hesselbach's triangle (inguinal triangle) is bordered laterally by the inferior epigastric vessels, medially by the rectus abdominis muscle, and inferiorly by the inguinal ligament.

TABLE 22-1. COMPARISON OF ADVANTAGES AND DISADVANTAGES OF TRANSVERSE AND MIDLINE INCISIONS

Transverse incision	Midline incision
Advantages	Advantages
Better cosmetic result	More exposure
Thirty times stronger	Less potential blood loss
Fewer hernias	Potentially more expedient in opening
Less prone to dehiscence	Improved upper abdominal exposure
Fewer wound eviscerations	Disadvantages
Less painful	Less cosmetic
Less interference with postoperative respirations	Weaker
	More hernias
Disadvantages	More prone to dehiscence
Less exposure	More wound eviscerations
More potential blood loss	More painful
Potentially more time consuming in opening	More interference with postoperative respirations
Poor upper abdominal exposure	

     c. The **deep circumflex iliac artery** lies between the internal oblique and transversus abdominis muscles.

II. **Types of incisions (Table 22-1)**

  A. **Transverse incisions.** In 1861, Langer described skin lines of minimal tension now called **Langer lines (lines of Langer)** (Fig. 22-4). An incision created parallel to these lines results in a better cosmetic result than an incision made perpendicular to these lines. Thus, a transverse abdominal incision tends to heal with less scarring than a midline incision.

    1. **Pfannenstiel ("bikini cut").** This incision is the most frequently used in obstetrics and gynecology.

      a. A transverse skin incision is made two fingerbreadths (3–4 cm) above the symphysis pubis and carried to the underlying anterior rectus sheath fascia.

      b. This fascia is nicked transversely in the midline to expose the underlying rectus muscle fibers.

      c. The fascial incision is extended laterally, usually with Mayo scissors. Two distinct layers of the anterior rectus sheath can be seen: the aponeurosis of the external oblique and the combined aponeuroses of the internal oblique and transversus abdominis.

      d. The rectus sheath is then dissected off the underlying rectus muscles superiorly and inferiorly. Of note, dissection of the rectus sheath off the underlying rectus muscles can result in cutaneous anesthesia, as this action may stretch the perforating nerves or result in nerve ligation during attempted hemostasis of perforating vessels. To minimize blood loss, the pyramidalis muscle is left attached to the fascia rather than dissected off.

      e. The rectus muscles are then separated in the midline, and the transversalis fascia and peritoneum are identified. The peritoneum is then entered off the midline and cephalad to avoid bladder injury.

      If more exposure is necessary, the preferred next step is to dissect the underlying rectus muscle off the anterior rectus sheath as far cephalad and caudally as possible. The incision can also be extended

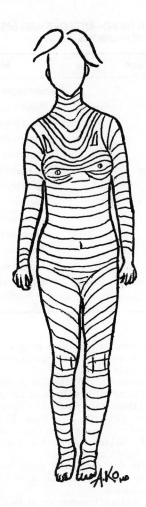

FIG. 22-4. Lines of Langer.

laterally on the skin and fascia, but this is not usually as effective as the previous step.

Once a Pfannenstiel incision is made, conversion to a Maylard incision cannot be performed, as the rectus abdominis muscles have already been dissected from the overlying fascia. In a true Maylard, the fascia remains attached to the muscle so that reapproximation of the fascia also reapproximates the rectus muscles. The best next step would be to convert to a Cherney incision (see later).

2. **Maylard.** The Maylard incision is considered the true transverse abdominal incision, as all the incisions made to enter the peritoneum are consistently transverse. It is generally more time consuming to perform but provides the best pelvic (not abdominal) exposure of all the incision types.

   a. The skin incision is classically made about the level of the anterior superior iliac spine.

b. The subcutaneous tissue and anterior rectus sheath are incised as in a Pfannenstiel incision. *The underlying rectus abdominis muscles are not dissected off the anterior rectus sheath.* Rather, they remain attached for future reapproximation.

c. Before the rectus muscles are transected, the inferior epigastric vessels are identified near or at the lateral border of the rectus muscles. These vessels are usually ligated before transecting the muscles.

d. The rectus muscles are transected with a knife or Bovie by placing the muscle bellies above an underlying finger or Kelly clamp.

e. The transversalis fascia and peritoneum are then transversely incised.

3. **Cherney.** The Cherney incision affords good exposure to the pelvis while sparing the transection of the rectus muscle bellies.

a. A low transverse incision through the skin and anterior rectus sheath is made similar to that in a Pfannenstiel incision.

b. The underlying rectus muscle is dissected off the anterior rectus sheath caudal to the incision until the symphysis pubis is reached.

c. The surgeon's finger is used to dissect under the tendinous insertion of the rectus muscles on the pubic bone, remaining medial to the inferior epigastric vessels. The tendons are cut approximately 0.5 cm above their insertion site. Care is exercised to leave enough tendon on the pubic bone but also enough tendon on the distal aspect of the rectus muscle so that these two ends may be reapproximated appropriately later.

d. The rectus muscles can then be carefully lifted off the underlying transversalis fascia and peritoneum, and the latter structures entered.

e. Repair of the tendinous insertions is performed with 2-0 delayed absorbable suture in a horizontal mattress fashion. The caudal aspect of the rectus muscles can be reapproximated to the tendon left on the pubic bone or sewn to the undersurface of the anterior rectus sheath directly above the symphysis pubis.

B. **Vertical incisions.** A midline or paramedian incision affords the best upper abdominal exposure, minimizes blood loss, and allows for expedient entry into the abdomen. Also, unlike in transverse incisions, there is minimal dead space created in a vertical incision.

1. The skin incision is usually made from the symphysis to approximately 1 cm below the umbilicus; however, this preference is operator dependent. This incision can be extended above the umbilicus, preferably in a circumferential fashion on the left aspect of the umbilicus.

2. The anterior rectus sheath is incised vertically.

3. The midline of the rectus muscles is identified by dissecting off the overlying rectus sheath. *Following the cephalad direction of the pyramidalis muscle fibers assists in locating the midline.*

4. The transversalis fascia and peritoneum are entered cephalad to avoid the bladder and incised vertically.

C. **Laparoscopic incisions.** In the majority of laparoscopic pelvic surgery, a maximum of three abdominal ports are made. These typically consist of an umbilical port and two lower quadrant ports. On occasion, a port located in the suprapubic region can be helpful. It is important to keep in mind the vascular supply of the abdominal wall when locating sites for trocar placement (Fig. 22-3).

1. **Positioning of the patient.** The patient should be placed in the dorsal lithotomy position. The buttocks should protrude slightly from the table, which allows for ease of placement and use of a uterine manipulator. The patient's thighs and knees should be in alignment with the plane of the body. Elevation of the thighs and knees can interfere with lower quadrant laparoscopic instrument manipulation. At least one of

the patient's arms, preferably on the surgeon's side, should be tucked by the side to afford the surgeon greater room for movement. *Great caution and attention should be shown to the patient's arm and hand in the tucked position, as the fingers can be injured during table manipulation.*

2. **Precautions.** Before steps are taken to place the primary trocar, it is of utmost importance to confirm that the longitudinal axis of the patient is parallel with the floor (and not in Trendelenburg or other deviated position). The sacral promontory should be identified, as the aortic bifurcation is located directly cephalad to this site. The anterior superior iliac spines should be identified because they serve as a point of reference for the lower half of the abdomen and the lower quadrant trocar sites. Taking these precautions assists in avoiding vessel and organ damage.

3. **Primary trocar insertion.** The most common primary trocar insertion site is at the umbilicus. A skin incision can be made in the umbilicus or immediately inferior to the umbilicus in a curved transverse or vertical fashion. The lower abdominal wall below the anterior superior iliac spines is grasped upward and the Veress needle or trocar is inserted perpendicular to the skin, aiming toward the hollow of the sacrum. The lower abdominal wall is tented upward for two purposes: to displace the entry site away from the bowel and to align the umbilical skin plane perpendicularly to the Veress needle or trocar as it is aimed toward the hollow of the sacrum. This allows the needle and trocar to traverse the shortest distance through the anterior abdominal wall without tunneling through the subcutaneum. *In obese patients a more vertical angle may be required to reach the peritoneum. Trocar insertions should generally be made at right angles to the skin.*

4. **Lower quadrant trocar insertion.** After placement of the umbilical trocar, initial survey of the abdomen and pelvis should include identification of the peritoneal folds, especially the lateral peritoneal fold containing the inferior epigastric vessels. The lower trocars should be placed lateral and cephalad to the operative site. A site 1–2 cm medial to the anterior superior iliac spine can be chosen as a starting point as well. The site to be entered should be indented with a finger under direct laparoscopic visualization to ensure avoidance of the inferior epigastric vessels. Transillumination of the site assists in avoiding the superficial epigastric vessels. The trocar should be placed under direct visualization perpendicular to the skin. One should keep in mind that the course of the deep epigastric and circumflex vessels usually parallels that of the superficial epigastric and circumflex vessels.

5. **Left upper quadrant entry.** Alternate routes of peritoneal entry should be considered for patients with prior abdominal or pelvic surgery, known adhesive disease, or a large pelvic mass, or in whom peritoneal entry via the umbilical route has failed. The left upper quadrant site of entry for a Veress needle is in the ninth intercostal space on the anterior axillary line; caution should be exercised to enter along the upper margin of the tenth rib to avoid the vascular bundle of the ninth rib. (A single "pop" should be felt here.) The trocar can then be inserted directly below the left costal margin on the midclavicular line (*Gynecol Endosc*, 4/141, 1995).

III. **Surgical spaces** (Fig. 22-5). The reproductive, urinary, and GI organ systems found in the pelvis have the ability to change their size and shape independently of each other. This is made possible by their loose attachment to each other via connective tissue planes comprised of fat and alveolar tissue. These planes are potential spaces that can become actual spaces only by surgical dissection. The spaces are divided by connective tissue septa that offer support and house the neurolymphovascular supply to the organs. *The nerves, lymphatics, and blood vessels remain in the septa only; therefore, the connective tissue spaces are avascular. Thus, careful dissection of surgical spaces can be*

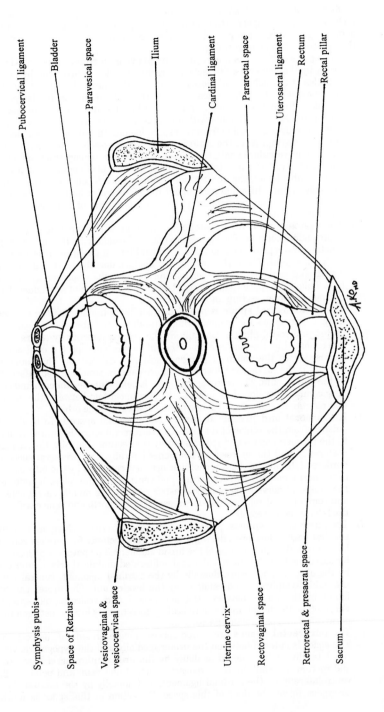

FIG. 22-5. Surgical spaces.

Pubocervical ligament

Bladder

Paravesical space

Ilium

Cardinal ligament

Pararectal space

Uterosacral ligament

Rectum

Rectal pillar

Symphysis pubis

Space of Retzius

Vesicovaginal & vesicocervical space

Uterine cervix

Rectovaginal space

Retrorectal & presacral space

Sacrum

performed bluntly and bloodlessly. There are eight surgical spaces, which include four paired spaces (the pararectal and paravesical spaces). Five of the eight surgical spaces are considered retroperitoneal: the presacral space and the paravesical and pararectal spaces.

A. The **space of Retzius (retropubic or prevesical space)** is bounded ventrally by the transversalis fascia and rectus muscles, ventrolaterally by the muscles of the pelvic wall, dorsolaterally by the cardinal ligament and the attachment of the pubocervical fascia to the arcus tendineus fasciae pelvis, and dorsally by the proximal urethra and bladder. It is possible to operate within the space of Retzius without entering the peritoneal cavity. Important structures accessible from this space include the dorsal clitoral vessels (under the symphysis), the obturator nerves and vessels (entering the obturator neurovascular canal), the nerves of the lower urinary tract (lateral to the bladder and urethra), the iliopectineal line (a fold of periosteum anterior on the pubic bone), the arcus tendinous fascia pelvis, and the arcus tendinous levator ani. Bleeding from injury to the obturator branch of the external iliac artery or from injury to the venous plexus of Santorini can be difficult to control.

B. The **vesicovaginal and vesicocervical spaces** are separated by a thin supravaginal septum. The spaces are bounded caudally by the fusion of the junction of the proximal one-third and distal two-thirds of the urethra with the vagina, ventrally by the urethra and bladder, dorsally by the vagina and cervix, and cephalad by the peritoneum forming the vesicocervical reflection. This is the space that is entered during the creation of a "bladder flap" during a cesarean section and hysterectomy.

C. The **rectovaginal space** is bounded caudally by the apex of the perineal body, 2–3 cm above the hymenal ring; laterally by the uterosacral ligament, ureter, and rectal pillars; ventrally by the vagina; dorsally by the rectum; and cephalad by the peritoneum of the cul-de-sac. This space should not be confused with the pouch of Douglas (posterior cul-de-sac). The pouch of Douglas is the cul-de-sac between the uterus and rectum bounded inferiorly by the peritoneum. The rectovaginal space is below this peritoneum and cul-de-sac, and is developed by incising the peritoneal fold between the uterus and rectum, in a line that extends from one ureter to the other.

D. **Retrorectal and presacral space.** The presacral space is to be distinguished from the retrorectal space. The retrorectal space is located caudal to the presacral space and is bordered by the rectum ventrally, the sacrum posteriorly, and the uterosacral ligaments laterally. The presacral space is bordered laterally by the internal iliac arteries, cephalad by the bifurcation of the aorta, dorsally by the sacrum, and ventrally by the colon. It contains the presacral nerve (superior hypogastric plexus), the middle sacral artery and vein (originating from the *dorsal* aspect of the aorta and vena cava) and the lateral sacral vessels.

E. The **paravesical spaces,** paired spaces adjacent to the bladder, are usually the first spaces developed during a radical hysterectomy for cervical cancer by entering the anterior leaf of the broad ligament. The paravesical space is bordered medially by the bladder and obliterated umbilical artery, laterally by the obturator internus, dorsally by the cardinal ligament, ventrally by the pubic symphysis, and caudally by the levator ani. The ureter can be found in the tissue between the paravesical and vesicovaginal spaces. Parametrial tissue obtained in a radical hysterectomy is located between the paravesical and pararectal spaces.

F. The **pararectal spaces** are paired spaces along each side of the rectum. The space is entered between the ureter medially and the hypogastric vessels laterally. It is bordered medially by the ureter, uterosacral ligament, and rectum; laterally by the hypogastric artery and vein, and pelvic wall; ventrolaterally by the cardinal ligament; and dorsally by the sacrum. The coccygeus forms the floor of this space. Dissection of this space is much more dangerous than dissection of the paravesical space as unskilled dissection can lead to bleeding. When dissection reaches the pelvic floor, care must be taken to avoid the lateral sacral and hemorrhoidal vessels. The pararectal spaces allow access to the sacrospinous ligaments.

IV. **Pelvic connective tissue and organs**

A. **Endopelvic fascia.** This fascia is comprised of a meshwork of collagen and elastin forming the fused adventitial connective tissue of the pelvic organs. It provides support to the pelvic organs by connecting the viscera to the pelvic wall, and it contains the neurovascular supply of the organs from the pelvic wall.

B. **Vagina.** The vagina is shaped like a flattened tube with the anterior and posterior walls in contact. It begins from the hymenal ring and extends to the fornices surrounding the cervix. Its average length is 8 cm; however, this varies considerably depending on age, parity, and surgical history. The anterior wall, which accommodates the cervix, is approximately 3 cm shorter than the posterior wall. Midline longitudinal ridges called the anterior and posterior columns are created by the urethra and rectum, respectively. The vaginal sidewall creases are called the lateral vaginal sulci. The epithelial lining is nonkeratinized stratified squamous epithelium lacking mucous glands and hair follicles. Mesonephric duct remnants in the vaginal wall can result in Gartner's duct cysts. Deep to the epithelium is the vaginal smooth muscle, consisting of an inner circular and outer longitudinal layer. The lower third of the vagina is connected laterally to each levator ani by the fibers of Luschka, anteriorly to the urethra and posteriorly to the perineal body. The middle third of the vagina is attached to the levator ani laterally, the vesical neck and trigone anteriorly, and the rectum posteriorly. The upper third of the vagina is attached to the cardinal ligaments laterally, bladder and ureters anteriorly, and cul-de-sac posteriorly.

C. **Uterus.** The uterus is a fibromuscular organ that contains the corpus, cervix, and isthmus, which joins the prior two.

1. **Corpus.** The fundus is the portion of the corpus that is located cephalad to the endometrial cavity. The uterine cornu is the portion that contains the interstitial portion of the fallopian tube. The endometrium is the innermost lining of the uterus and is comprised of columnar epithelium and specialized stroma. The superficial layer of endometrium contains hormonally sensitive spiral arterioles distinct to this layer. Spasms of these arterioles result in shedding of this layer after each menstrual cycle. The deeper basal layer has a different arterial supply and is preserved with each cycle. The myometrium contains interlacing smooth muscle fibers. The serosal surface of the uterus is formed by peritoneal mesothelium.

2. **Cervix.** The cervix is generally 2–4 cm in length and has two parts: the portio vaginalis (protruding into the vagina) and the portio supravaginalis (lying above the vagina). The cervix is made up of dense fibrous connective tissue and is surrounded in a circular fashion by a small amount of smooth muscle into which the cardinal and uterosacral ligaments and pubocervical fascia insert. This layer is dissected off the fibrous cervix during an intrafascial hysterectomy. The cylindrically shaped cervix contains a central longitudinal canal connecting the endometrial cavity with the vagina called the endocervical canal. It is lined with columnar epithelium that extends into the stroma as endocervical glands. The internal os of the cervix marks the beginning of the endocervical canal from the endometrial cavity. The external os marks the distal opening of the cervical canal and contains the new squamocolumnar junction. This squamocolumnar junction marks the transition from the squamous epithelium of the ectocervix to the columnar epithelium of the endocervical canal. The transformation zone is the area of metaplastic epithelium bordered distally by the old squamo-

columnar junction and proximally by the new squamocolumnar junction. The ectocervix is the portion of the cervical canal that is lined with squamous epithelium.

3. **Ligaments of the uterus.** These ligaments are formed by thickenings of endopelvic fascia or ridges of peritoneum.

a. The **round ligament** contains the **artery of Sampson** and courses from the anterior aspect of the uterus through the inguinal canal to insert into the labia majora. The round ligament has fibromuscular elements and can give rise to leiomyomas in this region. It is not supportive but helps to keep the uterus anteverted. *It is the homolog of the gubernaculum testis.*

b. The **utero-ovarian ligament** contains the anastomotic vasculature of the ovarian and uterine arteries. In a hysterectomy without salpingo-oophorectomy, this ligament, rather than the infundibulopelvic ligament, is clamped and ligated.

c. The **infundibulopelvic ligament (IP ligament, suspensory ligament of the ovary)** contains the ovarian vessels. During a hysterectomy, this vascular pedicle should be sutured first with a free tie on the proximal end and then suture ligated on the distal aspect. The peritoneal fold directly below the ovarian vessels is called the **avascular space of Graves.** A transfixion suture should not be the first ligation suture, as this can create a hematoma.

d. Bilaterally, the **cardinal ligaments (Mackenrodt's ligaments)** are thickenings of endopelvic fascia that extend from the lateral pelvic walls and insert into the lateral portion of the vagina, uterine cervix, and isthmus. The cardinal ligaments play a significant supportive role and prevent pelvic organ prolapse. Although they are described as extending laterally, in the standing position these ligaments are almost vertical. They contain the uterine artery and veins.

e. Bilaterally, the **uterosacral ligaments** are thickenings of endopelvic fascia that extend from the sacral fascia and insert into the posterior portion of the uterine isthmus. They are comprised predominantly of smooth muscle and contain the autonomic sympathetic and parasympathetic nerves of the pelvic organs. The cardinal and uterosacral ligaments are two parts of a single body of suspensory tissue that provides the major support for the uterus. The parametrium is the suspensory tissue that attaches to the uterus and is made up of the cardinal and uterosacral ligaments.

f. The **broad ligament** is comprised of peritoneum that covers the uterus and tubes bilaterally and has no supportive function. It forms folds creating a mesentery around the uterine ligaments with distinct names.

(1) **Mesoteres:** the broad ligament fold containing the round ligament.

(2) **Mesosalpinx:** the broad ligament fold containing the fallopian tube. This is the area through which a defect is created typically during a postpartum tubal ligation.

(3) **Mesovarium:** The broad ligament fold containing the utero-ovarian ligament.

D. **Adnexa.** The fallopian tubes and ovaries together constitute the uterine adnexa.

1. The **fallopian tubes** are bilateral tubular structures that connect the endometrial cavity to the peritoneal cavity and measure approximately 10 cm. Medially, each tube arises from the uterus at a point superior and dorsal to the round ligament and ventral to the utero-ovarian ligament. Distally, it has a fimbriated end providing a wide surface area to receive an ovum. Its lumen is lined by folds of ciliated columnar epithelium. The luminal opening to the endometrial cavity is termed the

tubal ostia. The fallopian tube has four portions (from proximal to distal): interstitial, isthmic, ampullary, and infundibular. The most common site of an ectopic pregnancy is the ampullary portion of the fallopian tube. During ovulation, the fimbria ovarica, a smooth muscle band attachment between the fimbria and ovary, brings these structures together.

2. The **ovaries** are bilateral white flattened oval structures that can measure 2.5–5.0 cm long, 1.5–3.0 cm thick, and 0.7–1.5 cm wide during reproductive life. Each ovary is suspended from the pelvic sidewall by the IP ligament laterally and from the uterus by the utero-ovarian ligament medially. The ovaries receive their blood supply from the ovarian arteries and some from the uterine arteries. Each ovary typically rests in the ovarian fossa **(fossa of Waldeyer)**, which is bordered by the hypogastric artery dorsomedially and the external iliac artery ventrolaterally. It is important to note that the ureter runs under the base of the fossa. Thus, in an ovarian ectopic pregnancy, endometriosis, or salpingo-oophoritis, the ovaries may be densely adherent to the ureter. The ovary has a fibromuscular and vascular medulla and an outer cortex containing specialized stroma with follicles, corpora lutea, and corpora albicantia. It is covered by a cuboidal epithelium.

E. **Vermiform appendix.** The appendix averages 10 cm in length and usually lies deep to McBurney's point, a point located one-third of the distance in a line from the anterior superior iliac spine to the umbilicus. Its position is usually retrocecal (65%) or pelvic (32%). The appendix has its own mesentery called the **mesoappendix** that suspends it from the mesentery of the terminal ileum and contains the appendicular artery. The main blood supply to the appendix is the **appendicular artery,** which is a branch of the ileocolic artery.

V. **Structures of the abdomen and pelvis** (Fig. 22-6A and B)

A. **Vasculature**

1. **Aorta.** From cephalad to caudad, the arteries that stem from the aorta below the diaphragm are the inferior phrenic, celiac trunk, middle suprarenal, superior mesenteric, renal, ovarian, inferior mesenteric, and middle sacral. The aorta then bifurcates into the common iliac arteries about the level of the fourth lumbar vertebra.

2. **Ovarian vessels.** The ovarian arteries stem from the anterior aspect of the aorta caudal to the renal arteries and course toward the pelvis, crossing laterally over the ureter at the level of the pelvic brim, during which path they pass branches to the ureter and fallopian tube. They then cross the proximal aspect of the external iliac vessels lateral to medial, and run medially in the IP ligament to supply the ovary. The left ovarian vein drains into the left renal vein. The right ovarian vein drains directly into the vena cava.

3. **Hypogastric artery (internal iliac artery).** After approximately 5 cm, the common iliac artery bifurcates into the external iliac and internal iliac (hypogastric) arteries at the level of the sacroiliac joint. The hypogastric artery then divides into an anterior and posterior division 3–4 cm after leaving the common iliac artery.

a. The **anterior division of the hypogastric artery** varies in its branching pattern. The branches that stem from the anterior division are the obturator, umbilical, uterine, vaginal, inferior and superior vesical, middle rectal, internal pudendal, and inferior gluteal arteries. The vessels that are derived from the anterior division can be classified into by tissues they primarily supply. The obturator, internal pudendal, and inferior gluteal primarily supply muscles. The uterine, superior and inferior vesical, vaginal, and middle rectal vessels supply the pelvic organs. During the classic hypogastric artery ligation, it is the anterior division of the hypogastric artery that should be ligated.

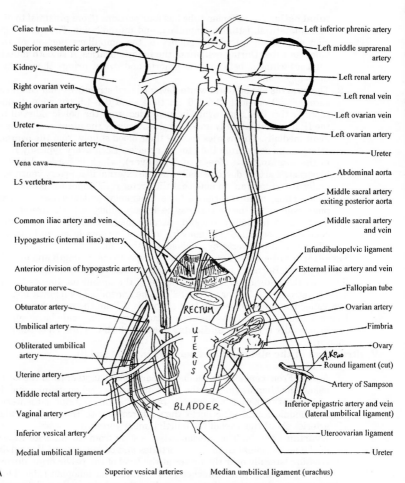

A

FIG. 22-6. A: Vasculature of the pelvic organs (frontal view). (*Continued.*)

The artery should be ligated at a site 2.5–3.0 cm distal to the bifurcation of the common iliac to preserve the posterior division of the hypogastric artery. This avoids necrosis of the gluteal muscles.

    b. The **posterior division of the hypogastric artery** leaves the hypogastric artery from the lateral surface and has three branches ("ILS"): the iliolumbar, the lateral sacral, and the superior gluteal.

  4. **External iliac artery.** Just before the external iliac artery travels under the inguinal ligament through the femoral canal to become the femoral artery, the deep epigastric artery and deep circumflex iliac artery branch from the external iliac. During hypogastric artery ligation, these vessels should be avoided as well.

B. **Ureteral course.** The ureter measures 25–30 cm from the renal pelvis to the bladder. Starting from the bladder, the ureter travels toward the pelvis along the anterior surface of the psoas muscle. It crosses medially under the ovarian vessels at the pelvic brim and travels medial to the ovarian vessels and then

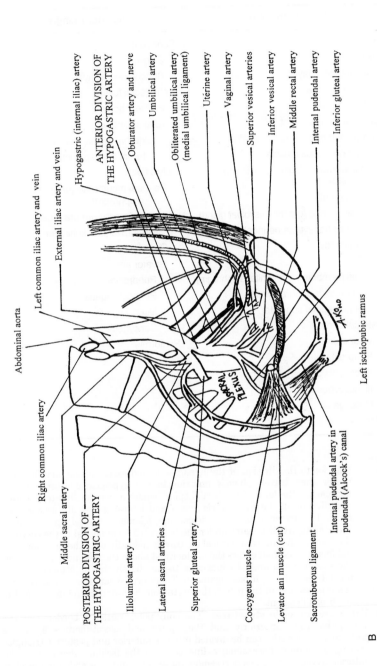

Abdominal aorta

Left common iliac artery and vein

External iliac artery and vein

Hypogastric (internal iliac) artery

ANTERIOR DIVISION OF
THE HYPOGASTRIC ARTERY

Obturator artery and nerve

Umbilical artery

Obliterated umbilical artery
(medial umbilical ligament)

Uterine artery

Vaginal artery

Superior vesical arteries

Inferior vesical artery

Middle rectal artery

Internal pudendal artery

Inferior gluteal artery

Left ischiopubic ramus

Internal pudendal artery in
pudendal (Alcock's) canal

Sacrotuberous ligament

Levator ani muscle (cut)

Coccygeus muscle

Superior gluteal artery

Lateral sacral arteries

Iliolumbar artery

POSTERIOR DIVISION OF
THE HYPOGASTRIC ARTERY

Middle sacral artery

Right common iliac artery

SACRAL PLEXUS

B

FIG. 22-6. *Continued.* **B:** Vasculature of the pelvic organs (sagittal view).

TABLE 22-2. LAYERS OF THE PERINEUM AND PELVIC FLOOR

Anterior triangle	Posterior triangle
Vulva	Perineum
Skin	Skin
Subcutaneous layer	Subcutaneous layer
Camper's fascia	Ischiorectal fossa
Colles' fascia	Perineal body
Superficial compartment	Anal sphincter
Clitoris and crura	External anal sphincter
Ischiocavernosus muscle	Internal anal sphincter
Bulbocavernosus (bulbospongiosus) muscle	Pelvic floor
Vestibular bulb	Perineal membrane (urogenital diaphragm)
Bartholin's gland (greater vestibular gland)	Compressor urethra muscle
Superficial transverse perineal muscle	Urethrovaginal sphincter
Perineal body	Perineal body
Pelvic floor	Levator ani
Perineal membrane (urogenital diaphragm)	Puborectalis
Compressor urethra muscle	Pubococcygeus
Urethrovaginal sphincter	Iliococcygeus
Perineal body	Coccygeus
Levator ani	Pyriformis
Puborectalis	
Pubococcygeus	
Iliococcygeus	
Coccygeus	
Pyriformis	

anterior to the division of the hypogastric and external iliac arteries. The ureter then travels slightly anterior to the hypogastric artery until it approaches the level of the ischial spine, where it runs medial to the anterior division of the hypogastric artery and lateral to the uterosacral ligament. The ureter then enters the cardinal ligament "tunnel," passes under the uterine artery ("water under the bridge") 1.5 cm lateral to the cervix at the level of the internal cervical os, travels medially over the anterior vaginal fornix, and then enters the bladder just above the trigone. In the pelvis, the ureter has a special connective tissue sheath that is attached to the medial leaf of the broad ligament. Therefore, when the retroperitoneal space is entered in the pelvis, the ureter can be found in the medial leaf of the broad ligament.

VI. **Vulva and erectile structures.** The bony pelvic outlet is bordered by the ischiopubic rami anteriorly and the coccyx and sacrotuberous ligaments posteriorly. The outlet can be divided into the anterior and posterior triangles sharing a common base along a line between the ischial tuberosities. The anterior triangle tissue layers resemble those of the anterior abdominal wall as follows (Table 22-2).

A. **Skin and subcutaneous layer.** The subcutaneous tissue is similar to that of the anterior abdominal wall with two nondiscrete layers: Camper's fascia and Colles' fascia.

1. **Camper's fascia of the vulva** includes the continuation of this layer from the anterior abdominal wall.

2. **Colles' fascia** is similar to Scarpa's fascia of the anterior abdominal wall. *It fuses* posteriorly with the perineal membrane and laterally with the ischiopubic rami; its anterior aspect is continuous with the anterior abdominal wall. This configuration prevents hematomas in this compartment from spreading posterolaterly but allows the hematomas to spread into the anterior abdominal wall.

3. **Structures of the skin and subcutaneous layer** (Fig. 22-7)
   a. The **mons (mons pubis, mons veneris)** is hair-bearing skin overlying adipose tissue lying on the pubic bones.
   b. The **labia majora** extend from the mons posteriorly and contain similar hair-bearing skin overlying adipose tissue. The labia majora contain the insertion of the round ligaments. Camper's fascia in the labia majora includes the continuation of fat from the anterior abdominal wall called the **digital process of fat,** which is used as a Martius fat pad graft to cover vaginal fistulas.
   c. The **labia minora** are hairless skin folds that split anteriorly to form the prepuce and frenulum of the clitoris. These labia overlie not adipose tissue but loosely organized connective tissue, which allows for mobility during intercourse. This loose attachment also permits ease of dissection of this layer during a skinning vulvectomy.
   d. **Gland duct openings**
      (1) The **greater vestibular gland duct** opening is seen on the posterolateral aspect of the vestibule 3–4 mm lateral to the hymenal ring.
      (2) The **minor vestibular gland duct** opening is seen in a line above the greater vestibular gland duct opening toward the urethra.
      (3) The **Skene duct openings** are located inferolateral to the urethral meatus at approximately 5 and 7 o'clock.
   e. **Specialized glands** located in the vulvar skin can enlarge and require surgical therapy.
      (1) **Holocrine sebaceous glands** located in the labia majora are associated with hair shafts.
      (2) **Apocrine sweat glands** located lateral to the introitus and anus produce increased secretions premenstrually. **Hydradenitis suppurativa** *can occur if these glands become chronically infected.* **Hidradenomas** *are neoplastic enlargements of these glands.*
      (3) **Eccrine sweat glands** are also located lateral to the introitus and anus. They can enlarge and form a **syringoma.**

B. **Superficial compartment of the vulva** (Fig. 22-8). This compartment lies between the subcutaneous layer and the perineal membrane.

1. The **clitoris** consists of the **glans,** a **shaft** that is attached to the pubis by a **subcutaneous suspensory ligament,** and **paired crura** that stem from the shaft and attach to the inferior aspect of the pubic rami.

2. **Ischiocavernosus muscles** overlie the crura of the clitoris. They originate at the ischial tuberosities and free surfaces of the crura and insert into the upper crura and clitoral shaft.

3. **Bulbocavernosus (bulbospongiosus) muscles** originate in the perineal body and insert into the clitoral shaft. They overlie the centrolateral aspects of the vestibular bulbs and Bartholin's gland. The ischiocavernosus and bulbocavernosus muscles act to pull the clitoral shaft caudally.

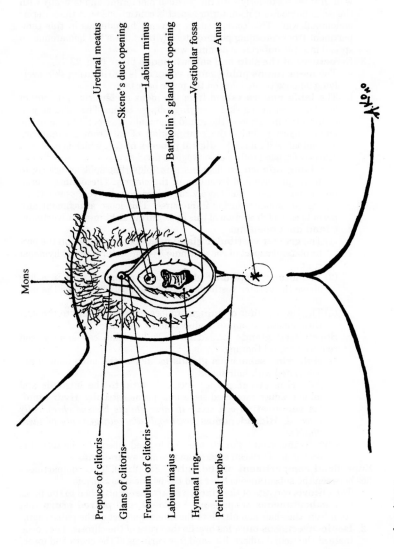

FIG. 22-7. Vulva and perineum.

Mons

Prepuce of clitoris
Glans of clitoris
Frenulum of clitoris
Labium majus
Hymenal ring
Perineal raphe

Urethral meatus
Skene's duct opening
Labium minus
Bartholin's gland duct opening
Vestibular fossa
Anus

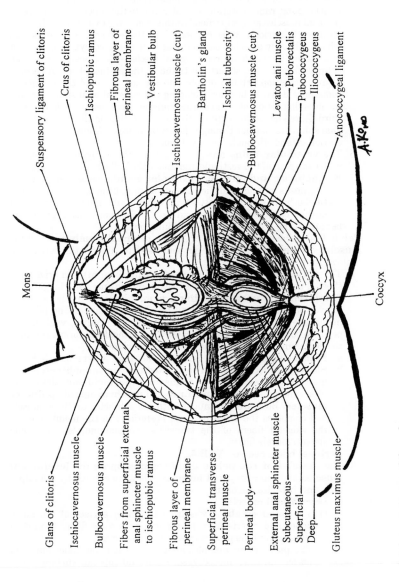

Glans of clitoris

Ischiocavernosus muscle

Bulbocavernosus muscle

Fibers from superficial external
anal sphincter muscle
to ischiopubic ramus

Fibrous layer of
perineal membrane

Superficial transverse
perineal muscle

Perineal body

External anal sphincter muscle
Subcutaneous
Superficial
Deep

Gluteus maximus muscle

Mons

Coccyx

Suspensory ligament of clitoris

Crus of clitoris

Ischiopubic ramus

Fibrous layer of
perineal membrane

Vestibular bulb

Ischiocavernosus muscle (cut)

Bartholin's gland

Ischial tuberosity

Bulbocavernosus muscle (cut)

Levator ani muscle
Puborectalis
Pubococcygeus
Iliococcygeus

Anococcygeal ligament

FIG. 22-8. Superficial compartment of the vulva.

4. **Superficial transverse perineal muscles** originate from the ischial tuberosities and insert into the perineal body.

5. The **perineal body (central tendon of the perineum)** (Fig. 22-9) is connected anterolaterally with the bulbocavernosus muscle. Anteriorly it is connected with the perineal membrane, which attaches it to the inferior pubic rami. Laterally it is attached to the superficial transverse perineal muscles and, superficial to this, some muscles of the pelvic diaphragm. Posteriorly, it is connected to the external anal sphincter, which indirectly attaches the perineal body to the coccyx. Superiorly it is attached to the distal rectovaginal fascia. A first-degree laceration extends through the superficial tissue of the perineal body. A second-degree laceration extends deeply into the soft tissue of the perineum, sometimes down to but not including the external anal sphincter, and involves disruption of some of the transverse perineal muscle fibers. A third-degree laceration extends through a portion or all of the external anal sphincter but not through the rectal mucosa. A fourth-degree laceration extends through the rectal mucosa.

6. The **vestibular bulbs** are paired erectile tissues lying immediately under the skin of the vestibule and under the bulbocavernosus muscles.

7. **Bartholin's gland (greater vestibular gland)** lies between the bulbocavernosus muscles and the perineal membrane at the tail end of the vestibular bulb. Its duct empties into the vestibular mucosa. Removal of a Bartholin's gland duct cyst can be a very hemorrhagic procedure because of the proximity of the vestibular bulb.

C. **Pelvic floor.** The pelvic floor comprises the **perineal membrane** and the **muscles of the pelvic diaphragm** and helps to support the pelvic contents above the pelvic outlet.

1. The **perineal membrane (urogenital diaphragm)** is a triangular sheet of dense fibromuscular tissue spanning the anterior triangle. Previously called the **urogenital diaphragm,** this was formerly viewed as a layer of skeletal muscle between two layers of fascia. The perineal membrane provides **support** by attaching the urethra, vagina, and perineal body to the ischiopubic rami. The perineal membrane contains the dorsal and deep nerves and vessels of the clitoris.

   a. **Fibrous layer.** This layer is superficial to the skeletal muscle layer.

   b. **Skeletal muscle layer.** The striated **urogenital sphincter** (formerly known as the **deep transverse perineal muscles**) comprises the **compressor urethrae** and **urethrovaginal sphincter muscles.** Both are continuous with the sphincter urethrae muscle and compress the distal urethra. Posteriorly in the membrane are the skeletal fibers of the transverse vaginal muscle with some smooth muscle fibers.

2. **Perineal body.** See sec. VI.B.5.

3. The **muscles of the pelvic diaphragm** comprise the **levator ani muscles** and the **coccygeal muscles.** They are covered by the **superior and inferior fasciae.**

   a. **Levator ani muscles**

      (1) The **puborectalis** arises from the inner surface of the pubic bones and inserts into the rectum, with some fibers forming a sling around the posterior aspect of the rectum.

      (2) The **pubococcygeus** also arises from the pubic bones but then inserts into the anococcygeal raphe and superior surface of the coccyx.

      (3) The **iliococcygeus** arises from the **arcus tendineus levator ani** and inserts into the anococcygeal raphe and coccyx. The **arcus tendineus fascia pelvis (white line)** is formed from a fibrous thickening of the obturator internus and pubocervical fasciae.

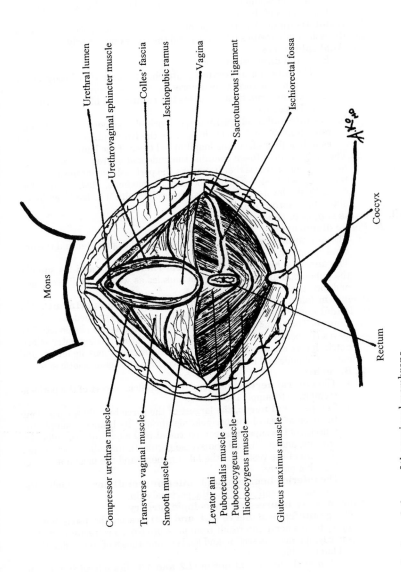

FIG. 22-9. Skeletal muscle layer of the perineal membrane.

Urethral lumen

Urethrovaginal sphincter muscle

Colles' fascia

Ischiopubic ramus

Vagina

Sacrotuberous ligament

Ischiorectal fossa

Coccyx

Rectum

Mons

Compressor urethrae muscle

Transverse vaginal muscle

Smooth muscle

Levator ani
Puborectalis muscle
Pubococcygeus muscle
Iliococcygeus muscle

Gluteus maximus muscle

   (4) The **urogenital hiatus** is the area within the levator ani through which the urethra, vagina, and rectum pass. The **levator plate** is the region of the levator ani where the anococcygeal raphe lies.

  b. The **coccygeus muscle** arises from the ischial spine, lies cephalad to the sacrospinous ligament, and inserts into the coccyx and the lowest area of the sacrum.

D. **Posterior triangle.** The three points surrounding the posterior triangle are the ischial tuberosities bilaterally and the coccyx posteriorly.

 1. **Anal sphincters**

  a. **External anal sphincter**

   (1) The **superficial portion** is attached to the perineal body anteriorly and the coccyx posteriorly.

   (2) The **deep portion** encircles the rectum and blends in with the puborectalis.

  b. The **internal anal sphincter,** comprised of smooth muscle, is separated from the external sphincter by the **intersphincteric groove** as well as fibers from the longitudinal layer of the bowel.

 2. The **ischiorectal fossa** contains the pudendal neurovascular trunk. It has an anterior recess that lies above the perineal membrane and a posterior portion that lies above the gluteus maximus. Medially, it is bordered by the levator ani muscles. Anterolaterally, it is bordered by the obturator internus muscles.

VII. **Nervous supply of the pelvis**

 A. **Pelvic diaphragm**

  1. The **pudendal nerve** supplies the external anal sphincter and the urethral sphincter.

  2. The **anterior branch of the ventral ramus of S3 and S4** supplies the puborectal and pubococcygeus muscles as well as the iliococcygeal and coccygeal muscles.

 B. **Perineum (skin, subcutaneum, and superficial compartment).** The **pudendal nerve** is the sensory and motor nerve of the perineum.

  1. **Course.** The pudendal nerve originates from the sacral plexus (S2–S4), leaves the pelvis with the pudendal vessels through the greater sciatic notch, hooks around the ischial spine and sacrospinous ligament, and enters the pudendal canal (canal of Alcock) in the lesser sciatic notch.

  2. **Branches**

   a. The **clitoral nerve** runs along the superficial aspect of the perineal membrane to supply the clitoris.

   b. The **perineal nerve,** the largest of the three branches, runs along the deep aspect of the perineal membrane. Its branches supply the muscles of the superficial compartment (ischiocavernosus, bulbocavernosus, and superficial transverse perineal), the subcutaneum, and the skin of the vestibule, the labia minora, and the medial aspect of the labia majora.

   c. The **inferior hemorrhoidal (inferior rectal) nerve** supplies the external anal sphincter and the perianal skin.

 C. **Common nerve injuries in gynecologic surgery**

  1. The **genitofemoral nerve (L1 and L2)** lies on the psoas muscle. Injury to this nerve can result from pressure from a retractor or during pelvic lymph node dissection and leads to anesthesia of the medial thigh and lateral labia.

  2. The **femoral cutaneous nerve (L2 and L3)** lies lateral to the genitofemoral nerve and psoas muscle. It can be damaged by hyperflexion of the hip in lithotomy position or also by a retractor; injury results in anterior thigh anesthesia.

  3. **Femoral nerve (L2, L3, L4) injury** can result in both sensory and motor symptoms. Hyperflexion of the thighs with external rotation and

abduction can cause compression of the nerve under the inguinal ligament and local ischemia of the nerve. Pressure from a retractor on the
psoas muscle and underlying femoral nerve can also result in injury.
Sensory deficits can involve the anterior thigh (anterior femoral cutaneous nerve), medial thigh (medial femoral cutaneous nerve), and tibial
thigh (long saphenous nerve). Motor deficits involve the quadriceps,
pectineus, and sartorius. Clinically, the patient usually falls when
attempting to walk after surgery and has a loss of the patellar reflex. This
condition is self-limited, with complete resolution in 3–60 days. Active
and passive quadriceps exercise for management is recommended.

4. **Sciatic nerve (L4, L5, S1, S2, S3) injury** can result from a stretch
injury due to incorrect positioning by extensive external hip rotation in
the dorsal lithotomy position or from sudden knee extension from a
flexed thigh when candy-cane stirrups are used. Foot drop and numbness are the usual manifestations of the affected side. This condition is
also self-limited, with complete resolution within 90 days.

5. **Obturator nerve injury** can result from deep pelvic surgery in the
area (i.e., pelvic node dissection) and results in medial thigh anesthesia
and thigh adduction weakness.

6. **Pudendal nerve (S2, S3, S4) injury** can result from a sacrospinous
vaginal vault suspension and leads to perineal paresthesia and urinary
and fecal incontinence.

VIII. **Lymphatic drainage** of the pelvis is an extensively interconnected system
with somewhat unpredictable flow; however, the following generalizations are
helpful. Vulva and lower vagina drain toward the inguino-femoral lymph nodes
and then toward the external iliac chains. The lymphatic drainage of the cervix
is through the cardinal ligaments, to the pelvic (hypogastric, obturator, and
external iliac) nodes, and to the common iliac and para-aortic nodes. The
lymphatic drainage of the endometrium is through the broad ligament and IP
ligament to the pelvic and para-aortic nodes. The lymphatic drainage of the
ovaries is through the IP ligament to the pelvic and para-aortic nodes.

23. PERIOPERATIVE CARE AND COMPLICATIONS OF GYNECOLOGIC SURGERY

Sven Becker and Alfred Bent

I. **Preoperative care.** Most gynecologic surgery is elective and low risk, except that in oncology and geriatric patients, who may have multiple medical problems. The main objective of the preoperative assessment is to make sure that the patient is fit for the appropriate surgery and that the patient understands the indications, benefits, risks, and alternatives for the planned procedure.
   A. **Medical issues**
      1. **Preoperative evaluation.** In the office setting, the history and physical examination are key in evaluating the patient's fitness for surgery and the need for further testing or consultation. Positive findings need to be evaluated with ECG, pulmonary function tests, or cardiac testing as appropriate. A history of alcoholism needs to be specifically elucidated and followed up with liver function tests. Complex preexisting conditions must be co-managed together with the appropriate physician. Preoperative consultation with an anesthesiologist is important for the medically compromised patient.
      2. **Preoperative testing.** Preoperative testing is guided mostly by positive findings on the history and physical examination. The patient should have current results of Pap smear and mammography. A pregnancy test is standard for women of reproductive age. For patients younger than 40 years, a CBC is usually required. Patients older than 40 years are evaluated with a CBC, basic metabolic panel, and ECG. For patients older than 60 years, a routine chest radiograph is added.
      3. **Preoperative management**
         a. **Deep venous thrombosis (DVT) prophylaxis.** The best DVT prophylaxis is early ambulation after surgery. For patients undergoing gynecologic surgery, below-the-knee elastic stockings and pneumatic compression devices are used. In high-risk patients (oncologic patients, obese patients, patients with a history of previous DVT or pulmonary embolism, or patients for whom prolonged pelvic surgery is anticipated), 5000 U of unfractionated heparin is given subcutaneously (SC) 30 minutes before surgery and every 8 hours postoperatively until the patient is mobile. Alternative regimens include the use of low-molecular-weight heparin formulations such as enoxaparin sodium (Lovenox) 40 mg/day SC starting 2 hours preoperatively or postoperatively, or dalteparin sodium (Fragmin) 2500–5000 U/day SC postoperatively.
         b. **Antibiotic prophylaxis.** For abdominal and vaginal hysterectomy, preoperative antibiotic prophylaxis often consists of a first- or second-generation cephalosporin, most commonly cefazolin sodium (1 g), cefotetan disodium (1 g) or cefoxitin sodium (2 g). Another good choice is ampicillin/sulbactam sodium (3 g). Postoperative antibiotic prophylaxis has not been shown to be effective. Anaerobic coverage (e.g., with metronidazole hydrochloride) should be added before anticipated colorectal surgery.
         c. **Prophylaxis for subacute bacterial endocarditis.** In 1997 the American Heart Association revised the recommendations for prophylaxis for subacute bacterial endocarditis. Patients are divided into high-, moderate-, and negligible-risk categories (Table 23-1). Prophylaxis is recommended only for those in the high- and moderate-risk categories.

TABLE 23-1. AMERICAN MEDICAL ASSOCIATION RISK CATEGORIES FOR PROPHYLAXIS FOR SUBACUTE BACTERIAL ENDOCARDITIS

High risk (prophylaxis recommended)
  Prosthetic valves
  History of bacterial endocarditis
  Complex cyanotic congenital heart disease, surgically constructed shunts or conduits
Moderate risk (prophylaxis recommended)
  Mitral valve prolapse with valvular regurgitation and/or thickened leaflets
  Hypertrophic cardiomyopathy
  Most other cardiac malformations
Negligible risk (no prophylaxis recommended)
  Surgically repaired atrial septal defect or ventricular septal defect (longer than 6 mos after surgery)
  Coronary artery bypass graft
  Physiologic, functional, or innocent heart murmurs
  Cardiac pacemakers, implanted defibrillators

High-risk patients should receive the old regimen of ampicillin (2 g IV within 30 minutes of starting the procedure and 6 hours afterward) and gentamicin hydrochloride (1.5 mg/kg up to 120 mg IV with first dose of ampicillin) or vancomycin (1 g IV over 1–2 hours) and gentamicin in case of penicillin allergy.

Moderate-risk patients should receive one dose of ampicillin/amoxicillin or vancomycin only. Gentamicin is no longer required.

Patients with mitral valve prolapse require prophylaxis only in the presence of regurgitation. In the absence of an echocardiography report, however, prophylaxis is usually indicated.

   d. **Bowel preparation.** Reduction of GI contents provides additional room in the pelvis and abdomen and facilitates surgery. Reduction in the number of pathogenic flora in the colon reduces the risk of infection if bowel surgery is performed. Mechanical bowel preparation with oral gut lavage using an agent such as polyethylene glycol electrolyte solution (Golytely) and a clear liquid diet for 24 hours the day before surgery is commonly used. Alternative regimens include sodium phosphate (Fleet Phospho-Soda) and magnesium citrate, with or without enemas. Table 23-2 gives practical recommendations.

TABLE 23-2. BOWEL PREPARATION OPTIONS

Planned surgery	Bowel preparation
Total abdominal hysterectomy, total vaginal hysterectomy	Magnesium citrate (1–2 bottles)
Severe endometriosis, risk of small bowel surgery, etc.	Fleet Phospho-Soda (sodium phosphate) 45 mL at 3 pm and 6 pm the day before surgery
Colorectal surgery, posterior repair, etc.	Fleet Phospho-Soda as above *and* enema on the morning of surgery

TABLE 23-3. RISK OF ACQUIRING VIRAL DISEASE WITH A UNIT OF BLOOD

Hepatitis C virus	1:30,000
Hepatitis B virus	1:100,000
Human immunodeficiency virus	1:500,000

e. **Autologous blood donation.** Information regarding the possibility and risk of a blood transfusion must be part of the informed consent procedure (Table 23-3). In healthy adult patients, blood loss up to 500–700 mL can usually be tolerated.

f. **Medications.** Antihypertensive medications and alpha-blockers should be taken with a sip of water on the morning of surgery. Diabetic patients are co-managed with their own physicians. Patients who were treated with steroids within 12 months of surgery usually receive stress doses of steroids intraoperatively. Two options are hydrocortisone 100 mg IV or methylprednisolone 100 mg IV at the time of surgery. No taper is necessary.

B. **Counseling**

1. **Informed consent** means that the physician has explained the need for the surgery, the risks, and possible alternatives, and that the patient has comprehended these facts and agreed to the surgery. All discussions about indications, risks, and alternatives as well as the patient's response must be documented in the chart.

2. **Risks and rates of complications.** The most important causes of perioperative death are myocardial infarction, pulmonary embolus, infection, and heart failure. The risk of dying from anesthesia alone is low, at approximately 1 in 10,000 and is related to preoperative risk category (Table 23-4).

II. **Intraoperative complications**

A. **Hemorrhage.** The management of catastrophic intraoperative hemorrhage includes aggressive fluid resuscitation and blood transfusions. Rarely does a patient require more than 4 U of packed red blood cells (PRBC). In such an event, 2 U of fresh frozen plasma should be given for every 6–8 U of PRBC. Also, for every 10 U of PRBC, 10 U of platelets should be given. Consultations should be readily sought.

B. **Ureteral injury.** Although much feared, ureteral injury is rare in gynecologic surgery, occurring in 0.3% to 0.5% of cases. Risk factors include pregnancy and the presence of malignant tumors, endometriosis, uterine procidentia, and pelvic hematomas. Areas in which injuries occur at the

TABLE 23-4. AMERICAN SOCIETY OF ANESTHESIOLOGISTS' PHYSICAL STATUS CLASSIFICATION AND ASSOCIATED RISK OF DEATH FROM ANESTHESIA

	Class	Mortality rate (%)
I	Healthy	0.08
II	Mild systemic disease	0.3
III	Severe systemic disease with functional limitation	1.8
IV	Severe systemic disease that is a constant threat to life	7.8
V	Severe illness, patient unlikely to survive 24 hrs without surgery	10

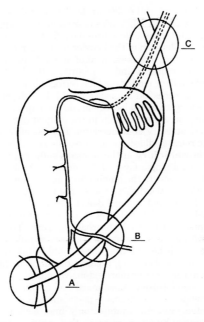

FIG. 23-1. Common sites of ureteral injury associated with hysterectomy are ureterovesical junction (A), junction of uterine artery and ureter (B), and infundibulopelvic ligament (C). (Adapted from Shingleton HM. Repairing injuries to the urinary tract. *Contemp Obstet Gynecol* March 1984;76, with permission.)

time of hysterectomy are (1) the pelvic brim (near the infundibulopelvic ligament), (2) the paracervical area (near the uterine artery), and (3) near the ureterovesical junction. Intraoperative cystoscopy with indigo carmine is an excellent test for ureteral integrity and allows immediate corrective surgery to be undertaken if an injury is detected (Fig. 23-1). For some injuries to the sheath and clamping and suturing injuries, stenting the ureter and placing a drain at the site of injury may be sufficient therapy. If there is no obvious severe damage or leakage, the ureteral sheath may be approximated with several 5-0 Vicryl sutures. Reimplantation into the bladder (ureteroneocystostomy) is the procedure of choice if the injury is within 6 cm of the bladder. Mobilization of the bladder and psoas muscle hitching can be used to bridge the gap when the ureter is short. Ureteroureterostomy is the procedure of choice when a ureter is injured in the upper pelvis (approximately 7 cm or more from the bladder).

Transureteroureterostomy is potentially hazardous to both renal units and should be considered a last resort. Percutaneous nephrostomy is rarely needed when an injury is discovered intraoperatively. Delayed diagnosis may require retrograde pyelography with cystoscopy and stent placement or percutaneous nephrostomy with antegrade stent placement.

The recovery potential of the kidney depends on the duration of the obstruction, the degree of obstruction, the degree of backflow, the presence or absence of infection, and the extent to which each kidney was functional before the injury.

C. **Bladder injury** occurs typically in the dome of the bladder at the time of the laparotomy or cesarean section and at the base of the bladder during hysterectomy. Development of the bladder flap by sharp dissection is the single best preventive measure. Small injuries (1–2 cm) can be repaired with continuous or interrupted 3-0 absorbable suture (i.e., Vicryl, Polysorb). Major lacerations may require mobilization of the bladder for tension-free repair. Any injury to the bladder base requires assessment of ureteral function. A two-layer closure with 3-0 Vicryl is required, and the security of this layer should be assessed by placing sterile milk or methylene blue retrograde into the bladder. A Foley or suprapubic catheter is left in place for 7–14 days, depending on the kind and extent of the surgery. Small lacerations do not require drainage.

D. **Bowel injury** occurs most often in the context of previous abdominal surgery or severe stage IV endometriosis. The use of blunt rather than sharp dissection to release adhesions increases the risk of bowel laceration.

   1. **Small bowel injury.** If the serosa is sufficiently injured to expose the muscularis, a single layer of 3-0 delayed absorbable suture should be placed transverse to the longitudinal axis of the lumen to avoid luminal constriction. If the defect exposes the lumen, the loop should be mobilized and inspected. A small defect may be closed transverse to the longitudinal axis of the bowel with the placement of full-thickness interrupted 3-0 delayed absorbable suture. This suture line is reinforced with a second layer of seromuscular imbricating interrupted 3-0 delayed absorbable stitches. Care should be taken to avoid injury to the mesenteric vessels during repair. Consultation should be requested in cases of uncertainty or more extensive injury.

   2. **Large bowel injury.** Mechanical and antibiotic bowel preparation is recommended when extensive pelvic disease is present or dissection is anticipated. Subtotal hysterectomy may be a prudent alternative to some planned hysterectomies, so that injury to the rectosigmoid colon can be avoided.

   Injuries to the rectosigmoid colon are closed in much the same way as injuries to the small intestine. If the defect is large, if there is significant fecal contamination and the bowel is unprepared, or if the bowel wall is unhealthy or previously irradiated, a diverting loop colostomy or ileostomy may be appropriate.

   Injury to the rectum may occur during vaginal procedures. The defect should be closed by placing a row of 3-0 delayed absorbable sutures through the rectal mucosa and then reinforcing this with a two-layered closure of overlying tissue. Colostomy is rarely necessary.

   The lower rectum and perineum may be injured during delivery of a large infant, during a difficult forceps delivery, or when an episiotomy is extended. Recognition and proper repair are essential. Continuous 3-0 or 4-0 delayed absorbable suture should be used to approximate rectal mucosa. This should be reinforced with several interrupted 3-0 delayed absorbable sutures. Repair must go beyond the superior apex of the defect in the mucosa. If the anal sphincter is involved, it should be approximated with several interrupted 2-0 delayed absorbable sutures. Finally, vaginal mucosa, perineal muscles, fascia, and skin should be approximated.

E. **Nerve injury.** Common peroneal nerve injury is most often caused by compression from the stirrups and may result in a transient foot drop postoperatively. Lateral femoral cutaneous nerve injury can result from placement of self-retaining retractors and results in anterior lateral thigh anesthesia. One should be aware of the location and the exact pressure exerted by the lateral side-wall retractors. Motor or sensory injury or both can occur to the femoral nerve when the thighs are severely flexed on the abdomen in the lithotomy position. Passing below the relatively firm inguinal ligament, the femoral nerve is vulnerable to compression at that point. Postoperatively the patient may experience weakness in the quadriceps muscle and difficulty walking.

The sciatic nerve can be injured when the thigh is flexed and the knee is suddenly straightened. This tends to happen more commonly with free hanging ("candy cane") stirrups. As with common peroneal nerve injury, this injury typically leads to foot drop.

Most neural injuries resolve completely. Early physical therapy reassures the patient and hastens the recovery, which can sometimes take up to 2–3 months.

F. **Complications specific to laparoscopy**

1. **Extraperitoneal insufflation of CO_2.** Misplacement of a Veress needle causes this complication. In most cases, CO_2 can be allowed to escape and needle placement attempted again. If this is not successful, open laparoscopy is performed. Mediastinal emphysema is an uncommon complication that requires observation for respiratory compromise and in severe cases may require ventilation.

2. **Vessel injury.** The Veress needle or trocar may traumatize omental, mesenteric, or major abdominal or pelvic vessels. Elevating the anterior abdominal wall and directing the needle or trocar toward the pelvis during insertion reduces the risk of injury. Injury of epigastric vessels with accessory trocar placement can generally be avoided. Superficial epigastric vessels can generally be identified by transillumination. The inferior epigastric vessels are deeper, which makes transillumination difficult; direct laparoscopic visualization of the vessels and insertion of trocars lateral to the edge of the rectus muscle (6–7 cm lateral to the midline) decreases risk of vessel laceration. Control of bleeding is accomplished by cautery, suture ligation, or even tamponade with a Foley catheter balloon.

3. **Bowel injury** may occur during insertion of a Veress needle or trocar or during operative procedures. Injury is more common in patients with a history of abdominal or pelvic surgery. Thermal injury can be caused by inadvertent contact between electrical, thermal, or laser energy and an organ or tissue. With electrical injury, the full extent of the damage may not be obvious immediately.

   A perforation with the Veress needle may remain undiagnosed and heal spontaneously. If perforation is suspected, the needle should be withdrawn and insufflation attempted at another site. Once the laparoscope is placed, the site of penetration must be carefully examined. Injury to the serosa does not need to be repaired provided there is hemostasis. Trocar insertion may result in injury that must be surgically corrected. If the laparoscope enters the lumen, it should be left in place to limit soiling and to facilitate identification of the injured site. Repair may be accomplished by laparoscopic or open techniques.

4. **Bladder injury.** All patients should have their bladders drained after anesthesia has been induced. Injury during trocar insertion may still occur. Injury may be detected by the presence of air in the drainage bag of an indwelling Foley catheter or by the presence of blood in the urine. The size of the injury dictates treatment. Needle perforations can be managed expectantly. Lacerations less than 10 mm long will heal spontaneously if the bladder is drained continuously for 3–4 days postoperatively. Larger injuries require suturing. This can be performed laparoscopically by surgeons experienced in laparoscopic suturing technique.

5. **Ureteral injury.** There is an increased risk of ureteral injury with adhesions or endometriosis involving the pelvic side walls. Preoperative stent placement may help locate the ureters and thus prevent inadvertent injury. If ureteral injury is suspected postoperatively, an IVP should be obtained.

6. **Trocar hernia.** Trocars larger than 7 mm carry increased risk of herniation, and fascial defects should be sutured.

G. **Complications specific to hysteroscopy.** At the time of hysteroscopy, fluids are often delivered into the uterine cavity with sufficiently high pres-

TABLE 23-5. MANAGEMENT RECOMMENDATIONS FOR SORBITOL- OR MANNITOL-RELATED FLUID DEFICITS IN HYSTEROSCOPY

Fluid deficit (mL)	Recommendation
500	Check sodium level, continue operative hysteroscopy.
1000	Check sodium level.
	Give furosemide, 20 mg IV.
	Stop procedure if sodium level is <125 mEq/L.
2000	Check sodium level.
	Give furosemide, 20 mg IV.
	Stop procedure and monitor patient closely.

sure to allow a flow reversal into the open blood vessels of the endometrium and myometrium. Hyskon is a 32% solution of dextran 70. In the bloodstream, it acts as a volume expander. Absorption of 200 mL of Hyskon will increase the intravascular volume by 2 L, potentially leading to acute noncardiogenic pulmonary edema. Also, dextran molecules can trigger disseminated intravascular coagulation and anaphylaxis. In an acute setting, dextran molecules must be removed from the circulation with plasmapheresis. Three percent sorbitol and 1.5% glycine are alternative solutions. These are hypotonic solutions. When absorbed into the bloodstream, they cause hyponatremia, which in turn can lead to arrhythmias, cerebral edema, coma, and death. Automated fluid-monitoring systems have made the exact measurement of input and output of the distending medium much easier. The surgeon should be aware of any deficit at all times (Table 23-5).

III. **Postoperative complications**
   A. **Infection**
      1. **Risk factors and prophylaxis.** The risk of postoperative infection can be lessened with shorter operative time, careful dissection, meticulous hemostasis, and adequate drainage. Antibiotic prophylaxis has been shown to decrease the incidence of infection for cesarean sections (in the case of ruptured membranes more than 6 hours before surgery) and for abdominal and vaginal hysterectomies.

      Closed suction drainage should be considered intraperitoneally in cases of contamination or less than perfect hemostasis and in the subcutaneous fat if the depth of the adipose layer exceeds 2 cm.

      2. **Evaluation.** Potential sites of postoperative infection include the lungs, the urinary tract, and the sites of surgery (including pelvic side wall and vaginal cuff), incisions, and IV catheters.
         a. **Fever.** A common definition of infection requires a temperature at or above 38°C (100.4°F) that appears after the first 24 hours postsurgery on two occasions at least 4 hours apart. Febrile morbidity within the first 48 hours of surgery has been estimated to occur in up to 50% of gynecologic surgery patients. It often resolves without therapy and usually does not require a fever workup. Fever after 24 hours postsurgery should be considered a sign of infection.
         b. **Examination.** Evaluation for infection should include a review of the patient's history and a thorough examination with specific attention to sites at risk, for example, pulmonary examination, palpation of kidneys and costovertebral angles, evaluation of incision and catheter sites, extremity examination to evaluate for DVT or thrombophlebitis, and pelvic examination to evaluate the vaginal cuff for cellulitis, hematoma, or abscess.

c. **Testing.** Laboratory and radiologic assessment should be tailored to the individual patient. Hematocrit, WBC with differential, and urinalysis and urine culture should be performed. Blood cultures seldom yield positive results but are helpful in patients with high fever or risk factors for endocarditis. Imaging studies may include chest and abdominal radiographs, IVP, ultrasonographs of pelvis and kidneys, contrast bowel studies, and CT scan.

3. **Sources**

a. The **urinary tract** is a common site of infection in surgical patients, with indwelling Foley catheters as the cause of contamination. Pyelonephritis is a rare complication. The treatment is hydration and antibiotic therapy tailored to the pathogen.

b. **Lungs.** Atelectasis secondary to hypoventilation is a potential cause of febrile morbidity and can predispose to the development of postoperative pneumonia, particularly in the elderly and debilitated patient. The best preventive measures are early ambulation, intensive respiratory therapy (incentive spirometry), and reversal of hypoventilation and atelectasis. Patients at risk of postoperative pneumonia have an American Society of Anesthesia status of 3 or higher, preoperative hospital stay of 2 days or longer, surgery lasting 3 hours or longer, surgery in the upper abdomen or thorax, nasogastric suction, postoperative intubation, or a history of smoking or obstructive lung disease. Treatment should be based on risk factors, fever, the presence of purulent sputum, positive sputum or blood culture results, leukocytosis, and physical and radiographic findings consistent with pneumonia. The antibiotics chosen to fight the pneumonia should be effective against both Gram-positive and Gram-negative organisms.

c. **Indwelling catheters.** Central lines (e.g., subclavian catheters or Hickman catheters) can be a source of febrile morbidity. Peripheral blood samples should be sent for culture. In the case of sepsis without obvious source, the central line should be changed to a new site. In the case of unexplained fever (but no sepsis), change of the catheter over a wire and culture of the intracutaneous segment is indicated. If the same organism (more than 15 colony-forming units) is isolated from the catheter and the peripheral blood cultures, the catheter site should be changed.

d. **Wound infection.** Table 23-6 defines the frequency of wound infection for different degrees of contamination. Wound infections occur late in the postoperative period, usually after the fourth postoperative day. Fever, erythema, induration, tenderness, and purulent drainage may be present. Management consists of opening, cleaning, and débriding the infected portion of the wound. Wet to dry dressing changes to keep the wound clean are indicated. Wound care has recently shifted away from an aggressive cleaning approach to one that emphasizes a clean but moist environment and minimizes the mechanical irritation caused by too-frequent dressing changes. Hydrogel applications play an important role. Clean granulating wounds can often be closed secondarily. Delayed primary closure should be used in high-risk cases. The wound is left open above the fascia, and sutures are placed through the skin and subcutaneous tissues 3 cm apart but are not tied. Wound care is begun immediately postprocedure and continued until the wound is granulating well. The sutures can then be tied to approximate the skin edges. Using this technique, the wound infection rate in high-risk patients may be decreased from 23% to 2%.

e. **Pelvic cellulitis.** Cuff cellulitis is most often self-limited and does not require treatment. Fever, leukocytosis, and pain localizing to the pelvis

TABLE 23-6. FREQUENCY OF WOUND INFECTION AS A FUNCTION OF DEGREE OF CONTAMINATION IN SURGERY

Degree of contamination	Examples	Wound infection (%)
Clean case (infection not present, aseptic technique, no hollow viscus entered)	Salpingo-oophorectomy	1–5
	Tubal ligation	
Clean-contaminated case (entry of genital, GI, urinary tract)	Abdominal hysterectomy	3–11
	Vaginal hysterectomy	
Contaminated case (major break in sterile technique, gross spillage from GI tract)	Accidental entry into colon	10–17
Dirty case (prior infection present)	Surgery for tubo-ovarian abscess	>27
	Ruptured appendicitis	

GI, gastrointestinal.

may accompany a severe cellulitis in which adjacent pelvic tissues are involved. Broad-spectrum antibiotic therapy covering Gram-positive, Gram-negative, and anaerobic organisms should be initiated. If an abscess is suspected at the cuff, drainage is indicated. Intra-abdominal abscesses are characterized by persistent fever and increased WBC. Radiologic confirmation with ultrasonography or CT scan is usually needed for diagnosis. Treatment involves surgical evacuation, drainage, and parenteral antibiotics. CT scan–guided drain placement has obviated the need for surgical exploration in many circumstances.

    f. **Necrotizing fasciitis** is a serious soft tissue infection. It is generally caused by group A streptococci but can also be caused by gas-forming anaerobic bacteria such as *Bacteroides fragilis, Clostridium perfringens,* and *Peptostreptococcus.* Clinically, the infection results in extensive soft tissue destruction, including necrosis of skin, subcutaneous tissue, and muscle. Extensive and aggressive surgical débridement until clean, viable, bleeding margins are obtained, together with broad-spectrum antibiotic therapy, is needed as quickly as possible. Treatment delay increases an already high mortality rate. This infection can occur after a simple skin abrasion becomes secondarily infected, but it is also encountered postoperatively.

B. **Deep venous thrombosis and pulmonary embolism**
1. **Incidence.** The incidence of venous thrombosis in gynecologic patients is 15% (range, 5–45%, depending on procedure and associated risk factors). Table 23-7 shows the risk categories for thromboembolism in gynecologic surgery.
2. **Prevention.** All large prospective trials have documented the necessity of initiating prophylactic techniques before surgery and continuing them for the duration of the postoperative stay. A number of methods of prevention are available.
    a. Low-dose heparin has been shown to reduce the risk of thrombi and pulmonary embolism (PE) in at-risk patients. Studies indicate that a regimen of 5000 U preoperatively and every 12 hours for 5 days postoperatively may be efficacious. These regimens do not significantly alter clotting time or increase operative or postoperative bleeding.
    b. Low-molecular-weight heparin has also been recognized as an effective preventive therapy. Dosing is as follows: enoxaparin 40 mg SC daily, dalteparin 2500–5000 U SC daily.

TABLE 23-7. RISK CATEGORIES OF THROMBOEMBOLISM IN GYNECOLOGIC SURGERY

Factor	Risk category		
	Low risk	Medium risk	High risk
Age	<40 yrs	≥40 yrs	≥40 yrs
Contributing factors			
Surgery	Uncomplicated or minor	Major abdominal or pelvic	Major, extensive malignant disease involved
			Prior radiation treatment
Weight	Normal	Moderately obese (75–90 kg or >20% above ideal weight)	Morbidly obese (≥115 kg or >30% above ideal weight)
Medical diseases	None	None	Previous venous thrombosis
			Varicose veins (severe)
			Diabetes (insulin dependent)
Thromboembolism			
Calf vein thrombosis	2%	10–30%	30–60%
Iliofemoral vein thrombosis	0.4%	2–8%	5–10%
Fatal pulmonary embolism	0.2%	0.1–0.5%	1%

Adapted from Rock JA, Thompson JD, eds. *Telinde's operative gynecology,* 8th ed. Philadelphia: Lippincott–Raven Publishers, 1997, with permission.

    c. Compression techniques have also been used for prophylaxis. The use of graduated compression stockings combined with early ambulation is thought to provide sufficient prophylaxis in the low-risk patient. Studies support the use of external intermittent pneumatic compression devices as a prophylactic measure in patients at moderate and high risk. Efficacy is similar to that of low-dose heparin.

    d. A combination of pharmacologic therapy and external pneumatic compression may be considered in patients at high risk, such as those with morbid obesity or malignancy.

  3. **Diagnosis of venous thromboembolism**

    a. **Deep venous thrombosis.** Unilateral lower-extremity swelling, pain, erythema, and palpable cord may be seen. Venography is the most definitive but also the most invasive method of diagnosis. Duplex Doppler ultrasonographic imaging combines Doppler ultrasonographic examination and real-time ultrasonography, which enables the radiologist to visualize the thrombus and measure blood flow through the vessels. Because of the high sensitivity (92%), high specificity (100%), and noninvasive nature of this technique, it has replaced venography as the gold standard for diagnosing DVT.

    b. **Pulmonary embolism.** The signs and symptoms of PE include anxiety, shortness of breath, tachypnea, chest pain, hypoxia, tachy-

TABLE 23-8. SIGNS AND SYMPTOMS OF PULMONARY EMBOLISM (PE)

Clinical finding	Frequency in patients with PE (%)
Tachypnea	89
Dyspnea	81
Pleuritic pain	72
Apprehension	59
Cough	54
Tachycardia	43
Hemoptysis	34
Temperature >37°C	34

cardia, and even mental status changes. Table 23-8 delineates their frequencies in patients with proven PE. Even when there is only a suspicion of PE, evaluation should be prompt and thorough: chest radiograph, ECG, and arterial blood gas assessment are the first line of diagnostic tests.

The chest radiograph helps distinguish between pneumonia and embolism. ECG findings are usually nonspecific except for tachycardia but helps rule out an ischemic cardiac event. Laboratory evaluation with arterial blood gas test results that show a low partial pressure of oxygen and a normal or slightly decreased partial pressure of carbon dioxide (indicating hyperventilation) are highly suggestive of PE.

Both radionucleotide imaging (i.e., ventilation-perfusion, or $\dot{V}/\dot{Q}$, scan) and spiral CT scan are useful imaging studies. $\dot{V}/\dot{Q}$ scans have a high sensitivity (negative scan results almost exclude PE) but a low specificity. Spiral CT scanning is rapid, easily accessible in most larger hospitals, and less prone to interference from other underlying pulmonary disease. Its sensitivity decreases for small, peripheral PEs, and its diagnostic quality is highly dependent on the familiarity of the radiologist with this test. In many institutions, the spiral CT has replaced the $\dot{V}/\dot{Q}$ scan as the first-line diagnostic imaging study. If all tests are normal and the suspicion of PE remains high, two options are available: in patients with weak cardiopulmonary reserve, pulmonary angiography may be performed. In ambulatory patients with good cardiopulmonary reserve, repeat spiral CT scans and $\dot{V}/\dot{Q}$ scans can be used to further rule in or rule out PE.

4. **Therapy.** Unfractionated heparin is accepted treatment for DVT and PE. The level of anticoagulation should be closely monitored. Oral therapy with Coumadin (a preparation of warfarin sodium) is started as early as possible, as the patient cannot be discharged until a therapeutic international normalized ratio value is reached. Anticoagulation should be continued for 6 months after the initial diagnosis (Table 23-9). Low-molecular-weight heparin formulations have several advantages over unfractionated heparin and may replace it in the treatment of venous thromboembolism. The half-lives of low-molecular-weight heparins are longer, the dose response is more predictable so that less monitoring is required, and they may cause less bleeding while producing an equivalent antithrombotic effect. Thrombolytic therapy is reasonable in some patients with extensive proximal vein thrombosis or PE. It has many contraindications and is rarely used in the immediate postoperative period. Placement of a vena caval filter may be necessary in patients with acute

TABLE 23-9. ANTICOAGULATION DOSAGES FOR HEPARIN THERAPY

Patient weight (kg)	Bolus dose (U)	Initial maintenance dose
40–50	3750	18 U/kg/hr
50–75	5000	18 U/kg/hr
>75	7500	18 U/kg/hr, not to exceed1600 U/hr initially

Activated partial thromboplastin time (aPTT) must be measured 6–8 hours after administration of the bolus. Target range for the aPTT ratio is 1.5–2.5; adjustments should be made accordingly.

thromboembolism and active bleeding or a high potential for bleeding, patients with a history of multiple venous thrombi who are on medical therapy, and patients with a history of heparin-induced thrombocytopenia. Bleeding that occurs after the use of heparin-related compounds can be reversed with protamine sulfate; Coumadin-related bleeding can be reversed with vitamin K or with plasma or factor IX concentrates.

C. **Ileus and bowel obstruction**

1. **Diagnosis.** Infection, peritonitis, electrolyte disturbances, extensive manipulation of the GI tract, and prolonged procedures increase the risk of ileus. The most common cause of obstruction of the small bowel after major gynecologic surgery is adhesions at the operative site, which occur in 1% to 2% of cases. Risk factors for both ileus and obstruction include infection, malignancy, and a history of radiation therapy. Nausea, vomiting, and distension may be present with both. Abdominal pain from obstruction is characterized by progressively more severe abdominal cramps. Absent and hypoactive bowel sounds are more likely to occur with ileus; borborygmi, rushes, and high-pitched tinkles are more characteristic of postoperative obstruction. Abdominal radiographs show distended loops of large and small bowel, with gas present in the colon in the setting of ileus. Single or multiple loops of distended bowel (most often the small bowel) with air-fluid levels are seen in postoperative obstruction.

2. **Treatment.** Ileus is treated with bowel rest, administration of intravenous fluids, and nasogastric suction if indicated. Lack of improvement within 48–72 hours requires a search for other causes of ileus, such as ureteral injury, pelvic infection, unrecognized GI tract injury, or persistent fluid and electrolyte abnormalities. In most cases of obstruction, the obstruction is partial and will respond to conservative management with bowel rest and nasogastric decompression. Increasing abdominal pain, progressive distension, fever, leukocytosis, or acidosis should be evaluated with the potential need for surgical exploration and treatment in mind. Parenteral nutrition should also be considered in patients with prolonged GI compromise.

D. **Diarrhea** is not common after abdominal and pelvic surgery, as the GI tract returns to its normal function and motility. Prolonged or multiple episodes, however, may represent a pathologic process, such as impending small bowel obstruction, colonic obstruction, or pseudomembranous colitis. *Clostridium difficile*–associated colitis may result from exposure to any antibiotics; stool testing can confirm clinical suspicions. Extended oral metronidazole therapy is needed for adequate treatment.

E. **Genitourinary fistulas.** In the United States, most genitourinary fistulas are the result of pelvic surgery, with the majority occurring after an abdominal hysterectomy for benign conditions. In contrast, in the developing world most fistulas are due to obstetric trauma secondary to absent or poor obstetrical care. The most simple initial test for a genitourinary fistula is the tampon test. A tampon or cotton ball is inserted completely into the vagina. The bladder is then filled with methylene blue through a Foley catheter. The appearance of dye at the urethral end of the tampon suggests urethral urinary loss. Dye at the vaginal apex end of the tampon suggests a vesicovaginal fistula. A wet but undyed tampon is suggestive of a ureteralvaginal fistula. Further workup may include cystoscopy, voiding cystourethrogram, and IVP.

IV. Routine postoperative care

A. **Diet.** Most randomized studies indicate that early feeding is both appropriate and beneficial.

B. **Fluids.** For healthy, young patients, 125 mL/hour of 5% dextrose in lactated Ringer's solution, 5% dextrose in normal saline, or 5% dextrose in half-normal saline (with 20 mEq potassium chloride) while NPO is sufficient for fluid maintenance. This quantity needs to be adjusted according to intraoperative fluid loss, third space loss, and presence of fever.

C. **Pain control.** Patient-controlled analgesia with intravenous or intrathecal opiates provides the best pain control postoperatively after open abdominal surgery. Protocols need to be strictly observed to prevent opiate overdose and respiratory arrest. Administration of 30 mg of ketorolac tromethamine (Toradol) every 6 hours for 24–48 hours postoperatively may improve paincontrol and decrease the opiate doses. Intramuscular injection of opiates can provide sufficient pain control as well. The main goal of pain control is to allow the patient to move around as soon as possible. As soon as the patient tolerates oral intake, oral opiates should be prescribed.

24. INFECTIONS OF THE GENITAL TRACT

Carolyn J. Alexander and Jeffrey Smith

I. **Infections of the lower genital tract.** Symptoms caused by infections of the lower genital tract are among the most common presenting complaints of gynecologic patients.

A. **Vulvar infections.** Normal vulva is composed of the following: skin with stratified squamous epithelium containing sebaceous, sweat, and apocrine glands, and underlying subcutaneous tissue, including Bartholin's glands. Vulvar itching or burning accounts for approximately 10% of gynecologic visits.

1. **Condyloma acuminatum** (genital or venereal warts) is a lesion of the vulva, vagina, or cervix caused by the human papillomavirus (HPV), which infects and transforms epithelial cells. HPV infection is the most common sexually transmitted disease and is associated with cervical, vaginal, and vulvar intraepithelial lesions, as well as squamous cell carcinoma and adenocarcinoma. The subtypes that cause exophytic condylomata (HPV types 6 or 11) are usually not associated with the development of carcinoma (HPV types 16, 18, 31, 33, and 35). More than 20 types of HPV can infect the genital tract.

   a. Peak **incidence** is among 15- to 25-year-olds. Pregnant, immunosuppressed, and diabetic patients are at increased risk.

   b. **Signs and symptoms** include soft, pedunculated lesions on any mucosal or dermal surfaces that range in size and formation. Lesions are usually asymptomatic unless they are traumatized or secondarily infected, which causes bleeding, pain, or both.

   c. **Diagnosis** is made primarily by gross inspection. Colposcopic examination may aid in identification of cervical or vaginal lesions. Histologic recognition of HPV changes in biopsy specimens or Pap smears can confirm the diagnosis. DNA typing may also be performed. The most important infection that must be differentiated from genital warts is the condyloma lata of secondary syphilis.

   d. **Treatment** consists of removing lesions surgically or through topical applications if they are symptomatic or if desired for cosmesis. There is no therapy for complete eradication of the virus (Table 24-1).

2. **Molluscum contagiosum** is a benign infection of the skin by poxvirus and is spread by sexual or nonsexual contact and autoinoculation. The incubation period ranges from several weeks to months. The frequency of this disease is increasing in the United States and United Kingdom.

   a. **Signs and symptoms** include the appearance of dome-shaped papules with central umbilication ranging from 1 to 5 mm in diameter. Multiple lesions may arise but generally fewer than 20. The lesions are usually asymptomatic but occasionally are pruritic. They are usually self-limited and may last for 6–9 months.

   b. **Diagnosis** is made by gross inspection or microscopic examination of white, waxy material expressed from a nodule. Wright or Giemsa staining for intracytoplasmic molluscum bodies confirms diagnosis.

   c. **Treatment** consists of evacuation of the white material, excision of the nodule with a dermal curette, and treatment of the base with ferric subsulfate (Monsel's solution) or 85% trichloroacetic acid. Cryotherapy with liquid nitrogen can also be used. Sexual partners should be examined and treated as well.

3. **Parasites**

   a. **Pediculosis pubis** (due to the crab louse) is among the most contagious sexually transmitted diseases, with approximately 3 million

TABLE 24-1. TREATMENT OPTIONS FOR GENITAL WARTS, INCLUDING CLEARANCE AND RECURRENCE RATES AND USAGE DURING PREGNANCY

Therapy	Application	Clearance rate (%)	Recurrence rate (%)	Use in pregnancy
Imiquimod 5% cream	Apply three times a week at bedtime for up to 16 wks. Wash area 6–10 hrs after application.	40–77	13	Permitted, class B
Podophyllotoxin 0.5% solution or gel	Apply bid for 3 days, no treatment for 4 days, repeat cycle 4–6 times.	68–88	16–34	Contraindicated
Podophyllin resin in a 10–25% concentration in benzoin	—	38–79	21–65	Contraindicated
Surgical excision	—	89–93	19–22	Not recommended
Electrodesiccation	—	94	25	Not recommended
CO_2 laser excision	—	72–97	6–49	Not recommended
Cryotherapy	—	70–96	25–39	Not recommended
Interferons	Inject at the edge of and beneath the wart with a 26- to 32-gauge needle.	36–53	21–25	Not recommended
Topical trichloroacetic acid (50–85% solution)	Apply small amount q1–2wks until wart sloughs off. Typical course is 6 treatments.	81	36	Permitted

cases treated in the United States each year. It is transmitted through sexual or nonsexual contact, including fomites such as towels or bedsheets. It is usually restricted to the pubic, perineal, and perianal areas but may infect eyelids and other body parts. The parasite deposits eggs at the base of the hair follicle. The adult feeds on human blood and moves relatively slowly (10 cm/day). The incubation period is 30 days.

   (1) **Symptoms** of infection include intense itching in the pubic area due to an allergic sensitization, accompanied by maculopapular lesions on the vulva. Occurrence of a large number of bites over a short period of time may lead to systemic manifestations such as mild fever, malaise, or irritability.

   (2) **Diagnosis** is made by gross visualization of lice, larvae, or nits in the pubic hair or microscopic identification of crab-like lice under oil.

  b. **Scabies** (due to the "itch mite") is transmitted via close contact (sexual or nonsexual) and may infect any part of the body, especially flexural surfaces of the elbows, wrists, finger webs, axillae, genitals, and buttocks. The adult female burrows beneath the skin, lays eggs, and travels quickly across the skin.

   (1) **Symptoms** of infection include an insidious onset of severe but intermittent itching that may worsen at night. It may present as papules, vesicles, or burrows.

   (2) **Diagnosis** is made by microscopic examination of skin scrapings under oil.

  c. **Treatment** for pediculosis pubis and scabies requires an agent that kills adult organisms and eggs.

   (1) Permethrin (Nix) cream
      (a) Pediculosis pubis. Apply permethrin 1% crème rinse to affected areas, wash off after 10 minutes, and comb the infested areas with a fine-toothed comb.
      (b) Scabies. Apply permethrin 5% cream to all areas of the body from the neck down and wash off after 8–14 hours.
      (c) Infants, young children, and pregnant or lactating women may be treated with permethrin.

   (2) Gamma-benzene hexachloride 1% or lindane (Tradename Kwell) lotion, cream, or shampoo
      (a) Pediculosis pubis. Apply for 4 minutes to affected area then thoroughly wash off.
      (b) Scabies. In adults apply 30–60 mL of lotion thinly over the entire body surface, paying particular attention to the hands and feet. Leave the lotion on for 8–12 hours. Pruritus may persist for several days and may be treated with antihistamines. Lindane resistance has been reported.
      (c) Toxic effects of lindane include seizures and aplastic anemia, and it is not recommended for use in pregnant or lactating women, children younger than 2 years, or patients with extensive dermatitis.

   (3) Clothes and linens should be laundered in hot water and heat dried or removed from body contact for at least 72 hours. Sexual partners should be treated.

B. **Genital ulcers**
  1. **Genital herpes** is a recurrent, sexually transmitted infection by the herpes simplex virus (HSV) (80% of cases are due to type II) that results in genital ulcers. Infection with genital herpes has reached epidemic proportions, with an incidence in the United States of 500,000 to 2 million cases per year. The prevalence is 10 million to 30 million cases per year. The incubation period is 3–7 days.

a. **Signs and symptoms**

(1) **Primary infection** may result in systemic as well as local manifestations. The patient may experience a virus-like syndrome with malaise and fever, then paresthesias of the vulva that are followed by vesicle formation. These are often multiple, resulting in shallow, painful ulcers that may coalesce. Multiple crops of vesicles and ulcers can occur in a 2–6 week period. The symptoms last for approximately 14 days, peaking at approximately day 7. The outbreak is self-limited, and lesions heal without scar formation. Viral shedding can continue for 2–3 weeks after the appearance of lesions. Cervical lesions are common in true primary infections.

(2) **Recurrent herpetic outbreaks** are usually shorter in duration (averaging 7 days), with less severe symptoms. They are often preceded by a prodrome of itching or burning in the affected area. Systemic symptoms are usually absent. Fifty percent of infected women experience their first recurrence within 6 months and have an average of 4 recurrences in the first year. Thereafter, the rate of recurrence is quite variable. Latent herpes virus resides in the dorsal root ganglia of S2, S3, and S4. Its reactivation can be triggered by an immunocompromised state such as pregnancy.

b. **Complications** include herpes encephalitis (rare) and infection of the urinary tract, which results in retention or severe pain or both.

c. **Diagnosis** is usually by inspection alone; however, if a definitive diagnosis is needed, a viral culture can be obtained. The vesicle should be opened, then vigorously swabbed. Sensitivity of a viral culture is approximately 90%. Immunologic or cytologic tests are not as sensitive. Polymerase chain reaction (PCR) has potential use as a rapid and sensitive diagnostic technique but needs further testing.

d. **Treatment** (Table 24-2)

(1) Goals of treatment are to shorten the clinical course, decrease transmission, and prevent complications and recurrence.

(2) The virus cannot be completely eradicated.

(3) An effective HSV vaccine is not yet available.

e. **Counseling.** Patients should be advised to remain abstinent from the onset of prodromal symptoms until complete reepithelialization of lesions. HSV infection may facilitate human immunodeficiency virus (HIV) infection. There is no probable association with the development of squamous intraepithelial lesions.

f. **During pregnancy,** women with primary HSV should be treated with antiviral therapy. Cesarean delivery is recommended for women with active lesions or prodromal symptoms of HSV at delivery. Refer to Chap. 40, Benign Vulvar Lesions, for further details.

2. **Syphilis** is a chronic systemic disease caused by *Treponema pallidum* that has a multitude of clinical manifestations. The disease is contagious during the primary and secondary stages and through the first year of the latent stage. The organism can penetrate skin or mucous membranes, and the incubation period is 10–90 days.

a. **Primary syphilis.** Signs and symptoms include a hard, painless chancre that is usually solitary and that may appear on the vulva, vagina, or cervix. Commonly, lesions occur on the cervix or in the vagina and go unrecognized. Extragenital lesions may occur. Nontender inguinal lymphadenopathy frequently is present. Even without treatment, the primary chancre resolves within 2–6 weeks.

b. **Secondary syphilis** is a systemic disease that occurs 6 weeks to 6 months after the primary infection through hematogenous spread of the organism. Patients in this stage present with skin and mucous

TABLE 24-2. TREATMENT OPTIONS FOR THE VARIOUS STAGES OF GENITAL HERPES

Stage	Treatment	Duration
Severe cases: disseminated infection, meningitis, encephalitis, or immuno-suppressed status	Acyclovir, 5–10 mg/kg IV q8h	5–7 days
Primary outbreaks in outpatients	Acyclovir, 400 mg PO tid	7–10 days
	Acyclovir, 200 mg PO 5×/day	
	Famciclovir, 250 mg PO tid	
	Valacyclovir hydrochloride, 1 g PO bid	
	Acyclovir cream, 3–4×/day to affected area (less effective than PO)	
Episodic recurrences	Acyclovir, 400 mg PO tid	5 days
	Acyclovir, 200 mg PO 5×/day	
	Acyclovir, 800 mg PO bid	
	Famciclovir, 125 mg PO bid	
	Valacyclovir hydrochloride, 500 mg PO bid	
Daily suppressive therapy	Acyclovir, 400 mg PO bid	prn
	Famciclovir, 250 mg PO bid	
	Valacyclovir hydrochloride, 500 mg PO qd	
	Valacyclovir hydrochloride, 1 g PO qd	

membrane lesions. Signs and symptoms are generalized maculopapular rash involving the palms and soles, mucous patches, condyloma latum (large, raised gray-white lesions), and generalized lymphadenopathy. These symptoms spontaneously clear in 2–6 weeks.

c. **Latent-stage syphilis** follows untreated secondary stage disease and can last 2–20 years. Signs and symptoms of the early latent phase (less than 1 year) include exacerbations of secondary syphilis in which the mucocutaneous lesions are infectious. The late latent phase (longer than 1 year) is not infectious by sexual transmission, but the spirochete may infect the fetus transplacentally.

d. **Tertiary syphilis** develops in up to one-third of untreated or inadequately treated patients. Signs and symptoms include involvement of the cardiovascular system (e.g., endarteritis, aortic aneurysms, and aortic insufficiency) and involvement of the CNS and musculoskeletal system, which results in varied disorders. Gummata of skin and bones occur in late tertiary syphilis. The CNS manifestations may include generalized paresis, tabes dorsalis, changes in mental status, optic atrophy, and Argyll Robertson pupil, which is pathognomonic of tertiary syphilis. Neurosyphilis must be ruled out in those with more than 1 year's duration of disease. Cerebrospinal fluid should be tested for fluorescent treponemal antibody absorption (FTA-ABS) reactivity.

e. **Diagnosis** is made definitively by dark-field examinations and direct fluorescent antibody tests of lesion exudate or tissue. After screening with nonspecific serologic tests such as the Venereal Disease Research Laboratory (VDRL) and rapid plasma reagin (RPR) tests, clinicians can then use specific tests to confirm the diagnosis. The specific serologic tests are FTA-ABS and microhemagglutination assay for antibody to *T. pallidum.* False-positive results may be seen in 1% of the nonspecific serologic tests. Biologic false-positive results, usually of low titers, may be caused by pregnancy, autoimmune disorders, chronic active hepatitis, intravenous drug use, febrile illness, and immunization. Serologic tests become positive 4–6 weeks after exposure, usually 1–2 weeks after appearance of the primary chancres.

  f. **Treatment** options are listed in Table 24-3.

  g. **Follow-up.** After treatment of early syphilis, VDRL or RPR titers should be obtained every 3 months for 1 year (all tests should be conducted by the same laboratory). Titers should decrease by fourfold in 1 year. If not, retreatment is required. If the patient has been infected for longer than 1 year, titers should be followed for 2 years. The specific FTA-ABS test remains positive indefinitely.

 3. **Other ulcerative lesions.** Granuloma inguinale, lymphogranuloma venereum, and chancroid are other infections that cause genital ulcers. They are rare in the United States but should be considered in any patient with ulcers that do not appear to be related to syphilis or HSV.

C. **Vaginitis** is characterized by pruritus, discharge, odor, dyspareunia, or dysuria. Odor is one of the most common complaints encountered by the gynecologist in office practice.

   The vagina is normally colonized by a number of organisms, including *Lactobacillus acidophilus,* diphtheroids, *Candida,* and other flora. Its physiologic pH is approximately 4.0, which inhibits overgrowth of pathogenic bacteria. There is also a physiologic discharge composed of bacterial flora, water, electrolytes, and vaginal and cervical epithelium. It is typically white, floccular, odorless, and seen in dependent areas of the vagina (Table 24-4).

   Diagnosis of vaginitis usually requires microscopic examination of vaginal discharge. There are three major types, as follows.

 1. **Bacterial vaginosis** (BV) is the most common cause of vaginitis. There is no single infectious agent, rather a shift in the composition of normal vaginal flora with an up to tenfold increase in anaerobic bacteria, including *Prevotella* species, *Gardnerella vaginalis,* and *Mobiluncus* species, and a decrease in the concentration of *Lactobacilli* species. It is not considered to be sexually transmitted.

  a. **Signs and symptoms.** The characteristic discharge of bacterial vaginosis is thin, homogeneous, and gray-white and has a fishy odor. The discharge can be copious and is adherent to vaginal walls on speculum examination. Vulvar or vaginal pruritus or irritation is rare.

  b. **Diagnosis** is made by the following methods.

   (1) Microscopic identification of clue cells (constituting more than 20%) on a wet smear. Clue cells are vaginal epithelial cells with clusters of bacteria adhering to the cell membrane, which creates a stippled appearance. Few inflammatory cells or lactobacilli should be noted.

   (2) The pH of the discharge should be equal to or greater than 4.5.

   (3) Positive "whiff" test, in which an amine-like (or fishy) odor is released with the addition of KOH solution (10% to 20%) to the discharge.

   (4) Erythema of the vagina is rare.

   (5) Pap smear results sometimes suggests a shift in vaginal flora. The Pap smear, however, is not a useful diagnostic tool for vaginitis.

  c. **Treatment.** Treatment regimens recommended by the Centers for Disease Control and Prevention are shown in Table 24-5.

TABLE 24-3. CENTERS FOR DISEASE CONTROL AND PREVENTION RECOMMENDED TREATMENT FOR SYPHILIS

Phase	Medication	Dosage	Duration
First- and second-degree syphilis	Benzathine penicillin G	2.4 million U IM	1 dose
Penicillin allergy (nonpregnancy)	Doxycycline OR	100 mg PO bid	2 wks
	Tetracycline	500 mg PO qid	—
Early latent syphilis (<1 yr)	Benzathine penicillin G	2.4 million U IM	1 dose
Penicillin allergy (nonpregnancy)	Doxycycline OR	100 mg PO bid	2 wks
	Tetracycline	500 mg PO qid	—
Late latent syphilis (>1 yr)	Benzathine penicillin G	2.4 million U IM (7.2 million U total)	q wk for total of 3 wks
Penicillin allergy (nonpregnancy)	Doxycycline OR	100 mg PO bid	4 wks
	Tetracycline	500 mg PO qid	4 wks
Late syphilis without neurosyphilis	Benzathine penicillin G	2.4 million U IM (7.2 million U total)	q wk for total of 3 wks
Penicillin allergy (nonpregnancy)	Doxycycline OR	100 mg PO bid	4 wks
	Tetracycline	500 mg PO qid	4 wks
Neurosyphilis	Aqueous crystalline penicillin G	3–4 million U IV q4h (18–24 million U total)	10–14 days
Alternate regimen (if compliance assured)	Procaine penicillin PLUS	2.4 million U IM qd	10–14 days
	Probenecid	500 mg PO qid	—
Syphilis during pregnancy	Penicillin	Regimen appropriate for the pregnant woman's stage of syphilis	—
Penicillin allergy (pregnancy)	Penicillin after desensitization	—	1 dose
Primary and secondary syphilis, HIV⁺ patient	Benzathine penicillin	2.4 million U IM	1 dose
Latent syphilis (normal cerebrospinal fluid examination), HIV⁺ patient	Benzathine penicillin G	2.4 million U IM (7.2 million U total)	q wk for total of 3 wks
Penicillin allergy (HIV⁺ patient)	Penicillin after desensitization	—	—

HIV⁺, positive for human immunodeficiency virus infection.

TABLE 24-4. DISTINGUISHING CHARACTERISTICS OF VAGINITIS

	Bacterial vaginosis	*Trichomonas* vaginitis	Candidal vaginitis
Vaginal pH	≥ 4.5	5.0–7.0	—
Type of discharge	Thin, white, adherent	Thin, frothy, white, gray, yellow	Thick, white, curd-like
Wet smear	Clue cells, no WBCs	Trichomonads, WBCs	Hyphae and buds, WBCs

WBCs, white blood cells.

    d. **Follow-up.** Recurrence of bacterial vaginosis is not unusual. A test of cure should be performed in 1 month for high-risk pregnant women. No long-term maintenance regimen is recommended.

  2. ***Trichomonas* infection** is a sexually transmitted infection by the protozoon *Trichomonas vaginalis*. It accounts for approximately 25% of infectious vaginitis. *Trichomonas* is a hardy organism, able to survive on wet towels and other surfaces, and thus can be nonsexually transmitted. Its incubation period ranges from 4 to 28 days.

    a. **Signs and symptoms** may vary greatly. The classic discharge is frothy, thin, malodorous, and copious. It may be gray, white, or yellow-green. There may be erythema or edema of the vulva and vagina. The cervix may also appear erythematous and friable.

    b. **Diagnosis**

      (1) A wet smear preparation reveals the unicellular fusiform protozoon, which is slightly larger than a WBC. It is flagellated, and motion can be observed in the specimen. Many inflammatory cells are usually present.

      (2) The vaginal discharge should have a pH of 5.0–7.0.

TABLE 24-5. CENTERS FOR DISEASE CONTROL AND PREVENTION RECOMMENDED TREATMENT FOR BACTERIAL VAGINOSIS

Medication	Dosage	Duration	Use in pregnancy
Metronidazole (Flagyl)	500 mg PO bid	7 days	Second and third trimesters
Clindamycin phosphate cream 2%	1 full applicator (5 g) intravaginally qhs	7 days	First trimester
Metronidazole (MetroGel) gel 0.75%	1 full applicator (5 g) intravaginally qhs	7 days	Not recommended Does not reduce preterm delivery rate
Metronidazole	2 g PO	7 days	Second and third trimesters
Clindamycin hydrochloride	300 mg PO bid	7 days	First trimester
Metronidazole	250 mg PO tid	7 days	Second and third trimesters Regimen minimizes exposure to the fetus but may result in poorer compliance

(3) In asymptomatic patients, the infection may first be recognized with detection of *Trichomonas* on a Pap smear specimen.

   c. **Treatment** consists of metronidazole 2 g by mouth (PO) (one dose) or metronidazole 500 mg PO twice daily (bid) for 7 days. The patient's sexual partners should be treated as well. This treatment should be avoided during the first trimester of pregnancy according to the American College of Obstetricians and Gynecologists. Patients who are infected with HIV should receive the same treatment regimen as earlier.

   d. **Follow-up** is unnecessary for asymptomatic women. Most organisms are susceptible to metronidazole, but if treatment failure occurs, a single dose of 2 g of metronidazole once a day for 3–5 days is recommended. Sexual partners must be treated and patients should be instructed to avoid intercourse until treatment is completed and symptoms have resolved.

3. **Candidal vaginitis** is not a sexually transmitted infection. *Candida* is a normal vaginal inhabitant in up to 25% of women and is found in the rectum and oral cavity in an even greater percentage. *Candida albicans* is the pathogen in 80–95% of cases of vulvovaginal candidiasis, with *Candida glabrata* and *Candida tropicalis* accounting for the remainder. Risk factors for infection include immunosuppression, especially HIV infection, diabetes mellitus, hormonal changes (e.g., pregnancy), broad-spectrum antibiotic therapy, and obesity.

   a. **Signs and symptoms.** The severity of symptoms does not correlate with the number of organisms. The predominant symptom is pruritus, which is often accompanied by vaginal irritation, dysuria, or both. The classic vaginal discharge is white, curd-like, and without an odor. Speculum examination often reveals erythema of the vulva and vaginal walls, sometimes with adherent plaques.

   b. **Diagnosis** is made when a KOH preparation of the vaginal discharge reveals hyphae and buds (a 10% to 20% solution of KOH lyses red and white blood cells, which facilitates identification of the fungus). The clinician may need to view many fields to find the pathogen. A negative finding on KOH preparation does not necessarily rule out the infection. The patient can be treated based on the clinical picture. A specimen can be obtained for culture, with results made available within 24–72 hours.

   c. **Treatment.** Symptomatic patients, including pregnant women, should be treated.

     (1) For intravaginal agents, refer to Table 24-6.

     (2) An oral agent (not recommended during pregnancy) is fluconazole (Diflucan) 150 mg PO (one dose).

     (3) In addition, clinicians can recommend consumption of yogurt, which may help replenish lactobacilli to reestablish the normal vaginal flora.

   d. **Follow-up.** If symptoms persist or recur, patients should return for follow-up. An alternative regimen that has been effective is the use of the oral azole agents; however, the toxicity of these systemic agents must be considered.

   e. **Treatment of male partners** is usually not necessary unless the partner has symptoms of yeast balanitis or is uncircumcised.

D. **Cervicitis** is characterized by an inflammation of the mucosa and submucosa of the cervix. Histologically, one may see infiltration by acute inflammatory cells as well as occasional necrosis of the epithelial cells. The primary pathogens of mucopurulent cervicitis are *Chlamydia trachomatis* and *Neisseria gonorrhoeae*, both of which are transmitted sexually. Mucopurulent cervicitis can be diagnosed by gross inspection. Gram stain testing can be used to confirm the diagnosis.

TABLE 24-6. CENTERS FOR DISEASE CONTROL AND PREVENTION RECOMMENDED TREATMENT FOR YEAST INFECTIONS

Intravaginal medication	Dosage	Duration	Use in pregnancy
Butoconazole nitrate 2% cream	1 applicator (5 g) qhs	3 days	Second and third trimesters
Clotrimazole 1% cream	1 applicator (5 g) qhs	7–14 days	
Clotrimazole	100 mg vaginal tablet	7 days	
Clotrimazole	10 mg vaginal tablet, 2 tablets	3 days	
Clotrimazole	500 mg vaginal tablet	1 dose	
Miconazole nitrate 2% cream	1 applicator (5 g) qhs	7 days	
Miconazole nitrate	200 mg vaginal suppository	3 days	
Miconazole nitrate	100 mg vaginal suppository	7 days	
Nystatin	100,000 U vaginal tablet	7 days	
Tioconazole 6.5% ointment	1 applicator (5 g) qhs	1 dose	
Terconazole 0.4% cream	1 applicator (5 g) qhs	7 days	
Terconazole 0.8% cream	1 applicator (5 g) qhs	3 days	
Terconazole	80 mg vaginal suppository	3 days	

Clinicians must remind patients that these creams and suppositories are oil-based and may weaken latex condoms and diaphragms.

1. ***C. trachomatis*** is the most common sexually transmitted organism in the United States.
   a. **Demographics.** There are approximately 4 million new infections per year. The prevalence of chlamydial cervicitis is 3–5% but may be as high as 15–30% in some populations. Twenty percent to 40% of sexually active women have positive findings on microimmunofluorescent *Chlamydia* antibody titer. Risk factors include age younger than 24 years, low socioeconomic status, multiple sex partners, and unmarried status.
   b. **Microbiology.** *C. trachomatis* is an obligatory intracellular organism that preferentially infects the squamocolumnar cells and thus the transition zone of the cervix.
   c. **Signs and symptoms.** Chlamydial infection is asymptomatic in 30–50% of cases and may persist for several years. Patients with cervicitis may complain of vaginal discharge or spotting or postcoital bleeding. On examination, the cervix may appear eroded and friable. A yellow-green mucopurulent discharge may be present. Gram staining should reveal more than ten polymorphonuclear leukocytes per oil immersion field.
   d. **Diagnosis** is by a culture, the direct fluorescent monoclonal antibody staining of chlamydial elementary bodies test, enzyme-linked immunosorbent assay for detection of chlamydial antigen in specimens, a DNA probe assay, or PCR testing. A culture specimen should be obtained by swabbing the endocervix. The synthetic swab should be rotated for 15–20 seconds to ensure that epithelial cells are obtained. Sensitivity is approximately 75%.

**TABLE 24-7. CENTERS FOR DISEASE CONTROL AND PREVENTION TREATMENT
RECOMMENDATIONS FOR *CHLAMYDIA TRACHOMATIS***

Medication	Dosage	Duration	Use in pregnancy
Azithromycin	1 g PO	1 dose	Recommended
Doxycycline	100 mg PO bid	7 days	—
Erythromycin base	500 mg PO qid	7 days	—
Erythromycin ethylsuccinate	800 mg qid	7 days	—
Ofloxacin	300 mg PO bid	7 days	Contraindicated

A rapid slide test (monoclonal antibody test) provides quicker, cheaper results. This test has a sensitivity of 86–93% and a specificity of 93–99%.

DNA probe tests use nucleic acid hybridization to identify *C. trachomatis* DNA directly from swab specimens. This test has a sensitivity of 86.1% and a specificity of 99.2%.

PCR testing is a simple, accurate, and reliable method for identifying chlamydial infections even in low-prevalence, asymptomatic patients and has a sensitivity of 97% and a specificity of 99.7%.

  e. Table 24-7 lists **treatment** recommendations of the Centers for Disease Control and Prevention for *C. trachomatis* infection.

   (1) Treatment for coinfection with gonorrhea is recommended using azithromycin dihydrate 2 g PO (one dose). Sexual partners should be referred to a clinic for treatment.

   (2) A test of cure is necessary only in pregnant patients or if symptoms persist.

 2. **Gonorrhea**

  a. **Demographics.** In the United States, each year 600,000 new infections with *N. gonorrhoeae* occur. The age group most affected is 15- to 19-year-olds, who constitute 80% of infected individuals. Prevalence ranges from 1–2% to as high as 25% in some populations. Risk factors are essentially the same as those for *Chlamydia* cervicitis. Although the incidence of gonorrhea in the total population is higher in men by a ratio of 1.5 to 1, the risk of transmission from man to woman is 50–90% in a single sexual encounter, whereas the risk of transmission from woman to man is 20–25%.

  b. **Microbiology.** *N. gonorrhoeae* is a Gram-negative diplococcus that infects columnar or pseudostratified epithelium; thus, the urogenital tract is a common site of infection. Pharyngeal and disseminated gonorrhea are other manifestations of this infection. The incubation period is 3–5 days.

  c. **Signs and symptoms.** As with chlamydial infections, patients are often asymptomatic; however, they may present with vaginal discharge, dysuria, or abnormal uterine bleeding. The most common infected site is the endocervix.

  d. **Diagnosis.** Culture with selective medium is the best test for gonorrhea. A sterile cotton swab is inserted into the endocervical canal for 15–30 seconds; the specimen is then plated on Thayer-Martin medium containing vancomycin, colistin sulfate, and nystatin, which will inhibit growth of contaminants. A Gram stain preparation demonstrating intracellular diplococci is diagnostic, but sensitivity is only approximately 60%. DNA probes are also available.

TABLE 24-8. CENTERS FOR DISEASE CONTROL AND PREVENTION TREATMENT RECOMMENDATIONS FOR *NEISSERIA GONORRHOEAE*

Medication	Dosage	Duration	Use in pregnancy
Cefixime	400 mg PO	1 dose	—
Ceftriaxone sodium	125 mg IM	1 dose	Recommended
Ciprofloxacin	500 mg PO	1 dose	Contraindicated
Ofloxacin PLUS	400 mg PO	1 dose	—
Azithromycin	1 g PO	1 dose	—
Doxycycline	100 mg PO bid	7 days	—

      e. Treatment options are listed in Table 24-8. Because coinfection with *Chlamydia* is common, azithromycin, 2 g PO (one dose), is recommended to treat both, and sexual partners should be referred for treatment.

  E. **Cystitis and urethritis.** Infections of the lower urinary tract are the most common bacterial infections in adult women and the most common medical complication of pregnancy (refer to Chap. 4 for more details). A woman's lifetime risk of experiencing one urinary tract infection is 20%. Women are more susceptible than men because of the shorter urethral tract and the colonization of distal urethra by bacteria from the vulvar vestibule. These infections are characterized by dysuria, urinary frequency, and urinary urgency and possible suprapubic tenderness. Findings include more than 10^5 organisms per milliliter of urine. The most common pathogens are *Escherichia coli* and *Staphylococcus saprophyticus*.

    1. **Diagnosis.** A clean-catch, midstream urine specimen should be obtained for microscopic examination, culture, and sensitivity testing (the specimen should be cultured or refrigerated within 2 hours of collection). The gold standard for diagnosis is a finding of more than 10^5 organisms per milliliter; however, as few as 10^5 organisms per milliliter can confirm cystitis. A pelvic examination should be performed to rule out vulvovaginitis, cervicitis, and other causes.

    2. **Lower urinary tract infection** should be treated with the following 3-day regimens:
      a. Trimethoprim, 100 mg every 12 hours, or
      b. Trimethoprim plus sulfamethoxazole (Bactrim), 160/800 mg every 12 hours, or
      c. Nitrofurantoin, 100 mg every 12 hours

    3. **Treatment.** The American College of Obstetricians and Gynecologists recommends that the use of quinolones, such as ciprofloxacin, 250 mg PO bid for 7–10 days, be reserved for strains resistant to the regimens listed earlier.

    4. **Prevention.** For women with recurrent postcoital urinary tract infections, prophylactic antibiotic therapy and voiding immediately after intercourse may be recommended. Postmenopausal women not receiving estrogen replacement therapy are at increased risk for urethritis and cystitis. Estrogen replacement may prevent recurrent infection. Drinking cranberry juice has been shown to decrease the incidence of recurrent urinary tract infections.

II. **Infections of the upper genital tract**
  A. **Pelvic inflammatory disease (PID)** is an infection of the upper genital tract. The disease process may include the endometrium, fallopian tubes, ovaries, myometrium, parametria, and pelvic peritoneum. It is the most significant and one of the most common complications of sexually transmitted infection.

1. **Demographics.** Approximately 1 million patients are treated for PID annually, of whom 250,000–300,000 are hospitalized and 150,000 undergo a surgical procedure for a complication of PID. PID is the most common serious infection of women aged 16–25 years.

   There has been a rise in the incidence of PID in the past two to three decades resulting from a number of factors, including more liberal social mores, increasing incidences of sexually transmitted pathogens such as *C. trachomatis*, and more widespread use of nonbarrier contraceptive methods such as the intrauterine device (IUD).

   Approximately 15% of cases of PID occur after procedures such as endometrial biopsy, curettage, hysteroscopy, and IUD insertion. Eighty-five percent of cases occur as spontaneous infections in women of reproductive age who are sexually active.

2. **Pathophysiology and microbiology.** Like endometritis, PID is caused by the spread of infection via the cervix. Although PID is associated with sexually transmitted infections of the lower tract, it is a polymicrobial process.

   One theory of the pathophysiology is that a sexually transmitted organism such as *N. gonorrhoeae* or *C. trachomatis* initiates an acute inflammatory process that causes tissue damage and thereby allows access by other organisms from the vagina or cervix to the upper genital tract. These organisms then can become predominant, which leads to clinical infection.

   Menstrual flow may facilitate infection of the upper tract by causing loss of cervical mucous plug, causing loss of the endometrial lining with its possible protective effects, and providing a good culture medium (menstrual blood) for bacteria.

   A positive endocervical culture result for a particular pathogen does not necessarily correlate with positive intra-abdominal culture findings.

   A variety of bacteria have been isolated directly from the upper genital tract, including *C. trachomatis*, *N. gonorrhoeae*, and multiple other aerobic and anaerobic bacteria (Table 24-9).

TABLE 24-9. MICROORGANISMS ISOLATED FROM THE FALLOPIAN TUBES OF PATIENTS WITH PELVIC INFLAMMATORY DISEASE

Type of agent	Organism
Sexually transmitted	*Chlamydia trachomatis*
	Neisseria gonorrhoeae
	Mycoplasma hominis
Endogenous agent, aerobic or facultative	*Streptococcus* species
	Staphylococcus species
	Haemophilus species
	Escherichia coli
Anaerobic	*Bacteroides* species
	Peptococcus species
	Peptostreptococcus species
	Clostridium species
	Actinomyces species

From Weström L. Introductory address: treatment of pelvic inflammatory disease in view of etiology and risk factors. *Sex Transm Dis* 1984;11(4)[Suppl]:437–440, with permission.

3. **Prevention.** Emphasis must be placed on aggressive treatment for lower genital tract infection and early aggressive treatment of upper genital tract infection. This helps reduce the incidence of long-term sequelae. Treatment of sexual partners and education are important in reducing the rate of recurrent infections.

   Both clinical and laboratory studies have shown that the use of contraceptives changes the relative risk of developing PID. Barrier methods of contraception provide a mechanical obstruction, whereas nonoxynol 9, the chemical used in spermicidal preparations, which is lethal to both bacteria and viruses, provides a chemical barrier.

   Oral contraceptive use is associated with a lower incidence of PID and with a milder course of infection when it does occur. The reason for this protective effect is unclear but may be related to change in cervical mucus consistency, shorter menses, or atrophy of the endometrium.

4. **Risk factors**
   a. Previous history of PID.
   b. Multiple sex partners, defined as more than two partners in 30 days. (Increased risk is not seen with serial monogamy.)
   c. Infection by a sexually transmitted organism. Fifteen percent of patients with uncomplicated anogenital gonorrhea develop PID at the end of or just after menses.
   d. Use of an IUD can increase the risk of PID by three to five times. The greatest risk of PID is at the time of insertion of the IUD and in the first 3 weeks after placement.

5. **Signs and symptoms.** The most common presenting symptom is abdominopelvic pain. Other complaints are variable, including vaginal discharge or bleeding, fever and chills, nausea, and dysuria. Fever is seen in 60–80% of patients.

6. **Diagnosis** of PID is difficult because the presenting signs and symptoms vary widely. In patients with cervical, uterine, or adnexal tenderness, PID is accurately diagnosed only approximately 65% of the time. Because of the sequelae of PID, especially infertility, ectopic pregnancy, and chronic pelvic pain, PID should be suspected in at-risk women and treated aggressively. Diagnostic criteria outlined by the Centers for Disease Control and Prevention help improve the accuracy of the diagnosis and the appropriateness of treatment.
   a. Minimum criteria for clinical diagnosis (all three should be present) are as follows:
      (1) Bilateral lower abdominal tenderness
      (2) Cervical motion tenderness
      (3) Bilateral adnexal tenderness
   b. Additional criteria for a diagnosis. Routine criteria are those that can be ascertained by simple procedures and support or confirm the presence of an acute inflammatory process. Specialized criteria are those whose verification requires more elaborate procedures that should be reserved for clinical situations in which the patient presents with more severe clinical findings and in which other serious diagnoses must be ruled out.
      (1) Routine
         (a) Oral temperature higher than 38°C
         (b) Abnormal cervical or vaginal discharge
         (c) Elevated erythrocyte sedimentation rate, elevated C-reactive protein level, or both
         (d) Laboratory documentation of cervical infection with *N. gonorrhoeae* or *C. trachomatis*
      (2) Specialized
         (a) Histopathologic evidence of endometritis
         (b) Tubo-ovarian abscess on sonograph or other imaging study
         (c) Laparoscopic evidence

TABLE 24-10. CENTERS FOR DISEASE CONTROL AND PREVENTION RECOMMENDATIONS FOR OUTPATIENT MANAGEMENT OF PELVIC INFLAMMATORY DISEASE

Medication	Dosage	Duration
Regimen A		
Ofloxacin PLUS	400 mg PO bid	14 days
Metronidazole	500 mg PO bid	
Regimen B		
Ceftriaxone sodium	250 mg IM	1 dose
Cefoxitin PLUS	2 g IM	1 dose
Probenecid	1 g PO	
Third-generation cephalosporin PLUS	IM	1 dose
Doxycycline	100 mg PO bid	14 days

Patients treated with an outpatient regimen should be reevaluated in 48 hours to assess the success of treatment.

7. **Treatment** for PID should have as its goal prevention of tubal damage that leads to infertility and ectopic pregnancy and prevention of chronic infection. Many patients can be successfully treated as outpatients, and early ambulatory treatment should be the initial therapeutic approach. Antibiotic choice should target the major etiologic organisms (*N. gonorrhoeae* and *C. trachomatis*) but should also address the polymicrobial nature of the disease (Tables 24-10 and 24-11).

   Conservative practitioners may consider hospital admission for all cases of acute PID, especially in nulligravidas or patients thought to be unable to adhere to the outpatient regimen (Table 24-12).

8. **Sequelae.** Approximately 25% of PID patients experience long-term sequelae. Infertility affects up to 20%. Women with a history of PID have a 6–10 times higher risk of ectopic pregnancy. Chronic pelvic pain and dyspareunia have been reported.

   Fitz-Hugh and Curtis syndrome is the development of fibrous perihepatic adhesions resulting from the inflammatory process of PID. This can cause acute right upper quadrant pain and tenderness. It does not, however, cause alterations of liver enzyme levels.

TABLE 24-11. CRITERIA FOR HOSPITALIZATION OF PATIENTS WITH ACUTE PELVIC INFLAMMATORY DISEASE

Suspected pelvic or tubo-ovarian abscess

Pregnancy

Temperature >38°C

Inability to tolerate PO intake

Peritoneal signs

Failure to respond to oral antibiotics within 48 hrs

Adolescent patient

Nulliparous patient

Uncertain diagnosis

TABLE 24-12. CENTERS FOR DISEASE CONTROL AND PREVENTION RECOMMENDED TREATMENT SCHEDULES FOR INPATIENT TREATMENT OF PELVIC INFLAMMATORY DISEASE

Medication	Dosage	Duration
Regimen A		
Cefotetan disodium PLUS	2 g IV q12h	Continue PO for a total of 14 days
Doxycycline	100 mg IV or PO q12h	
Cefoxitin sodium PLUS	2 g IV q6h	Continue PO for a total of 14 days
Doxycycline	100 mg IV or PO q12h	
Regimen B		
Clindamycin PLUS	900 mg IV q8h	
Gentamicin PLUS	Loading dose 2 mg/kg IV or IM	
	Maintenance dose 1.5 mg/kg q8h	
Doxycycline OR	100 mg PO bid	Total of 14 days
Clindamycin	450 mg PO 5×/day	Total of 10–14 days

The regimen should be continued for at least 48 hours after the patient improves. Patients should be discharged on an oral regimen and should be seen for follow-up as outpatients after approximately 7 days.

B. **Endometritis (nonpuerperal)**
   1. **Pathophysiology.** Endometritis is caused by the ascension of pathogens from the cervix to the endometrium. Pathogens include *C. trachomatis, N. gonorrhoeae, Streptococcus agalactiae,* cytomegalovirus, HSV, and *Mycoplasma hominis.* Organisms that produce bacterial vaginosis may also produce histologic endometritis, even in women without symptoms. Endometritis is also an important component of PID and may be an intermediate stage in the spread of infection to the fallopian tubes.
   2. **Signs and symptoms**
      a. **Chronic endometritis.** Many women with chronic endometritis are asymptomatic. The classic symptom of chronic endometritis is intermenstrual vaginal bleeding. Postcoital bleeding and menorrhagia may also be present. Other women may complain of a dull, constant lower abdominal pain. Chronic endometritis is a rare cause of infertility.
      b. **Acute endometritis.** When endometritis coexists with acute PID, uterine tenderness is common. It is difficult to determine whether inflammation of the oviducts or of the endometrium produces the pelvic discomfort.
   3. **Diagnosis.** The diagnosis of chronic endometritis is established by endometrial biopsy and culture. The classic histologic findings of chronic endometritis are an inflammatory reaction of monocytes and plasma cells in the endometrial stroma (five plasma cells per high-power field). A diffuse pattern of inflammatory infiltrates of lymphocytes and plasma cells throughout the endometrial stroma or even stromal necrosis is associated with severe cases of endometritis.
   4. **Treatment.** The treatment of choice for chronic endometritis is doxycycline, 100 mg PO bid for 10 days. Broader coverage of anaerobic organisms may also be considered, especially in the presence of bacterial vaginosis. When endometritis is associated with acute PID, treatment should focus on the major etiologic organisms, including *N. gonorrhoeae* and *C. trachomatis,* and should also include broader polymicrobial coverage.

25. ECTOPIC PREGNANCY

Julie Pearson and Julie Van Rooyen

I. **Definition.** Ectopic pregnancy (EP) is defined as implantation of the blastocyst anywhere other than in the endometrial cavity.

II. **Incidence.** Approximately 2% of pregnancies are ectopic. The incidence more than quadrupled between 1970 and 1987 (from 1 in 200 live births to 1 in 43). EP accounts for 9% of all maternal mortality and is the leading cause of maternal death in the first trimester. One-third or more of pregnancies occurring after failure of tubal sterilization procedures are likely to be EPs.

The implications of EP for future fertility are significant: The overall conception rate after an EP is 60–80%. Among pregnancies occurring after the initial ectopic pregnancy, 10–28% are recurrent EPs. Only one-third of women with a history of EP eventually deliver a liveborn infant. Heterotopic pregnancy (combined intrauterine and extrauterine gestation) is an uncommon event: 1 in 4000 to 1 in 30,000–40,000 pregnancies. The incidence of heterotopic pregnancy has risen significantly due to the use of ovulation-inducing agents for treatment of infertility and may be as high as 1 in 100.

III. **Etiology.** The increase in incidence of EP has been correlated with an increase in the incidence of pelvic inflammatory disease and improved treatment for this disorder, which in the past would have rendered the patient infertile; the use of intrauterine devices, especially those that contain progesterone; the increase in surgical procedures for the treatment of fallopian tube disease; an increase in use of elective sterilizations; improved diagnostic techniques; and miscellaneous other contributing factors, including diethylstilbestrol exposure, endometriosis, and the use of ovulation-inducing agents.

The vast majority of EPs are tubal. Most tubal pregnancies are found in the distal two-thirds of the tube. The ampulla is the most common site of implantation, accounting for 78% of EPs; 12% are located in the isthmus, 5% are in the fimbriae, and 2% are cornual or interstitial. The remainder are abdominal, cervical, or ovarian.

IV. **Diagnosis.** EP may present as a surgical emergency, and therefore timely diagnosis is essential (Fig. 25-1).

A. **Clinical manifestations** are diverse. Patients typically present with complaints of bleeding and lower abdominal pain. Both symptoms may vary in severity and may occasionally be accompanied by syncope, dizziness, or neck and shoulder pain.

1. The classic triad of signs and symptoms of EP (present in less than 50% of patients) includes history of a missed menstrual period followed by abnormal vaginal bleeding, abdominal or pelvic pain, and a tender adnexal mass.

2. The most frequently experienced **symptoms** of EP are pelvic and abdominal pain (95%) and amenorrhea with vaginal bleeding (60–80%).

a. **Pain.** The early pain from an EP is usually colicky in nature and is believed to result from tubal distention. Pain may be perceived anywhere in the abdomen but is usually confined to the lower abdomen and is more severe on the side of the EP. With a large hemoperitoneum, pleuritic chest pain or shoulder pain reflecting diaphragmatic irritation may be present. Exquisite tenderness is noted during abdominal palpation and vaginal examination; cervical motion tenderness occurs in 75% of women with ruptured or rupturing tubal pregnancies.

b. **Vaginal spotting** occurs when endocrine support [trophoblastic human chorionic gonadotropin (hCG)] for the endometrium declines, and presents as scanty, dark brown bleeding, either intermittent or continuous. The uterus grows during the first 3 months

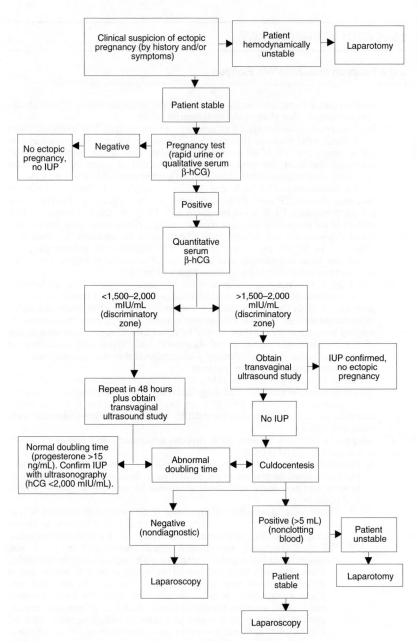

FIG. 25-1. Algorithm for ectopic pregnancy diagnosis and management. β-hCG, human chorionic gonadotropin β-subunit; IUP, intrauterine pregnancy.

of tubal gestation as a consequence of stimulation by placental and ovarian hormones and is slightly enlarged in 25% of cases. Uterine decidual casts are passed in 5–10% of cases; this passage is accompanied by cramps similar to those of a spontaneous abortion.

3. **Physical examination** elicits abdominal or pelvic tenderness in most cases. Tenderness in patients with EP may be generalized (45%), located bilaterally in the lower quadrants (25%), or located unilaterally in the lower quadrant (30%). Rebound tenderness may or may not be present. Cervical motion tenderness resulting from peritoneal irritation is usually present but is nonspecific for EP. A palpable **adnexal mass** or mass in the cul-de-sac is reported in approximately 40% of cases; however, absence of a palpable mass does not rule out EP. Conversely, a corpus luteum cyst accompanying an intrauterine pregnancy (IUP) may result in a palpable adnexal mass, which can be mistaken for an EP. Additional signs include shoulder pain (15%) and low-grade fever (less than 10%).

B. **Differential diagnosis**
   1. **Salpingitis** presents with similar symptoms and examination findings but negative pregnancy test results, an elevated WBC, and temperature elevation.
   2. **Threatened abortion.** Bleeding is usually heavier, pain is localized to the lower mid abdomen, and cervical motion tenderness may be absent. The presence of corpus luteum cyst may confuse the diagnosis.
   3. **Appendicitis.** Amenorrhea or abnormal vaginal bleeding is usually absent. Persistent right lower quadrant pain, with fever and GI symptoms, suggests appendicitis. Cervical motion tenderness is usually less severe but still may be present. Pregnancy test results are negative.
   4. **Ovarian torsion.** Pain initially is intermittent and later becomes constant as vascular supply is compromised. Findings may include an elevated WBC and a palpable adnexal mass, but pregnancy test results are negative .
   5. Other differential diagnoses include dysfunctional uterine bleeding (usually painless and heavier than with an EP), persistent corpus luteum cyst, and intrauterine device use associated with pain and severe dysmenorrhea (pain is often localized to the midline and pregnancy test results are negative). Gastroenteritis, urinary tract infection, or calculus early in pregnancy may also mimic an EP.

C. **Laboratory tests**
   1. **Pregnancy tests**
      a. **Urine.** Urinary pregnancy tests for hCG are usually latex agglutination inhibition slide tests, which can give positive results at levels of 25 mIU/mL or more. They are qualitative and are read as either positive or negative, and provide rapidly available results.
      b. **Serum.** For distinguishing EP or other abnormal pregnancies from normal IUPs, the most sensitive test is the serum human chorionic gonadotropin β-subunit (β-hCG) radioimmunoassay, a quantitative test that gives positive results at levels of 5 mIU/mL [International Reference Preparation (IRP)]. Serial measurements allow comparison with normal doubling times of approximately every 48 hours until 6 weeks' gestation. Approximately 85% of normal pregnancies fall within these limits; EPs are generally associated with lower overall β-hCG levels than normal IUPs. Pregnancies near 6 weeks demonstrating a less than 66% increase in hCG within a 48-hour period are either EPs or nonviable IUPs that are likely to abort.
   2. **Hemoglobin and hematocrit.** Baseline levels should be obtained. Serial measurements are useful if the diagnosis is uncertain. An acute drop in hemoglobin or hematocrit over the first few hours of observation is more important than the initial reading. After acute hemorrhage, initial readings may at first be unchanged or only slightly

decreased; a subsequent decline represents restoration of depleted blood volume by hemodilution.

3. **Leukocyte count** varies considerably in ruptured EPs. It is normal in 50% of EPs but has been reported to rise as high as 30,000 cu mm.

4. **Progesterone level.** Although a single level cannot predict whether a patient has an EP, levels can often be used to establish that there is an abnormal pregnancy (either incomplete abortion or EP). A serum progesterone level of 25 ng/mL or higher indicates a normal pregnancy with a 97.5% sensitivity. Conversely, less than 2% of EPs and no more than 4% of abnormal IUPs have progesterone levels of more than 25 ng/mL. A level of 5 ng/mL or less is consistent with an abnormal pregnancy.

D. **Ultrasonography (US)** allows the clinician to rule out an IUP when an EP is suspected. A positive US diagnosis can be made by identifying an extrauterine fetus, but this is an uncommon finding. In practice, an IUP sac or fetus seen on US essentially excludes the presence of an EP.

1. **Abdominal US.** An IUP is usually not recognized using abdominal US until 5–6 weeks' gestation or 28 days after timed ovulation and with serum hCG concentration greater than 6000 mIU/mL (IRP). Although an adnexal mass seen on US is suggestive of EP, fetal heart motion outside the uterus is diagnostic. At serum hCG concentrations of 6000–6500 mIU/mL (IRP), a normal IUP can be visualized by transabdominal US 94% of the time. At the time of initial evaluation, however, less than 25% of patients with EPs have hCG levels of more than 6000 mIU/mL (IRP).

   US findings suggestive of early IUPs may be apparent in some cases of EP. A structure appearing to be a small sac or collapsed sac may actually be a blood clot or decidual cast.

2. **Vaginal US.** Vaginal US is more sensitive and specific; however, 10% of EPs are still missed by this procedure. Earlier and more specific diagnoses are made with the following diagnostic criteria for IUP: identification of a gestational sac of at least 1–3 mm, a sac eccentrically placed in the uterus and surrounded by a decidual-chorionic reaction, and presence of a fetal pole within the sac, especially when accompanied by fetal heart motion. A point of differentiation between false and genuine sacs is the presence of a yolk sac. When vaginal US is used, a gestational sac can usually be seen when serum hCG concentrations are as low as 1500 mIU/mL.

E. **US and β-hCG levels.** In hemodynamically stable patients, evaluation of suspected EP involves serial determinations of serum β-hCG levels in conjunction with vaginal or abdominal US.

1. If the β-hCG level is more than 6000 mIU/mL and an intrauterine sac is seen by abdominal US, an EP may be ruled out, except for rare cases of heterotopic pregnancy.

2. If the β-hCG level is higher than 6000 mIU/mL and no intrauterine sac is seen on abdominal US, or if the β-hCG level is above 1500–2500 mIU/mL and no intrauterine sac is seen on a vaginal US, an EP is very likely, although a spontaneous abortion may also give this picture.

3. If the β-hCG level is less than 6000 mIU/mL and a definite intrauterine gestational sac is visualized on abdominal US (or the level is 1500–2500 mIU/mL and an intrauterine gestational sac is seen on vaginal US), a spontaneous abortion is likely, but an EP must be ruled out. A serum progesterone level determination may be useful.

4. With β-hCG levels of less than 6000 mIU/mL and no intrauterine sac on abdominal US (or levels less than 1500–2500 mIU/mL and no intrauterine sac on vaginal US), no diagnosis can be made. A determination of serum β-hCG level can confirm a pregnancy 8 days after fertilization. An intrauterine gestational sac cannot be conclusively identified even with vaginal US until 28 days after conception; the time between 8 and 28 days results in a "20-day window." A progesterone level determination may be useful, but it is not always rapidly available in most institu-

tions and the normal range is variable. Serial β-hCG measurements and follow-up ultrasonography are used to resolve the diagnosis.

F. **Culdocentesis** is a simple technique for identifying hemoperitoneum. The cervix is elevated with a tenaculum, and a 20-gauge spinal needle is passed through the posterior vaginal fornix into the cul-de-sac. The presence of old blood clots or bloody fluid that does not clot suggests hemoperitoneum. Clotting of blood obtained via culdocentesis suggests aspiration from an adjacent blood vessel or brisk bleeding from a ruptured EP. Culdocentesis may be unsatisfactory in patients with a history of previous salpingitis and pelvic peritonitis because of cul-de-sac obliteration. Presence of purulent fluid points to a diagnosis of salpingitis.

G. **Curettage** is useful in differentiating between threatened or incomplete abortions and tubal pregnancies. Stovall et al. recommend that curettage be carried out in cases in which the progesterone level is less than 5 ng/mL, β-hCG titers are rising abnormally and are less than 2000 mIU/mL, and no IUP has been visualized by transvaginal US. If curettings yield placental or fetal tissue, a simultaneous EP is unlikely. If curettings yield decidual tissue but no villi, careful follow-up is needed with serial hCG determinations and US. The presence of decidua alone on pathologic examination implies extrauterine pregnancy, although it may be seen in patients with a complete abortion.

V. **Treatment.** The initial management decision is based on the patient's stability. Patients in shock or with a surgical abdomen should be taken to the operating room as soon as possible, resuscitated with intravenous fluids using two large-bore intravenous cannulas, and an indwelling catheter placed in the bladder to monitor urine output. Blood should be obtained for a type and crossmatch for packed red blood cells, CBC, prothrombin time, partial thromboplastin time, and renal panel.

A. **Surgical management.** The operative procedure is selected based on the rate of bleeding, patient stability, the extent of damage to the fallopian tube, and the desire for future fertility. There are two primary approaches.

1. **Laparoscopy.** Laparoscopy has become the preferred surgical approach in the hemodynamically stable patient. Its advantages are that it is less invasive than laparotomy and generally enables a quicker recovery and earlier return to work. It usually provides definitive diagnosis, although early ectopic pregnancies are missed 4–8% of the time. Disadvantages include difficulty in controlling hemorrhage. Not all physicians are comfortable with operative laparoscopy and some patients are not ideal candidates (e.g., patients with large body habitus or previous abdominal surgeries).

2. **Laparotomy.** Laparotomy is an appropriate choice for a patient with obvious hemorrhage and hemodynamic compromise. After hemostasis is obtained, the treatment of choice is complete or partial salpingectomy. With a ruptured interstitial or cornual pregnancy, cornual resection may be required. Laparotomy is also indicated when adhesive disease precludes adequate visualization through the laparoscope or in circumstances indicated previously.

B. **Surgical technique.** Once the approach (laparoscopy versus laparotomy) has been decided on, a variety of surgical techniques are possible.

1. **Salpingostomy** involves incision of the fallopian tube to create a new opening (stoma). It is used to remove a small pregnancy in the distal third of the tube. A linear incision is made on the antimesenteric border over the pregnancy, which usually extrudes from the incision and may be removed. Bleeding points are cauterized with laser or needle-point cautery, and the incision is left to heal by secondary intention.

2. **Salpingectomy** involves removal of the entire tube on the affected side. This is done when the size and extent of the EP are such that salvage of the tube is not possible or in some cases of recurrent EP in the same tube.

3. **Segmental resection (partial salpingectomy)** involves excising the involved portion of fallopian tube. The remaining ends may be anastomosed at a later date if indicated. It is recommended for unruptured EPs located in the isthmus because salpingostomy in this narrow region may result in scarring and further narrowing. Segmental resection may also be done for ruptured ampullary EPs in an unstable patient, when hemostasis must be rapidly obtained and childbearing potential preserved. The mesosalpinx is incised, the EP is excised, and the mesosalpinx is sutured.

4. **Fimbrial evacuation** involves squeezing the EP out of the fimbriated end of the tube. The milking, or suctioning, of the ectopic mass from distally implanted tubal pregnancies is not recommended because it results in a doubling in recurrence rates of EPs compared to treatment with salpingostomy and a high rate of surgical reexploration for recurrent bleeding secondary to persistent trophoblastic tissue.

5. **Cornual resection,** which involves excision of the cornu, is reserved for the very rare occurrence of a cornual EP. In this procedure, a wedge of the outer one-third of the interstitial portion of fallopian tube, together with the EP, is removed to avoid recurrence of EP in the tubal stump without creating a defect in the uterus, where rupture would be a concern. Laparotomy is usually required for this procedure.

VI. **Complications**

A. **Persistent trophoblastic tissue.** With conservative approaches, there is a 4–8% risk that not all trophoblastic tissue is evacuated, so that close follow-up is required postoperatively. With persistent or increasing hCG values, reexploration or chemotherapy with methotrexate sodium (MTX) may be chosen based on the patient's stability and hCG level.

B. **Persistent EP** is the most common complication and the major reason for secondary intervention after initial conservative surgical treatment of an EP. There is limited information concerning reproductive outcome after treatment of this complication. Salpingectomy appears to be the most dependable treatment, offering the greatest assurance for complete resolution of persistent EP (less than 1% risk of persistent EP with salpingectomy). Issues regarding further fertility often influence the decision to defer salpingectomy and select repeat salpingostomy or MTX.

Conservative surgery should be followed by weekly determinations of β-hCG level until nonpregnant levels are reached. An hCG clearance occurs in two phases: an initial phase, with a half-life of 5–9 hours, and a second, longer phase, with a half-life of 22–32 hours. When removal of tissue is fairly complete, serum hCG levels will be 20% or less of intraoperative or preoperative levels within 72 hours after surgery. If hCG levels continue to fall, expectant management with serial hCG determinations is sufficient. If they plateau or rise, further treatment options (salpingectomy, partial salpingectomy, or MTX therapy) should be considered.

VII. **Medical management**

A. **Systemic methotrexate.** MTX, a folic acid analog, inhibits dihydrofolate reductase and DNA synthesis and has been used in the treatment of unruptured EP. MTX targets rapidly dividing cells, including fetal cells, trophoblast, bone marrow cells, and cells of the buccal and intestinal mucosa. Its repeated use is limited by dose- and duration-dependent side effects: severe leukopenia, bone marrow aplasia, thrombocytopenia, ulcerative stomatitis, diarrhea, liver cell necrosis, and hemorrhagic enteritis. Death has been reported from intestinal perforation. The current single-dose MTX protocol, developed by Stovall et al. for treatment of an unruptured EP, is summarized in Table 25-1. Stovall recommends that patients with subnormally rising hCG titers of less than 2000 mIU/mL undergo dilation of the cervix and curettage of the uterus. The hCG titer is measured again the following day, and if it is rising, MTX (50 mg/m^2) is given intramuscularly. For patients

TABLE 25-1. SINGLE-DOSE METHOTREXATE SODIUM PROTOCOL FOR ECTOPIC PREGNANCY TREATMENT

Day	Therapy and tests
0[a]	hCG, D&C, CBC, AST, BUN, creatinine, blood type (including Rh)
1	MTX, hCG
4[b]	hCG
7[c]	hCG

AST, aspartate aminotransferase; BUN, blood urea nitrogen; CBC, complete blood cell count; D&C, dilation of the cervix and curettage of the uterus; hCG, quantitative β-human chorionic gonadotropin (mIU/mL); MTX, intramuscular methotrexate sodium, 50 mg/m²; Rh, rhesus factor.

[a]In patients not requiring D&C before MTX initiation (hCG of 2000 mIU/mL and no gestational sac on transvaginal ultrasonography), day 0 and day 1 are combined.

[b]The hCG titer on day 4 is usually higher than the hCG titer on day 1.

[c]If there is a <15% decline in titer between days 4 and 7, give second dose of methotrexate, 50 mg/m² on day 7. If there is a ≥15% decline in hCG titer between days 4 and 7, follow weekly until hCG is <10 mIU/mL.

Adapted from Stovall TG, Ling FW. Single-dose methotrexate: an expanded clinical trial. *Am J Obstet Gynecol* 1993;168:1759–1762.

with rising hCG titers of more than 2000 mIU/mL, dilation and curettage is not required, and MTX can be administered on day 0.

Before treatment, all patients should have a normal platelet and WBC count, normal liver function test results, and normal renal function. A blood type/Rhesus test should be done to assess the need for Rh_O (D) immune globulin (RhoGAM). An hCG titer is measured on days 4 and 7, although the level will usually be higher on day 4 than on day 1. If the titer on day 7 is less than that on day 4, hCG levels are measured weekly until negative. If not, or if the level is not declining, a second dose of MTX (same dosage) is given, and the titers are measured days 4 and 7, as earlier.

Patients should be informed that the failure rate after MTX treatment varies based on the level of hCG and the size of the EP, although success rates are generally in the 70% range with one dose and up to 85% with two or more doses. The majority of patients have an increase in abdominopelvic pain during treatment, which may be difficult to distinguish from pain due to rupture of the EP. Patients should be followed clinically and managed surgically if there is evidence of rupture. US examination is *not* necessary and may increase the likelihood of additional unnecessary intervention.

1. **Strict criteria** must be met for initiating MTX therapy (Table 25-2). The most important selection criterion for medical management involves patient stability. The presence of fetal cardiac activity is a relative contraindication because it is associated with a significantly higher failure rate (14%) than in the absence of cardiac activity (5%).

2. **Contraindications** to MTX therapy are listed in Table 25-3.

3. **Disadvantages** of single-dose systemic MTX include prolonged time for the hCG titers to decline and the EP to resolve (70–120 days) and the need for close monitoring of outpatients for rupture and MTX side effects, which makes compliance an important consideration in patient selection.

B. **Local (transvaginal/laparoscopic) treatment**

1. Transvaginal intratubal MTX therapy has been undertaken but has a significant failure rate (30%). Laparoscopic intratubal MTX treatment has not been found to be successful and has been abandoned because of the need for surgery for persistence of EP.

TABLE 25-2. CRITERIA FOR METHOTREXATE THERAPY

Stovall and Ling, 1993[a]

    Hemodynamic stability

    Increase in hCG titers after curettage

    Transvaginal ultrasonography showing an unruptured ectopic pregnancy of <3.5 cm in greatest diameter

    Desire for future fertility

American College of Obstetricians and Gynecologists, 1990[b]

    Ectopic pregnancy size of ≤3 cm

    Desire for future fertility

    Stable or rising hCG levels with peak values of <15,000 mIU/mL

    Intact tubal serosa

    No active bleeding

    Ectopic pregnancy fully viable at laparoscopy

    Cervical and cornual pregnancy (in selected cases)

---

hCG, human chorionic gonadotropin.

[a]Adapted from Stovall TG, Ling FW. Single-dose methotrexate: an expanded clinical trial. *Am J Obstet Gynecol* 1993;168:1759–1762.

[b]From American College of Obstetricians and Gynecologists. *Ectopic pregnancy.* Washington: American College of Obstetricians and Gynecologists, 1990. ACOG Technical Bulletin No. 150.

    2. Laparoscopic intratubal prostaglandin and hyperosmolar glucose injections have been used but have been found to be no more effective than salpingostomy; these approaches are not recommended.

    3. **Cervical EPs.** MTX, as well as other substances such as actinomycin D, have also been used in the treatment of cervical EPs. Direct injection of various agents has been reported using laparoscopy or US-directed

TABLE 25-3. CONTRAINDICATIONS TO METHOTREXATE THERAPY

Stovall and Ling, 1993[a]

    Hepatic dysfunction: aspartate aminotransferase level >2 times normal

    Renal disease: serum creatinine level >130 mmol/L (1.5 mg/dL)

    Active peptic ulcer disease

    Blood dyscrasia: leukocyte count <3000 cells/μL or platelet count 100,000/μL

American College of Obstetricians and Gynecologists, 1990[b]

    Contraindications listed above, plus:

        Poor patient compliance

        History of active hepatic or renal disease

        Presence of fetal cardiac activity

---

[a]Adapted from Stovall TG, Ling FW. Single-dose methotrexate: an expanded clinical trial. *Am J Obstet Gynecol* 1993;168:1759–1762.

[b]From American College of Obstetricians and Gynecologists. *Ectopic pregnancy.* Washington: American College of Obstetricians and Gynecologists, 1990. ACOG Technical Bulletin No. 150.

transvaginal injection. Injection of MTX under US guidance is associated with a success rate of less than 80%. Although MTX injection with US avoids surgery, it carries a lower success rate than systemic MTX therapy (92%).

4. RU-486 (mifepristone, Mifeprex), a progesterone receptor blocker, has been used but has shown limited effectiveness.

VIII. **Fertility after EP.** The choice of surgical procedure in the management of an EP is not a significant determinant of fertility outcome in women with EPs. A history of previous infertility is the single most important factor influencing future fertility. It is recommended that conservative surgery be performed in women desiring subsequent pregnancy. A recent population-based study reported in the *British Journal of Obstetrics and Gynaecology* showed differences in subsequent fertility (with treatment by salpingectomy versus salpingostomy versus MTX) only in women with preexisting infertility; subsequent fertility rates were higher after medical and conservative management than after salpingectomy. For women with no infertility factor, there was no significant difference among treatments. A recent Cochrane Database System Review compared treatment success rates, tubal patency, and future fertility and found similar tubal patency rates and subsequent IUP for radical surgical, conservative surgical, and medical means of management.

A. When outcomes after salpingostomy and salpingectomy are compared in women with a history of infertility, a slightly higher subsequent pregnancy rate and EP rate is found in women who have had salpingostomy than in those undergoing salpingectomy. Fertility is improved, however, in patients with contralateral adhesive disease or history of infertility when conservative management is chosen instead of salpingectomy (76% versus 44%). Data on later pregnancies after salpingostomy in patients with a tubal pregnancy in a sole patent oviduct (20% ectopic recurrence) suggest that the risk of repeat EP in a conserved tube is similar to that in a diseased contralateral tube that was not operated on.

B. The risk of recurrence increases in patients who have had two or more EPs. Only one out of three will conceive, and 20–57% of these will have EPs.

C. The fact that patients with badly damaged fallopian tubes and those whose tubes have been removed can conceive through in vitro fertilization should be factored into the decision-making process in treating EP.

IX. **Follow-up.** Patients should be advised to take birth control pills or use other reliable contraceptive methods until initial inflammation resolves (6–12 weeks). Contraception will avoid confusion between rising hCG levels from a new pregnancy and those from a persistent EP, should conception occur in the immediate postoperative period. Patients should undergo extensive counseling regarding their risk for recurrence of EP and the absolute necessity for early medical care, which should include serial determinations of hCG levels until an early US examination can document an IUP or EP. It is important to give RhoGAM (300 µg) postoperatively to an Rh-negative woman to prevent Rh alloimmunization in a future pregnancy.

26. CHRONIC PELVIC PAIN

Lara Burrows and J. Courtland Robinson

I. **Introduction.** Although chronic pelvic pain (CPP) is common in clinical practice, the exact prevalence of this condition is unknown; however, it has been estimated to range from 14.7% to 39% in young women of reproductive age.

There is no universally accepted definition of CPP. Most, however, would agree that the characteristics of the CPP syndrome include pain of more than 6 months' duration, incomplete relief by previous treatments, pain out of proportion to tissue damage, loss of physical function, vegetative signs of depression, and altered family dynamics.

CPP has been shown to negatively affect a woman's quality of life because it can limit normal exercise patterns, cause loss of time at work, increase the use of medications, lead to sexual dysfunction, and limit normal home life.

II. **Pain theories.** Most chronic pain states begin with a nociceptive event or process, although that event may go unrecognized or unremembered. Cartesian theory (the specificity theory) states that pain signals are conducted in one direction along nerves to the brain, where they are perceived and interpreted as pain. Gate control theory states that signals from a nociceptive stimulus from the periphery are conducted to the spinal cord and may be modulated by various feedback loops; they may then stop completely in the spinal cord or may continue via lateral spinothalamic tracts. This theory also allows for the fact that neurotransmitter states in the brain may chemically mediate the ability of the spinal cord to block the transmission of nociceptive signals. Thus, higher brain centers can modulate spinal cord activity, and it implies that information is transmitted in both directions, not just in a single direction, that is, from injured tissue to the brain.

III. **Causes**

A. **Gynecologic.** There are no symptoms that uniquely identify genitourinary structures as the source of a patient's pain.

1. **Extrauterine**

a. **Chronic pelvic infection.** Tuberculosis is the only cause of chronic pelvic infection.

b. **Pelvic adhesive disease** is the result of previous surgery or infection. The role of adhesions in CPP is controversial. The prevalence ranges from 6–51%. The observation of adhesions in patients with CPP is not proof of a cause-and-effect relationship. Studies have shown that the density of adhesions does not correlate with the severity of the pain; however, the pain location correlates highly with the location of limited adhesions found on laparoscopy. Some authors feel that adhesions may cause pain by direct nerve damage from tissue destruction and scar formation, or by devitalization and ischemia of parts of internal pelvic organs secondary to damage of the blood supply. Clinical examination and imaging studies are unreliable in identifying patients with adhesions.

c. **Endometriosis** is among the most common morbidities associated with CPP. Grossly evident endometriosis is diagnosed in 30–50% of women who undergo laparoscopy for CPP. Endometriosis can present in a variety of ways, including dysmenorrhea (the most common symptom reported in those with CPP), dyspareunia, and chronic noncyclic pain. Mechanisms theorized to be responsible include inflammation, pressure, adhesions, neuronal involvement, increased prostaglandin production, and psychological factors. The depth of infiltration of endometriosis has been recognized to correlate with the presence of pelvic pain.

d. **Ovarian remnant syndrome** is found in patients who are thought to have had their ovaries removed. Cyclic pelvic pain caused by an ovarian remnant is most commonly associated with the development of ovarian follicles within hormonally active ovarian tissue. This diagnosis should be suspected when serum levels of follicle-stimulating hormone and luteinizing hormone are normal in a woman who gives a history of a previous oophorectomy. Surgical treatment usually requires extensive intraperitoneal adhesiolysis and retroperitoneal dissection to remove all of the ovarian tissue. Studies of postoperative pain relief are limited but show cure rates as high as 90%.

e. **Vulvar vestibulitis** is a chronic syndrome of uncertain etiology characterized by severe pain on vestibular touch or attempted vaginal entry, tenderness to light pressure within the vulvar vestibule, and gross physical findings limited to vestibular erythema. Colposcopic examination of the vulvar vestibule adds little to the diagnosis. Histopathologic findings are consistent with chronic nonspecific inflammation. With regard to treatment, spontaneous remissions do occur, especially in women with symptoms of less than 6 months' duration. Mild cases should be managed conservatively; local irritants and potential allergens should be avoided. For treatment of severe cases, the best results are obtained with surgery, specifically, **U-shaped vestibulectomy with perineoplasty.**

2. **Uterine**

a. **Adenomyosis.** The reported prevalence of adenomyosis ranges from 10% to 26%. This condition typically affects women in the fourth and fifth decades of life, and approximately 35% of women with adenomyosis are asymptomatic. The most common presenting complaint is abnormal uterine bleeding, but dysmenorrhea, metrorrhagia, nonmenstrual pelvic pain, and dyspareunia may also be present. The diagnosis is made histopathologically when endometrial stroma and glands are observed at least 2–3 mm below the endometrial surface within the myometrium. The cause of the pain associated with this condition is not known. Ultrasonography and hysterosalpingography are not useful in the diagnosis of adenomyosis. MRI, however, can be used to diagnose adenomyosis. Hysterectomy has consistently been shown to be successful in treating and controlling the symptoms associated with adenomyosis.

b. **Chronic endometritis or cervicitis.** Chronic infection of the endometrium or cervix may contribute to CPP and dyspareunia. Cultures of the cervix are frequently negative for the usual pathogens, including *Chlamydia*. Nevertheless, treatment with antibiotics such as tetracyclines or erythromycin for 2–4 weeks may be successful in improving symptoms.

c. **Leiomyomata** are the most common tumors found in the female genital tract. Degeneration of a leiomyoma can cause pain due to alteration in the blood supply such as occurs with rapid growth, torsion, or atrophy with menopause. The pain associated with degeneration is usually gradual in onset and intermittent in nature. Leiomyomata are also associated with a sense of pelvic pressure because their bulk rests on adjacent pelvic organs. The contribution of a leiomyoma requires further evaluation. Surgery for the removal of large leiomyomata is successful in decreasing uterine bulk and diminishing pressure on adjacent organs. The long-term results in managing CPP are achieved in 70–80% of cases.

d. **Pelvic vein incompetence** occurs in the setting of pelvic varicosities. This syndrome is thought to be caused at least in part by incompetent valves in the pelvic veins and other variations from normal. This leads to venous stasis and can cause pain in a fashion similar to varicosities in the lower extremities. Patients with this syndrome are typically in their late twenties or early thirties and have variable parity. They typically describe the pain as brought on or exacerbated by any stimulus that increases intra-abdominal pressure, such as prolonged walking, standing, or lifting; lying down provides relief. The pain is described as a dull aching pain in the pelvis. Cyclic changes in the intensity of the pain have been reported. Dyspareunia may be a symptom, although patients more commonly describe a postcoital ache. On physical examination, the cervix is often blue as a result of engorgement, and on bimanual examination, cervical motion tenderness is common. The most useful physical sign is marked ovarian tenderness elicited by gentle compression on bimanual vaginal examination. However, the combination of ovarian point tenderness on abdominal examination and a history of a postcoital ache is 94% sensitive and 77% specific. The diagnosis of pelvic congestion syndrome is difficult to make based on history and physical examination alone. Testing aimed at assessing the pelvic vasculature is needed to establish the diagnosis. Laparoscopy is not a very effective means of diagnosing pelvic congestion syndrome because the dilated veins are frequently retroperitoneal and decompress when the patient is supine or in the Trendelenburg position and therefore cannot be seen. Direct venography in a cardiovascular diagnostic setting is required to establish the finding of incompetent pelvic veins. Embolization, the appropriate therapy, can be done at the same time, all in an outpatient setting. Patients with a diagnosis of Ehlers-Danlos syndrome need special attention, because abnormal pelvic veins are common in this disease.

B. **Urologic**

1. **Chronic urinary tract infection (UTI)** is one of the most common causes of irritative voiding symptoms in women. Women older than 65 years are especially susceptible to UTIs and have a higher recurrence rate than premenopausal women. Estrogen replacement therapy may lower the vaginal pH, decrease vaginal colonization with *Escherichia coli,* and decrease the frequency of UTIs.

2. **Interstitial cystitis** is a symptom complex presenting as urinary frequency, nocturia, urgency, and suprapubic pain, which is often relieved by voiding. Approximately 60% of patients also have dyspareunia. Interstitial cystitis has also been referred to as **urethral syndrome, urethrotrigonitis, urgency-frequency syndrome,** and **pseudomembranous trigonitis.** It is mostly seen in white women and can be chronic and debilitating. Thirty percent of these patients report that they are unable to work, and their scores are lower on quality-of-life assessments. The etiology of interstitial cystitis is unknown but is believed to be multifactorial. Suggested causes include infections, autoimmune disorders, neurogenic factors, lymphatic obstruction, endocrinologic factors, and alterations of the glycosaminoglycan layer. Accurate diagnosis can be made only by cystoscopy and hydrodistension under anesthesia. After distension, the typical cystoscopic findings are **glomerulations** that resemble petechial hemorrhages or fissures called **Hunner ulcers.** Finally, a bladder biopsy must be performed to rule out other causes of the patient's symptoms, such as endometriosis or chronic or eosinophilic cystitis. With regard to treatment, hydrodistension has been shown to relieve symptoms in 30–60% of patients. Other therapies include amitriptyline hydrochloride 20–75 mg orally at bedtime, which has been shown to produce a 90% improvement in the patient's symptoms; however, it is not curative. Those with urinary frequency as their chief complaint tend to benefit more from dimethyl sulfoxide therapy, which has a response

rate of 50–90%. It is given via a small urethral catheter after anesthetization of the urethra with lidocaine jelly.

3. **Suburethral diverticulitis** should be suspected in women with persistent lower urinary tract symptoms that are unresponsive to traditional treatment. The classic triad of symptoms is dysuria, dyspareunia, and postvoid dribbling. Diagnosis is frequently made on physical examination when a mass is seen on the anterior vaginal wall or when milking the anterior wall of the vagina produces purulent discharge or urine. The optimal treatment is surgical.

4. **Urethral syndrome** is a symptom complex that can include dysuria, urinary frequency, urgency, suprapubic discomfort, and **stranguria,** which is the slow and painful discharge of urine. First, the possibility of an infection must be ruled out. If sterile pyuria is found in association with symptoms consistent with the urethral syndrome, *Chlamydia trachomatis* infection should be suspected and a urethral culture should be obtained. Empiric therapy with antibiotics is indicated when pyuria is identified and bacterial cystitis has been ruled out. Treatment options include estrogen supplementation in postmenopausal women, which should be considered especially when atrophic changes are present. Other treatments include dimethyl sulfoxide, anti-inflammatory agents, skeletal muscle relaxants, or alpha-antagonists such as terazosin hydrochloride or doxazosin mesylate. Some advocate biofeedback techniques. The best results (85–100%) often occur with observation alone.

C. **Gastrointestinal**

1. **Chronic appendicitis.** Patients with chronic appendicitis generally present with localized right lower quadrant pain unresponsive to conservative treatment. These patients should undergo laparoscopy with preparations made for performing an appendectomy should the appendix appear abnormal and no other pathology be found. Relief of their symptoms supports the diagnosis. Appendiceal perforation with subsequent pelvic abscess formation can also cause CPP.

2. **Diverticular disease.** The incidence of diverticular disease increases with age. Diverticuli are commonly found in the sigmoid colon. Infection of the diverticuli and microabscess formation create an ongoing indolent inflammatory process with subsequent abdominal pain and tenderness.

   Which diagnostic tests to use depends on the severity of symptoms. CT scans are the diagnostic test of choice. Barium enema examinations can also be used; however, they are contraindicated in the acute phase. Management depends on the severity of the disease, and GI consultation is required.

3. **Inflammatory bowel disease.** Inflammation of the colon and rectum due to ulcerative colitis or Crohn's disease may be associated with CPP. Symptoms include bloating, abdominal distension, and a sense of incomplete evacuation, all of which are similar to those of irritable bowel syndrome (see later); however, the symptoms tend to be more severe and sometimes disabling. In a young patient who presents with intermittent cramping, lower abdominal pain, and chronic bloody diarrhea, **ulcerative colitis** should be strongly suspected. The diagnosis is usually made by sigmoidoscopy, in which the typical findings are friable mucosa and pseudopolyps.

   Crohn's disease generally presents with pain, which may be intermittent and cramping or continuous. Crohn's disease commonly involves the terminal ileum, which often lies in the pelvis; therefore, these patients frequently present with pelvic pain. Other symptoms include bloody diarrhea and fever, which is often associated with perforation or the presence of an abscess. Management requires referral to a gastroenterologist.

4. **Irritable bowel syndrome** is characterized by a complex of symptoms associated with abnormal GI motility. The symptom criteria for the dis-

ease are called the **Rome criteria.** The three common clinical presentations are (1) chronic abdominal pain and constipation, or a spastic colon, (2) intermittent painless diarrhea, and (3) alternating constipation and diarrhea with associated abdominal pain. Other associated symptoms include abdominal distension, bloating, fatigue, headaches, and irritability. Unfortunately, there are no good diagnostic tests for this syndrome, and it is generally a diagnosis of exclusion after other causes of the patient's complaints have been excluded. Again, for the gynecologist, management by a gastroenterologist is reasonable.

5. **Neoplasia.** Cancers of the colon and rectum should be included in the differential diagnosis of CPP.

D. **Musculoskeletal**

1. **Coccydynia.** A fall or any trauma to the coccyx can cause coccygeal pain. The coccyx is innervated by S1–S4 and may cause referred pain throughout the pelvic floor. One of the more common causes of coccydynia is childbirth-related damage to the sacrococcygeal ligaments during vaginal delivery. The most common symptom is pain in the tail bone, and the pain may be worsened with hip extension activities, such as stair climbing or prolonged sitting. This condition is associated with spasm of the pelvic floor muscles, and the inflammation associated with a traumatic coccygeal injury can cause a **tension myalgia** as a secondary response. Most cases respond to injections of local anesthetics and steroids into the sacrococcygeal and other surrounding ligaments.

2. **Sacroiliac dysfunction** may occur in response to the strain of poor posture or trauma. The trauma of labor and delivery can sprain or displace the sacroiliac articulation. Sensory innervation of the sacroiliac joints arises from L4–S4, which includes the posterior thigh and leg as well as the ventral surface of the foot.

3. **Degenerative joint disease** is thought to begin with alterations in range of motion that disturb the normal nutrition and lubrication processes of the joint and cause destruction of the articular cartilage. People with degenerative joint disease should be referred for physical therapy; nonsteroidal anti-inflammatory drugs can be used to manage associated pain.

4. **Thoracolumbar syndrome** includes anterior abdominal and lateral hip pain referred from the thoracolumbar area and is caused by hypermobility at the thoracolumbar junction in patients who have had a lumbar fusion. The pain resolves with stabilization exercises and use of anti-inflammatory agents and cold compresses.

5. **Peripheral entrapment neuropathies** can be associated with mechanical impingement of neural tissue, usually by the surrounding musculoskeletal tissue. The abdominal muscles are commonly associated with entrapment sites of the ilioinguinal and iliohypogastric nerves. Poor posture, trauma, and surgery can create fibrous tissue or muscle length changes and cause an entrapment neuropathy. More commonly, surgical resection of the nerve with neuroma formation is a cause of an ilioinguinal or iliohypogastric neuropathy. The obturator nerve as it enters and exits the obturator foramen is closely related to the abdominal musculature and the obturator internus. Tension in these muscles can potentially contribute to entrapment of the obturator nerve with subsequent pain in the groin and anterior thigh. Similarly, the genitofemoral, ilioinguinal, and iliohypogastric nerves all lie in close proximity to the iliopsoas muscle.

   Nerve blocks can provide temporary relief or diagnostic information. If there is anatomic distortion or compromise, **transcutaneous neurolysis** can then be performed. When mechanical stretching of a given nerve is thought to be the cause of the pain, **myofascial release techniques** directed at the involved tissues may alleviate the pain.

6. **Levator ani syndrome** can be diagnosed when a patient has chronic or recurrent rectal or vaginal pain, aching, or dyspareunia in the absence of another explanation for their pain. It is thought to be caused by spastic pelvic floor muscles. Pain is usually reproduced by palpating the pelvic floor during a rectal or vaginal examination. Patients generally describe the pain as an ache or feeling of stool in the rectum that is worse when they sit, and the discomfort may be relieved by the application of heat. Muscle relaxants may be of use temporarily; however, the mainstay of treatment is manual massage by a physical therapist along with use of relaxation methods.

7. **Myofascial pain syndrome** is a disorder of the muscles characterized by the presence of trigger points that, when stimulated, give rise to localized pain, a referred pain in an area away from the anatomic location, or both. Trauma leads to formation of trigger points in the muscle, which stimulate the CNS to produce local referred pain or pelvic pain. In addition, visceral disease can produce hyperalgesia in a dermatomal distribution.

To diagnose a myofascial pain syndrome, a physical examination directed toward eliciting trigger points and evidence of cutaneous hyperalgesia is important. Cutaneous hyperalgesia of the abdominal wall can be assessed by pinching the skin of each dermatome and comparing the sensation with that of the contralateral dermatome. Trigger points can be assessed by applying single fingertip pressure to each abdominal wall dermatome to reproduce the patient's symptoms. Careful palpation of the vulva, vagina, cervix, paracervical tissue, and dorsal sacral area should be carried out in a similar fashion.

Treatment is based on the concept that pain is a symptom complex of reflex mechanisms provoked by trigger points. Once initiated, it is perpetuated by self-exciting chains of internuncial neurons in the CNS. One method of eliminating trigger points entails penetrating the trigger point with a needle with or without injection of lidocaine or saline. The second technique consists of "stretching and spraying" the muscle affected by the trigger point.

IV. **Evaluation**

A. **History.** The goal of taking a complete history is twofold: to understand the patient's problem in search of a diagnosis and to establish a physician-patient relationship. Questionnaires can help patients express feelings and concerns that they might not feel comfortable verbalizing in an interview. All post–surgical operation notes and pathology reports are important, as well as the patient's understanding of these events. The intensity, location, and distribution of the pain must be characterized. In addition, the onset and duration of the pain as well as any associated events (i.e., menses or intercourse) and factors that relieve or worsen the pain should be understood. A complete history should include a review of GI, urologic, and musculoskeletal systems and their possible relationship to the patient's pain. The possibility of physical or sexual abuse as well as domestic discord, parental loss, divorce and other psychosocial stresses should be explored. The internalization of stress as physical symptoms is called **somatization disorder.** Finally, the patient's mental health history should be assessed. Depression or other mood disorders can compound the physical pain experienced by the patient and complicate the diagnosis and management of CPP.

B. **Physical examination.** The patient should be fully informed as to what will take place, which will promote her cooperation and comfort. The physical examination should begin with a general physical and a neurologic assessment. The patient should be asked to indicate where her pain is located. Generally, if she uses a single finger to indicate the location, it is more likely that the pain has a discrete source than if she uses a broad, sweeping motion of the whole hand. When the abdomen is examined, the presence of scars or hernias must be noted. An attempt should be made to elicit **trigger points,** which are hyperirritant spots within a taut band of a muscle or the muscle's fascia. Trigger points are areas overlying muscles that induce spasm or pain. Alterations in the patient's musculoskeletal system can be evaluated by viewing the spine while the patient sits, stands, walks, and bends at the waist (with a check for scoliosis). A thorough neurologic examination including evaluation of sensation, muscle strength, and reflexes should be performed.

In addition to performing a complete gynecologic examination, the physician should pay close attention to pain reproduction during the physical examination. Systematic palpation of the external genitalia can be facilitated with a cotton-tipped swab, as hyperesthesia may be present despite normal-appearing vulvar skin.

Internal discomfort may be exacerbated by insertion of a speculum or the examining hand. Trigger points in the myofascial layers of the pelvic side wall or floor may be elicited. The obturator internus and levator ani muscles are common sites of these trigger points and should be palpated. Sometimes palpation of a specific organ can reproduce a patient's pain; however, this does not mean that removal of that organ will provide relief. **Conscious pain mapping** is a new technique for assessing patients with CPP. It is performed by microlaparoscopy in the office under local anesthesia. The pelvis is systematically inspected and the major structures are probed or grasped in a standard fashion. Patients are asked to rate the pain on a scale of 1 to 10.

C. **Laboratory studies** should be tailored to the individual patient. If the patient's history or physical examination indicates the need for cultures, serum chemistry analysis, or electrolyte measurement, they should be performed. Erythrocyte sedimentation rate should be measured if a chronic disease state is suspected.

D. **Diagnostic studies** should be tailored to the patient's symptoms and presumptive diagnoses. Ultrasonography and other imaging studies are not always necessary and should be used to supplement an inadequate or inconclusive examination. MRI may be helpful when considering peripheral vascular insufficiency. Depression and sleep disorders are common in patients with CPP and can complicate diagnosis and treatment. Although psychological factors should be explored, their presence does not rule out an organic cause for the pain. In addition, if the patient feels that her physician thinks her pain is "all in her head," this can be frustrating to her and can disrupt the physician-patient relationship. The Beck Depression Inventory is useful as a screening test for depression. In selected cases, a diagnostic laparoscopy may aid in the evaluation and treatment of these patients. Laparoscopy is most helpful when the pelvic examination is abnormal or initial therapy fails.

E. **Consultations.** The patient's symptoms may necessitate a consultation with other specialists such as anesthesiologists, orthopedists, neurologists, gastroenterologists, interventional radiologists, clinical psychologists, or physical medicine specialists.

V. **Principles of pain management.** It is generally accepted that patients with CPP represent a complex and challenging group of patients to treat. Frequently solutions to the patient's problem are not easily found, and this can be frustrating to both the clinician and the patient. The goal of the integrated approach to treating these patients, as described by J. F. Steege, is to (1) understand the interactions among disease states, physical sensations, and psychological processes that exist in a given patient and (2) understand how the pain problem started and evolved into its present condition in each of these three dimensions. The fact that it is an integrated approach does not necessarily mean that it is a multispecialty approach. The treatment of a given patient may be carried out by one clinician or by several, depending on the patient and the complexity of her problem, but a single physician should be involved in coordinating the overall flow.

The management of CPP has several components.

A. **Patient education.** Given that there are so many possible causes of pelvic pain, these should be explained to the patient, if possible with family members present. A patient's pain over time can affect other family members and alter interpersonal dynamics. Therefore, the importance of involving family and close friends, especially the spouse, in the treatment process cannot be overemphasized.

As the potential causes of CPP are many, a list should be made of the possible causes for a given patient's pain and the patient should be given a copy. Generally, "physical" causes are more readily accepted by patients. Discussing a patient's mood or other psychosocial factors is important but may be best accomplished after a rapport has been established. Once the physician and patient have decided together which are the most likely causes of the patient's pain, they can decide together which treatment options would be the most important and cost effective to try. This approach not only empowers the patient, it also helps the patient and her family to understand that working through the treatment of different components of the pain takes time. Scheduling regular appointments, instead of asking the patient to call if the pain continues, also aids in this process.

B. **Medications.** The patient and her family should be taught that analgesics usually will partially alleviate the pain instead of providing complete relief. In addition, these medications should be taken on a regular basis, not as needed. This regimen provides the greatest degree of pain relief over time. This method of taking medication is called **noncontingent** scheduling. Taking the medication is not contingent on voicing a complaint of pain and then receiving medication. Such behavior tends to reinforce the patient's disability to both the patient and her family. Noncontingent scheduling removes the patient's family from the role of having to acknowledge her pain, which can be reinforcing.

   1. **Analgesics**
      a. **Nonnarcotic.** Commonly used medications include ibuprofen, 400 mg q4–6h, 600 mg q6–8h, or 800 mg q8–12h. Long-term use can result in GI toxicity such as ulceration. Naproxen (Naprosyn), 250–500 mg twice daily, and nabumetone, 1000 mg daily, have a side-effect profile similar to that of nonsteroidal anti-inflammatory drugs; the incidence of GI ulceration is lower and the most common side effect is diarrhea or dyspepsia.
      b. **Narcotic.** The judicious use of narcotics is reasonable and can greatly improve a patient's ability to function. Commonly used medications include hydrocodone, 5–10 mg q6–8h, with acetaminophenoxycodone hydrochloride, 5 mg with 325 mg acetaminophen (Percocet) q6–8h; oxycodone (OxyContin), 10–40 mg q12h; or Tylenol No. 3 (acetaminophen), one to two tablets q6–8h. Side effects of these medications include lightheadedness, dizziness, sedation, nausea, and constipation. When narcotics are used, it is advisable to sign a joint letter indicating the risks and benefits.
   2. **Antidepressants.** Low-dose tricyclic antidepressants have been the mainstay of chronic pain management for decades. The mechanism of action is thought to be alteration of the pain threshold of a person with chronic pain. Treatment with antidepressants is clinically reasonable, especially when there are signs of depression. Amitriptyline hydrochloride, 50 or 75 mg, at bedtime is commonly used. Side effects include constipation and morning drowsiness.
   3. **Organ-specific medications.** Muscular problems such as levator ani spasm, piriformis muscle spasm, and vaginismus are best treated with physical therapy, as the sedative side effects from muscle relaxants limit their use. Many causes of CPP can have a negative impact on sexual function and sexual response may be diminished, with the development of new discomfort due to insufficient vaginal lubrication. Sometimes,

the response progresses to the point at which levator or introital muscular spasm takes place with the ensuing problem of vaginismus. Therapeutic measures to manage this part of the problem can include supplemental vaginal lubrication with an agent such as KY jelly or Astroglide, or change in sexual position.

C. **Physical therapy.** Some physical therapists are skilled and knowledgeable about pelvic floor musculoskeletal function and can be very helpful in evaluating and treating problems originating from pelvic floor structures. Ideally, the physical therapist will collaborate and communicate frequently with the clinician to ensure that all aspects of the pain are addressed. Tools frequently used by physical therapists include **transcutaneous electric nerve stimulation** and **biofeedback.** Transcutaneous electric nerve stimulation units are generally used to treat somatic pain that is located in a well-defined anatomic area. **Massage therapy** has been successful for patients who have musculoskeletal problems. With regard to pelvic pain specifically, it is efficacious because the levator plate can be massaged transvaginally. Some clinicians also feel that **acupuncture** can be beneficial for these patients.

D. **Psychotherapy.** The discussion of emotional issues at the beginning of the discussion of the pain problem conveys to the patient that her emotional and psychological well-being are an integral part of the evaluation and management of the problem. Should a mental health evaluation be warranted, it should be included on the list the physician and patient have created. As with a physical therapist, there should be frequent communication between the mental health worker and the primary care provider. Those with a history of sexual or physical abuse should be offered psychological counseling regardless of how much this abuse is thought to contribute to the given patient's pelvic pain syndrome.

In addition to participating in the evaluation, mental health workers can also help the patient and family to cope with some of the needs that may arise in patients with CPP. Marital and family therapy may have a pivotal role in the treatment of women with CPP, as family dynamics and interpersonal relationship are often altered.

27. UROGYNECOLOGY AND RECONSTRUCTIVE PELVIC SURGERY

Lara Burrows and Geoffrey W. Cundiff

I. **Introduction.** A urogynecologist and reconstructive pelvic surgeon are involved in the management of women with complex benign pelvic conditions, lower urinary tract disorders, and pelvic floor dysfunction.

II. **Urinary incontinence** is the involuntary loss of urine that is objectively demonstrable and is a social or hygienic problem.

  A. **Etiology of urinary incontinence**

    1. **Genuine stress incontinence (GSI)** is the most common type of urinary incontinence among ambulatory incontinent women, accounting for 50–70% of cases. GSI occurs when the bladder neck and urethra fail to maintain a watertight seal under conditions of increased abdominal pressure (such as coughing, sneezing, and laughing) or even at rest. Most commonly, GSI occurs due to loss of integrity of the musculofascial attachments that support the bladder neck and urethra. This compromises the backboard against which the urethrovesical junction (UVJ) is compressed during increases in intra-abdominal pressure. This type of GSI is often referred to as **urethral hypermobility,** as the UVJ is unsupported and rotates in a posterior and inferior direction with increased abdominal pressure. The hypermobility and descent of these structures under conditions of increased intra-abdominal pressure leads to impaired pressure transmission to the urethra with resultant incontinence of urine. GSI can also occur due to **intrinsic sphincter deficiency** (ISD), which is sometimes called **low-pressure urethra** or **type III incontinence.** In this condition, the sphincteric mechanism is compromised and fails to close the UVJ. These patients are unable to maintain a watertight seal even at rest. They are often severely incontinent and can leak urine with minimal exertion. ISD can occur with or without urethral hypermobility.

    2. **Urge incontinence** is incontinence in which loss of urine is associated with the urge to void. This refers to symptoms of frequency (defined as more than eight voids per day) and urgency with or without urge incontinence. Some women have only frequency or urgency and do not experience urinary incontinence. Recent studies suggest that this may be a less severe variant of the same condition that causes urge incontinence. This has led to the use of the term **overactive bladder** (OAB), which is defined as urgency or frequency with or without urge incontinence. OAB often results from inappropriate contraction of the detrusor muscle. These involuntary contractions can be demonstrated on cystometrogram during urodynamic testing and are referred to as detrusor instability (DI). DI is a urodynamic diagnosis, whereas OAB is a diagnosis based on symptoms. The term **detrusor instability,** also referred to as **unstable bladder,** has been used interchangeably with the term **urge incontinence.** Unstable detrusor contractions may be asymptomatic or they may elicit feelings of urgency, frequency, or both, and urge incontinence. **Detrusor hyperreflexia** is detrusor instability that is attributable to a neurologic disturbance. **Detrusor overactivity** is the preferred term for both DI and detrusor hyperreflexia. Estimates of the prevalence of detrusor instability range from 38% to 61% of institutionalized elderly women. **Nocturia** is defined as being awakened from sleep with the urge to urinate more than two times per night.

Patients may or may not experience enuresis or urge incontinence on the way to the bathroom.

3. **Mixed incontinence** is used to describe symptoms of both stress and urge incontinence. The diagnosis of mixed incontinence refers to the presence of GSI and OAB. Fifty percent to 60% of patients have symptoms of mixed urinary incontinence. Detrusor abnormalities and mixed incontinence are more common in younger ambulatory women, occurring in 29–61% of cases of incontinence. Approximately 30% of women with mixed incontinence become dry after nonsurgical therapy alone.

4. **Detrusor sphincter dyssynergia.** Normal voiding requires coordinated relaxation of the urethral sphincter during contraction of the detrusor muscle. Failure of this coordination is referred to as *detrusor sphincter dyssynergia.* This may be caused by a high spinal cord lesion or inability to relax the pelvic floor musculature. It can present similarly to overflow incontinence.

5. **Overflow incontinence** is the involuntary loss of urine associated with overdistension of the bladder due either to outlet obstruction or to bladder atonicity. This condition is frequently associated with diabetes, neurologic diseases, severe genital prolapse, or postsurgical obstruction. Patients have high postvoid residuals as well as unconscious urinary incontinence.

6. **Functional incontinence** is associated with cognitive, psychological, or physical impairments that make it difficult to reach the toilet or interfere with appropriate toileting. Examples include limitations of mobility, presence in an unfamiliar setting, joint abnormalities, muscle weakness, or a urinary tract infection. These impairments do not cause incontinence directly but prevent normal compensatory mechanisms from countering mild insults to the continence mechanism. A useful mnemonic to remember the possible causes of urinary incontinence is **DIAPPERS: D**elirium, **I**nfection, **P**harmacology, **P**sychology, **E**ndocrinopathy, **R**estricted mobility, **S**tool impaction.

7. **Bypass continence mechanisms** include the presence of a **urinary fistula,** an ectopic ureter, or a **urinary diverticulum.**

B. **Risk factors** for the development of urinary incontinence include the following.

1. **Gender.** Urinary incontinence is two to three times more common in women than in men.

2. **Race.** There is literature to suggest differences in the frequency of different causes of incontinence, with a higher proportion of incontinence attributable to OAB in African-American women than in white women.

3. **Age.** The prevalence of urinary incontinence increases with age. Bladder capacity, ability to postpone voiding, bladder compliance, and urinary flow rate decrease with age in both sexes. In addition, although younger people excrete most of their ingested fluid before bedtime, this pattern reverses with age. One or two episodes of nocturia per night may be normal in older women; however, urinary dysfunctions such as frequency, urgency, and incontinence are not a normal result of aging, even though urinary symptoms are found in over half of institutionalized elderly people.

4. **Hypoestrogenism.** Estrogen deficiency can result in urogenital atrophy with resultant changes in the urogenital epithelium, including thinning of the submucosa and decrease in the functional urethral length. At the same time, randomized trials have shown no association between estrogen deficiency and urinary incontinence.

5. **Parity.** There is a higher incidence of urinary incontinence in parous women than in nulliparous women. Stress incontinence has an especially high association with parity, whereas the incidence of OAB is higher with nulliparity.

6. **Childbirth.** Damage to the pelvic tissues during a vaginal delivery is thought to be a key factor in the development of stress urinary incontinence and other pelvic support abnormalities. Women who have undergone cesarean deliveries have greater pelvic muscle strength during and after the postpartum period than women who delivered vaginally. Nevertheless, cesarean section has not been shown to be protective, and pregnancy in and of itself may be detrimental to the pelvic floor, regardless of the route of delivery. Vaginal deliveries can cause nerve damage due to stretch injury or compression. Vaginal delivery has been shown to lead to prolongation of nerve conduction in the pelvic floor, although this resolves in approximately 80% of women.

7. **Neuromuscular injury** to the pelvic floor due to chronic straining from constipation or heavy lifting or lumbar disk disease has been associated with urinary incontinence.

8. **Underlying medical conditions** with resultant increases in intra-abdominal pressure such as obesity and chronic obstructive pulmonary disease with coughing are risk factors for stress urinary incontinence.

9. **Prior pelvic surgery** with resultant scar formation can alter the function of certain structures such as the urethral sphincter.

10. **Pharmacologic agents** such as diuretics, caffeine, anticholinergics, and alpha-adrenergic blockers can affect urinary tract function.

C. **Evaluation of urinary incontinence**

1. **Medical history.** In addition to taking a thorough medical, surgical, gynecologic, and obstetric history, the clinician should gain an understanding of the duration, frequency, and severity of the patient's symptoms. The clinical type and severity of urinary incontinence as well as how much fluid the patient drinks per day should be established. The patient's mobility and living environment should be assessed. A complete list of the patient's medications should be obtained. A history of any previous therapies should be elicited as well.

2. **Urinary diary.** The patient records the volume and frequency of fluid intake and voiding as well as symptoms of frequency and urgency and episodes of incontinence for a period of 1–7 days.

3. **Physical examination.** A comprehensive physical examination should be performed at the first visit. As urinary incontinence may be the presenting symptom of neurologic disease, a screening neurologic examination to evaluate mental status and sensory and motor function of the lower extremities should be performed. A mental status examination aids in the evaluation of functional incontinence. In addition, sacral nerve roots and the **sacral reflex** (also called the **bulbocavernosus reflex**) should be evaluated. If the sacral reflex is intact, then, when the labia are scratched, there should be an ipsilateral contraction of the anal sphincter. If this reflex is present, it signifies that afferent and efferent pathways are intact. In older patients, this reflex may be absent even though the patient is neurologically intact. This does not mean that there is a neurologic basis for the patient's incontinence.

The pelvic examination is an important part of the evaluation, and particular attention should be given to urethral anatomy, overall support, tender areas, estrogen status, and the presence of scarring. The speculum examination is helpful to assess estrogen status and the presence of scarring. A Sims or broken speculum permits evaluation of the apical, posterior, and anterior support individually. The International Continence Society and the National Institutes of Health recommend the Pelvic Organ Prolapse Quantitation system of grading support defects, but other staging systems are in common use. Which system is used is not as important as using a consistent system to document support defects. The **Q-tip test** should be performed to evaluate urethral support. In this test, a cotton swab is placed in the urethra to the level of the vesical neck, and the change in axis on straining is measured with a goniometer to assess urethral hypermobility. Angular measurements of more than 30 degrees are generally considered abnormal. The strength of the pelvic diaphragm should be assessed by asking the patient to squeeze as if she were trying to prevent flatus. This is performed on bimanual examination by placing one or two fingers in the vagina and asking the patient to squeeze. A rectal examination can further assess pelvic pathology as well as evaluate the presence of fecal impaction, which may be associated with voiding dysfunction. A positive result on a **stress test** is essential to the diagnosis of GSI. The stress test is performed by looking for urine leakage from the urethral meatus when abdominal pressure is increased.

4. **Diagnostic tests.** Urinary tract infection should be ruled out in all patients either by urine culture, urinalysis, or microscopic evaluation of the urine; this is especially important in the elderly, as a urinary tract infection can cause or contribute to the patient's symptoms. Measurement of postvoid residual can aid in diagnosing overflow incontinence and eliminating it from the differential diagnosis.

  a. **Urodynamic studies** are a group of tests that assess the physiologic function of the bladder. The tests evaluate the three functions of the lower urinary tract: bladder filling, urethral closure, and bladder emptying. This is accomplished by measuring pressure within the bladder, urethra, and abdominal cavity during maneuvers that reproduce normal physiologic function. In addition to the three measured pressures, two pressures are calculated by subtraction. **Detrusor pressure** represents the pressure generated by contraction of the detrusor muscle itself and is calculated by subtracting abdominal pressure from the vesicular pressure. **Urethral closure pressure** represents the vesical pressure that must be exceeded to overcome urethral pressure and cause incontinence. It is calculated as the bladder pressure subtracted from the urethral pressure.

    The different components of bladder function are investigated by different urodynamics tests.

    (1) **Bladder filling.** Urethrocystometry evaluates filling of the bladder. The pressures are measured during sequential filling of the bladder. Measured parameters include the volume of first sensation, volume of initial urge to void, and maximum capacity, as well as bladder compliance.

    (2) **Urethral function.** Urethral function is evaluated with several tests. In urethral pressure profilometry, a pressure transducer is pulled through the urethra at a fixed rate, providing a sequential graph of pressure variations across the length of the urethra. There is normally a rise in pressure in the functional part of the urethra (functional urethral length is 3–4 cm). Values of less than 20 cm H_2O have been shown to indicate a weak sphincter. This test has become less popular in recent years due to questions about the reproducibility of the results.

    (3) **Bladder emptying.** Uroflowmetry evaluates voiding by measuring the urine volume voided over time. The patient voids on a special commode and urine is funneled into a flowmeter that records the voided volume versus time. The maximum flow rate should be at least 20 mL/second, and the patient should finish voiding in less than 40 seconds. In healthy patients, the postvoid residual should be less than 50 mL. The indications for urodynamic testing are listed in Table 27-1.

  b. **Cystourethroscopy.** Just as urodynamic testing provides a physiologic evaluation of the bladder, cystourethroscopy is used to assess the anatomy of the lower urinary tract.

TABLE 27-1. INDICATIONS FOR URODYNAMIC STUDIES

Failed previous surgical therapy

Abnormal neurologic examination

Immobile urethrovesical junction

Severe or continuous incontinence

Urinary retention

Unexplained incontinence

Failed conservative therapy

D. **Treatment**
  1. **Nonsurgical**
     a. **Pharmacologic**
        (1) **Medications for OAB** include anticholinergics and tricyclic antidepressants. Anticholinergic agents inhibit involuntary detrusor contractions. **Oxybutynin chloride** is an anticholinergic with antispasmodic properties. Although oxybutynin is also associated with a high incidence of side effects, recent extended-release versions have better side-effect profiles. Another new anticholinergic, **tolterodine tartrate,** is a competitive muscarinic receptor antagonist. It is far more selective for muscarinic receptors in the bladder and is better tolerated. The most common side effects include constipation and dry mouth. Tricyclic antidepressants can also be used, for example, **imipramine** 12.5–25.0 mg orally two or three times per day. This medication improves bladder hypertonicity and compliance. Drugs and dosages are listed in Table 27-2.
        (2) The limited available **medications for stress urinary incontinence** are aimed toward increasing urogenital sphincter tone. In women with a urinary tract atrophy, combining **estrogen** with an alpha-sympathetic agonist can produce an additive effect in the treatment of stress urinary incontinence. **Imipramine** can improve symptoms in some women with stress urinary incontinence.
     b. **Behavioral**
        (1) **Bladder retraining drills** are a program of scheduled voiding with progressive increases in the interval between voids. Therapy is based on the assumption that conscious efforts to suppress sensory stimuli will reestablish cortical control over an uninhibited bladder and thus reestablish a normal voiding pattern.

TABLE 27-2. PHARMACOLOGIC TREATMENT OF URINARY INCONTINENCE

Medication	Dosage
Tolterodine tartrate	2 mg PO bid
Propantheline bromide	1–30 mg PO tid or qid
Oxybutynin chloride	5 mg tid
Oxybutynin chloride extended release	5–10 PO q day
Imipramine	10–20 mg PO q day

(2) **Biofeedback** is a form of patient reeducation in which a closed feedback loop is created so that one or more of the patient's normally unconscious physiologic processes is made accessible to her by auditory, visual, or tactile signals. While the bladder is being filled, the patient visualizes the urodynamic tracing and attempts to inhibit detrusor contractions.

(3) **Functional electrical stimulation** works by stimulating the afferent limb of the pudendal reflex arc, which results in an increase in pelvic floor and urethral striated muscle contractility.

(4) **Sacral nerve root stimulation** is indicated for patients with urinary retention or urgency and frequency syndromes not responsive to other forms of therapy. An implanted neurostimulation system delivers small electrical impulses to the appropriate sacral nerve that controls bladder function.

2. **Surgical**

   a. **Procedures to treat genuine stress urinary incontinence**

      (1) **Intraurethral bulk injections** are best used in patients with urinary incontinence secondary to a poorly functioning urethral sphincter (ISD) in the absence of urethral hypermobility. The mechanism of action of intraurethral injections is to coapt the urethral lumen at the bladder neck and re-create normal sphincteric competence. Injectable materials include collagen, polytetrafluoroethylene, autologous fat, and silicone. Complications include transient urinary retention and irritative voiding symptoms; 5% of patients develop urinary tract infections.

      (2) **Retropubic urethropexy procedures** are indicated for women with the diagnosis of GSI and a hypermobile proximal urethra and bladder neck. In the **Burch** procedure, sutures are placed in the periurethral fascia lateral to and on each side of the bladder neck and proximal urethra, and the UVJ is elevated by attaching the suture to Cooper's ligament. The 5-year success rate is 85–90%. The **Marshall-Marchetti-Krantz** procedure is less popular. This operation is similar to the Burch procedure, except that the sutures are attached to the symphysis pubis. The most common postoperative complication is urinary retention. Frequently these patients need to learn **intermittent self-catheterization** before going home. Other less common postoperative complications include urinary tract infections and detrusor instability.

      (3) **Sling procedures** are performed to support the urethra or bladder neck in a hammock that provides static stabilization of the urethra at rest and dynamic compression of the urethra with increased abdominal pressure. A sling procedure has traditionally been recommended for patients with stress urinary incontinence caused by ISD or failure of the urethral sphincter to maintain a watertight seal. Suburethral slings can be created using a variety of materials, including fascia lata, rectus fascia, cadaveric fascia, or AlloDerm.

      (4) **Tension-free vaginal tape procedures.** In this type of suburethral sling procedure, polypropylene mesh is placed at the *distal* urethra. This procedure is one of the newest for treating genuine stress urinary incontinence.

   b. **Procedures to restore urinary continence. Urethrolysis** can be performed after bladder neck surgery that has resulted in voiding dysfunction and urinary retention. These symptoms are generally attributable to obstruction. After conservative therapy with intermittent self-catheterization has failed, transvaginal or transabdominal urethrolysis may be performed.

c. **Other procedures for treating urinary incontinence**
   (1) **Artificial urinary sphincters** are rarely used for severe stress incontinence secondary to urethral damage.
   (2) **Augmentation cystoplasty** has been used for resistant cases of DI. The bladder is bisected almost completely and a patch of gut, usually ileum, is sewn in place. This operation often cures the symptoms of DI but results in inefficient voiding.
   (3) **Urinary diversion via an ileal conduit** may be considered for women with severe DI or hyperreflexia in whom all other methods of treatment have failed. This treatment may be especially helpful for young disabled women with severe neurologic dysfunction.

III. **Urinary diverticulum.** A suburethral diverticulum is a fluid-filled mass along the anterior portion of the vagina that has a direct communication with the urethra. The cause is usually infection of a furuncle in a urethral gland. Other causes include birth trauma, instrumentation injury, and urethral stones. Suburethral diverticula are not common and can easily be overlooked; therefore, a high index of suspicion is important. Patients usually have vague complaints. They experience dysuria and dyspareunia, leak frequently, have some urgency, and have recurrent urinary tract infections. Some patients complain of a tender vaginal mass. On examination, one-third of patients have a suburethral mass, which is diagnostic. Sometimes, pus can be expressed from the mass via the urethral orifice. Other means of diagnosing a suburethral diverticulum are positive-pressure urethrography and cystourethroscopy. Treatment is usually surgical. The most common operation is a diverticulectomy. If the diverticulum is located in the proximal urethra near the bladder neck, a partial ablation is usually performed to minimize the risk of damaging the bladder neck and urethral sphincter.

IV. **Fistulas.** Urinary fistulas are rare. In the United States, gynecologic surgery is the most common cause of a urogenital fistula. They are a complication in 0.1% of hysterectomies. Radiation therapy is another cause. In Third World countries, obstetric injuries are the most common cause, usually resulting from operative deliveries. The common history of a patient who has a fistula is painless and continuous vaginal leakage of urine, usually within the context of recent pelvic surgery. Instillation of methylene blue dye into the bladder will stain a vaginal pack if a **vesicovaginal fistula** is present, and such staining is diagnostic. Cystourethroscopy should be performed to determine the site and number of fistulas. Most posthysterectomy vesicovaginal fistulas are located anterior to the vaginal vault. IVP should be performed to locate a **ureterovaginal fistula.**

Postsurgical fistulas are usually repaired 3–6 months after diagnosis to allow inflammation to resolve and to attain optimal tissue vascularity. To repair a vesicovaginal fistula, the **Latzko operation** is the most commonly used. In this operation, a 1.5- to 2.0-cm area around the vaginal opening of the fistula is denuded of vaginal mucosa. The fistula is then closed with interrupted sutures in multiple layers.

The treatment of a ureterovaginal fistula depends on its location. If it is close to the UVJ, a **ureteroneocystostomy** can be performed, in which the ureter proximal to the fistula is implanted into the bladder. If the fistula is several centimeters from the bladder, a bladder hitch or a segment of ileum may be interposed between the proximal ureter and the bladder. Small fistulas occasionally may close after placement of a ureteric stent.

V. **Fecal incontinence**
   A. **Etiology of anal incontinence**
      1. **Congenital anomalies** are only rarely the cause of fecal incontinence. One in 5000 newborn girls who have an imperforate anus can have associated fecal incontinence through a congenital rectovaginal or retroperitoneal fistula.

2. **Trauma.** By far, the most common type of trauma leading to fecal incontinence is obstetric injury to the pelvic floor. Forceps deliveries are particularly likely to result in sphincter defects. In addition, even after a successful anatomic repair of the anal sphincter, denervation injury to the sphincter muscle may cause persistent incontinence. Fecal incontinence may also result from the trauma of operative procedures such as a posterior repair or extensive vulvectomy for cancer.

3. **Acquired factors.** The most common cause of fecal incontinence is fecal impaction with overflow incontinence. In addition, 40–60% of patients with rectal prolapse have fecal incontinence.

4. **Colorectal diseases.** Inflammatory bowel diseases, particularly Crohn's disease and subsequent fistula formation, have been associated with fecal incontinence. Malignant tumors that involve the rectovaginal septum and subsequently are irradiated can also create a fistula that leads to incontinence.

5. **Aging.** The normal aging process results in decreased efficiency of the sphincter. With increasing age, the sphincter generates a lower pressure and the proportion of fibrous tissue increases. Older age is also associated with increasing pudendal nerve terminal motor latencies and increased rectal and anal sensory thresholds.

6. **Idiopathy.** Fecal incontinence may be idiopathic in approximately 10% of women.

B. **Evaluation**

1. **History.** The evaluation of a patient with fecal incontinence begins with a thorough history taking. The clinician must ascertain the effects of incontinence on the patient's daily life. Pertinent issues to be addressed include duration of the problem, frequency of incontinence, time of day of incontinent episodes, quality of stool lost (i.e., liquid versus solid), the ability to control flatus, frequency of bowel movements, and problems with constipation or diarrhea. It is important to ensure that the patient distinguishes between diarrhea and fecal incontinence. In addition, it is important to identify the quality of the material being lost, as flatus is more difficult to control than liquid stool, and solid stool is the most easily controlled. Finally, the clinician should obtain a thorough obstetric history, including the number of vaginal deliveries, the use of forceps in delivery, and previous episiotomy or perineal tears.

2. **Physical examination** begins with inspection of the anal area for evidence of skin irritation or stool on the skin. One should also note the presence of gaping muscles or scarring. The patient should be asked to squeeze and simulate holding in a bowel movement so that the examiner can look for uniform, circular contraction of muscle. Asking the patient to strain may show perineal descent or prolapsing hemorrhoids. The **anocutaneous** reflex should be evaluated. This is done by rubbing the perianal skin gently with a cotton swab and looking for reflex contraction of the anal sphincter. This procedure gives a general assessment of sphincter innervation. The sphincter should be palpated with a digital examination; the initial tone should be noted and the patient should be asked to squeeze as if holding a bowel movement. Strength, defects in the muscle, and the length of time the patient is able to maintain the contraction are assessed.

C. **Diagnostic techniques**

1. **Enema.** Approximately 100 mL of tap water is given. The clinician notes whether the patient can hold this for more than a few minutes. If the patient can hold a tap water enema, she probably does not have significant incontinence.

2. **Anal manometry** provides quantitative information regarding the resting and squeeze pressures of the sphincter muscles. Resting pressures reflect the constant tone of the internal sphincter muscle.

Squeeze pressures reflect the pressure generated by the external sphincter muscle. Normal findings do not exclude incontinence.

3. **Rectal compliance testing.** Rectal compliance can be determined by inserting a balloon and determining the minimal volume the rectum can sense, then progressively inflating the balloon to a volume that cannot be tolerated.

4. **Electromyography** is used to study the innervation of the external sphincter complex and to examine for the reinnervation seen in pelvic neuropathy.

5. **Pudendal nerve terminal motor latency** can be determined using an electrode attached to a glove inserted into the anal canal. A prolonged conduction in the pudendal nerve may signal damage to the innervation of the external sphincter and puborectalis muscle.

6. **Defecography** is indicated if rectal prolapse or internal intussusception is suspected.

7. **Anoscopy, proctoscopy, sigmoidoscopy, or colonoscopy** is appropriate for patients who have diarrhea or bloody stool.

8. **Endosonography.** A probe is inserted into the rectum allowing a 360-degree visualization of the internal and external anal sphincters. This technique allows the clinician to visualize defects in the sphincter muscle that might be surgically correctable.

D. **Treatment**
   1. **Nonsurgical**
      a. **Dietary change.** For patients who do not have severe incontinence, the use of bulking agents, such as psyllium preparations (Metamucil), can change the consistency of stool, making it firmer and more easily controlled.
      b. **Medications.** Agents that slow motility may help some patients exercise more control over their stool. **Loperamide hydrochloride** (Imodium) can be prescribed for this reason. **Diphenoxylate hydrochloride** (Lomotil) can also be used, especially if diarrhea is a contributor to the incontinence.
      c. **Biofeedback** requires a substantial time commitment from the patient as well as a dedicated therapist. A balloon is placed in the rectum to simulate stool. Anal sphincter contraction is measured with another balloon in the rectal canal or by perianal surface electrodes. The final goal is to increase sphincter strength and to teach patients how to sense and respond to smaller volumes of the stool in the rectum. Improvement is seen in 63–90% of patients.
      d. **Pelvic muscle–strengthening exercises.** Although there are no data to support a benefit from these exercises for patients with fecal incontinence, they are safe and cost nothing. These exercises may be helpful to patients who have early fatigability of the sphincter muscle, which can be noted on physical examination when the patient is asked to squeeze.
      e. **Enema.** For some people, daily enemas in the morning and after eating induce bowel motility and facilitate emptying of the rectum.
   2. **Surgical**
      a. **Sphincteroplasty** is performed when there is a defect in the anal sphincter. The two ends of the sphincter muscle are reunited. The ends can be reapproximated, or they can be overlapped.
      b. **Colostomy** is indicated for patients with severe fecal incontinence. An end colostomy sometimes can provide an improvement in quality of life when previous repairs have failed or have little chance of success.
      c. **Muscle transposition** is performed when patients have lost their sphincter muscle or when repair of the sphincter does not relieve their symptoms. Transposition of the gracilis muscle has been used. These operations, when performed by experienced surgeons, can

produce excellent results, especially because the alternative for many patients is a stoma.

d. An **artificial anal sphincter** is indicated for patients in whom conventional management has failed. This is an implantable device containing a balloon that, when fully inflated, occludes the anus.

VI. **Pelvic organ prolapse** can occur when normal pelvic organ supports are chronically subjected to increases in intra-abdominal pressure or when defective genital support gives way under the influence of normal increases in intra-abdominal pressure. (See Chap. 22 for a detailed discussion of pelvic anatomy.)

A. **Anatomic support defects**

1. **Cystocele** is present when there is descent of the anterior vaginal wall. It is generally caused by separation of the paravaginal attachment of the pubocervical fascia from the arcus tendineus fasciae pelvis or tearing of the pubocervical fascia, which results in herniation of the bladder.

2. **Rectocele** is caused by a defect in the rectovaginal septum. This results in herniation of the posterior wall of the vagina and the anterior wall of the rectum, so that they are in direct apposition to vaginal epithelium.

3. **Loss of perineal body integrity** occurs when the perineal body becomes detached from the rectovaginal septum and becomes mobile. Loss of perineal body integrity can lead to an inferior rectocele and perineal descent.

4. **Uterovaginal prolapse** occurs secondary to damage of the cardinal-uterosacral ligament complex and endopelvic fascia that normally support the uterus and upper vagina over the pelvic diaphragm. **Vaginal vault prolapse** refers to descent of the vaginal apex below its normal position in the pelvis after a woman has had a hysterectomy.

5. **Enterocele** is a hernia in which the normal anatomic endopelvic fascia is absent so that small bowel fills the hernia sac and peritoneum is in contact with vaginal mucosa. Enteroceles are the result of separation of the pubocervical and rectovaginal fasciae, which allows a peritoneal sac with its contents to protrude through the fascial defect.

B. **Etiology of pelvic floor damage.** There are several factors that contribute to the development of pelvic organ prolapse. The intrinsic strength of the connective tissue and muscles of the pelvic floor in a given individual, damage that may occur to these structures during childbirth, deterioration with age, and stresses that they are subjected to over the course of a lifetime play a role in the development of pelvic organ prolapse. Heavy lifting, obesity, chronic coughing, and chronic diseases, especially those accompanied by neuropathy, are associated with pelvic organ prolapse. The hypoestrogenic state of menopause is also thought to contribute to the weakening of pelvic tissues. In addition, there seems to be a genetic predisposition to the development of prolapse. For example, whites are more likely to develop prolapse than African-Americans or Asians.

C. **Evaluation**

1. **History.** Patients with vaginal prolapse commonly describe aching in the groin or lower back. This is caused by traction on the uterosacral ligaments. This discomfort typically resolves when the patient lies down. Sometimes, there is ulceration on the vaginal wall. The symptoms of urethral support are generally those of stress urinary incontinence. When patients have defective support of the upper anterior vaginal wall, they often complain of difficulty voiding and a sense of incomplete emptying. Sometimes, these patients report that they must strain or perform a Valsalva maneuver to empty the bladder.

Patients with a rectocele may complain of the sensation of pelvic pressure or the feeling that there is a mass or bulge in the vagina. They may also complain of inability to evacuate the distal rectum without straining or splinting (applying pressure between the vagina and the rectum to elevate the rectocele and facilitate defecation). Unfortunately, as the woman bears down to empty the rectum, stool is pushed into the rectocele, and the harder she strains, the larger the rectocele becomes.

2. **Physical examination.** When a patient with pelvic organ prolapse is being evaluated, there are four "compartments" that should be systematically assessed: the anterior vaginal wall, the uterus and vaginal apex, the posterior vaginal wall, and the presence or absence of an enterocele should be determined. The physical examination should be performed with the patient in the lithotomy position. Pelvic organ prolapse defects are best identified using a Sims speculum or the posterior blade of a Graves speculum. While the other compartments are supported, the patient is asked to strain forcefully or cough vigorously. During this time, descent of the pelvic organs is systematically observed. The **Pelvic Organ Prolapse Quantitation** system is commonly used to quantify the degree of pelvic organ prolapse seen during the physical examination. It describes nine measured segments of a patient's pelvic organ support. The prolapse of each segment is evaluated and measured relative to the hymenal ring, which is a fixed anatomic landmark.

Examination of the anterior vaginal wall should evaluate the support of the urethra and bladder. With the speculum used to depress the posterior vaginal wall, the patient is asked to strain, and any descent of the anterior vaginal wall is observed. Then, ring forceps may be used to support the midline of the anterior vaginal wall and elevate the anterior sulci so that each upper corner of the vagina is supported to the pelvic side wall. This can differentiate between defects caused by tearing of the pubocervical fascia with resultant bladder herniation and defects caused by lateral detachments of the pubocervical fascia from the arcus tendineus fasciae pelvis **(paravaginal defects)**.

As the vagina and cervix are attached to each other, prolapse of the cervix is invariably accompanied by prolapse of the upper vagina, and this is called **uterovaginal prolapse.** The location of the cervix is usually used to gauge the severity of uterine prolapse. Its position in relation to the hymeneal ring should be noted while the prolapse is at its greatest. In patients who have undergone hysterectomy, descent of the vaginal apex is called **vaginal vault prolapse;** when the vagina turns completely inside out, it is called **vaginal eversion.**

The posterior vaginal wall is where rectoceles and enteroceles occur. An enterocele may occur in association with a rectocele. With a speculum retracting the anterior vaginal wall, the posterior wall of the vagina can carefully be inspected. A **rectocele** is present when the anterior rectal wall and overlying vagina protrude below the hymeneal ring on straining. Anterior displacement of the rectal wall on rectovaginal examination is diagnostic. An **enterocele** exists when the cul-de-sac becomes distended with small bowel and causes a bulging of the posterior vaginal wall outward. Anatomically, there is a hernia in which peritoneum is in contact with vaginal mucosa, with the normal intervening endopelvic fascia absent. On examination, small bowel can be palpated between the vagina and rectum during a rectovaginal examination with the patient straining.

Evaluation of the perineum includes determining the presence or absence of perineal descent (descent of the perineum with straining).

3. **Diagnostic studies.** The evaluation of pelvic organ prolapse relies primarily on the clinical examination and Pelvic Organ Prolapse Quantitation staging. If multiple systems are involved, it can be challenging to assess simultaneously the function of the pelvic floor and of the organs it supports. Especially if the patient has defecatory complaints, a **dynamic MRI** can be useful. A **defecating proctogram** (quadruple-

contrast study), which is performed under fluoroscopy, allows visualization of the small bowel, bladder, vagina, and rectum during defecation.

D. **Treatment.** Treatment of prolapse depends on how severe it is, whether or not symptoms are present, and whether or not physiologic complications have arisen that are attributable to the prolapse. The decision to treat medically or surgically depends on the patient's overall state of health as well as the wishes of the patient.

1. **Nonsurgical**

   a. **Hormone replacement therapy.** Estrogen replacement therapy affects postmenopausal urogenital symptoms. Hormone replacement therapy alone will not relieve a patient's prolapse. However, hormone replacement before a surgical repair is performed is beneficial because it promotes vaginal cellular maturation and improves symptoms of atrophy.

   b. **Pelvic muscle exercises.** Because the bladder and other pelvic organs are supported by the levator ani muscles, **Kegel exercises,** which are aimed at improving muscle tone, can alleviate the symptoms of prolapse. After appropriate training, most women are able to contract their levator ani muscles correctly.

   c. **Pessaries** are the oldest effective treatment for prolapse. There are many varieties, but one of the most commonly used for prolapse is the doughnut-shaped pessary. Pessaries are placed in the vagina and are retained above the pelvic floor musculature, which prevents the smaller uterine cervix from passing through the introitus. Having the patient remove the pessary at night minimizes the vaginal discharge that is commonly associated with pessary use. In addition, treatment with estrogen, either locally or systemically, helps the vaginal mucosa tolerate the foreign body. Because pessaries can cause erosion and ulceration, patients should be examined periodically.

2. **Surgical**

   a. **Abdominal**

      (1) **Enterocele repair.** There are three techniques for the abdominal repair of an enterocele. The **Moschcowitz procedure** is performed by placing concentric purse-string sutures around the cul-de-sac, including the posterior vaginal wall, right pelvic side wall, the serosa of the sigmoid, and the left pelvic side wall. The **Halban procedure** obliterates the cul-de-sac using sutures placed sagittally between the uterosacral ligaments. Transverse **plication of the uterosacral ligaments** can also be used to obliterate the cul-de-sac. In all three of these procedures, care must be taken to avoid kinking a ureter.

      (2) **Abdominal sacral colpopexy** is a procedure used to suspend the vagina to the sacral promontory as a treatment for uterovaginal prolapse and vaginal eversion. It is the procedure of choice for patients who have other indications for abdominal surgery. Although many different materials can be used for the graft, synthetic materials such as polypropylene or polytetrafluoroethylene mesh are most commonly used.

      (3) **Paravaginal repair.** This repair is performed for anterior vaginal wall prolapse and can be accomplished using an abdominal (retropubic) or vaginal approach. The presence of concomitant vaginal or abdominal pathology as well as the experience of the surgeon determine which approach is taken. The goal of this repair is to reattach the anterolateral attachments of the vagina, including the overlying endopelvic fascia, to the arcus tendineus fasciae pelvis.

   b. **Vaginal**

      (1) **Transvaginal hysterectomy with or without anteroposterior colporrhaphy** is the operation most commonly performed

for the treatment of uterovaginal prolapse. Each patient has different degrees of prolapse in the anterior and posterior compartments. Should there be significant prolapse in either of these compartments, simply removing the uterus will not correct prolapse of the vaginal walls.

(2) **Anterior colporrhaphy.** The objective of anterior colporrhaphy is to reduce the protrusion of the bladder and vagina. In this procedure, the layers of the vaginal muscularis and adventitia overlying the bladder (pubocervical fascia) are plicated.

(3) **Posterior colporrhaphy** is the plication of the pararectal and rectovaginal fasciae over the rectal wall. In the past, levator plications were frequently performed for the treatment of rectoceles; however, they had a tendency to decrease the caliber of the vagina with subsequent dyspareunia.

(4) **Rectovaginal fascia defect repair** is a procedure in which isolated defects in the rectovaginal fascia are identified and reapproximated, so that normal anatomy is restored.

(5) **Perineorrhaphy** is the identification and reconstruction of the elements of the perineal body.

(6) **Enterocele repair.** In the **McCall culdoplasty** procedure, an enterocele is surgically corrected at the time of a vaginal hysterectomy. The advantage of this procedure is that it not only repairs the enterocele, but it provides apical support for the vagina. Some have recommended performing this procedure with every vaginal hysterectomy to prevent future enterocele formation and vaginal vault prolapse.

(7) **Vaginal vault suspension.** Many techniques have been described to suspend the vagina.

   (a) **Sacrospinous ligament suspension** anchors the vaginal apex to the sacrospinous ligament. Complications of this procedure include hemorrhage, nerve injury, and buttock pain.

   (b) **Iliococcygeus fascia suspension** can be performed in patients who have suboptimal uterosacral ligaments. This procedure entails attaching the vaginal apex to the iliococcygeal fascia just below the ischial spine.

   (c) **High uterosacral ligament suspension with fascial reconstruction** suspends the apex of the vagina to the hollow of the sacrum while reestablishing the continuity of the endopelvic fascia, which restores the integrity of the anterior and posterior vaginal walls.

(8) **Colpocleisis** is performed to obliterate the vagina. A **LeFort partial colpocleisis** is performed to reduce uterovaginal prolapse and apposes the anterior and posterior vaginal walls. It is considered to be an operation of last resort, and the patient should understand that she will not have a functional vagina. Advantages are that the procedure can be performed quickly and under regional anesthesia. This procedure is commonly used in elderly patients who are poor surgical candidates. Other obliterative procedures used for vaginal vault prolapse include **partial colpectomy** and **total colpectomy.**

28. FERTILITY CONTROL

Julia Cron, Katie Todd, and George Huggins

I. **Introduction.** According to the Alan Guttmacher Institute, 64% of the more than 60 million women aged 15–44 in the United States practice contraception. Thirty-one percent of reproductive-age women do not need a method because they are pregnant, postpartum, or trying to become pregnant; have never had intercourse; or are not sexually active. Thus, only 5–7% of women aged 15–44 in need of contraception are not using a method. The 3 million women who use no contraceptive method account for almost half of unintended pregnancies (47%), whereas the 39 million contraceptive users account for 53% (Table 28-1). The majority of unintended pregnancies among contraceptive users result from inconsistent or incorrect use. The most common contraceptive method currently relied on is female sterilization, followed by oral contraceptive pills, male condoms, and male sterilization (Table 28-2).

II. **Contraceptive methods**

  A. **Voluntary sterilization**

    1. **Tubal ligation** is a surgical procedure in which the fallopian tubes are altered, so that sperm is prevented from reaching the ova and causing fertilization. Tubal ligation is the most frequently used method of fertility control. A variety of procedures can be performed to occlude the tube: segmental resection or partial salpingectomy, devascularization, or crush injury (Table 28-3).

      a. **Effectiveness.** Pregnancy rate of 0.5 per 100 women in first year after surgery. The Collaborative Review of Sterilization (CREST) study compared the long-term effectiveness of bipolar coagulation, unipolar coagulation, silicone rubber band application, spring clip application, interval partial salpingectomy, and postpartum partial salpingectomy. Results are shown in Table 28-4.

      b. **Advantages.** Highly effective, no long-term side effects.

      c. **Disadvantages.** Requires a surgical procedure and anesthesia with its associated risks; is permanent; offers no protection against sexually transmitted diseases (STDs); if pregnancy occurs, there is an increased risk of ectopic pregnancy.

    2. **Vasectomy** is a surgical procedure in which the vas deferens is occluded, which prevents sperm from being ejaculated. Up to 20 ejaculations are required before the procedure becomes effective (as judged by two negative results on semen analysis).

      a. **Effectiveness.** Pregnancy rate of 0.10–0.15 per 100 women in the first year after surgery.

      b. **Advantages.** Highly effective, no long-term side effects, less expensive and fewer complications than tubal ligation.

      c. **Disadvantages.** Requires a surgical procedure, is permanent, offers no protection against STDs, is not immediately effective.

  B. **Hormonal contraceptives**

    1. **Combined oral contraceptives** (COCs) consist of synthetic estrogen and progestin preparations that prevent pregnancy by suppressing ovulation, thickening the cervical mucus, and altering the endometrium (Table 28-5). Besides providing contraception, COCs may be used to manage dysmenorrhea, menorrhagia, and metrorrhagia. COC use is not recommended for breast-feeding women until at least 6 months postpartum (see Chap. 20). Non–breast-feeding women should wait 3 weeks postpartum before beginning COC use because of the increased risk of

TABLE 28-1. PERCENTAGE OF WOMEN EXPERIENCING A PREGNANCY WITHIN THE FIRST YEAR OF USE FOR VARIOUS CONTRACEPTIVE METHODS

Method	Perfect use	Average use
No method	85.0	85.0
Periodic abstinence	9.0	25.0
Cervical cap	9.0, 26.0[a]	20.0, 40.0[a]
Spermicide	6.0	26.0
Diaphragm	6.0	20.0
Withdrawal	4.0	19.0
Male condom	3.0	14.0
IUD (Copper T)	0.6	0.8
Tubal sterilization	0.5	0.5
Injectable contraceptive	0.3	0.3
Oral contraceptive	0.1	5.0
Vasectomy	0.10	0.15
Implanted contraceptive	0.05	0.05

[a]Parous women.

Adapted from Hatcher RA, Trussell J, Stewart F, et al. *Contraceptive technology*, rev. 17th ed. New York: Ardent Media, 1998:216.

TABLE 28-2. PERCENTAGE OF WOMEN AGED 15–44 USING PARTICULAR CONTRACEPTIVE METHODS

Method	Percentage of reproductive-age women using method
Female sterilization	25.6
Oral contraceptive	24.9
Male condom	18.9
Male sterilization	10.1
Withdrawal	2.9
Injectable contraceptive	2.7
Periodic abstinence	2.2
Diaphragm	1.7
Implanted contraceptive	1.3
Spermicide	1.3
Intrauterine device	0.7
Other	0.1

Adapted from Hatcher RA, Trussell J, Stewart F, et al. *Contraceptive technology,* rev. 17th ed. New York: Ardent Media, 1998:213.

TABLE 28-3. DIFFERENT METHODS OF TUBAL LIGATION

Occlusion method	Example of method
Segmental resection	Uchida technique
	Parkland technique
	Pomeroy-Prichard technique
	Irving technique
Devascularization	Unipolar coagulation
	Bipolar coagulation
Crush injury	Spring clip (Hulka clip)
	Silastic band (Fallope ring)
	Silicone clip (Filshie clip)

thromboembolic disease. If one pill is missed in a cycle, two pills should be taken at the next scheduled time, and the pack should be completed as usual. If two or more consecutive pills are missed, the package of pills should be completed as prescribed, and an alternative contraceptive method should be used for the remainder of the cycle. There are several contraindications to COC use (Table 28-6) and several side effects (Table 28-7).

   a. **Effectiveness.** Pregnancy rate of 0.1–5.0 per 100 women in first year of use.

   b. **Advantages.** Highly effective, protect against ovarian and endometrial cancer, decrease menstrual irregularities and anemia associated with menses, and are associated with improvement in mild acne. It is not clear whether oral contraceptive use is positively or negatively associated with the risk of breast cancer.

   c. **Disadvantages.** Not recommended during breast feeding, rare but serious side effects such as thromboembolism may occur, offer no protection against STDs, must be taken daily, require a prescription.

2. **Progestin-only oral contraceptives** are synthetic progestin preparations that are thought to prevent pregnancy by suppressing ovula-

TABLE 28-4. CUMULATIVE PROBABILITY OF PREGNANCY AFTER 10 YEARS (PER 100 PROCEDURES)

Tubal ligation method	Pregnancy probability
Spring clip	3.7
Bipolar coagulation	2.5
Interval partial salpingectomy	2.0
Silicone rubber band	1.8
Unipolar coagulation	0.8
Postpartum partial salpingectomy	0.8
All methods	1.9

Adapted from Peterson HB, Xia Z, Hughes JM, et al. The risk of pregnancy after tubal sterilization: findings from the US collaborative review of sterilization. *Am J Obstet Gynecol* 1996;174(4):1161–1170.

TABLE 28-5. COMBINED ORAL CONTRACEPTIVES CURRENTLY AVAILABLE IN THE UNITED STATES

Ethinyl estradiol dose (µg)	Progestin type	Progestin dose (µg)	Brand name
35	Norgestimate	250	Ortho-Cyclen
35		180, 215, 250	Ortho Tri-Cyclen
30	Desogestrel	150	Desogen
			Ortho-Cept
20, 10		150	Mircette
30	Levonorgestrel	150	Levlen
			Levora
			Lo/Ovral
			Nordette
20		100	Alesse
			Levlite
30, 40, 30		50, 75, 125	Tri-Levlen
			Triphasil
			Trivora
20	Norethindrone	1000	Loestrin 1/20
30		1500	Loestrin 1.5/30
35		400	Ovcon 35
35		500	Brevicon
			Modicon
35		1000	Necon
			Norethin 1/35E
			Norinyl 1/35
			Ortho-Novum1/35
35		500, 750, 1000	Ortho-Novum 7/7/7
35		500, 1000	Ortho-Novum 10/11
			Jenest
35		500, 1000, 500	Tri-Norinyl
20, 30, 35		1000	Estrostep
35	Ethynodiol diacetate	1000	Demulen 1/35
			Zovia 1/35

Adapted from Hatcher RA, Trussell J, Stewart F, et al. *Contraceptive technology,* rev. 17th ed. New York: Ardent Media, 1998:430–432; and Nelson AL, Hatcher RA, Zieman M, et al. *Managing contraception.* Tieger, GA: Bridging the Gap Foundation, 2000:87–93.

tion, thickening the cervical mucus, altering tubal motility, and altering the endometrium (Table 28-8). They have advantages over COCs because they may be used by breast-feeding women, they are not thrombogenic, and they are not associated with liver disease. However, because protective changes to cervical mucus begin to decrease 22 hours

TABLE 28-6. CONTRAINDICATIONS TO USE OF COMBINED ORAL CONTRACEPTIVES

World Health Organization Class 3 (not recommended unless other methods are not available)	World Health Organization Class 4 (method should not be used)
Unexplained vaginal bleeding	Liver disease, including liver tumors
BP >160/100 but <180/110	BP >180/110
History of breast cancer but no evidence of current disease	Breast cancer
Women taking phenytoin, barbiturates, carbamazepine, rifampin, or griseofulvin[a]	Thromboembolic disease
	Ischemic heart disease or stroke
	Diabetes for >20 years or diabetes with complications
	Migraine headaches with focal neurologic symptoms
	Major surgery requiring prolonged bed rest
	Smoker older than 35 years

[a]There is limited support that antibiotics (besides rifampin and griseofulvin) decrease the effectiveness of combined oral contraceptives. However, some authorities (e.g., Planned Parenthood) recommend using an alternative method of contraception for the first 2 weeks of broad-spectrum antibiotic use.

Adapted from Blumenthal PD, McIntosh N. *Pocket guide for family planning service providers*, rev. 2nd ed. Baltimore: JHPIEGO Corp, 1996:92–99.

after the pill is taken, effectiveness is decreased if the pill is not taken at the same time every day.
   a. **Effectiveness.** Pregnancy rate of 0.5–5.0 per 100 women in first year of use.
   b. **Advantages.** Rapidly effective (within 24 hours of initiation of use) with immediate return of fertility when the pill is discontinued, decrease menorrhagia and associated anemia, offer some protection against endometrial cancer and protection against some causes of pelvic inflammatory disease, do not have some of the serious side effects associated with estrogen.
   c. **Disadvantages.** High incidence of intermenstrual bleeding, must be taken at the same time every day, less effective than COCs, require a prescription.
3. **Progestin-only injectable contraceptives** are synthetic progestin preparations that prevent pregnancy via the same mechanisms as oral progestins but are injected intramuscularly. The most commonly used injectable is medroxyprogesterone acetate (Depo-Provera), 150 mg given every 3 months.
   a. **Effectiveness.** Pregnancy rate of 0.3 per 100 women in first year of use.
   b. **Advantages.** Rapidly and highly effective, long-acting.
   c. **Disadvantages.** Return of fertility is delayed 5–7 months; may cause lipid abnormalities; require administration by a health care provider; offer no protection against STDs; associated with weight gain, hair loss, reversible bone loss, and menstrual irregularities including menometrorrhagia and amenorrhea.
4. **Progestin-only implants** are thin, flexible capsules filled with levonorgestrel that are inserted under the skin of a woman's arm. They prevent

TABLE 28-7. MANAGEMENT OF SIDE EFFECTS OF COMBINED ORAL CONTRACEPTIVES

Side effect	Management strategy
Amenorrhea	Rule out pregnancy.
	Make sure pills are being taken correctly.
	Consider increasing the estrogen dose.
	Consider decreasing the progestin dose.
Breast fullness or tenderness	Perform breast examination.
	Counsel that this usually resolves by fourth month of use.
	Consider possible mammography or ultrasonography.
	Consider lowering estrogen dose.
Depression	Consider other method of contraception.
Vascular headache or severe migraine	Consider continuous hormone administration with only occasional withdrawal bleeding.
	Avoid phasic formulations.
	May need to consider other method of contraception.
	Discontinue use if migraines are newly diagnosed after patient begins combined oral contraceptives.
Spotting or intermenstrual bleeding	Reassure patient that this usually decreases by fourth month of use.
	Consider increasing estrogen dose.
	Consider lowering progestin dose.
Missed pills	If one pill is missed, patient should take two pills at the next scheduled time and complete the package as usual.
	If two or more consecutive pills are missed, patient should finish the package of pills and use an alternative contraceptive method for the remainder of the cycle.

Adapted from Blumenthal PD, McIntosh N. *Pocket guide for family planning service providers*, rev 2nd ed. Baltimore: JHPIEGO Corp, 1996:102–109.

pregnancy by suppressing ovulation, thickening the cervical mucus, altering the endometrium (atrophy), and changing tubal motility. The Norplant system is the only implant system currently available. The implants are effective within 48 hours of placement and may be left in place for 3–5 years. Fertility returns within the first month after removal of the capsules.

TABLE 28-8. PROGESTIN-ONLY ORAL CONTRACEPTIVES CURRENTLY AVAILABLE IN THE UNITED STATES

Progestin type	Progestin dose (µg)	Brand name
Norgestrel	75	Ovrette
Norethindrone	350	Micronor
		Nor-Q D

Adapted form Nelson AL, Hatcher RA, Zieman M, et al. *Managing contraception*. Tieger, GA: Bridging the Gap Foundation, 2000:88.

    a. **Effectiveness.** Pregnancy rate of 0.05 per 100 women in first year of use.

    b. **Advantages.** Highly effective, very long-acting.

    c. **Disadvantages.** Require a minor surgical procedure for capsule placement and removal; offer no protection against STDs; associated with breast tenderness, weight gain, lipid abnormalities, hirsutism, hair loss, and menstrual irregularities including menometrorrhagia and amenorrhea.

C. Barrier methods

  1. **Condoms (male and female)** are a barrier method in which semen is collected in the condom and thus prevented from entering the female genital tract. The male condom should be applied before each vaginal penetration and should cover the entire length of the erect penis. It should not be applied tightly (a reservoir should be left to retain the ejaculate). Adequate lubrication should be used, and the condom should be removed immediately after ejaculation. Female condoms consist of a latex sheath with two flexible rings at either end. The closed end and upper ring is applied against the cervix, and the open end and ring rest against the labia minora outside the introitus. Condoms may be used with or previously treated with spermicide to increase effectiveness.

    a. **Effectiveness.** Pregnancy rate of 3–14 per 100 women in first year of use.

    b. **Advantages.** No method-related health risks, fairly effective in preventing pregnancy if used properly, may be used during breast feeding, the only contraceptive method that provides protection against STDs (only synthetic condoms protect against hepatitis B virus and human immunodeficiency virus).

    c. **Disadvantages.** High failure rate if not used properly, latex type may not be used if either partner has a latex allergy (only vinyl or natural type may be used).

  2. **Diaphragm and cervical cap** are barrier devices that are inserted into the vagina and prevent sperm from entering the upper genital tract. The diaphragm is a rubber or latex cup with a flexible ring. The diaphragm should lie just posterior to the symphysis pubis and deep into the cul-de-sac so that the cervix is completely covered and behind the center of the diaphragm. The largest diaphragm that fills this space comfortably should be selected. Spermicide should be applied to the inside of the rubber cup before each coitus, and the diaphragm should be left in place for a minimum of 6 hours after the last coital act. Women with uterine prolapse or structural abnormalities of the reproductive tract may not be able to use a diaphragm if it does not remain in position during use. The cervical cap is a round cap with an inside rim that fits snugly against the outer cervix adjacent to the vaginal fornix. Cervical caps are made of rubber and are designed to form a seal between the inner rim of the cap and the outer cervix. The cap may be left in place for up to 48 hours, as reapplication of spermicide is not necessary between coital events.

    a. **Effectiveness.** Pregnancy rate of 6–40 per 100 women in first year of use.

    b. **Advantages.** User controlled, may be used during breast feeding, no method-related health risks, may offer some protection against bacterial STDs and cervical neoplasia (although a normal Pap smear result should be confirmed before starting use).

    c. **Disadvantages.** Relatively high failure rate; slight increase in risk of infections, including toxic shock syndrome and urinary tract infections; require initial evaluation by a physician, may be considered inconvenient.

D. Spermicides are agents that cause destruction of the sperm cell membrane and thereby decrease motility. Types of spermicides include aerosol foams, creams, vaginal suppositories, jellies, films, and sponges. All contain a spermicidal agent, usually nonoxynol 9.

1. **Effectiveness.** Pregnancy rate of 6–26 per 100 women in first year of use.
2. **Advantages.** No method-related health risks, serve as a lubricant, may provide some protection against bacterial STDs.
3. **Disadvantages.** Relatively high failure rate; recent studies by the Centers for Disease Control and Prevention have found evidence that nonoxynol 9 may increase transmission rates of human immunodeficiency virus; effective for only 1–2 hours.

E. **Intrauterine devices (IUDs)** are flexible, medicated, plastic devices that are inserted into the uterus and cause an alteration in the uterine environment, which consequently decreases fertilization or implantation. Three types are currently commercially available in the United States: copper-containing (Paraguard T380A) and two progestin-releasing (Mirena and Progestasert). Copper-releasing devices interfere with the ability of the sperm to pass through the uterine cavity and may remain in place for up to 10 years. Progestin-releasing devices thicken the cervical mucus and thin the endometrial lining. The Progestasert IUD is effective for 1 year. IUDs can be used for emergency postcoital contraception (see sec. **II.H.2** on emergency contraception). IUDs should not be used if pregnancy is suspected, if there is current or recent pelvic infection, if there is unexplained vaginal bleeding, or if pelvic malignancy is suspected. Women at risk for sexually transmitted infection and immunocompromised women should consider another method because of the increased risk of infection.

1. **Effectiveness.** Pregnancy rate of 0.3–0.8 per 100 women in first year of use.
2. **Advantages.** Highly effective at preventing pregnancy, immediately effective after insertion with prompt return of fertility after removal, offer long-term protection.
3. **Disadvantages.** The risk of pelvic inflammatory disease is minimally increased (seen in women at risk of genital infection, mostly at time of insertion or removal), high occurrence of dysmenorrhea and menorrhagia (usually) within the first few months after device insertion, risk of uterine perforation with insertion, higher risk of ectopic pregnancy if pregnancy does occur.

F. **Natural family planning (rhythm method)** is a method in which a couple voluntarily avoids or interrupts sexual intercourse during the fertile phase of the woman's menstrual cycle.

The menstrual cycle may be divided into three phases for the purpose of assessing fertility (Table 28-9).

TABLE 28-9. THREE PHASES OF THE MENSTRUAL CYCLE

	Phase I	Phase II	Phase III
Fertility	Relatively infertile	Fertile	Infertile
Time of cycle	Onset of menses until preovulation	Several days pre-ovulation to 48 hrs postovulation	48 hrs postovulation until menses
Cervical mucus	Scant, thick, breaks easily	Abundant, clear, stretches	Scant, thick, breaks easily
Temperature		Sustained rise of 0.2°C to 0.6°C indicates ovulation	The morning of third temperature elevation begins phase III

1. **Effectiveness.** Pregnancy rate of 9–25 per 100 women in first year of use.
2. **Advantages.** No physical side effects, economical, immediate return to fertility on cessation of use, no method-related health risks.
3. **Disadvantages.** High failure rate, no protection against STDs, inhibits spontaneity, requires regular menstrual cycles.

G. **Lactational amenorrhea method.** During breast feeding, suckling causes hormonal changes at the level of the hypothalamus that interrupt the pulsatile release of gonadotropin-releasing hormone. This, in turn, impairs the luteinizing hormone surge and ovulation does not occur, so that pregnancy is prevented.

This is an effective method only if strict criteria are followed. Feedings must be every 4 hours during the day and every 6 hours at night. Supplemental feedings should not exceed 5–10% of the total.

1. **Effectiveness.** Pregnancy rate of 2 per 100 women in first 6 months postpartum, 6 per 100 women from 6 to 12 months postpartum.
2. **Advantages.** Protection against pregnancy starts immediately postpartum, economical method, encourages breast feeding with all of its advantages.
3. **Disadvantages.** Not highly effective, requires strict adherence to criteria, provides no protection against STDs.

H. **Emergency contraception**

1. **Hormonal emergency contraception.** High-dose estrogen or progestin is given within 72 hours of unprotected intercourse; it prevents ovulation and causes changes in the endometrium that make implantation less likely. Dosing options include the following: four COC pills containing 30–35 µg ethinyl estradiol by mouth, repeated in 12 hours; two COC pills containing 50 µg ethinyl estradiol (Préven), repeated in 12 hours; one 0.75 mg levonorgestrel pill (Plan B), repeated in 12 hours. Absence of any preexisting pregnancy must be confirmed before administering. Use is contraindicated in women who cannot take hormonal contraception (see sec. **II.B** on hormonal contraception). This method should not be used as routine contraception.
   a. **Effectiveness.** Pregnancy rate of 2 per 100 women if taken within 72 hours.
   b. **Advantages.** A highly effective method to use in emergency situations.
   c. **Disadvantages.** High incidence of nausea and irregular bleeding.
2. **Intrauterine device as emergency contraception.** IUDs may be inserted within 5 days of unprotected intercourse to decrease chance of implantation.
   a. **Effectiveness.** Pregnancy rate of less than 1 per 100 women if inserted within 5 days.
   b. **Advantages.** See sec. **II.E.**
   c. **Disadvantages.** See sec. **II.E.**

I. **New developments in contraception.** There are several contraceptive devices that are in the development stage and may even be available on the market at the time of publication.

1. **Combined injectable contraceptives** consist of a combined estrogen-progestin preparation that is injected intramuscularly. Injections must be given every month. Its advantage over current progestin-only injectables is that the progestin-associated side effects are reduced.
2. **Continuous-dose combined oral contraceptives** are COCs in which menses occurs every 3 months during use. They may reduce menses-related anemia and may be viewed as more convenient by some patients.
3. Combined transdermal hormonal contraceptive (Ortho Evra).
4. Combined estrogen-progestin vaginal ring (Nuva Ring).
5. Combined estrogen-progestin monthly injection (Lunelle).

III. **Elective termination**
   A. **Epidemiology.** In the United States, 49% of all pregnancies are unintended; approximately one-half of these unintended pregnancies end in abortion. This results in over 1 million abortions per year in the United States. The abortion rate in 1996 was 22.9 per 1000 women. This rate has been steadily decreasing since 1980. In 1990, approximately 50% of pregnancy terminations were performed on patients less than 25 years old. Ninety percent of abortions took place in the first 12 weeks after the last menstrual period, and nearly all were performed using suction or instrumental evacuation.

   Abortion data are subject to underreporting, as not all states require official documentation and the sensitive nature of this procedure may result in decreased disclosure by both physician and patient. With the advent of medical abortion, it is speculated that underreporting will increase because no surgical procedure will be recorded.

   B. **Law and policy.** In 1973, the *Roe v. Wade* decision ruled that women, in consultation with their physicians, have a constitutional right to abortion up until the time of fetal viability. In 1992, the court upheld the right to abortion dictated in *Planned Parenthood v. Casey* but gave states the right to enact restrictions that do not create an "undue burden" for women seeking abortion. For minors, thirty-one states require parental involvement (notification or consent) for abortion. The U.S. Congress prohibits the use of federal Medicaid funds to pay for abortion, except when the woman's life is at risk or in cases of rape or incest. Sixteen states use state funds to pay for abortions for poor women. On June 28, 2000, in *Stenberg v. Carhart*, the Supreme Court ruled that Nebraska's law which restricted late-term abortions was unconstitutional, as it was too broad and did not contain an exception to protect the health of the mother.

   C. **First trimester termination**
      1. **Medical termination.** Mifepristone (RU-486) and methotrexate sodium with misoprostol have been used to induce first trimester abortion with a success rate (complete abortion, no suction curettage needed) of approximately 93% when the gestational age is less than 7 weeks. Success rates of abortion are inversely related to gestational age, and accurate dating is essential. Mifepristone works as a progesterone antagonist and alters endometrial blood supply. Methotrexate inhibits DNA synthesis and affects rapidly dividing cells, including trophoblastic cells. Mifepristone generally works faster and is associated with fewer side effects. Misoprostol is a prostaglandin agonist that is used to induce uterine contractions after administration of either mifepristone or methotrexate.

      Protocols include the following: mifepristone 200–600 mg orally, followed 36 hours later by 400–800 µg of misoprostol orally or vaginally; methotrexate 50 mg/m^2 intramuscularly, followed in 5–7 days by 800 µg of misoprostol vaginally.

      Mifepristone is the first abortifacient approved by the U.S. Food and Drug Administration for pregnancy termination (approved September 2000); the use of methotrexate as an abortifacient is well documented, although there is not a Food and Drug Administration protocol for this purpose. It is essential that women who have medical abortions can ensure follow-up and have access to a medical facility.

      2. **Surgical termination (suction dilation and curettage).** The surgical procedure of choice for early pregnancy termination is suction curettage of the uterus. It is imperative that adequate, slow cervical dilation be performed to avoid cervical injury and excessive blood loss. Cervical dilation may be accomplished before surgery by using osmotic or medical agents.

      Osmotic agents derived from *Laminaria* (genus of seaweed) are inserted into the cervix between 4 and 16 hours before the procedure.

TABLE 28-10. COMPLICATIONS OF INDUCED ABORTION

Complication	Rate per 100,000 induced abortions
Major complications requiring hospitalization	
Retained tissue	27.7
Sepsis	21.2
Uterine perforation	9.4
Hemorrhage	7.1
Inability to complete	3.5
Intrauterine plus ectopic	2.4
Major complications managed on outpatient basis	
Mild infection	462.0
Reaspiration same day	180.8
Reaspiration later	167.8
Cervical stenosis	16.5
Cervical tear	10.6
Underestimated gestation	6.5
Convulsive seizure	4.0

Adapted from Speroff L, Darney PD. *A clinical guide for contraception,* 2nd ed. Baltimore, Williams & Wilkins, 1996.

They slowly absorb water and expand, which allows the cervix to soften and dilate. They also cause the release of prostaglandin, which ultimately disrupts the stroma of the cervix and results in a soft, flaccid cervix that is easy to dilate.

Medical dilating agents, including misoprostol (50–200 μg taken 12–24 hours before the procedure orally or 4–6 hours vaginally) and mifepristone (100 mg taken orally 24–36 hours before the procedure) work to both soften and dilate the cervix. Intraoperatively, the cervix is dilated by serial insertion of tapered rods that increase progressively in size (Pratt, Hegar, or Denniston dilators). Evacuation of the uterus is most often accomplished by using a suction curette attached to a vacuum. The cannula of the curette should be approximately the same diameter (in millimeters) as the weeks of gestation. After aspiration with the suction curette is completed, the tissue should be inspected to verify that products of conception consistent with the gestational age are present. Sharp curettage can be used to ensure that all uterine contents have been evacuated. Fewer than 1% of all abortion patients experience a major complication (Table 28-10). Antibiotics (usually doxycycline) may be administered for prophylaxis. Aspirin and acetaminophen should not be used for analgesia because their antipyretic properties may mask the early signs of uterine infection. Persistent fever within 7 days of the procedure is strong evidence for retained products of conception and should be treated with repeat curettage and antibiotics. If left untreated, complications of retained products can lead to sepsis and possible death. Patients with an Rh-negative blood type should receive Rhogam.

D. **Second trimester termination**
   1. **Medical termination** offers several advantages over dilation and extraction as it does not require anesthesia (however, analgesia is usu-

ally necessary) and a skilled operator is not required. Disadvantages, compared with dilation and extraction, include the following: the procedure can take 24 hours or longer, major complications and mortality are higher, and fever and severe GI side effects are common when prostaglandins are used.

The overall goal is to administer medications that cause uterine contractions which lead to expulsion of the products of conception. Medications include high-dose intravenous oxytocin and different preparations of vaginally administered prostaglandins [prostaglandin E_2 (Prostin E_2) and misoprostol (Cytotec)]. Hypertonic solutions (saline or urea) are also administered intra-amniotically to induce second trimester abortions.

The major complications of second trimester medical termination are uterine atony with subsequent hemorrhage, retained placental tissue, and electrolyte imbalance leading to disseminated intravascular coagulation in cases in which hypertonic solutions are used. For this reason, second trimester medical abortions comprise only 0.7% of abortions performed annually.

2. **Surgical termination (dilation and extraction).** The procedure for surgical termination between 14 and 22 weeks' gestation is similar to the first trimester procedure, with several caveats.

Ultrasonographic confirmation of gestational age is essential.

Preoperative cervical preparation is mandatory and is often carried out over the 1–2 days before the procedure to maximize cervical dilation. Sequential insertion of osmotic dilators is most frequently used.

Amniotomy is sometimes performed before vacuum aspiration, because it allows the uterus to contract, which reduces blood loss and brings the products of conception closer to the cervical os. In addition to application of the vacuum aspirator, instrumental removal of the products of conception is usually required. It is essential to examine and account for all fetal parts and a volume of placental tissue consistent with the gestational age.

Complications such as cervical trauma, uterine perforation, hemorrhage, and retained products are more common after 18 weeks' gestation and may result in significant morbidity.

29. SEXUAL ASSAULT AND DOMESTIC VIOLENCE

Ginger J. Gardner and Catherine A. Sewell

I. **Epidemiology.** Violence against women is a diverse and disturbing problem in our society. The violence includes abuse by family members and strangers, and physical and sexual assault. It occurs to women of all ages, races, incomes, and educational backgrounds. Overall, domestic violence is the single most common cause of injury to women. Nearly 25% of women in the United States (more than 12 million) will be abused by a current or former partner sometime during their lives. Five million women are abused each year, and 1.7 million are subjected to severe violence.

Violence against women often results in acute as well as long-standing physical and emotional pain. Women may present to gynecologists directly or they may be referred with chronic conditions such as pelvic pain. Battering may begin or escalate during pregnancy and can result in poor pregnancy outcomes, including miscarriage, preterm labor, or low birth weight. Violence occurs in up to 20–37% of pregnancies and is more prevalent than common disorders such as preeclampsia, gestational diabetes, and placenta previa.

As health care providers for women, we are often the first and sometimes the only professionals that victims of violence may encounter. It is our responsibility to identify patients with a history of abuse, understand the potential physical and emotional consequences, and provide appropriate treatments and resources.

II. **Rape crisis evaluation and treatment.** Rape crisis typically involves an acute attack that leads the patient to present to the emergency department. The evaluation and treatment approach are as follows.
   A. **Report patient statement.**
      1. Make sure a chaperon who is the same sex as the patient is present at all times for the history taking and examination.
      2. Ask about the patient's injuries.
         a. What was the nature of the sexual violation?
         b. What has the patient done since the event—for example, has she showered, changed clothes?
      3. Do not impose interpretation on the description—document the patient's exact description of the event.
      4. Document medically relevant information only. Do not include the time and place of the event, as such descriptions will be covered in the police report. Any description of such events by the physician may only increase the possibility of a discrepancy in the patient's report of attack when reviewed later.
      5. Do not use legal terms such as "sexual assault" or "rape." It is acceptable to comment on findings "consistent with the use of force."
      6. Take a thorough sexual and gynecologic history, including history of infections, pregnancy, use of contraception, and last consensual intercourse.
      7. Obtain informed consent to proceed with examination. This should be done for legal purposes and because it may help the victim begin to regain her autonomy.
   B. **Examine the patient and collect evidence.**
      1. Be sensitive and gentle.
      2. Document the patient's emotional condition.
      3. Be thorough and systematic and record all evidence of injury; use drawings and photographs as needed.

4. Collect appropriate clothing from the patient (if she has not yet changed) and give it to the proper personnel.
5. Perform a full skin examination and evaluate all orifices for evidence of laceration, bruising, bite marks, or use of foreign objects. A Wood's lamp, if available, can be used to identify semen on the body.
6. Perform an overall general examination for any other injuries, such as abdominal trauma or broken bones.
7. Collect dry and wet swabs of secretions to evaluate for semen and hair (evidence of coitus will be present in the vagina for up to 48 hours after attack, in other orifices only for up to 6 hours). Perform wet preparation to identify sperm. Collected samples are sent for acid phosphatase testing to identify semen, or DNA in situ hybridization to identify a Y chromosome.
8. Collect oral, cervical, and rectal culture specimens for testing for sexually transmitted diseases (STDs). Perform a wet preparation for *Trichomonas* testing.
9. Perform irrigation of the vaginal vault; examine samples immediately and send to the crime laboratory to evaluate for sperm.
10. Take samples of and perform combings of the patient's genital hair.
11. Obtain fingernail scrapings.
12. Obtain baseline test specimens for herpes simplex virus, hepatitis B virus, syphilis, human immunodeficiency virus (HIV), cytomegalovirus, and pregnancy.
13. Maintain the chain of evidence collection—give samples directly to rape crisis personnel.
14. Report to authorities as required.

C. **Treat the patient.**
 1. **Suture lacerations as needed.**
 2. **Treat presumptively for STDs.** Approximately 43% of sexual assault victims have at least one preexisting STD. The risk of acquiring an STD from a sexual assault is as follows: gonorrhea, 6–12%; syphilis, 3%; HIV infection, <1%.
    Treatment options include
    a. Ceftriaxone sodium, 125 mg intramuscularly; metronidazole, 2 g orally (one dose); and doxycycline, 100 mg orally twice daily for 7 days. This provides coverage for gonorrhea, trichomoniasis, and *Chlamydia* infection.
    b. Azithromycin, 1 g orally (one dose), may be substituted for doxycycline for pregnant patients and can improve patient compliance.
 3. **Provide emergency contraception.** The chance of pregnancy after an assault is reported to be 2–4% in victims not protected by some form of contraception at the time of attack. The available options include the following.
    a. Oral contraceptive tablets containing ethinyl estradiol, 50 µg, two pills orally immediately; repeat in 12 hours. This method is at least 75% effective and can be given up to 72 hours after the incident. Acceptable treatment regimens include two pills/dose of Ovral, or four pills/dose of Lo/Ovral, Nordette, Levlen, Triphasil, or Tri-Levlen.
    b. Ethinyl estradiol, 5 mg/day for 5 days.
    c. Conjugated equine estrogen, 20–30 mg/day for 5 days.
    d. Intrauterine device placement.
 4. **Provide hepatitis B immune globulin,** 0.06 mL/kg, as soon as possible, but within 14 days of the attack.
 5. **Provide follow-up.**
    a. Follow up at 1–2 weeks for psychological evaluation and pregnancy test.
    b. Follow up at 3–4 weeks for repeat hepatitis B testing, collection of culture specimens for test of cure, and a repeat pregnancy test.

    c. Follow up at 3–6 months for repeat HIV, hepatitis B, and syphilis testing.

    d. Provide 24-hour hotline numbers and social work resources.

III. **Domestic violence evaluation and treatment.** Although some women are victims of an acute attack or rape, others find themselves in long-standing abusive and destructive relationships. Such relationships tend to develop a cycle of behavior in which a violent episode is followed by a period of apologies and promises of hope and change. A tension-building phase soon begins and culminates in a repeat violent attack. The cycle then begins again. Over time, these relationships are progressive and the degree of violence escalates. Escape from the relationship is difficult for the victim because of the fear, shame, powerlessness, and social isolation imposed by the batterer. Domestic violence is all-encompassing. Muelleman defines it as "the exercise of emotional intimidation, psychological abuse, social isolation, deprivation, nonconsensual sexual behavior, physical injury by a competent adult to maintain coercive control in an intimate relationship with another competent adult/adolescent" (*An Emergency Medicine Approach to Violence Throughout the Life Cycle*, Vol. 7/708–715, 1996).

Women are more likely to be injured, raped, or even killed by a current or former male partner than by all other types of assailants combined. Women who are injured as a result of domestic violence are more likely to suffer serious injury or loss of consciousness than are victims of violence by strangers. Up to 12% of American women in an ongoing relationship experience some type of violence each year, and 30% of all female murders are the result of domestic disputes.

The clinical approach to addressing domestic violence involves screening, assessment, and patient empowerment, as described in what follows.

A. **Screening**

1. **Ask about domestic violence** as part of a routine patient evaluation during office visits and emergency room evaluations. Abuse crosses all ethnic, religious, and socioeconomic divides—ask as frequently as possible.

2. **Ask periodically.** Studies show that women asked about violence more than once during detailed in-person interviews or asked more than once during pregnancy report higher prevalence rates.

3. **Interview the patient in private** without her partner, children, or other relatives present. Be aware that the batterer often accompanies the woman to the appointment and wants to stay close at hand to monitor what she says to the physician. Find a way for him to be excused from the room to allow for a private patient-physician interview.

4. **Assure patient confidentiality.** Never ask what she did wrong or why she has not left her partner—avoid being judgmental. Avoid value-laden terms such as "abused" and "battered." You can begin with an objective statement that demonstrates that your screening is universal and necessary to provide comprehensive health care. For example: "Because violence is so common in many women's lives and there is help available for women being abused, I now ask every patient about domestic violence." Then follow with some direct questions.

    a. Have you ever been hit, slapped, kicked, or otherwise physically hurt by anyone?

    b. Are you in a relationship with anyone who threatens or physically hurts you?

    c. Has anyone forced you to engage in sexual activities that made you uncomfortable?

    d. Are you ever afraid of your partner?

    e. Does your partner treat you well?

    f. Does your partner criticize you or your children a lot?

    g. Has your partner ever hurt or threatened you or your children?

    h. Has your partner ever hurt pets or destroyed objects in your home or something you especially cared about?

    i. When you argue or fight with your partner, what happens?

    j. Does your partner throw or break objects during arguments?

    k. Is your partner jealous?

    l. Has your partner ever tried to keep you from taking medication you needed or from seeking medical help?

    m. Does your partner make it difficult for you to find or keep a job or go to school?

    n. Does your partner ever withhold money when you need it?

    o. Has your partner ever forced you to do something you did not want to do?

    p. Does your partner abuse drugs or alcohol? What happens?

5. Ask about a history of **previous trauma, chronic pain, or psychological distress.**

6. Most important, regardless of the method, **make time to screen.** According to Dr. Richard Jones of the University of Connecticut, "If you ask about domestic violence early on, it probably takes less time than the multiple visits for PMS or pelvic pain you face with many patients. Long range, in fact, it's probably a very good use of your time and the patient's" (*Contemporary OB/Gyn*, 78–110, 1997).

B. **Assessment.** Typically, a battered woman has numerous emergency room visits for injury. Her injuries classically involve multiple sites (such as three or more body parts); affect the head, back, breast, and abdomen (accidental injuries are more likely to be peripheral); and are in various stages of healing. The patient may say she is accident prone or give a vague or inconsistent description of the mechanism of injury in relation to the bodily damage.

    In contrast, the patient may report a variety of somatic complaints. Patients may have headaches, insomnia, musculoskeletal discomfort, choking sensations, hyperventilation, palpitations, or back and chest pain. Abused women may have GI disturbance, and they are twice as likely as nonabused women to report a history of functional bowel disorder. Rather than describe or show evidence of physical pain, some patients may present with mood changes, anxiety, eating disorders, drug abuse, or suicidal thoughts. Battered women account for 25% of women who attempt suicide, and a suicide threat on the part of the batterer or the victim may be a warning that homicide will occur. Somatic or psychological complaints certainly warrant a full assessment for underlying disease. They should also be considered as a possible indicator of domestic violence (Fig. 29-1).

1. **Symptoms and signs** specifically seen by obstetricians and gynecologists that may be associated with domestic violence include the following:

    a. Gynecologic

        (1) Chronic pelvic pain

        (2) Severe premenstrual syndrome

        (3) Multiple or recurrent STDs or recurrent vaginitis

        (4) Medical noncompliance

        (5) Sexual dysfunction

        (6) Abdominal complaints

    b. Obstetric

        (1) Unintended pregnancy

        (2) Late registration for prenatal care, no prenatal care, missed appointments

        (3) Fetal or maternal injury (violence is often directed toward the woman's abdomen during pregnancy)

        (4) Spontaneous abortion or stillbirth

        (5) Vaginal bleeding in the second or third trimester

        (6) Preterm labor

        (7) Infection

        (8) Anemia

General presentations
Statement "I've been beaten"
Vague description of cause
Inconsistent description of
   cause
Time delay from occurrence
Multiple injuries
Various stages of healing
Depression and attempted
   suicide
Anxiety and panic disorders
Repetitive somatoform dis-
   orders
Substance and alcohol
   abuse
Eating disorders
Hostile, uncooperative
   behaviors

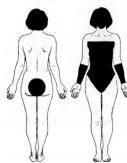

Indirect clues
Accident prone
Immature personality
Hysteric
Psychosomatic complaints
Diffuse anxiety disorder
Help-rejecting behaviors
Masochistic

**Physical examination
   demeanor**
Flat affect
Embarrassed
Hesitant
Eye contact avoided
Frightened
Evasive
Hostile
Disassociation or zoning out
   during examination

**Gynecologic presenta-
   tions**
Sexually transmitted dis-
   eases, including human
   immunodeficiency virus
Unintended pregnancy
Chronic pelvic pain
Sexual dysfunction
Recurrent vaginal infections
Premenstrual stress syn-
   drome

Obstetric presentations
Late prenatal care, missed
   appointments
Substance use and abuse
Multiple, repeated com-
   plaints
Poor weight gain and
   nutrition
Preterm labor
Low birth weight
Fetal injury and death
Maternal injury

FIG. 29-1. Indicators of domestic violence. (From American College of Obstetricians and gynecologists, Family Violence Work Group. *Domestic violence: the role of the physician in identification, intervention, and prevention.* ACOG slide lecture presentation, 1995, with permission.)

   (9) Poor weight gain
   (10) Low-birth-weight infants
2. Alternatively, the patient may directly reveal that she has been battered. If the patient reports she is a victim, or if you suspect battering without her disclosure, ask the following to assess the degree of the risk to the patient.
   a. How were you hurt?
   b. Has this happened before?
   c. When did it first happen?
   d. How badly have you been hurt in the past?
   e. Have you ever needed to go to the emergency room for treatment?
   f. Have you ever been threatened with a weapon, or has a weapon ever been used on you?
   g. Have you ever tried to get a restraining order against a partner?
   h. Have your children ever seen or heard you being threatened or hurt?
   i. Do you know how you can get help for yourself if you are hurt or afraid?
   j. Is the violence getting worse? Are there threats of suicide or homicide? Is there a gun at home?
C. **Empowerment of the patient**
   1. Discuss the seriousness of the situation and assess immediate safety needs.

The following exit plan has been proposed for a woman who feels that she or her children are in danger from her male partner:

1. Have a change of clothes packed for herself and her children, including toilet articles, necessary medications, and an extra set of house and car keys. These can be placed in a suitcase and stored with a friend or neighbor.

2. Cash, a checkbook, and a savings account book may also be kept with the individual chosen.

3. Identification papers, such as birth certificates, social security cards, voter registration card, utility bills, and a driver's license should be kept available because children will need to be enrolled in school and financial assistance may be sought. If available, financial records, such as mortgage papers, rent receipts, or an automobile title, should be taken.

4. Something of special interest to each child, such as a book or toy, should be taken.

5. A plan of exactly where to go, regardless of the time of day or night, should be decided on. This may be a friend or relative's home or a shelter for battered women and children.

FIG. 29-2. Exit plan for abused women. (Modified from Helton A. Battering during pregnancy. *Am J Nurs* 1986;86:910–913.)

    2. Reinforce the fact that the patient is not to blame.

    3. Treat the patient's injuries and assess emotional status for suicidal tendencies, depression, and substance abuse.

    4. Empower the woman to be able to better protect herself and her children. Most women feel unable to leave an abusive relationship because of lack of financial resources or fear that the batterer will follow them.

    5. Discuss court restraining orders and laws against stalking.

    6. Provide the patient with phone numbers of resource agencies.

    7. Review an exit plan or exit drill (Fig. 29-2).

    8. Provide continued ongoing support and offer referrals for counseling and therapy.

    9. Provide documentation, including direct quotations and photographs. Information in the medical record cannot be used as discrimination against the patient, such as for insurance coverage.

IV. **Pediatric and geriatric abuse**

    A. **Childhood physical abuse.** While screening women for current abusive encounters, it is important to recognize that their risk factors include prior childhood sexual or physical abuse. The abused woman and her children may have a history of or be at risk for injuries such as circumferential soft tissue injuries, or show scars or bruises in various stages of healing, which indicates repetitive abuse.

    B. **Childhood sexual abuse.** The majority of childhood sexual abuse occurs between the ages of 6 and 14, especially between the ages of 12 and 14. The victim is typically a girl who sustains vaginal, anal, or oral penetration, and the perpetrator is usually a relative or an acquaintance. Unlike in cases of physical abuse, there are rarely physical or laboratory findings of the trauma. It is the child's word that is the indicator of the abuse.

        Some signs, however, can be used as diagnostic clues for childhood sexual abuse, especially if the abuse is recent or repetitive and leaves physical stigmata. These include the following:

        1. Genital findings

            a. Thickening or hyperpigmentation of labia majora, labia minora, or introitus

            b. Irregular or enlarged hymenal orifice

            c. Bruises, bleeding, and abrasions in the vulvovaginal area

     d. Vaginal discharge and pruritus

     e. Laxity of the anal sphincter, anal fissures or lacerations, or perianal scarring

     f. Positive acid phosphatase findings on the body or in the clothes; sperm in the child's urine

         Refer to Chap. 30, Pediatric Gynecology, for additional information on the gynecologic examination of a child. The textbook *Pediatrics* (vol. 89, 1992:359), is also useful, especially for its pictures. A visual reference can be helpful to make the sometimes subtle distinction between normal versus abused prepubescent genitalia.

  2. **Childhood STDs.** Although only 2–10% of abused children become infected, a finding of childhood syphilis, gonorrhea, condylomata acuminata, or *Chlamydia* infection should alert the clinician to evaluate for sexual abuse.

  3. **Behavioral problems.** Abused children may demonstrate anxiety, sleep disturbances, withdrawal, somatic complaints, increased sex play, inappropriate sexual behavior, school problems, acting-out behaviors, self-destructive behaviors, depression, or low self-esteem.

  4. **Adolescent pregnancy.** Former victims of childhood sexual abuse are at increased risk for conception during adolescence.

  5. **Child's parent is in an abusive relationship.** Forty-five percent to 59% of mothers of abused children have been abused or raped themselves.

      Unlike in cases of partner violence, evidence of child abuse must be reported to the police or specified social agencies in all 50 states.

C. **Adolescent sexual abuse.** More than 75% of adolescent rapes are committed by an acquaintance of the victim. These include date rape, statutory rape, and incest. Teenagers are still learning to establish social boundaries, and they bring a variety of expectations to dating situations. Some adolescents believe that violence is acceptable in some social situations. Further, adolescents frequently use alcohol and illicit drugs, which alter judgment. A history of nonvoluntary sexual activity has been associated with early initiation of voluntary sexual activity, unintended pregnancy, poor use of contraceptives, and involvement with a significantly older man (defined as at least 5 years older).

  1. As part of **routine screening,** all teenagers should be asked direct questions regarding their sexual experiences and any incidence of coercion. This is an opportunity for the physician to identify adolescent victims and initiate a discussion of contraception and STDs.

  2. Physicians can provide adolescents with education, counseling referrals, community resource information, and prevention messages. Some teenage **empowerment messages** include the following:

     a. You have the right to say no to sexual activity.

     b. You have the right to set sexual limits and insist that your partner honor them.

     c. Be assertive.

     d. Stay sober and watch out for dates or anyone else who doesn't.

     e. Recognize and avoid situations that may put you at risk.

     f. Never leave a party with someone you don't know well.

     g. No one should ever be raped or otherwise forced or pressured into engaging in any unwanted sexual behavior.

D. **Elder and disabled adult abuse.** Elder abuse is a type of domestic violence, typically at the hands of adult family members or caregivers, that affects as many as 2 million Americans. Disabled adults are also at risk. Physicians should apply the same criteria in assessing older or disabled individuals as they would in assessing a younger woman for domestic violence.

V. **Abuse in lesbian, gay, and bisexual relationships.** Less is known about medical issues regarding the gay, lesbian, and bisexual community; however, domestic violence appears to be as common in same-sex relationships as in heterosexual relationships. The victims encounter the same spectrum of abusive behavior as do their heterosexual counterparts, and they may face additional obstacles to disclosing the abuse, accessing care, and achieving safety. Physicians should approach screening, diagnosis, and treatment with special sensitivity.

30. PEDIATRIC GYNECOLOGY

Andrea C. Scharfe and Catherine A. Sewell

I. **Gynecologic evaluation of a child**
  A. **Introduction.** Pediatric gynecology presents many challenges to the general obstetrician-gynecologist unfamiliar with these cases. Most of the obstacles may be overcome by communicating effectively and allowing the patient to feel "in control." The interview is the most important aspect in determining the true reason for the visit. Due to differing levels of maturity of each age group of children, it is important to consider different approaches to communication. Including the parental figure in the discussions is key. This chapter describes how to perform an appropriate history taking and physical examination as well as some of the common situations an obstetrician-gynecologist will be called on to evaluate.
  B. **Examination.** The examination presents another set of difficulties, which can be overcome by giving the patient a **sense of control.** If the child or adolescent is undergoing her first gynecologic examination, she should be treated with particular care, as her initial evaluation can set the tone for all future examinations. If the examination is extremely painful or of there is a lack of rapport between the examiner and physician, the child may suffer lasting psychological consequences. It is vital that a gentle, caring attitude be displayed at all times with these patients. Very young patients or those traumatized by sexual abuse who refuse to cooperate may have to be examined under anesthesia. Otherwise, gaining the confidence of the patient through a series of outpatient visits is advisable. The child should be told that the examination is permitted by her caregiver. It should also be made clear that if anyone else attempted or attempts to touch her genital area, she should tell her parent or caregiver.
    1. **Method.** A detailed and labeled sketch of the external genitalia should be included in the medical record. A diamond-shaped space can be used to represent the vestibule of a child in the supine position, with the clitoris positioned at 12 o'clock and the posterior fourchette at 6 o'clock. The ideal positioning of the pediatric patient is in a "frog-leg" posture. Sometimes, a knee-chest position with a Valsalva maneuver allows assessment of the introital area. Use of the supine lateral-spread method is often sufficient to allow the vestibular structures to be visualized. This involves placing the index finger of each hand or the index and middle finger or thumb and index finger of one hand on both labia majora, lateral to the vestibule and slightly posterior to the vaginal orifice. The tissues are then spread gently until visualization is adequate.
    2. **Prepubertal examination.** The examination should begin with a general pediatric physical. Abdominal examination can be facilitated by placing the child's hand over the examiner's hand. Inguinal examinations may reveal a hernia or gonad. Rectoabdominal examinations may aid in examining the uterus of a patient who does not tolerate a vaginal examination. Inspection of the external genitalia is followed by visualization of the vagina and cervix using the smallest-sized Cusco speculum. Other methods include use of a Cameron-Myers vaginoscope or an otoscope. The Tanner classification of the external genitalia and breast development should be used to quantify pubertal changes (Fig. 30-1). Note should be made of perineal hygiene, presence of pubic hair, hymenal configuration, and size of the clitoris. Introital estrogenization also should be noted. From the toddler years until age 9 or 10, the unestrogenized vaginal mucosa of the prepubertal child appears thin, red, and atrophic. Capillary beds appearing like roadmaps can be seen and are

Tanner stage

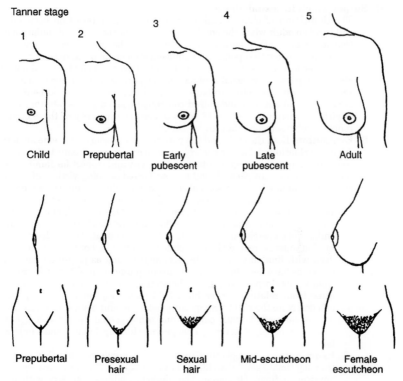

FIG. 30-1. Tanner stages of development. (From Beckmann CR, et al. *Obstetrics and gynecology*, 2nd ed. Baltimore: Williams & Wilkins, 1995:8, with permission.)

often mistaken for inflammation, especially around the sulcus of the vestibule and periurethral area. In areas of inflammation, the capillary beds are obscured by erythema and thickened edematous tissue.

3. **Peripubertal examination.** The estrogenized mucosa of the peripubertal child and of the newborn infant until approximately 3 years appears moist with a whitish pink color. Capillary beds cannot be visualized. The tissue is pliable and easily distended. Careful inspection of the hymen must be completed before pelvic examination. The examining index finger should be placed through the introitus before use of a speculum. A Huffman adolescent speculum or Pederson speculum can be used only if indicated. Dropping the knees outward allows the perineal body to relax. Use of the "extinction of stimuli" phenomenon can greatly facilitate a first pelvic examination. This involves using a primary distracting stimulus to draw attention from a second stimulus, such as pressing the nonexamining finger into the patient's perineum before touching the introitus and having the patient acknowledge the presence of its pressure. Many times a rectal examination may be equally informative and easier to perform. In early puberty, a thick, white, cloudy discharge is often present. This is often a physiologic leukorrhea, a result of unopposed estrogen causing vaginal and cervical secretions. This usually occurs before menarche. Proper perineal hygiene should be stressed, as *Escherichia coli* colonization is the most common cause of adolescent vulvovaginitis.

II. Suspected child sexual abuse

A. The **definition** of child sexual abuse is contact or interaction between a child and an adult when the child is being used for the sexual stimulation of that adult or another person. Abuse may also be committed by another minor either when that person is significantly older than the victim or when the abuser is in a position of power or control over the child. Sexual abuse also encompasses nonsexual contact such as pornography or exhibitionism. In addition, any girl found to have a vaginal foreign body should be evaluated for sexual abuse. Randomized controlled trials demonstrate that 38% of girls are victimized before 18 years of age. The majority of these occurrences involve someone they know socially.

B. **Evaluation.** Both the child and the parent may experience extreme anxiety during evaluation. A lack of control or security can make both feel victimized. Such encounters require utmost sensitivity and respect for family concerns and privacy. In general, children suspected of being victims of abuse should be evaluated by professionals trained in conducting interviews, documenting questions and responses, and collecting necessary evidence.

1. **History.** Communication is of utmost value. Questions should be open-ended. Sufficient time should be allowed to establish rapport with the child, and a coercive quality to the evaluation should be avoided. Information must be recorded in the child's own words. For very young children with limited verbal skills, techniques such as play-interviews or drawings have been used to promote communication. When it is impossible to obtain a history from the victim, the information then must come from relatives, other household members, neighbors, or police officers. Note the child's composure, behavior, and mental state, as well as the interactions with parents and other people. Nonspecific symptoms include night terrors, changes in sleeping habits, and clinging behavior.

2. **Examination.** A repeating theme in distinguishing abusive events from legitimate genital accidents is a mismatch between the history and physical findings. Of course, the physical findings will vary with the degree of trauma the victim has experienced and the time that has elapsed since the incident. The examination should be complete, extending from head to toe, allowing the child to become accustomed to the touch of the evaluator and establishing trust. Table 30-1 lists sites and findings on examination. Table 30-2 lists nonspecific versus definitive findings of sexual abuse. Unfortunately, unless vaginal penetration has taken place, the absence of physical findings is common, because healing often is complete (2–3 weeks) by the time the child is evaluated.

3. **Collection of evidence.** If the assault occurred within 72 hours of the examination, samples should be collected for the forensic laboratory and handled separately. All collected specimens must be individually packaged, labeled, sealed with special evidence tape, and signed by the appropriate people. A routing slip must be attached. Each label must include patient identification, the specimen, the site from which the specimen was collected, the date and time of collection, and the examiner's initials. The specimen package must be given to the police investigator, who signs it and a routing slip. Anyone handling the specimen must sign a routing slip, as this chain of evidence is crucial for admissibility in court. Items that can be collected for evidence include the clothing that was worn at the time of the assault and combings of the pubic hair for the perpetrator's hair. An examination for semen on the skin and clothing should be done. A Wood's light can be used to examine the body for secretions. Positive-appearing areas can be swabbed with saline-moistened swabs, which should be air-dried and put into sterile tubes or clean paper envelopes. Depending on the local forensic laboratory, the swabs may be immediately frozen instead. Several enzymes in semen can be detected to demonstrate its presence. The most commonly

TABLE 30-1. EXAMINATION IN CASES OF SUSPECTED CHILD ABUSE

Mouth, gums, mucosa	Swab samples may reveal sperm or pubic hair.
Body	Bruising in patterns (thumb print, palm print) and bruises of different ages
	Cigarette burns
	Fingernail scratches
	Bite marks on thighs or genitalia
Genital region	Damage to 6 o'clock regions rather than the classic 12 o'clock regions of straddle injuries
Vagina	Hymenal-vaginal tears
	Enlarged hymenal opening (>1 cm)
	Sexually transmitted disease
Anus	Resting dilation in absence of stool (>2 cm)
	Fixed opening
	Thickening, smoothing, or asymmetry of skin of anal verge

used marker is the enzyme acid phosphatase. The activity of this enzyme decreases rapidly in the vagina, and it becomes indistinguishable from normal vaginal enzymes after 72 hours. Motile sperm can be recovered up to 8 hours after an assault. Nonmotile sperm can be found up to 26 hours after an incident. If oral sex was forced, separate swabs should be taken from the perioral skin, gums, tongue, and pharynx. Drops of fluid mixed with swab material can then be air-dried on a slide and either stained or processed as a cytopathology specimen.

  C. **Treatment** for the victim consists of addressing the immediate medical needs as well as providing protection against further abuse and psychological support for the victim and her family.

    1. **Injuries.** Repair of injuries depends on the type of injury sustained. Good perineal hygiene with sitz baths should be emphasized. Superficial injuries will resolve within a few days. Any evidence of infection requires use of antibiotics. Small hematomas can be controlled by pressure with an ice pack. Hematomas that continue to expand should be excised, the clots removed, and the bleeding area ligated. Large tears require suturing under anesthesia. Suspected vaginal or rectal lacerations also should be repaired under anesthesia. Bite wounds should be irrigated. Most of these wounds should be left open. A noninfected fresh wound can be primarily closed. Any necrotic tissue should be débrided. After 3–5 days, a secondary débridement may be required. If the child is not already immunized, she should be given a tetanus immunization.

TABLE 30-2. DEFINITIVE VERSUS NONSPECIFIC FINDINGS OF SEXUAL ABUSE

Definitive	Pregnancy, presence of sperm, or presence of a sexually transmitted disease vaginally, orally, or in the rectoanal area.
Nonspecific findings	Poor local hygiene causing superficial lesions must be interpreted with caution; findings include redness, irritations, abrasions, friability of the posterior fourchette, labial adhesions, hymenal tags or bumps, bruising of the external genitalia, and nonspecific infections.

2. **Infection.** The patient should be screened for gonorrhea, syphilis, *Chlamydia*, *Trichomonas*, human immunodeficiency virus, and hepatitis B. Treatment for a sexually transmitted disease should be deferred until the results of cultures and serologic tests for syphilis are known. Antibiotic therapy should be instituted only if the child is symptomatic on the initial visit. A repeat Venereal Disease Research Laboratory test should be performed in 6 weeks to rule out seroconversion. Human immunodeficiency virus and hepatitis B surface antigen testing should also be considered at 6 weeks.

3. **Safety.** All suspected victims of child abuse should be referred to **child protective services.** Occasionally it is necessary to admit a child to the hospital for safety. Until the question of protection can be answered, it is advisable to provide temporary placement for the child.

4. **Counseling.** An essential part of any evaluation for suspected abuse includes provision of intensive day-to-day counseling, support, and guidance. A trained therapist should be available to help the victim cope with the evaluation process, including the medical treatment and encounters with child protection services and law enforcement agencies. The family also should be offered treatment.

5. **Pregnancy.** If the child is peripubertal, the option of emergency contraception should be addressed. A follow-up pregnancy test may be appropriate.

III. **Traumatic injuries.** The period of highest incidence is between 4 and 12 years of age. Because of the differences in anatomy between a child and an adult, a seemingly innocuous lesion can result in a serious injury. Six common injuries are outlined in the following subsections.

A. **Straddle injuries.** Straddle injuries account for approximately 75% of all genital injuries in young girls. These may present as an area of ecchymosis or hematoma with painful swelling over the labia. Injuries often involve the mons, clitoris, urethra, or anterior portions of the labia minora and labia majora. Hymenal injuries extending to the vaginal opening are rarely seen. If hematuria accompanies a perineal lesion, a voiding cystourethrogram to rule out bladder or urethral injury may be warranted. To treat blunt perineal injuries, observation and cold compresses are used for the first 6 hours. If the hematoma remains the same size or becomes smaller, warm sitz baths often are all that is required. Urethral catheterization, analgesics, and prophylactic antibiotics can be used when a hematoma at the urethral orifice is causing pain and poor urination.

B. **Accidental penetration.** Accidental penetration is often the result of falling on a sharp object, usually a pen or pencil. The age most often affected is 2–4 years. Presentation can include hematuria, vaginal discharge, or bleeding, because a puncture wound may not be obvious. In fact, it may be intraperitoneal with rectal pain or bleeding as the presenting complaint. The child should also undergo a thorough examination with abdominal radiography, roentgenography, anoscopy, and sigmoidoscopy. Microscopic hematuria warrants a very careful urethral catheterization. Resistance is an indication to perform voiding cystourethrography instead. In cases of gross hematuria, catheterization should not be attempted.

C. **Foreign bodies.** Retained foreign bodies in the vagina often present with bloody or purulent discharge, and this is a common presentation at age 2–4 years. Other symptoms include genital pruritus, abdominal pain, or fever. The presence of a vaginal foreign body may be a previously unrecognized indicator of sexual abuse. The foreign bodies can vary from wads of toilet paper, buttons, or coins to peanuts and crayons. Persistent vaginal discharge in a toddler warrants an examination under anesthesia. Antibiotics should be started before removal. If the object remains undetected, peritonitis can develop from the ascension of purulent secretions to the fallopian tubes. A careful examination of the vaginal wall for any defects or additional embedded foreign bodies should be performed after the object has been removed. If the rectovaginal septum is involved, a temporary colostomy with delayed repair of the vaginal and rectal tissues may be indicated.

D. **Sex-related trauma.** Most often sited at the perineal area, sex-related trauma can be difficult to diagnose, especially if the patient is embarrassed or coerced into not revealing it in the history.

E. **Lacerations.** Forceful abduction of the legs can result in lacerations of the vaginal orifice that can frequently extend into the fornix. This may also result from gymnastic exercise, waterskiing, or a major motor vehicle accident. An examination under general anesthesia must be performed to determine the extent of the injury. Involvement of the rectovaginal septum or extension of the laceration into the peritoneal cavity must be ruled out.

F. **Clitoral strangulation** or ischemia can be a difficult diagnosis, as it often results when a hair from a caretaker accidentally becomes wrapped around the base of the organ. Symptoms are irritability, engorgement, and possible cellulitis. The outcome depends on the degree of ischemia.

IV. **Urinary tract infection (UTI).** Urologic complaints often go hand in hand with gynecologic complaints. Obtaining a careful history with regard to voiding patterns, day and night frequency, urgency or stress, quality of the stream, bed wetting, and previous infections and treatments is very important. Physical examination entails a complete abdominal and external genitalia evaluation; vaginal inspection if indicated; a neurologic assessment, including evaluation of reflexes, perineal sensation, and sphincter tone; and inspection of the lower back for evidence of a spinal abnormality.

A. The **prevalence of asymptomatic bacteriuria** is influenced by age, sex, and method of diagnosis. Lack of symptoms is due to the low virulence of the bacterial strains, which do not have the ability to adhere to and ascend the uroepithelium. Because asymptomatic bacteriuria in children can be a marker for a renal abnormality, it is recommended that these children be evaluated thoroughly.

B. **Clinical presentation**

1. **Cystitis.** Very young children often present with irritability, poor feeding, failure to grow, vomiting, or abdominal distention. Fever may be absent in the neonate. Young children present with failure to be toilet trained at the appropriate age, enuresis, incontinence, frequency, and dysuria. Symptoms recur in approximately 10% of these girls. Adolescents present with symptoms similar to those of adults. Hemorrhagic cystitis is more common in adolescents.

2. **Pyelonephritis.** Young children with pyelonephritis present with high fevers, abdominal or flank pain, chills, nausea, vomiting, and myalgia. They are often very ill, requiring hospitalization. Young infants, however, usually present with nonspecific findings associated with high fever. Unlike cystitis, a leukocytosis with a left shift can be present. The most common risk factor is vesicoureteral reflux (VUR), estimated to have a prevalence of 1% in healthy children. In those with UTIs who have fevers higher than 38.5°C, reflux has been found in 90%. The cause of reflux in the majority of children with VUR is congenital maldevelopment of the ureterovesical junction. In those with severe bladder dysfunction, the normal valve mechanism can be overcome by high pressure. Acute cystitis may produce a transient reflux. In children with a normal bladder and without infection, VUR is a benign condition. Other predisposing factors for pyelonephritis are obstruction and severe malformation of the urinary tract. Pyelonephritis can lead to renal scarring in 25–30% of children. In this setting, renal scarring usually develops during the first 5 years of life and occurs predominantly at the renal poles with hypertrophy of normal parenchyma. Increasing number of episodes of pyelonephritis increases the incidence of renal scarring. Early and aggressive antibiotic treatment is indicated.

C. **Evaluation** of the child should be undertaken after the first documented UTI. Reinfection occurs within 18 months in up to 40–60% of all children. Evidence of an upper UTI warrants a complete radiographic evaluation. The diagnosis of reflux is made by voiding cystourethrography. In children with reflux, the most common urodynamic abnormality is uninhibited bladder contractions. Most low-grade reflux resolves spontaneously with improved bladder function. Renal ultrasonography also can be used to assess the upper urinary tract. In children, it has been found to be as sensitive as an IVP for the detection of significant renal abnormalities with the exception of uncomplicated duplication anomalies and focal scarring. Older adolescent girls with recurrent infection may best be evaluated by an IVP and cystoscopic evaluation with or without a voiding cystourethrogram.

D. **Bacteriology.** The majority of UTIs are caused by Gram-negative organisms, most often *Escherichia coli*, which is present in 60–80% of cases. The most common Gram-positive organisms are *Staphylococcus* and *Enterococcus*. The majority of uncomplicated UTIs involve only one organism. Lactobacilli, corynebacteria, and streptococci should be considered contaminants unless the urine was a specimen collected via catheter or suprapubic aspiration.

E. **Treatment** of an acute, uncomplicated lower UTI uses sulfonamides such as trimethoprim-sulfamethoxazole, nitrofurantoin, trimethoprim, and the cephalosporins. Fluoroquinolones are best avoided because they have demonstrated toxicity in cartilage. Although controversy exists regarding the duration of treatment, it is at present recommended that children be treated for 7–10 days because of the higher risk of anatomic anomalies. After the first UTI, a child should remain on prophylactic antibiotics until a radiographic evaluation is undertaken, usually within 2–3 weeks.

1. In managing reflux, the main goal is to prevent an ascending UTI and renal scarring. Low-grade reflux tends to resolve spontaneously over time. Most resolutions occur within the first few years after diagnosis. The rate of resolution remains constant at 10–15% per year. Reflux nephropathy is the most common disorder leading to hypertension in children. Management involves preventing UTIs with daily antibiotic prophylaxis, frequent voiding, and avoidance of constipation. A radiographic evaluation of the upper urinary tract should be performed annually until the reflux disappears.

2. Surgical management of reflux involves ureteral reimplantation. Indications are persistent or recurrent infection despite prophylaxis, noncompliance with medical therapy, development of new scarring or failure of renal growth, or persistent significant reflux in adolescent girls. Reimplantation is successful in more than 95% of children.

V. **Vulvovaginitis** is the most common gynecologic complaint in the prepubertal girl. Vulvovaginal inflammation accounts for 40–50% of visits to a pediatric gynecology clinic. Physiologic changes of the vagina include those resulting from the initial stimulation of maternal hormones in the newborn period, which results in a thickened vaginal mucosa and a physiologic leukorrhea. As estrogen levels decrease, the epithelium becomes smooth, thin, and atrophic, with a pH of 6.5–7.5. These changes usually take place by 6 weeks postnatally. Because of the neutral pH and lack of estrogenization, these delicate tissues are particularly susceptible to inflammation.

A. **Risk factors** contributing to increased susceptibility are the lack of antibodies that help fight infection, lack of protective hair and labial fat pads, proximity of the rectum to the vagina, relatively small labia minora, and lack of proper hygiene. Other potential risk factors for vulvovaginitis include a small hymenal opening, obesity, preexisting vulvar dermatoses, and systemic illness such as diabetes mellitus. The normal prepubertal vaginal flora include lactobacilli, α-hemolytic streptococci, *Staphylococcus epidermidis*, and diphtheroid and Gram-negative enteric organisms, especially *E. coli*.

B. **Signs and symptoms** include vaginal discharge that stains the under-clothing. On occasion, blood stains are noted. Genital pain, itching, irrita-tion, and dysuria are common. Vulvar burning or stinging may occur when urine comes into contact with irritated, excoriated tissues. On examination, erythema and discharge with an odor may be noted.

C. **Evaluation**

1. A **history** should be taken before a physical examination is conducted. The duration, consistency, quantity, and color of the discharge should be noted. Infections with anaerobic bacteria may be accompanied by the presence of a foul odor, and questions should be directed at eliciting behaviors such as inadequate hygiene, including back-to-front wiping; trauma associated with play; or any genital manipulation with a foreign body or contaminated hands. Wearing of close-fitting, poorly absorbent clothing or prolonged exposure to a wet bathing suit may predispose to vulvovaginitis. In younger children, the type of diaper and frequency of changes should be noted. Information about recent systemic infections, new medications or lotions, bed wetting, use of harsh soaps or bubble baths, dermatosis, and nocturnal perianal itching should be included in the history.

2. On **physical examination,** a sample of the discharge should be obtained for microscopic examination and culture. In nonrecurrent vul-vovaginitis with no suspicion of bleeding or a foreign body, a vaginos-copy is not necessary. Presentations for vulvovaginitis are extremely variable, ranging from no discharge to copious secretions. Erythema, edema, and excoriations are commonly noted. Evidence of poor perineal hygiene may be evident, with stool seen in the vulva or between the labia. The configuration of the hymen should be carefully noted and evaluated for any signs of trauma. The perianal skin should also be examined.

D. **Treatment** involves improving perineal hygiene. The majority of vulvovag-inal infections result in nonspecific vaginitis, which is often caused by dis-turbed bacterial homeostasis. This is often a result of suboptimal hygiene. These alterations in the flora or host defense mechanisms result in inflam-mation. A wet preparation of a discharge specimen shows a mixture of WBCs, bacteria, and other debris. Sitz or tub baths twice a day for half an hour help eliminate the vaginal discharge from vulvar areas. Nonirritating soaps and white cotton underpants should be recommended. Nylon tights, tight blue jeans, and bubble baths should be discouraged. Both the caregiver and child should be instructed about proper front-to-back wiping. The child should be instructed to urinate with her knees apart so that urinary reflux into the vagina is reduced with drying. In summer months, prolonged wear-ing of a wet bathing suit should be discouraged. If symptoms persist after 2 weeks of therapy, the child should be reexamined. Pinworms should be excluded and, if found, can be treated with a single dose of medication, which is repeated 2 weeks later. Mebendazole should not be given to chil-dren younger than 2 years. All family members may need to be treated. Vag-inoscopy should be considered to exclude a foreign body, neoplasm, or abnormal communication with the GI or urinary tract. In unusually persis-tent cases for which a specific cause has been ruled out, irrigation of the vagina with a 1% solution of povidone-iodine (Betadine) may be helpful. Another approach is to prescribe a 2-month course of a small dose of antibi-otic at bedtime or three times a week. Estrogen-containing creams can be tried, but only for 3–4 weeks at a time. Caution must be exercised, as sys-temic absorption of estrogen during prolonged use can result in iatrogenic precocious puberty. Recurrence often develops when the child has an upper respiratory infection or has failed to use proper hygiene. Obese girls are par-ticularly at risk for recurrences. Hymenotomy is curative for those whose vaginitis occurs secondary to a high hymenal opening that impairs vaginal drainage. Other causes include a pelvic abscess and an ectopic ureter.

TABLE 30-3. PATHOGENS CAUSING VULVOVAGINITIS

Pathogen	Symptoms	Treatment
Neisseria gonorrhoeae Sites: vagina, rectum, pharynx, and conjunctiva	Discharge Swelling	Lotions and sitz baths Ceftriaxone sodium IM injection Older children: doxycycline
Chlamydia Sites: Vagina, rectum Acquired by perinatal exposure or by sexual abuse (24–36 mos and older)	Perinatal infections may persist for up to 53–55 wks in the vagina/rectum	Erythromycin, 50 mg, divided qid for 10 days Older children: doxycycline, 100 mg PO, or azithromycin, 1 g PO
Herpes simplex virus type I or II Sites: vulva, oropharynx, rectum (Infection from transplacental passage usually presents in the first week of life)	Painful ulcerating vesicular lesions, fever, nausea, malaise, headache, and inguinal adenopathy Urinary retention	Acyclovir (controversial) Others prescribe symptomatic treatment with sitz baths and drying agents Antibiotics can be prescribed for bacterial superinfection
Human papillomavirus (genital warts) Sites: vulva, urethra, bladder, mouth, eye, perianal most common (Also presents as laryngeal papillomatosis by vertical transmission)	Aceto-white appearance of condyloma after application of 3–5% acetic acid to suspected lesions Usually associated with sexual abuse	Laser excision or cautery
Trichomonas vaginalis Rarely seen in patients under 9 yrs old	Copious yellow-gray frothy discharge and complaints of dysuria and vulvar itching	Metronidazole 15 mg/kg/day divided tid for 7 days
Mixed infection of *Gardnerella vaginalis,* anaerobes, and genital mycoplasmas (bacterial vaginosis)	Same symptoms as adults Usually associated with sexual abuse	No guidelines in pediatric population Metronidazole as above, or ampicillin or amoxicillin may also be beneficial
Treponema pallidum Hematogenous transplacental passage if less than 1 yr of age *Must rule out sexual abuse*	Congenital primary: painless oral or genital chancre Secondary: skin rash Tertiary: neurologic signs	Congenital/tertiary: penicillin G (200,000–300,000 U/kg/day) for 10–14 days Primary/secondary: 50,000 U/kg IM benzathine penicillin, single dose (not to exceed 2.4 million U)

E. **Pathogens.** Table 30-3 highlights the pathogens causing vulvovaginitis in the pediatric population that are often associated with sexual abuse. Other infectious causes of vaginitis usually involve secondary inoculation. Recovery of *Haemophilus influenzae* from vaginal secretions has unclear significance, and the infection may be treated with 20–40 mg/kg/day Amoxicillin by mouth (PO) for 7 days. Infection with group A β-hemolytic streptococci (e.g., *Streptococcus pyogenes*) is an important cause that often presents with vaginal bleeding 1 week after a sore throat. It is treated with penicillin V potassium, 125–250 mg PO four times per day for 10 days. Shigellosis results in a mucopurulent and malodorous vaginal discharge. Diarrhea occurs in less than one-fourth of individuals. Treatment is with trimethoprim, 8 mg/kg/day, and sulfamethoxazole, 40 mg/kg/day, divided into two doses PO for 7 days. *Staphylococcus aureus* can be part of the normal vaginal flora. When found in a symptomatic individual, it can be treated with cephalexin, 25–50 mg/kg/day PO for 7 days; dicloxacillin, 25 mg/kg/day PO for 7 days; or amoxicillin plus clavulanate potassium (Augmentin), 20–40 mg/kg/day PO for 7–10 days. Candidal vulvovaginitis occurs infrequently in prepubertal girls. The infection usually involves a child still in diapers with a history of recent use of an antibiotic, diabetes mellitus, or immunodeficiency. It is diagnosed by KOH wet preparation of a discharge specimen. If candidal vulvovaginitis is diagnosed in a child without a predisposing condition, an evaluation for diabetes or immunodeficiency should be undertaken. Treatment consists initially of application of a topical antifungal cream such as miconazole. If this is not successful, subsequent treatment consists of intravaginal nystatin liquid or antifungal suppositories of an appropriate size. One-fifth of girls with pinworms develop an associated vulvovaginitis. Symptoms include vulvar and perianal itching, particularly at night. The "Scotch tape test" can be used to diagnose pinworm infestation by recovering the characteristic eggs. Treatment of *Enterobius vermicularis* is with mebendazole, 100 mg PO for one dose, for all members of a household except pregnant women and children younger than 2 years.

F. **Congenital anomalies,** such as an ectopic ureter, may result in vulvovaginitis. Anomalous openings onto the perineum or into the vagina or urethra can result in a discharge of clear or infected urine. An IVP can be used to make the diagnosis.

G. **Chemical vaginitis** secondary to the use of new lotions, bubble baths, or harsh soaps can cause irritation of the perineal and vulvar skin. Treatment includes discontinuation of the causative agent, good perineal hygiene, and sitz baths.

H. **Systemic illnesses,** such as varicella, Crohn's disease, Stevens-Johnson syndrome, diabetes, Behçet's syndrome, or Kawasaki syndrome, can result in vaginitis.

VI. **Vaginal bleeding** in children is a cause for concern and requires thorough evaluation. It can be caused by vulvar or vaginal irritation or lesions, trauma or sexual abuse, or precocious puberty.

A. **Vulvovaginitis** may cause vaginal bleeding. The causes and management of vulvovaginitis are discussed in detail in sec. V.

B. **Urethral prolapse** can sometimes be the cause of bleeding. It is thought to occur after an episode of increased abdominal pressure. The urethral mucosa protrudes through the meatus, forming an annular, hemorrhagic mass that bleeds easily. The average age of onset is 5 years. A short-term course of therapy with estrogen cream is indicated in cases of asymptomatic prolapse. Sitz baths often can be of benefit. If the patient is symptomatic with urinary retention or if the mass is large and necrotic, resection of the prolapsed tissue with insertion of an indwelling catheter for more than 24 hours may be warranted. Antibiotic treatment is necessary if infection occurs. Other urologic disorders with similar presentations include urethral polyps, caruncles, cysts, and prolapsed uterocele.

C. **Dysfunctional uterine bleeding** is excessive, prolonged, or erratic bleeding from the endometrium that is not caused by anatomic lesions of the uterus. It is discussed in sec. **VII, Pubertal Disorders.**

D. **Endometrial shedding** resulting in vaginal bleeding is often associated with precocious puberty, which is defined as the onset of sexual maturation at an age younger than 2 standard deviations from the norm. In the United States, sexual precocity is the appearance of secondary sexual characteristics before the age of 8 years or the onset of menarche before the age of 10 years. Among African-American girls, breast development before 7 years of age is defined as precocious puberty. Causes of endometrial shedding include a physiologic neonatal withdrawal bleed in the first 2 weeks of life secondary to maternal estrogen withdrawal; isolated premature menarche, which is rare without other signs of precocious puberty; iatrogenic or factitious precocious puberty caused by medications containing exogenous estrogens; functional ovarian cysts; ovarian neoplasms; idiopathic precocious puberty; McCune-Albright syndrome; CNS lesions; or other hormone-producing neoplasms.

E. **Labial adhesions.** Estrogen is required to maintain normal tissue tone in the labia majora and minora. In the low-estrogen environment of childhood, the labia may fuse in response to any genital trauma, even diaper rash. Adhesive vulvitis involves fusion of the labia minora, likely caused by the chronic irritation associated with vulvitis. This is common between ages 2 and 6 years. Lichen sclerosis has also been known to cause adhesions secondary to low estrogen levels. Regardless of the cause, topical estrogen cream can be applied to the adhesion twice daily for 2–4 weeks.

F. **Genital tumors** are relatively uncommon in the prepubertal girl. They must be considered part of the differential diagnosis, however, when a patient is found to have a chronic genital ulcer, tissue protruding from the vagina, a malodorous bloody vaginal discharge, or an atraumatic swelling of the external genitalia. There are both benign and malignant tumors of the genitalia. This section describes the more common malignant growths.

1. **Sarcoma botryoides** (rhabdomyosarcoma) is a fast-growing, aggressive tumor of the genital tract. It is the most common malignant tumor of the genital tract in girls. The peak incidence is before age 2 years, with 90% of patients diagnosed before age 5 years. It arises in the submucosal tissue, spreading beneath an intact vaginal epithelium. The vaginal mucosa then is punctuated by polypoid growths. The hallmark sign is passage of a polypoid mass from the anterior vagina, vulva, or urethra. Symptoms include vaginal bleeding or discharge and abdominal pain. On examination, an abdominal mass can sometimes be palpated. Diagnosis is made by biopsy. Staging, including a chest radiograph and abdominopelvic CT scan, is necessary before treatment. Treatment involves chemotherapy using a combination regimen of vincristine sulfate, actinomycin D, and cyclophosphamide. If the tumor can be resected after chemotherapy, a radical hysterectomy and vaginectomy can be performed. If the tumor is unresectable, radiotherapy can be instituted. There is a tendency for this tumor to recur locally. Follow-up is mandatory.

2. **Embryonal carcinoma, mesonephric carcinoma, and clear cell adenocarcinoma** are often seen in the setting of maternal diethylstilbestrol exposure. Clear cell carcinoma may commonly present with abnormal vaginal bleeding and discharge. Clear cell carcinoma may also occur in absence of maternal diethylstilbestrol exposure. The youngest case reported was in a 7-year-old.

3. **Germ cell tumors** are the most common ovarian neoplasms in the pediatric population. They arise from primitive germ cells, which can further differentiate into two different tumors: dysgerminomas and embryonal carcinomas. They usually present with a complex mass in the pelvis and are often associated with the presence of tumor markers such as alpha-fetoprotein, human chorionic gonadotropin, and chorio-

TABLE 30-4. BASELINE HORMONAL LEVELS BY AGE

1–2 yrs	LH: 0.6–1.3 ng/mL	Estradiol: 11 and 18 pg/mL
	FSH: 1.9–3.2 ng/mL	
3–4 yrs	LH: 1.1–2.0 mIU/mL	Estradiol: 14–26 pg/mL
	FSH: 1.0–1.7 mIU/mL	
6 yrs	LH: 1.1–4.3 mIU/mL	Estradiol: 20 pg/mL
	FSH: 1.0–2.0 mIU/mL	
Pubertal levels	LH: 5.0–20.0 mIU/mL	Estradiol: 20–40 pg/mL
	FSH: 5.0–30.0 mIU/mL	

FSH, follicle-stimulyating hormone; LH, luteinizing hormone.

embryonic antigen. Surgical management usually involves a unilateral salpingo-oophorectomy and staging. The resultant pathology dictates therapy. Germ cell tumors respond well to chemotherapy except for dysgerminomas, which respond to radiation.

VII. **Disorders of puberty.** Abnormal puberty can be classified into three categories: delayed, asynchronous, and precocious.

A. **Delayed puberty.** Delay of puberty can be caused by anatomic abnormalities, chromosomal disorders, neoplastic growths, or nutritional deficiencies. On history and physical examination, the presence or absence of secondary sexual characteristics must be elucidated. In addition, a progestin challenge test can be performed by administering a progestin for 10 days to ascertain whether the patient experiences a withdrawal bleed after cessation of progestin. In addition, it is easy to classify them as to whether the disorder is associated with an increase or decrease in follicle stimulating hormone (FSH) levels. Baseline values of prepubertal hormones are given in Table 30-4.

1. **High follicle-stimulating hormone levels (higher than 30 mIU/mL)**

a. **Gonadal dysgenesis.** These are phenotypic females unable to fully develop. They present with primary amenorrhea, normal chromosomes, and streak gonads. They may have some secondary sex characteristics and spontaneous menstruation. Genotypes associated with this condition are 45,XO, its mosaics (45,X/46,XX; 45,X/46,XY), and 46,XY (Swyer's syndrome). Turner's syndrome is the most common type of gonadal dysgenesis. The karyotype associated is most often 45,X (Table 30-5).

TABLE 30-5. TURNER'S SYNDROME STIGMATA

Webbed neck

Lymphedema at birth

Horseshoe kidney

Multiple pigmented nevi

Coarctation of the aorta

Space-form blindness

Small hyperconvex fingernails

Endocrine and autoimmune disorders

Short stature at 2–3 yrs and older

b. **Ovarian failure.** In primary ovarian failure, the ovaries develop but do not contain oocytes. This may be associated with chemotherapy, galactosemia, gonadotropin resistance, autoimmune ovarian failure, or failure secondary to prior infection. Treatment is usually by administration of exogenous estrogen and progesterone to avoid osteoporosis and facilitate development of secondary sexual characteristics.

2. **Low follicle-stimulating hormone levels (less than 10 mIU/mL).** The following conditions produce gonadotropins in insufficient quantities to allow follicular development and, therefore, sex steroid production.

a. **Constitutional delay.** Delay in the gonadotropin-releasing hormone (GnRH) pulse generator.

b. **Syndromes. Kallmann syndrome** is a classical triad of anosmia, hypogonadism, and color blindness. The hypothalamus cannot secrete GnRH due to a dysfunction in the arcuate nucleus. Therefore, there are few or no secondary sexual characteristics. Other syndromes associated with delayed puberty include **Prader-Labhardt-Willi syndrome** and **Laurence-Moon-Biedl syndrome.**

c. **Hormone deficiencies.** Any aberration of growth hormone or thyroid hormone levels will affect puberty. Therefore, these levels should be investigated and treated appropriately. In addition, hyperprolactinemia can cause a decrease in levels of FSH and luteinizing hormone (LH) and thus delay puberty. These levels should be investigated as well.

d. **Neoplasms.** Both craniopharyngiomas and pituitary adenomas may cause delayed puberty. Visual symptoms are often associated with these tumors, as are short stature and diabetes insipidus. Diagnosis is by CT or MRI of the head. Treatment includes either surgical excision or radiotherapy.

e. **Malnutrition.** Both starvation and anorexia nervosa can cause pubertal delay.

3. **Anatomic causes of primary amenorrhea**

a. **Genital tract obstruction**

(1) **Imperforate hymen.** An imperforate hymen may be evident in a neonate and may regress as the girl enters childhood. After menarche, the imperforate hymen may become evident as an abdominal mass when accumulated menstrual blood forms a hematocolpos. This requires surgical intervention to incise the hymen and allow the stored debris to escape.

(2) **Transverse vaginal septum** is due to the failure of canalization of müllerian tubules and the sinovaginal bulb, which leaves a membrane present. If it is thin, it can be incised and dilated. The edges can be sutured to the vagina. If the membrane is thick, a split-thickness skin graft may be required for repair.

b. **Müllerian dysgenesis.** Disorders of the outflow tract are sometimes accompanied by renal and skeletal anomalies. These anomalies are classified along a spectrum from complete müllerian agenesis to simple hypoplasia.

B. **Asynchronous puberty**

1. **Androgen insensitivity.** Androgen insensitivity is caused by either the absence or the insensitivity of androgen receptors. Chromosome analysis must reveal 46,XY. Such patients, however, are phenotypically female with a blind-ending vagina and no fallopian tubes or uterus. Bilateral testes are present along the line of descent. These patients present with breast development to Tanner stage 5 and decreased pubic and axillary hair relative to their breast development. Diagnosis can be made by a finding of very high levels of testosterone with normal levels of LH and FSH. Gonadectomy should be performed and then exogenous estrogen supplied. Families must receive genetic counseling, as this disorder can be inherited in an X-linked fashion.

2. **Incomplete androgen insensitivity.** Infrequently, patients may have the findings described earlier as well as clitoral enlargement and labioscrotal fusion at puberty, thus demonstrating the presence of a few androgen receptors.

C. **Precocious puberty**

1. **Definition.** In North America, sexual precocity is defined as the appearance of any sign of secondary sexual characteristics at younger than 8 years of age (an age more than 3.0 standard deviations below the mean).

   a. **Central or true precocity.** Complete isosexual precocity, also known as **true** or **central precocious puberty,** is the result of premature activation of the pulsatile hypothalamic GnRH mechanism. **Isosexual** refers to secondary sexual characteristics appropriate for the child's sex.

   b. **Idiopathic precocious puberty** may manifest itself in infancy and is more common in girls (for whom age of onset is 6–7 years) than in boys. Inquiries should be made about a family history of early maturation, because true precocious puberty may be transmitted in an autosomal recessive fashion.

   Physical findings in girls include development of breasts and pubic hair, enlargement of the labia minora, and maturation of the vaginal mucosa. Usually, the development of secondary sexual characteristics progresses more rapidly than in normal puberty. The child may experience a course of development that fluctuates between progression and regression. Some girls may experience spontaneous regression, whereas in others secondary sexual characteristics may persist.

2. **CNS tumors** that result in true precocious puberty are equally prevalent among boys and girls. Astrocytomas; ependymomas; optic or hypothalamic gliomas or hamartomas, which are often associated with neurofibromatosis; tuberous sclerosis; suprasellar cyst; sarcoid granuloma; and craniopharyngiomas may result in true precocious puberty.

   a. **Pathophysiology.** The mechanism that causes precocious puberty is hypothesized to be either a mass effect of the growth, which impinges on the pathway that inhibits the GnRH pump in childhood; effects of the cranial radiation used to treat the tumor; or the presence of ectopic GnRH-secreting cells, which are usually associated with hamartomas. Accompanying features often include seizures, mental retardation, accelerated growth, headaches, visual changes, and dysmorphic syndromes. These masses are diagnosed by CT of the head.

   b. **Treatment.** The location of tumors leading to precocious puberty makes their surgical removal difficult. Management usually involves radiation therapy, chemotherapy, or both. Manifestations of precocious puberty can be treated with GnRH agonists depending on the age and psychological capabilities of the girl.

3. Other **CNS disorders** such as hydrocephalus, encephalitis, brain abscess, static cerebral encephalopathy, sarcoid granulomas, hypothalamic tuberculous granulomas, and head trauma (associated with cerebral atrophy or focal encephalomalacia) can result in true precocious puberty. Arachnoid cysts, which emerge de novo as a consequence of infection, can cause precocious puberty (possibly with an associated growth hormone deficiency).

4. **Congenital adrenal hyperplasia (CAH).** Patients with CAH who either have been undertreated or have started treatment late may undergo early puberty. Patients who have been treated for either CAH or virilizing tumors may develop precocious puberty after the lowering of androgen levels.

5. **Primary hypothyroidism** may result in premature breast development and galactorrhea. Both symptoms regress after the initiation of thyroid hormone replacement. The absence of a growth spurt may help to establish hypothyroidism as the cause of premature development.

D. **Pseudoprecocious puberty.** Incomplete isosexual precocity, also known as **pseudoprecocious puberty** or **GnRH-independent sexual precocity,** characterized by extrapituitary secretion of gonadotropins or gonadal steroid secretion that is independent of GnRH pulsatile stimulation.

1. **Autonomous ovarian follicular cysts** are the most common form of estrogen-secreting masses in children. Plasma levels of estradiol may be elevated. A sonogram may reveal ovarian cysts. Exploratory laparotomy or laparoscopy is sometimes necessary to differentiate between these benign cysts and a malignant ovarian neoplasm. Removal of a hormonally active cyst may result in correction of the precocity. Autonomously secreting cysts are not associated with increased LH pulsatile secretion or with a pubertal response of LH to GnRH.

2. **Ovarian tumors** (2%) may cause precocious puberty. Approximately 60% of ovarian tumors causing precocious puberty are granulosa cell tumors; the remainder are arrhenoblastomas, thecomas, or lipid cell tumors. Although LH and FSH levels usually are suppressed in patients with ovarian tumors, their plasma concentrations of estradiol are usually elevated. Sonography of the ovary facilitates the diagnosis. Subsequent to surgical removal of the tumor, measurements of plasma levels of estradiol may be used to screen for metastasis.

3. **Peutz-Jeghers syndrome** is characterized by mucocutaneous pigmentation and GI polyposis and is also associated with a rare sex cord tumor. The tumor's estrogen secretion may result in feminization and incomplete sexual precocity. Although rare, epithelial tumors of the ovary, dysgerminomas, or Sertoli-Leydig cell tumors have been found in patients with Peutz-Jeghers syndrome. Girls with Peutz-Jeghers syndrome should be evaluated with serial pelvic sonographic examinations for the presence of gonadal tumors.

4. **McCune-Albright syndrome** is characterized by irregular hyperpigmented macules (café au lait spots), polyostotic fibrous dysplasia (progressive bone disorder), and GnRH-independent sexual precocity. At least two of these three features must be present to make the diagnosis of McCune-Albright syndrome.

   a. **Pathophysiology.** Sexual precocity results from an autonomous luteinized follicular cyst. The pubertal pattern of LH pulses is initially absent, but when the bone age approaches 12 years, the GnRH pulse mechanism is activated and ovulation is established, which results in a progression from GnRH-independent to GnRH-dependent puberty.

   b. **Treatment.** GnRH agonists are not effective therapy for this disorder. Aromatase inhibitors [e.g., testolactone (Teslac)] have been shown to help to decrease symptoms.

5. **Adrenal disorders** such as adenomas can secrete estrogen alone and give rise to sexual precocity. Patients in whom CAH has been untreated may exhibit virilization as well as some breast development. Estrogen-secreting adrenal carcinomas may also produce other hormones that result in heterosexual precocity.

E. **Heterosexual puberty.** Contrasexual precocity results from increased androgen levels and leads to inappropriate virilization. In girls, virilization is an indicator of organic disease (with the exception of premature adrenarche).

1. **Congenital adrenal hyperplasia**

2. **Cushing disease** that results from an adrenal carcinoma may manifest as growth failure with or without virilization, obesity, striae, and moon facies.

3. **Ovarian tumors** such as arrhenoblastoma, lipoid cell tumor, and gonadoblastoma can be culprits in a virilizing girl. Arrhenoblastoma is the most common virilizing ovarian tumor.

a. **History.** Inquiries should be made about birth trauma, encephalitis, changes in personality, headaches, visual changes, seizures, abdominal pain, urinary or bowel changes, increased appetite, and use of medications or creams. In most cases, information about the age of onset of precocious puberty is not helpful in establishing a diagnosis. Also, the age of pubertal onset in the patient's mother, sisters, and grandmothers should be ascertained. Any family history of neurofibromatosis and tuberous sclerosis should be noted. The child's growth pattern should be recorded in a chart, because accelerated growth and bone age may help to distinguish between premature thelarche and true precocious puberty.

b. **Physical examination.** On examination, evidence of papilledema, visual field defects, or café au lait spots should be sought. The child's head circumference should be measured and recorded. The size and texture of the thyroid gland should be noted, and inquiries should be made about any hair or skin changes. The breasts and external genitalia should be closely inspected, and the degree of breast, pubic, and axillary hair growth and the appearance of the vaginal mucosa should be noted. Ovarian masses can often be palpated.

c. **Laboratory testing** depends on the initial evaluation. An extensive workup is indicated in the presence of vaginal estrogenization and acceleration of linear growth. If premature thelarche is found, however, a radiographic film of the wrist to document bone age and a vaginal smear to test for estrogen effect are indicated. A skeletal survey is indicated for patients in whom the McCune-Albright syndrome is suspected. Bone lesions may be detected by bone scan before they are apparent radiographically. A CT or MRI scan is often helpful in diagnosing CNS abnormalities. True precocity, gonadotropin-independent precocity, and premature thelarche may be differentiated with a GnRH-stimulation test. Patients with pituitary insufficiency show a diminished (prepubertal) response to GnRH. In patients with gonadotropin-independent precocity, ovarian tumors, or premature thelarche, a prepubertal response to the GnRH test can be expected.

d. **Findings.** In patients with precocious puberty, bone age is greater than height age. Both gonadotropin and gonadal steroid concentrations in the plasma, as well as the LH response to GnRH and the frequency and amplitude of LH pulses, are in the normal pubertal range. In fact, although affected children may initially be tall, they have a short final height as a result of early epiphyseal closure. High levels of estradiol (100–200 pg/mL) and low gonadotropin levels indicate an estrogen-secreting cyst or tumor. High LH levels may signal a gonadotropin-producing tumor or choriocarcinoma (which secretes human chorionic gonadotropin that cross-reacts with LH on the standard assay). A urine or serum pregnancy test would detect such a rise in human chorionic gonadotropin. Elevated LH alone does not lead to isosexual precocity in the absence of increased estrogen secretion. Elevated estradiol levels are seen in 50% of patients with theca-granulosa cell tumors.

e. **Treatment** varies according to the diagnosis. Ovarian tumors require surgical removal. Ovarian cysts may spontaneously regress or may require aspiration. In cases of recurrent cysts, cystectomy may be indicated. In patients with McCune-Albright syndrome, treatment of an ovarian cyst will fail to produce a regression of puberty. In central precocity, ovarian cysts should be followed with observation, because gonadotropin suppression is likely to result in their regression. GnRH agonists have been shown to suppress precocious puberty by selectively and reversibly suppressing LH and FSH secretion, restoring estradiol to its prepubertal level, and mediating the regression (or preventing progression) of breast development and the cessation of menses. GnRH-agonist therapy is also effective in treating patients with precocity secondary to hypothalamic hamartomas and optic nerve gliomas (associated with neurofibromatosis). It is important to inform patients that their development is *early*, not *abnormal*. GnRH agonists will not lead to a decrease in estradiol levels or regression of puberty in girls with the following disorders: McCune-Albright syndrome, gonadotropin-independent puberty, and cyclic gonadal steroid production.

    f. **Follow-up** depends on the diagnosis. Patients undergoing treatment with GnRH agonists require close monitoring of bone age, vaginal cytologic study (for maturation index), physical examination, and maintenance of growth records. A pediatric endocrinologist should be consulted in cases of accelerated growth rate, advanced bone age, and vaginal estrogenization. Patients whose onset of puberty occurs after age 6 and whose prognosis for adult stature is favorable without intervention may require only careful follow-up, reassurance, and counseling. Medroxyprogesterone (Depo-Provera) may be used to induce cessation of menses.

VIII. **Thelarche** is unilateral or bilateral breast development. Without other signs of sexual maturation, early breast development is referred to as **premature thelarche.** It commonly occurs by age 2 and is rare after age 4. Usually a regression of the breast enlargement occurs after a few months. It may persist for several years, however, or until the onset of puberty. In approximately 50% of patients, breast development lasts 3–5 years. Plasma estrogen levels may be elevated, and a urocystogram may demonstrate an estrogen effect on squamous epithelial cells in the urine. In affected patients, FSH serum concentrations may be in the pubertal range, with an FSH to LH ratio that is higher than in normal individuals or in girls with central precocious puberty. The LH response to GnRH is prepubertal. Ovarian sonography often reveals one or several cysts that appear and disappear with changes in the size of the breasts. The uterus, however, remains prepubertal in size.

    A. **Patient assessment** includes a review of medications or creams used recently. Application of topical conjugated estrogens (Premarin) for longer than 2–3 weeks may result in breast changes. On examination, the appearance of the vaginal mucosa, breast size, and presence of a pelvic mass on rectal examination should be noted. The uterus should not be enlarged, and growth charts should document a rate within the previously established percentile for height and weight. A vaginal smear or urocystogram to assess estrogenization and a pelvic ultrasonographic study should be obtained.

    B. **Treatment** is directed toward reassurance and follow-up to confirm that thelarche is not the first manifestation of precocious puberty. It is important to reassure the patient and her parents that, in most cases, pubertal development ensues at a normal, adolescent age.

IX. **Ambiguous genitalia** must be evaluated with a careful history taking, physical examination, and laboratory tests. Based on the karyotype, two groups of patients with ambiguous genitalia can be distinguished: XX neonates and XY neonates. Patient assessment must include measurement of the stretched phallus from the pubis to the tip, with attention to the location of the urethra (perineal versus penile), evaluation of the degree of labial-scrotal fold fusion, and determination of the presence or absence of gonads in the scrotum or inguinal rings. A digital rectal examination may reveal the presence of a cervix (usually easily palpable at birth due to stimulation by placental estrogen in utero).

    A. **Karyotype XX neonate**

       1. **Congenital adrenal hyperplasia** results from the excessive production of adrenal androgens caused by increased levels of adrenocorticotropic hormone. Sustained levels of adrenocorticotropic hormone cause

overstimulation of the adrenals and overproduction of adrenal andro-gens, which results in virilization. These disorders are autosomal reces-sive and manifest as varying degrees of virilization, depending on the degree of enzymatic block.

   a. **Etiology.** The most common cause of CAH (95% of cases) is 21-hydroxylase deficiency. Virilization is the result of production of 17-hydroxyprogesterone (an androgen precursor), which leads to excess secretion of adrenal androgens.

   b. **Diagnosis.** Patient assessment may reveal clitoromegaly, postvagi-nal fusion with wrinkling or pigmentation of the scrotal sac, and absence of a proper vesicovaginal septum (which results in a uro-genital sinus). A genetic female may show a penile urethra as well as fully male external genital phenotype, with the exception of tes-tes. The salt-losing form of CAH secondary to decreased aldoster-one secretion is usually associated with more severe virilization. A male neonate may be discharged before the diagnosis is made, before the onset of the life-threatening hyponatremia that can result in shock and death. Virilized female neonates who do not manifest salt loss may go undiagnosed for years, until hyponatre-mia and shock occur when they are stressed, or until pubic hair, lower voice, abnormal muscular hyperplasia, or excessive growth develops within the first year of life. The diagnosis of 21-hydroxy-lase deficiency should be considered in any child with ambiguous genitalia in the absence of palpable testes; in a phenotypic male without palpable testes; in a male child with ambiguous genitalia and a history of severe vomiting, hypoglycemia, and shock; in a boy with premature virilization; and in a girl of any age with any degree of virilization.

  2. **Female pseudohermaphroditism** is defined as the presence of nor-mally developed ovaries and müllerian structures with ambiguous external genitalia. In utero, the external genitalia feminize in the absence of testes. Therefore, a female fetus exhibits masculinization if exposed to androgens. Exposure to androgens after 12 weeks' gestation, after separation of the vagina and the urogenital sinus, results in clito-ral hypertrophy. Earlier exposure leads to retention of the urogenital sinus and labioscrotal fusion; a penile urethra from labial fusion forms if exposure occurs early enough in differentiation. The uterus and the fallopian tubes are normal, even with severe masculinization, because regression of the müllerian duct requires secretion of antimüllerian hormone, formally referred to as **müllerian inhibiting factor,** by the fetal testes, an event that is not mimicked by androgens.

B. **Karyotypes XX,XY or XX/XY** can exhibit true hermaphroditism. True her-maphroditism must include evidence of both ovarian and testicular tissue in either the same or the opposite gonad. The presence of gonadal stroma in the absence of oocytes is insufficient to designate the rudimentary gonad as an ovary. Evidence of a few oocytes in a streak gonad accompanying testicular tissue on the contralateral side is also insufficient to make this diagnosis.

  1. **Physical findings** may reveal evidence of either female or male exter-nal genitalia, often ambiguous. As a result of the size of the phallus, 75% of affected children are raised as males. Hypospadias is common, with a penile urethra seen in some cases. The patient may present with cryptorchidism and an inguinal hernia that may contain a uterus (seen in most cases) or gonad. Breast development is seen in puberty, with menses developing in approximately 50% of patients. Although sper-matogenesis is rare, ovulation often occurs; pregnancy and childbirth have been reported in patients with a 46,XX karyotype. In an ovotestis, ovarian function is often normal, with a normal cyclic pattern of FSH and LH production. Testicular function is usually abnormal.

2. **Diagnosis.** True hermaphroditism must be considered in any patient with ambiguous genitalia. Approximately 70% of patients are X chromatin positive. Approximately 60% are 46,XX, 12% are 46,XY, and 13% have a 46,XX/46,XY karyotype. A 46,XX/XY karyotype in conjunction with ambiguous genitalia is a strong indicator of true hermaphroditism, although the presence of a 46,XX or 46,XY karyotype does not rule it out. After all forms of pseudohermaphroditism have been excluded, the diagnosis of true hermaphroditism can be established with histologic evidence of both ovarian and testicular tissue.

3. **Treatment** is based on the patient's age at diagnosis and on evaluation of the internal and external genitalia. In infants without an established gender identity, either a female or a male assignment can be made. The testis or testicular tissue in an ovotestis has an increased risk of malignant transformation. All 46,XX true hermaphrodites raised as boys should undergo gonadectomy, prosthetic testes implants, and hormonal replacement at puberty. True hermaphrodites raised as girls must undergo removal of all testicular tissue. The risk of neoplastic transformation in retained ovarian tissue in such patients remains unclear. In older patients, gender identity assignment should be consistent with the sex of rearing. All dysgenetic and discordant tissue must be removed, with plastic repair of the external genitalia. Gonadal hormone treatment is recommended at puberty. Finally, it is vital to monitor the patient's electrolyte levels, as the salt-losing form of CAH may be life threatening if not monitored appropriately.

Section Four. REPRODUCTIVE ENDOCRINOLOGY AND INFERTILITY

31. INFERTILITY AND ASSISTED REPRODUCTIVE TECHNOLOGIES

Brandon J. Bankowski and Nikos Vlahos

I. **Infertility**
   A. **Definition.** Infertility is defined as the failure of a couple of reproductive age to conceive after at least 1 year of regular coitus without contraception. Primary infertility exists when a woman has never been pregnant. Secondary infertility occurs when a woman has a history of one or more previous pregnancies. Fecundability is the probability of achieving a pregnancy within one menstrual cycle. For a normal couple, this is approximately 25%. Fecundity is the ability to achieve a live birth within one menstrual cycle.
   B. **Incidence.** Recent data estimate that 10–20% of couples are infertile. In recent years, there has been an increasing demand for infertility services, especially in Western countries. The main reason for this is the tendency of women to delay childbearing because of career work. Other factors include an increase in the variety and effectiveness of assisted reproductive technology (ART) treatments, an increased public awareness of these treatments, an increase in tubal factor infertility as a consequence of sexually transmitted diseases, and a relative scarcity of babies placed for adoption because of effective contraception and increased availability of abortion services. In 1997 alone, 335 fertility clinics in the United States reported performing 71,826 ART treatment cycles that resulted in 17,054 deliveries of one or more living infants and a total of 24,582 babies born.
   C. **Differential diagnosis** (Table 31-1). The differential diagnoses of infertility encompass five principal categories: male factors, cervical factors, problems with the uterus or female pelvic organs or both, ovulatory problems, and unexplained causes. In addition, immunologic factors involving antiovarian or antisperm antibodies may adversely affect fertility by impairing fertilization, destroying gametes, and interfering with embryo cleavage or implantation. Their significance is controversial.
II. **Evaluation.** Successful reproduction requires proper structure and function of the entire reproductive axis, including hypothalamus, pituitary gland, ovaries, fallopian tube, uterus, cervix, and vagina. To assess this axis, the infertility evaluation comprises seven major elements:
   - History and physical examination
   - Semen analysis
   - Sperm–cervical mucus interaction (postcoital testing)
   - Testing for ovulation
   - Evaluation of tubal patency
   - Detection of uterine abnormalities
   - Determination of peritoneal abnormalities

   If these are properly coordinated, the evaluation can be completed in one menstrual cycle (Fig. 31-1). After the completion of the steps outlined in sec. **II.A–H,** no abnormality or cause of infertility can be identified in 15% of couples. This group comprises a category known as "unexplained infertility."
   A. **History and physical examination.** The initial assessment begins by obtaining an extended and complete history from both partners and performing a physical examination. A sexual history should include the frequency and timing of intercourse, as well as information regarding menstruation, impotence, dyspareunia, the use of lubricants, and sexually transmitted diseases.

TABLE 31-1. DIFFERENTIAL DIAGNOSIS OF INFERTILITY

Differential diagnosis	%	Basic evaluation
Male factors	30	Semen analysis
Tubal/uterine/peritoneal factors	25	Hysterosalpingogram, laparoscopy, chromopertubation
Anovulation/ovarian factors	25	Basal body temperature chart, midluteal progesterone level, endometrial biopsy, luteinizing hormone testing
Cervical factors	10	Postcoital test
Unexplained infertility	10	All of the above

B. **Semen analysis.** The semen sample should be collected after a period of abstinence of at least 48 hours and should be evaluated within 1 hour of ejaculation. The sample is obtained either by masturbation or by sexual intercourse with a silicone condom, as latex condoms are spermicidal. Normal parameters according to the World Health Organization are, per 1 mL volume: 20 million sperm or more, greater than 50% motility, greater than 30% normal morphology. If abnormalities are present, the patient should be referred to a urologist specializing in infertility to be evaluated for reversible causes of male-factor infertility.

C. The **postcoital test (PCT** or **Huhner test)** allows direct analysis of sperm and cervical mucus interaction and provides a rough estimate of sperm quality.

1. The test is done between days 12 and 14 of a 28–30 day menstrual cycle (after 48 hours of abstinence) when there is maximum estrogen secretion. The mucus is examined within 2–8 hours.

2. Because interpretation of the PCT is subjective, the validity of the test is controversial despite its long history of use. However, a finding of 5–10 progressively motile spermatozoa per high-power field and clear acellular mucus with a spinnbarkeit (the degree to which the mucus stretches between two slides) of 8 cm generally excludes a cervical factor. Fecundity rates do not correlate directly with number of motile sperm seen.

3. The most common cause of an abnormal PCT is poor timing. Other causes include cervical stenosis, hypoplastic endocervical canal, coital dysfunction and male factors. The sample can also be assessed for pH, mucus cellularity, WBC, ferning. Clumping and flagellation of sperm without progression are often suggestive of antisperm antibodies.

D. The **basal body temperature (BBT) chart** (Fig. 31-1) is a simple means of determining whether ovulation has occurred. The woman's temperature is taken daily with a thermometer on awakening, before any activity, and is recorded on a graph. After ovulation, rising progesterone levels increase the basal temperature by approximately $0.4°F$ ($0.22°C$) through a hypothalamic thermogenic effect. Because the rise in progesterone may occur anytime from 2 days before ovulation to 1 day after, the temperature elevation does not predict the exact moment of ovulation but may establish that it has occurred. A temperature elevation that persists for less than 11 days is suggestive but not diagnostic of a luteal phase defect.

E. **Midluteal phase progesterone level** is another test to assess ovulation. A concentration greater than 3.0 ng/mL in a blood sample drawn between days 19 and 23 is consistent with ovulation, whereas a concentration greater than 10 ng/mL implies adequate luteal support. Luteal phase deficiency is diagnosed histologically, because the progesterone level does not

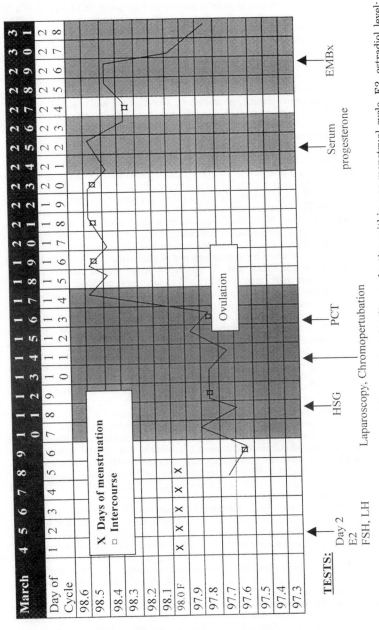

FIG. 31-1. Sample basal body temperature chart with complete infertility evaluation within one menstrual cycle. E2, estradiol level; EMBx, endometrial biopsy; FSH, follicle-stimulating hormone level; HSG, hysterosalpingogram; PCT, postcoital test.

indicate the cumulative response of the endometrium to progesterone during the luteal phase.

F. An **endometrial biopsy** evaluates the response of the endometrium to progesterone. The test is usually performed between days 24 and 26 of a 28 day menstrual cycle or 2–4 days before anticipated menstruation. The biopsy documents ovulation by histologic demonstration of decidualized stroma, allows for dating of the endometrium within 2–3 days, and assesses for endometritis. The date of the biopsy and the subsequent menstrual cycle are used to determine whether a luteal phase deficiency is present. Correlation of endometrial dating with the rise in BBT or luteinizing hormone (LH) surge or both is also helpful. A luteal phase defect may result from inadequate estrogen priming, progesterone secretion, or endometrial response. The risks of the procedure are minimal, but include infection, bleeding, interruption of pregnancy, and uterine perforation.

G. The **hysterosalpingogram (HSG)** assesses uterine and fallopian tube contour and tubal patency. It is performed in the early follicular phase, within 1 week of cessation of menstrual flow. This timing minimizes the chances of interrupting a pregnancy. The procedure is performed by injecting a radiopaque dye through the cervix. As more dye is injected, the dye passes through the uterine cavity into the fallopian tubes and peritoneal cavity. Permanent radiographic films are made under fluoroscopy to demonstrate patent or obstructed tubes. Nonsteroidal anti-inflammatory drugs may be given to prevent cramping. Prophylactic antibiotics (e.g., doxycycline, 100 mg orally twice daily) are advisable when the patient has a history of pelvic inflammatory disease or when hydrosalpinges are identified during the study. Cervical cultures for gonorrhea and *Chlamydia* infection should confirm negative results before instrumentation to avoid an iatrogenic peritonitis.

H. A **diagnostic laparoscopy** assesses peritoneal and tubal factors such as endometriosis and pelvic adhesions, and can provide access for simultaneous corrective surgery. Laparoscopy should be scheduled in the follicular phase, as with HSG, and is the final and most invasive step in the patient's evaluation, unless the HSG raised suspicion of abnormalities. Findings on HSG correlate with laparoscopic findings 60–70% of the time. Dye (usually a dilute solution of indigo carmine) should be instilled through the fallopian tubes (chromopertubation) during laparoscopy to visually document tubal patency. Hysteroscopy may also be included to ensure that no abnormalities were missed on the HSG.

III. **Treatment.** Before progressing to assisted reproductive technologies, an infertility patient should undergo treatment for reparable problems.

A. **Anovulation.** The agents most commonly used to stimulate multiple ovarian follicles are clomiphene citrate (CC), human menopausal gonadotropins (hMG), and purified follicle-stimulating hormone (FSH). CC, a synthetic, nonsteroidal estrogen agonist-antagonist, increases the release of gonadotropin-releasing hormone (GnRH) and subsequent LH and FSH release. CC is useful in women with oligomenorrhea and amenorrhea with intact hypothalamic-pituitary-ovarian axes. If the patient is anovulatory, CC is often used before diagnostic procedures continue. Patients who are overweight and hyperandrogenic are the least likely to respond to CC. GnRH, hMG, FSH, and bromocriptine mesylate are used primarily in women who fail to respond to CC or who have hypogonadotropic amenorrhea or unexplained infertility. Prescription of these expensive drugs, which are used in the more complicated protocols for in vitro fertilization (see later), should be left to specialists trained in their use.

B. **Hyperprolactinemia. Bromocriptine** is used to induce ovulation in patients with hyperprolactinemia. Bromocriptine is a dopamine agonist that directly inhibits pituitary secretion of prolactin, which restores normal gonadotropin release. The usual starting dose is 2.5 mg each bedtime to prevent dopaminergic side effects, which include nausea, diarrhea, dizziness, and headache. If oral administration cannot be tolerated, vaginal administration is recommended. A response is usually seen in 2–3 months, and 80% of hyperprolactinemic patients ovulate and become pregnant. CC is added if ovulation does not occur within 3 months after beginning treatment.

C. **Thyroid problems** should be treated appropriately, as both hypothyroidism and hyperthyroidism may lead to infertility.

D. **Hypothalamic-pituitary axis problems,** including extreme weight gain or loss, excessive exercise, and emotional stress, can all impact the secretion of GnRH from the hypothalamus and cause ovulatory dysfunction. These must be addressed by appropriate behavioral or psychological intervention.

E. **Male factor infertility.** Although the gynecologist does not treat male patients directly, therapies to treat male factor infertility often involve hormonal manipulation in the female partner. The evaluation is analogous to that in the woman, with examination of the hypothalamic-pituitary-testicular axis, outflow tract, and testicular function. Toxins, viruses, sexually transmitted diseases, varicoceles, and congenital problems can all influence infertility. Fortunately, the initiation of intracytoplasmic sperm injection has revolutionized treatment of male infertility. As long as viable sperm can be retrieved by ejaculation, epididymal aspiration, or testicular biopsy, successful fertilization and pregnancy can be achieved. The current fertilization rate is 95% and the pregnancy rate is comparable to that of in vitro fertilization (IVF).

F. **Endometriosis,** the ectopic growth of hormonally responsive endometrial tissue, may account for 15% of infertility in women; it is diagnosed and staged by laparoscopy. Endometriosis has a negative impact on fertility, and once diagnosed, it should be treated surgically before instituting infertility therapy. Laparoscopic resection or ablation of even minimal endometriosis may enhance fecundity in infertile women. If pregnancy fails to occur after surgical treatment, IVF or gamete intrafallopian transfer (GIFT) may be used. GnRH agonists, danazol, and continuous oral contraceptive pills may be used for the treatment of pain symptoms, but each will prevent pregnancy during its use.

G. **Luteal phase defects** occur in both fertile and infertile women, and treatment is controversial. Nevertheless, in a couple with documented infertility, it is prudent to treat luteal phase deficiency with intramuscular or intravaginal progesterone until the luteoplacental shift occurs at 8–10 weeks gestational age.

H. **Uterine factors** such as submucous leiomyomas, intrauterine synechia (Asherman's syndrome), and uterine deformities or septa cause approximately 2% of infertility. The mainstay of treatment for these conditions is surgical correction, usually via a hysteroscopic approach.

I. **Infections** of the female and male genital tracts have been implicated as causes of infertility. *Chlamydia* infection and gonorrhea are the major pathogens and should be treated appropriately. *Ureaplasma urealyticum* and *Mycoplasma hominis* have also been implicated, however. If *U. urealyticum* and *M. hominis* are identified by culture, the patient should be treated with doxycycline, 100 mg by mouth twice daily for 7 days. This has been shown to increase the pregnancy rate in patients with primary infertility.

J. **Tubal factor infertility** has become more prevalent with the increased incidence of salpingitis. The frequency of tubal occlusion after one, two, and three episodes of salpingitis is reported to be 11%, 23%, and 54%, respectively. Appendicitis, prior abdominopelvic surgery, endometriosis, and ectopic pregnancy can also lead to adhesion formation and damaged tubes. **Proximal** tubal obstruction is identified on HSG. Tubal spasm may mimic proximal obstruction, however, and obstruction should be confirmed by laparoscopy. Treatment consists of tubal cannulation, microsurgical tubocornual reanastomosis, or IVF. **Distal** tubal disease or distortion can be seen on HSG and laparoscopy. The success of corrective surgery (neosalpingostomy) depends on the extent of disease.

IV. **Assisted reproductive technologies.** Louise Brown, the first child successfully conceived by IVF, was born in 1978. Since then, several techniques have been developed that enhance our ability to overcome infertility. Among these are the ability to cryopreserve or freeze oocytes and use donor sperm and oocytes. Of all ART procedures nationwide, 29.5% resulted in pregnancy according to the 1997 National Fertility Clinic data. Over 50% of pregnancies resulted in single live births whereas 25.9% resulted in twins and 5.3% in triplets or higher multiples. Miscarriages occurred in 14.5%, ectopic pregnancies in 0.3%, and stillbirths in 0.6%. The following types of procedures, listed in chronologic order of their development, are currently used.

A. In **gamete intrafallopian transfer,** extraction of oocytes is followed by the transfer of gametes (sperm and oocyte) into a normal fallopian tube by laparoscopy. GIFT requires general anesthesia and does not allow for visual confirmation of fertilization. If pregnancy does not occur, there is no way to determine if the cause is failure of fertilization or failure of implantation. The overall 1997 live birth/retrieval rate was 29.8%. (The statistics presented here are all for fresh, nondonor cycles.)

B. **Zygote intrafallopian transfer (ZIFT)** refers to the placement of embryos into the fallopian tube after oocyte retrieval and fertilization. It combines features of in vitro fertilization and GIFT. The overall 1997 live birth/retrieval rate was 28.0%.

C. **In vitro fertilization** refers to controlled ovarian hyperstimulation, ultrasonographically guided aspiration of oocytes, laboratory fertilization with prepared sperm, embryo culture, and transfer of the resulting embryos into the uterus through the cervix. Although most IVF procedures use fresh oocytes from the patient, transfer of frozen oocytes and transfer of "donor eggs" are also options. The overall 1997 live birth/retrieval rate was 27.7%. For patients undergoing IVF, the pregnancy success rate varies little by cause of infertility, with a success rate approximating the overall national rate in women with most diagnoses. The cumulative pregnancy rates increase as patients complete more cycles (after three cycles, 38%; after four cycles, 47%; after five cycles, 49%; and after six cycles, 58%). Frozen embryos yielded a live birth rate/transfer of 18.6% compared to 29.7% for fresh embryos (Table 31-2).

D. In **intracytoplasmic sperm injection,** a single spermatozoon is injected into each oocyte, and the resulting embryos are transferred transcervically into the uterus. To date, no increased risk of congenital malformation has

TABLE 31-2. IN VITRO FERTILIZATION (IVF) SUCCESS RATES

Diagnosis of patients undergoing IVF	Percentage of total cases	Live births per cycle (%)
Pelvic (or tubal) factor	27.9	24.2
Male factor	26.0	25.5
Endometriosis	14.6	24.5
Ovarian	12.6	22.6
Unexplained infertility	8.5	24.8
Other (immunologic or serious illness)	8	19.9
Uterine	2.2	18.9

Adapted from Figures 6 and 14 of the National Summary and Fertility Clinic Report, 1997.

been seen. There is great concern, however, over the possibility of transmitting genetic defects to offspring during intracytoplasmic sperm injection, which may be responsible for infertility in the father.

E. **Indications for in vitro fertilization**
   1. **Tubal conditions**—large hydrosalpinges, absence of fimbria, severe adhesive disease, repeated ectopic pregnancies, or failed reconstructive surgical therapy.
   2. **Endometriosis** increasing as an indication for IVF, if other forms of treatment have failed.
   3. **Unexplained infertility**
   4. **Male factor infertility**—low sperm count, low sperm motility, and abnormal morphology are associated with reduction in fertilizing ability.
   5. **Uterine malformations** related to diethylstilbestrol exposure.

F. **Controlled ovarian hyperstimulation and protocols for in vitro fertilization.** The agents most commonly used to stimulate multiple ovarian follicles are CC, hMG, and purified FSH. The particular products and protocols used may be tailored as the treatment proceeds to boost the chances of an adequate response and increase the pregnancy rate.

G. **Clomiphene-only** regimens are given on days 5–9 of the menstrual cycle. Response may be followed by BBT measurement, ultrasonography, and measurement of LH and estradiol levels. CC is inexpensive and has a low risk of ovarian hyperstimulation syndrome (OHSS). However, it creates a low oocyte yield (one or two per cycle) with frequent LH surges that lead to high cancellation rates in IVF cycles and low pregnancy yield. Most treatment regimens start with 50 mg/day for 5 days. If ovulation fails to occur, the dose is increased to 100 mg/day. The maximum dose is 250 mg/day. Human chorionic gonadotropin (hCG), 5000 IU to 10,000 IU, may be used to simulate an LH surge. Eighty percent of properly selected couples will conceive in the first three cycles after treatment. Potential side effects are vasomotor flushes, blurring of vision, urticaria, pain, bloating, and multiple gestation (5–7% of cases, usually twins).

H. **Clomiphene/hMG combinations** are used to increase the number of recruited follicles. The hMG and purified FSH are useful in patients who do not achieve pregnancy with CC and in patients with endometriosis or unexplained infertility. The hMG, which is a combination of LH and FSH, is given for 2–7 days after the clomiphene. This treatment is more expensive and can lead to life-threatening OHSS. Trade names for hMG include Humegon, Pergonal, and Repronex. Follicle maturation is monitored using sonography and serial measurement of estradiol levels. To complete oocyte maturation, hCG needs to be given once the follicles have reached 17–18 mm in diameter. Aspiration of follicles should be timed 35–36 hours after the hCG injection. The disadvantages of this protocol include premature luteinization, spontaneous LH surges that result in high cancellation rates, and multiple gestations.

I. **Gonadotropin-releasing hormone analogs/agonists (GnRHa)** are used via a flare-up protocol or a luteal phase protocol. The flare-up protocol causes an elevation of FSH in the first 4 days, which increases oocyte recruitment. After 5 days of administration, the GnRH agonist then down-regulates the pituitary to prevent premature luteinization and a spontaneous LH surge. The luteal phase protocol involves starting GnRHa administration on the seventeenth to twenty-first menstrual day. GnRHa increase the number, quality, and synchronization of the oocytes recovered per cycle and thereby improve the fertilization rate, the number of embryos, and the pregnancy rate. Successful ovulation rates are 75% to 85%. GnRHa are expensive and more complex to use, however, and can lead to OHSS.

J. **GnRH analogs/antagonists** are the latest addition to the fertility drug armamentarium. They block LH secretion without causing a flare-up effect. They are administered in a single dose on the eighth menstrual day or in smaller doses over 4 days. Because they block the periovulatory LH surge, fewer gonadotropins are required to stimulate ovulation, and side effects are decreased.

K. **Oocyte retrieval, culture fertilization, and transfer**

1. The two major techniques of oocyte retrieval are ultrasonographically guided follicular aspiration and laparoscopic oocyte retrieval. The former is the most widely used technique. **Ultrasonographically guided oocyte retrieval** using a 17-gauge needle passed through the vaginal fornix is performed 34–36 hours after hCG injection. The procedure is done under heavy sedation. Potential complications include risk of bowel injury and injury to pelvic vessels.

2. **Oocyte fertilization.** Sperm are diluted, centrifuged, and incubated before 50,000–100,000 motile spermatozoa are added to each Petri dish containing an oocyte. Fertilization is documented by the presence of two pronuclei and extrusion of a second polar body at 24 hours. At that stage, most embryos are cryopreserved for an unlimited period, with a survival rate of 75%.

3. **Embryo transfer** is most commonly carried out 48–80 hours after retrieval at the four- to ten-cell stage. In general, no more than two embryos are transferred to limit the risk of multiple gestation and to optimize pregnancy rates. The actual number of embryos transferred depends on the individual's age and other risk factors for multiple pregnancy. It is common practice to supplement the luteal phase with progesterone given by vaginal suppository, beginning the day of oocyte release and continuing into the twelfth week of pregnancy.

4. **Retrieval and pregnancy results.** Most programs have delivery rates of approximately 20% for women under the age of 40 years who are not affected by male factor infertility. The risk of ectopic pregnancy is 4% to 5%, and the risk of heterotopic pregnancies is less than 1%. Multiple gestation rate is approximately 30% (25% twins and 5% triplets). Summary of national data for 1997 showed that the average age of the woman was 35 years. A woman's chances of success with ART using her own eggs decrease at every stage as her age increases. The likelihood of implantation of a fertilized oocyte depends on the age of the oocyte donor, not that of the receiver; therefore, older women commonly use donor oocytes to improve chances of success.

32. REPEATED PREGNANCY LOSS

Diane Clarke Boykin and Nikos Vlahos

I. **Definition.** Repeated pregnancy loss (RPL) is defined as three consecutive spontaneous abortions before 20 weeks' gestation. RPL affects 0.5–1.0% of pregnant women and can be divided into **primary,** in women without a previous liveborn infant, and **secondary,** in those women with at least one prior liveborn infant. It is generally accepted that 15–20% of all clinically documented pregnancies result in spontaneous abortion. Many factors affect the actual risk of miscarriage, including maternal age. For women younger than 20 years, miscarriage occurs in 12% of pregnancies. This number increases to 26% for women older than 40. When unrecognized pregnancies are factored into the equation, the loss rate for women over 40 is 75%. For most women who experience a miscarriage, the recurrence rate is below 30%. In fact, 80–90% of women will have a successful pregnancy after a spontaneous abortion. In cases of RPL, the chance of a live birth after three consecutive losses is 55–60%.

II. **Causes** of RPL include but are not limited to genetic, anatomic, endocrine, immunologic, infectious, and environmental factors.

  A. **Genetic**

    1. **Chromosomal abnormalities** are a common cause of spontaneous abortion. In up to 70% of first trimester miscarriages, a chromosomal abnormality is shown when fetal tissue is tested. These include aneuploidies, trisomies, monosomies, and so forth. Trisomies are the most common type and are detected in almost 50% of miscarriages. The most common trisomies are 13, 16, 18, 21, and 22. The next most common abnormality is 45X, which accounts for 25% of all chromosomal abnormalities.

    2. **Parental chromosomal abnormalities** may play a role in RPL. Studies have shown that the incidence of chromosomal abnormalities in couples experiencing RPL is 3–8%, five to six times higher than the incidence in the general population. Balanced translocation is the most common abnormality found in the karyotypes of parents with RPL. Often, the parent is phenotypically normal. The translocation may be passed on in one of three ways: normal karyotype, balanced translocation, or unbalanced translocation, which may be incompatible with life. Other parental chromosomal abnormalities include inversions and mosaicism.

  B. **Anatomic** reasons for RPL can be further divided into congenital and acquired problems.

    1. **Congenital problems** encompass a variety of conditions often involving müllerian development. These losses more commonly occur during the second trimester, although losses at earlier stages of gestation can occur. Common uterine abnormalities include septate, bicornuate, didelphic, and, less commonly, unicornuate uteri. Of these uterine abnormalities, septate uterus is the most common. Some studies have shown that 27% of women with a history of losses have some anatomic abnormality.

    A septate uterus results from failure of resorption of the paramesonephric ducts and is often associated with poor obstetric outcomes. Studies have reported 15–28% livebirth rates in women with this type of uterine abnormality. With surgical correction, however, successful pregnancy can occur in up to 80% of cases.

    2. **Acquired anatomic abnormalities** associated with RPL include leiomyomata, intrauterine synechiae, and in utero diethylstilbestrol (DES) exposure.

a. **Fibroids,** particularly submucosal, have been purported to cause RPL. These anatomic lesions may result in unfavorable implantation sites and may jeopardize the vascular supply to the placenta. Intramuscular and subserosal fibroids may also be problematic if they are large enough to distort the uterine cavity (see Chapter 33).

b. **Intrauterine synechiae** most often form after instrumentation of the uterus, although they may occur in cases in which there is an estrogen deficiency. Adhesions are said to account for 5% of RPL cases. Often, these occur after a dilation and curettage procedure in which there is direct trauma to the endometrial cavity. These adhesions may interfere with implantation and future vascular supply to the fetus.

c. **DES-exposed women** have been shown to have poor reproductive outcomes. One study reported a 42% livebirth rate for these women, with a majority of losses occurring in the first trimester. In utero exposure has been reported to cause multiple anatomic abnormalities, including a T-shaped uterine cavity, a widened lower uterine segment, midfundal constrictions, filling defects, and irregular margins. These defects can be seen on a hysterosalpingogram in 42–69% of DES-exposed women. It has been proposed that these abnormalities may result from DES binding to estrogen receptors during embryologic development of the müllerian system.

d. **Cervical incompetence** is another anatomic cause of RPL. This is a condition of painless cervical dilation and may be congenital or acquired. Acquired causes include previous cervical surgery (i.e., conization, traumatic delivery with cervical laceration, aggressive cervical dilation during dilation and curettage).

C. **Endocrine.** A defect with the corpus luteum known as **luteal phase deficiency** is a proposed cause of RPL. In this condition, a deficiency in progesterone causes the endometrial tissue to lag by 2 or more days behind the anticipated histologically determined age of the tissue. Progesterone production by the corpus luteum is needed to support a pregnancy until the eighth week, when the placenta starts to produce the majority of this hormone. Individuals with a luteal phase defect do not produce enough progesterone to support an early pregnancy. Losses tend to occur early, at 4–7 weeks' gestation. Although luteal phase defect is thought to be a cause of RPL, the meta-analysis of randomized trials in which pregnant women were treated with progestational agents failed to find any evidence of a positive effect on the maintenance of pregnancy.

Studies show that subclinical diabetes and thyroid disease are unlikely causes of RPL, although women with poorly controlled insulin-dependent diabetes are at an increased risk of spontaneous abortion.

D. **Immunologic** disorders associated with RPL can be further divided into those involving autoimmune and alloimmune factors.

1. In a compilation of studies on women with RPL, 15% were found to have recognizable **autoimmune factors.** The most common antibodies include anticardiolipin and lupus anticoagulant. In vitro, these factors cause thrombosis. In vivo, they may cause thrombosis and placental infarctions that in turn result in spontaneous abortion. The majority of these losses occur during the second trimester.

2. **Alloimmune factors,** meaning immunity against a foreign entity, are another possible cause of RPL. Some couples experiencing RPL share human leukocyte antigens. These antigens are thought to interfere with formation of maternal antibodies that coat fetal antigens and thus prevent rejection. The role of this mechanism is controversial, because the sharing of human leukocyte antigens does not always result in poor pregnancy outcome.

E. **Infectious.** Only a few microbiological agents have been related to RPL, but none have been demonstrated to have an effect in randomized trials. Women experiencing RPL have been shown to be infected with *Ureaplasma urealyticum.* Other organisms that have been implicated but whose role has not been substantiated include *Toxoplasma gondii, Listeria monocytogenes,* and *Mycoplasma hominis.* Overall, infection as a cause of RPL is controversial.

F. **Environmental.** It has been shown that use of tobacco, alcohol, and some drugs is related to RPL. Some chemotherapeutic agents are also a proven cause of pregnancy loss. Ionizing radiation, anesthetic gases, and some heavy metals are other possible causes of spontaneous abortion in women exposed to these agents. Many dermatologic preparations, especially those containing vitamin A derivatives, cause spontaneous abortions.

G. **Unknown.** In as many as 50–60% of women experiencing RPL, there is no identified cause.

III. **Diagnosis.** Although RPL is defined as three consecutive pregnancy losses, a physician need not wait for three losses to begin a diagnostic workup. In particular, for older couples without children, it may be wise to start a workup after two losses. Also, it is important to perform a complete workup, as in some couples there are multiple reasons for RPL.

A complete history and physical examination is the first step. A detailed family history should be taken, including reproductive outcomes and medical illnesses. An occupational history should also be elicited to determine exposure to various chemicals. This should be followed by a thorough examination, including cultures for *Chlamydia, Neisseria gonorrhoeae, Mycoplasma,* and *Ureaplasma.* Specific blood studies, including thyroid function tests, random or fasting glucose level, lupus anticoagulant level, and anticardiolipin antibody level should be ordered. A karyotype of each partner is helpful in locating translocations, inversions, and mosaicisms. Karyotypes of fetal tissue obtained from aborted material may also be obtained but may be of limited value.

To diagnose a luteal phase defect, a timed endometrial biopsy should be obtained in two consecutive cycles. A histologically determined lag of 2 or more days is considered significant. Some practitioners obtain a midluteal serum progesterone level, although the sensitivity is considered low by many. A serum progesterone level above 10 ng/dL points to a low probability of an out-of-phase endometrial biopsy. These results should be read carefully, as different pathologists may record varying results for biopsy dating. In addition, several studies have reported a histologically identified lag in endometrial tissue in women with no history of pregnancy loss.

To exclude anatomic abnormalities, several studies may be performed. Evaluation begins with a good physical examination and imaging studies, including hysterosalpingogram, sonohysterography, CT scan, or MRI. In the operating room, an examination under anesthesia, hysteroscopy, and a diagnostic laparoscopy may be performed.

IV. **Treatment.** As mentioned earlier, in as many as 50% of women, no cause is found for the RPL. For these patients, supportive measures are the best treatment.

A. When **genetic causes** of RPL are diagnosed, it is important to include genetic counseling as part of any treatment plan. The rate of recurrence of miscarriage often depends on the actual genetic abnormality discovered. Some couples with a known translocation or inversion can have a good pregnancy outcome. Others may need to turn to sperm or oocyte donation to avoid lethal abnormalities in their offspring.

B. Treatment for **anatomic abnormalities** often involves surgery. Hysteroscopic removal of uterine septa and synechiae has resulted in good pregnancy outcomes for many couples. Some physicians also insert an intrauterine device after resection of synechiae and place the patient on oral estrogen therapy to help prevent reformation of adhesions. If surgery is selected for uterine abnormalities, such as fibroids and unicornuate uterus, it should be clearly discussed with the couple that some studies have shown no difference in pregnancy outcome for patients treated surgically versus those not treated. Some women with anatomic abnormalities who are not treated have a fair to good rate of pregnancy success.

C. **Endocrine abnormalities** can often be treated with replacement therapy. Researchers are currently undecided as to whether luteal phase deficiency affects pregnancy outcome. Many studies have shown no benefit from treating luteal phase defects. Some physicians, however, administer progesterone either as intravaginal suppositories (25 mg twice daily starting the third day after ovulation and continuing for 8–10 weeks), as intramuscular injections, or as orally administered micronized progesterone. It should be mentioned that as many as 60–70% of women diagnosed with a luteal phase deficiency will carry a viable infant with the next pregnancy. Other endocrine abnormalities, such as thyroid disorders and diabetes, should be corrected.

D. When an **infection** is diagnosed, the appropriate antibiotic therapy should be instituted. Infections with *Mycoplasma* and *Ureaplasma* are treated with doxycycline, 100 mg twice daily by mouth for 10 days. Clindamycin 300 mg three times daily by mouth for 7–10 days can be used for patients who are pregnant or allergic to doxycycline. Both partners should be treated to prevent reinfection.

E. **Environmental factors.** Women who smoke or drink alcoholic beverages should be encouraged to abstain from these activities. If exposed to environmental toxins, individuals should try to eliminate or reduce exposure.

33. UTERINE LEIOMYOMAS

Kimberly A. Bernard and Edward E. Wallach

I. **Uterine leiomyomas** are the most common pelvic tumors in women. They are benign tumors in which malignant transformation is extremely rare. Leiomyomas originate from smooth muscle cells of the uterus and in certain instances from the smooth muscle cells of uterine blood vessels. They have traditionally been described as present in 20% of women over age 35, but their presence in 50% of postmortem examinations indicates a much higher frequency. Leiomyomas represent the single most common indication for hysterectomy and were the cause of 33% of such procedures in 1994, according to the American College of Obstetricians and Gynecologists. Twenty percent of women have had a hysterectomy by age 40 and one-third by age 65.

II. **Etiology and pathophysiology of uterine leiomyomas.** Leiomyomas are thought to be unicellular in origin. They range in size from seedlings only millimeters in diameter to large tumors not only filling the pelvis but also occasionally reaching the costal margin. These tumors may be solitary or multiple. Leiomyomas can be located within the uterine wall, can protrude into the endometrial cavity, or can be on the surface of the uterus, and are referred to as intramural, submucosal, and subserosal, respectively.

A genetic basis for the presence and growth of uterine leiomyomas appears likely. Abnormal gene expression of myomas suggests that they represent tumors of dysregulated differentiation and resemble myometrium of pregnancy. The incidence of leiomyomas is significantly greater among African-American women than among white women.

The growth of uterine leiomyomas is clearly related to their exposure to circulating estrogen. These tumors are most prominent and demonstrate maximal growth during the reproductive years, when ovarian estrogen secretion is maximal. With the onset of menopause, leiomyomas tend to regress in volume. The regression may be counterbalanced by hormone replacement therapy. Whenever leiomyomas grow after menopause, malignancy must be seriously considered.

The growth of leiomyomas during pregnancy is common. Growth is observed less frequently during the cyclic use of oral contraceptive pills and other estrogen-progestogen preparations. Progesterone and progestational compounds may exert an antiestrogen effect on the growth of leiomyomas. In view of the balance between estrogenic and progestational effects, gestational growth of leiomyomas is probably related to the enhanced uterine blood supply that accompanies pregnancy and edematous changes in these tumors.

The two most significant changes observed in leiomyomas are malignant change and degeneration. Malignant transformation of leiomyomas is probably in the order of approximately 0.04%. In a review of 13,000 leiomyomas by Montague et al. (*Am J Obstet Gynecol*, 92/421, 1965), 38 cases (0.29%) demonstrated malignant change. Corscaden and Singh (*Am J Obstet Gynecol*, 75/148, 1958) reported that malignant change developed in fewer than 0.13% of uterine leiomyomas. These figures may be unduly elevated considering the high prevalence of these tumors and the relative rarity of leiomyosarcomas. Only a small percentage of uterine leiomyomas are surgically removed; thus, the denominator is much higher than that based solely on surgical procedures in which leiomyomas are found. Some authors believe that leiomyosarcomas are a de novo neoplasm and are not the result of malignant change.

As leiomyomas grow, they risk diminution of blood supply, which leads to a continuum of degenerative changes, including calcium deposition. Calcific change can be appreciated radiographically as a diffuse honeycomb pattern, a series of concentric rings, or a solid calcific mass. Infection is commonly observed when a submucosal leiomyoma protrudes through the cervix into the vagina. Infection may also accompany puerperal endometritis and advance to endomyometritis with or without abscess formation. Necrosis and cystic changes are manifestations of compromised blood supply secondary to growth or to infarction from torsion of a pedunculated leiomyoma. Fatty degeneration with a yellow appearance macroscopically and fat demonstrated histologically represents another common form of necrosis.

Leiomyosarcomas are diagnosed on the basis of counts of ten or more mitotic figures per ten high-power fields (HPFs). Those tumors with five to ten mitotic figures per ten HPFs are referred to as **smooth muscle tumors of uncertain malignant potential.** Tumors with less than five mitotic figures per ten HPFs and little cytologic atypia are classified as **cellular leiomyomas.** In terms of prognosis, a high mitotic count indicates a poor outcome.

III. **Clinical manifestations and diagnosis of uterine leiomyomas.** Most patients with leiomyomas are symptom free. The most commonly experienced symptoms (pain, pressure, and menorrhagia), are related to the size and location of the leiomyoma or to compromise of blood supply with degeneration.

Excessive menstrual bleeding is often the only symptom produced by leiomyomas. Vascular alterations in the endometrium associated with leiomyomas have been correlated with hypermenorrhea. The obstructive effect on uterine vasculature produced by intramural tumors has been associated with the development of endometrial venule ectasia. As a result, leiomyomas give rise to proximal congestion of the myometrium and endometrium. The engorged vessels in the thin atrophic endometrium that overlies submucosal tumors contribute to excessive bleeding during cyclic sloughing. The increased size of the uterine cavity also gives rise to the increased volume of menstrual flow.

Pressure and increased abdominal girth are more commonly encountered than pain and are usually described vaguely by the patient. Pressure on the bladder customarily provokes urinary frequency. When the leiomyoma is adjacent to the bladder neck and urethra, acute urinary retention with overflow incontinence may occur. An enlarging leiomyoma over the cervix may cause protrusion of the base of the bladder and anterior wall of the vagina, which suggests pelvic relaxation. Urinary stress incontinence may also reflect leiomyomas located in the vicinity of the bladder neck. Ureteral obstruction is one of the most serious complications of chronic pressure on the ureter. Unless the kidney has suffered parenchymal damage, alleviation of the pressure will reverse any anatomic change. Chronic obstruction of the bladder neck leads to hydroureter and hydronephrosis. Rectal pressure is rare unless a large leiomyoma is located on the posterior surface of the uterus. Constipation or tenesmus may also be associated with a posterior leiomyoma.

Pain may be a consequence of torsion of the stalk of a pedunculated leiomyoma, cervical dilation by a submucosal leiomyoma protruding through the lower uterine segment, or degeneration of a leiomyoma. In each of these conditions, the pain is acute and requires immediate attention. Other pathologic conditions characterized by acute pain include ectopic pregnancy, accident in an ovarian cyst, appendicitis, and acute pelvic inflammatory disease.

IV. **Therapeutic approaches to leiomyomas.** The treatment options for leiomyomas are conservative follow-up with observation by serial examinations, hormonal therapy, surgical therapy, and radiologic intervention.

A. **Observation.** No standard size of an asymptomatic myomatous uterus has been invoked as an absolute indication for treatment. In a patient with a large asymptomatic myomatous uterus in whom dimensions have not increased and malignancy is unlikely, the patient's age, fertility status, and desire to retain the uterus or avoid surgery must be factored into the treatment plan. Physical and ultrasonographic examinations should be performed initially and repeated in 6–8 weeks to document size and growth pattern. If growth is stable, the patient may be followed at 3- to 4-month intervals.

B. **Hormonal therapy**
   1. **Progestins.** Progestational therapy using norethindrone, medrogestone, and medroxyprogesterone acetate has been successful. These compounds produce a hypoestrogenic effect by inhibiting gonadotropin secretion and suppressing ovarian function. Conversely, use of RU-486 (mifepristone), an antiprogestin, has been associated with decrease in size of leiomyomas.
   2. **Gonadotropin-releasing hormone analogs (GnRHa).** More recently, GnRHa have been used successfully to achieve hypoestrogenism in various estrogen-dependent conditions. Reduction in tumor size of approximately 50% on average has been observed with the use of GnRHa over a 3-month course of treatment. These agents are useful as a conservative therapy or as an adjunct to surgical treatment. Longer than 3 months of GnRHa therapy in young patients is neither practical nor desirable because of the possibility of bone loss as a consequence of hypoestrogenism.

      Concomitant treatment with a low dose of estrogen, referred to as **add-back therapy**, can be used to minimize the adverse affects of GnRHa on bone in patients who are found to benefit from continued therapy after the initial 3-month course. The dosage of leuprolide acetate (Lupron Depot) is 11.25 mg intramuscularly every 3 months.

      The effects of hormonal treatment are transient, and within several cycles after withdrawal of hormonal therapy, leiomyomas return to pretherapy state. Adjunctive therapy with a 3- to 4-month course of GnRHa should reduce tumor size and render surgery easier and reduce blood loss. GnRHa therapy may also be useful in perimenopausal women, in whom reduction in leiomyoma volume may stabilize when menopause occurs shortly thereafter. By producing amenorrhea, GnRHa therapy enables a patient to restore her own hemoglobin levels and to provide autologous blood preoperatively. It should be noted that common side effects of GnRHa include hot flashes, nausea, vomiting, diarrhea, constipation, rash, dizziness, acne, breast tenderness, and headaches.

C. **Surgical therapy**
   1. **Myomectomy.** Myomectomy should be considered whenever preservation of the uterus is desired for its childbearing function. It is the procedure of choice for a solitary pedunculated leiomyoma. Other indications for a myomectomy include interference with fertility or predisposition to repeated pregnancy loss due to the nature or location of leiomyomas.

      A myomectomy can be performed by abdominal, laparoscopic, laparoscopically assisted, transvaginal, and hysteroscopic techniques. The location and size of the myoma dictates the specific surgical approach.

      For patients who wish to conceive, a delay of 4–6 months before attempting pregnancy is advisable after the surgical procedure when the myometrium has been deeply entered and sutured, because the myometrium is significantly disrupted during deep myomectomy. Cesarean section is generally the procedure of choice for delivery of patients who have undergone a myomectomy with extensive myometrial dissection to decrease the risk of uterine rupture.

      Complications of a myomectomy should be considered in choosing a course of treatment. Multiple myomectomy is generally more difficult and time consuming than hysterectomy. Substantial blood loss may accompany myomectomy, leading to a greater need for blood replacement and a higher incidence of postoperative anemia, paralytic ileus, and pain. The need for future surgery due to recurrence of leiomyomas cannot be ignored. Roughly 20–25% of patients who have undergone a myomectomy ultimately require another surgical procedure for recurrence.
   2. **Hysterectomy.** With few exceptions, removal of the uterus is the procedure of choice whenever surgery is indicated for leiomyomas and when childbearing has been completed. Hysterectomy should also be

considered in the event of a rapidly enlarging tumor, in which there is a reasonable likelihood of malignancy. Hysterectomy may be performed vaginally in selected cases.

3. **Myolysis.** Laparoscopic coagulation of a leiomyoma, or myolysis, is performed with a neodymium:yttrium-aluminum-garnet laser through degeneration of protein and destruction of vascularity. Dense pelvic adhesions have been found on follow-up. Bipolar coagulation and cryomyolysis have also been used, but sufficient follow-up is not available to evaluate safety and future fertility.

4. **Uterine artery embolization (UAE)** was initially proposed for managing hemorrhagic complications of obstetrics. Recently, UAE has become an alternative treatment for leiomyomata. UAE works by occluding the uterine artery, which decreases the blood supply to the uterus and ultimately to the leiomyomata. The procedure is performed by placing a catheter into the femoral artery and accessing the hypogastric arteries. The substances used to occlude the arteries include Gelfoam, absolute alcohol, and Ivalon particles (polyvinyl alcohol). An angiogram is performed to assess the anatomy of the vessels and the success of the procedure. This technique requires that a trained interventional radiologist work in conjunction with the gynecologist. The benefits of UAE include the relatively short operating time and recovery time, use of local anesthesia, and minimal blood loss. The risks of the procedure include infection (4%), complications of angiography (3%), and uterine ischemia (one case reported). Premature ovarian failure secondary to compromise of the ovarian circulation has been reported. Patients typically experience cramping for the first 12–18 hours after the procedure. Postembolization syndrome (fever, nausea, vomiting, and at times severe abdominal pain) has been observed in approximately 30% of patients.

   Outcomes of UAE include 40–60% reduction in uterine size and decreased menstrual bleeding. The impact on fertility postprocedure has not been well defined, although there are reports of term pregnancies in women who have undergone UAE.

34. ENDOMETRIOSIS

Amy E. Hearne and Joseph Whelan

I. **Definition.** Endometriosis is the extrauterine presence of endometrial glands and stroma.

II. **Epidemiology.** The exact incidence of endometriosis is uncertain due to the fact that the disease process exists in several states from microscopic lesions to macroscopic disease, some of which are not apparent during evaluation. Three percent to 10% of reproductive-age women are afflicted with endometriosis, although the prevalence is much higher in infertility patients (25–35%). Studies have reported that the incidence of endometriosis in patients with chronic pelvic pain ranges from 20% to 90% and in patients with dysmenorrhea ranges from 40% to 60%. The mean age at diagnosis is 25–30 years.

III. **Etiology.** The exact cause of endometriosis is still unknown. Several theories regarding the histogenesis of endometriosis as well as immunologic and genetic factors have been postulated.

   A. **Transport (metastasis)**
      1. **Retrograde menstruation.** In 1927, Sampson's theory was published, suggesting that endometriosis was related to retrograde menstruation of endometrial tissue via the fallopian tubes into the peritoneal cavity. This theory has been supported by the following data: (1) blood flow from the fimbriated ends of fallopian tubes has been visualized during laparoscopy, (2) endometriosis is most often found in the dependent portions of the pelvis, (3) endometrial fragments can be retrieved from peritoneal fluid in menstruating women, (4) the incidence of endometriosis is higher in women with obstruction to normal outward menstrual flow, (5) endometriosis is increased in women with shorter menstrual cycles or longer duration of flow, which provides more opportunity for endometrial implantation. Because not all women who are observed to have retrograde menstruation develop endometriosis, other factors may also be involved in this pathologic process.
      2. **Other transport mechanisms.** Endometrial fragments may also be transported by means of hematogenous, lymphatic, or iatrogenic dissemination.
   B. **Coelomic metaplasia.** The transformation of coelomic epithelium into endometriotic tissue has been proposed but is not well supported by data.
   C. **Induction.** The induction theory proposes that undefined biochemical factors may induce undifferentiated peritoneal cell to transform into endometrial tissue. There are some animal data to support this theory; however, it has not been substantiated in humans.
   D. **Immunologic factors.** Factors at the site of the endometriotic implants may also play a role. An alteration of the peritoneal cell population volume, alteration in activity of the peritoneal cells, alteration in peritoneal fluid contents, and altered endometrium may all play a role. Data suggest that a change in peritoneal macrophage cytotoxicity and secretory activity occurs in women with endometriosis.
   E. **Genetic factors.** A genetic relationship would also be likely because chromosomal defects have been observed in endometriotic tissue, and women who have a primary relative with endometriosis have a sevenfold greater risk of developing endometriosis.

IV. **Symptoms.** Although some women with endometriosis are asymptomatic, the most common symptoms are pelvic pain, dysmenorrhea, dyspareunia, and infertility.

A. **Pelvic pain.** The pain associated with endometriosis is usually described as **deep** and often in the rectal area. More often it is **central** in location, but unilateral pain may be compatible with lesions in the ovary or pelvic side wall. **Dysmenorrhea** often starts before the onset of menstrual bleeding and continues throughout the menstrual period. **Dyspareunia** may occur, especially in the premenstrual or menstrual periods of the cycle. **Dysuria** or **dyschezia** can occur with urinary tract or intestinal tract involvement.

B. **Infertility.** The effect of endometriosis on fertility may be due to an altered environment that affects sperm and egg binding. In advanced disease, pelvic, tubal, or ovarian adhesions may interfere with gamete or embryo transport.

V. **Clinical findings.** Common findings on physical examination include nodularity of the uterosacral ligaments, which are often tender and enlarged; or tender adnexa; painful swelling of the rectovaginal septum; and pain with motion of the uterus and adnexa. A fixed retroverted uterus and large immobile adnexa are indications of severe pelvic disease. In many women with endometriosis, however, no abnormalities are found on clinical examination.

VI. **Diagnosis**

A. A definitive diagnosis can be made only through **histologic** examination, which reveals both endometrial glands and stroma. Hemosiderin-laden macrophages have been identified in 77% of endometriosis biopsy specimens. Laparoscopy can enable biopsy of tissue as well as evaluation for extent of disease. This may be impractical, however, and not always possible.

B. Experienced clinicians often presumptively diagnose endometriosis based on a **classic** blue-black powder-burn visual appearance. Endometriosis has also been identified in **nonclassic** lesions, which may appear as red, white, tan, nonpigmented, or vesicular lesions. Red lesions are considered to be the more active form of endometriosis. Symptoms, pelvic findings, and results of adjunctive procedures such as imaging and laboratory analysis often support the diagnosis. The presence of defects in the peritoneum, usually scarring overlying endometrial implants, is known as **Allen-Masters syndrome**. Endometriomas can also be visualized during laparoscopy and may be dubiously referred to as "chocolate cysts" based on their dark brown appearance.

C. **Imaging techniques. Pelvic ultrasonography** may be useful in suggesting the presence of endometriomas at a cost significantly less than that of CT or MRI. Ultrasonography is inadequate, however, to detect the more common superficial endometriotic lesions along the peritoneal lining.

D. **Laboratory findings.** Levels of cancer antigen 125 (CA-125) and cancer antigen 19-9 have been shown to be elevated in endometriosis. These antigens may also undergo physiologic elevations in the normal menstrual cycle, however. CA-125, which is elevated in other conditions including pelvic disease processes (ovarian neoplasia, uterine leiomyomas, pelvic inflammatory disease), has little specificity in the diagnosis of endometriosis. There may be a role for CA-125 measurement in tracking endometriosis that has undergone or is undergoing medical or surgical management.

VII. **Classification and staging.** The American Society for Reproductive Medicine revised classification of 1996 is the most widely used classification system in the medical literature. This system is based on appearance, size, and depth of peritoneal and ovarian implants; the presence, extent, and type of adnexal adhesions; and the degree of cul-de-sac obliteration. Parameters such as degree of pain and infertility are not included.

VIII. **Management.** Once the diagnosis of endometriosis has been made, management options may be based on extent of disease and patient needs. Both medical and surgical regimens exist. Treatment choice often requires attention to infertility, desire to relieve pain and maintain fertility, or desire for pain management alone.

A. **Medical management.** Implants of endometriosis react in a similar manner to intrauterine endometrial tissue in that estrogen stimulates growth. Medical therapy is aimed at suppressing ovarian estrogen stimulation by interrupting the hypothalamic-pituitary-ovarian axis. Inhibition of ovulation by gonadotropin suppression removes the stimulation of endometriosis by cycling sex steroids. Review of the data has shown that the various treatment agents are similar in terms of efficacy; therefore, cost and side effects should determine choice of agent.

1. **Gonadotropin-releasing hormone (GnRH) agonists,** when given over the long term, suppress pituitary function by down-regulating pituitary GnRH receptors. This interruption of the hypothalamic-pituitary-ovarian axis produces a "medical oophorectomy" or "pseudomenopause." Three available agents are leuprolide acetate (Lupron Depot), which is administered in a dose of 3.75 mg by intramuscular injection every month for 6 months, nafarelin acetate nasal spray, which is administered in a dose of 200 μg twice daily for 3 months, and goserelin acetate (Zoladex) 3.6 mg subcutaneous implants at 4 week intervals. The side effects (Table 34-1), which occur in approximately 11% of patients, are related to the hypoestrogenic state. Treatment is usually limited to 6 months to avoid the consequences of the hypoestrogenic state on bone metabolism and lipoprotein profile. If therapy is to be continued for longer duration, consideration should be given to add-back therapy. A postmenopausal estrogen-progesterone add-back regimen can be used, such as daily conjugated estrogen 0.625 mg together with medroxyprogesterone acetate 2.5 mg.

2. **Oral contraceptives** cause anovulation and decidualization, which results in atrophy of endometrial tissue. Symptomatic relief of pelvic pain and dysmenorrhea is reported in 60–95% of patients. The estrogenic component in oral contraceptive pills may potentially stimulate growth and increase pain during the first few weeks of treatment. Side effects are listed in Table 34-1.

3. **Progestins** have antiendometriotic effects by causing decidualization and atrophy of endometrial tissue. Progestins also inhibit ovulation by luteinizing hormone suppression and eventually may induce amenorrhea. Medroxyprogesterone acetate can be administered in a dosage of 150 mg intramuscularly every 3 months for 1 year or 30 mg orally (PO) every day (qd) for 90 days. Megestrol acetate 40 mg PO qd can also be used. Progesterone therapy can be continued for suppression of endometriosis symptomatology; however, health care providers should be aware of the potential for bone demineralization with long-term progesterone use. Other side effects are listed in Table 34-1.

4. **Danazol (Danocrine)** is a derivative of the synthetic steroid 17α-ethinyltestosterone. It suppresses the midcycle luteinizing hormone surge, inhibits steroidogenesis in the human corpus luteum, and produces a high-androgen and low-estrogen environment that does not support the growth of endometriosis. Regimens of 400–800 mg PO qd for 6 months have been described. Amenorrhea may be a better indicator of response than drug dose. One strategy is to start treatment with 400 mg/day (200 mg PO twice daily) and increase the dose as necessary to achieve absence of menstruation and relieve symptoms. Approximately 80% of patients experience relief or improvement in symptoms within 2 months of beginning danazol treatment. However, recurrence of symptoms is almost 50% within 4–12 months after discontinuation of therapy. Adverse side effects, listed in Table 34-1, occur in approximately 15% of women taking danazol. A 6-year prospective study found no difference in side effects with 400-mg and 800-mg doses. Danazol is metabolized in the liver and may cause hepatocellular damage and reversible alterations in cholesterol profile; thus, caution should be used in patients with liver disease. Caution should also be used in patients with hypertension, CHF, or impaired renal function, as danazol can cause fluid retention. Danazol use is contraindicated in pregnant patients because of the risk of masculinization of the fetus, and patients should also be encouraged to use a barrier form of contraception during

TABLE 34-1. MEDICAL MANAGEMENT OF ENDOMETRIOSIS

Drug	Mechanism	Dosage	Side effects
Gonadotropin-releasing hormone analogs	Down-regulation of pituitary receptors, inhibition of the hypothalamic-pituitary-ovarian axis leading to ovarian suppression	Leuprolide acetate (Lupron): 3.75–7.5 mg IM q mo ×6 Nafarelin acetate (Synarel): 200–400 µg intranasally bid ×6 mos Goserelin acetate (Zoladex): 3.6-mg implant SC q28d 10.8-mg implant SC q12wks ×6 mos	Hot flashes, vaginal dryness, bone demineralization, insomnia, libido changes, fatigue
Oral contraceptives	Anovulation, atrophy and decidualization of endometrial tissue	Monophasic pill	Weight gain, breakthrough bleeding, breast tenderness, bloating, nausea
Progestins	Atrophy and decidualization of endometrial tissue, suppression of gonadotropins, inhibition of ovulation, amenorrhea	Medroxyprogesterone acetate: 150 mg IM q3mos ×4 30 mg PO qd ×90 days Megestrol acetate: 40 mg PO qd ×6 mos	Weight gain, fluid retention, breakthrough bleeding, depression Possible bone demineralization with long-term use
Danazol	Anovulation by decreasing the midcycle luteinizing hormone surge Inhibition of steroidogenesis, creation of high-androgen and low-estrogen environment	400–800 mg PO qd ×6 mos	Amenorrhea, virilization, acne, hirsutism, atrophic vaginitis, decrease in breast size, hot flashes, deepening of voice

treatment. Preliminary data suggest that vaginal danazol rings may be effective in treating deep endometriosis with less androgenic side effects. Gestrinone, a 19-nortestosterone derivative used in Europe, is administered two times per week.

5. **Antiprogesterones** inhibit ovulation and disrupt the endometrium. They are currently investigational, and indications for their use in treating endometriosis are yet to be established.

6. **Pain control** with nonsteroidal anti-inflammatory drugs inhibits prostaglandin production by ectopic endometrium.

B. **Surgical management.** Medical therapy may be a management modality in patients whose goals are pain management or pain management in the presence of fertility. In patients with infertility, however, or those in whom symptoms do not improve or recur with medical treatment, surgical management is an option. Surgical management can be subdivided into definitive surgery and conservative surgery.

1. **Definitive therapy** entails total abdominal hysterectomy with bilateral salpingo-oophorectomy, excision of peritoneal surface lesions or endometriomas, and lysis of adhesions. This definitive treatment is not always an option, however, if the patient wishes to maintain reproductive capacity or conserve ovarian tissue. A "semidefinitive" procedure that preserves an uninvolved ovary is usually discouraged because of the sixfold increased risk of developing recurrent symptoms and a high reoperative rate to remove the remaining ovary if it develops recurrent disease. Patients who have undergone hysterectomy and bilateral saplingo-oophorectomy may receive replacement estrogen postoperatively. There is only a slight risk of recurrent growth of residual endometriotic implants during ERT.

2. **Conservative surgery** may include the following:
   a. Excision or destruction (via laser vaporization, electrocoagulation, thermal coagulation) directed at surface lesions or endometriomas
   b. Lysis of pelvic adhesions
   c. Adjunctive pain management procedures (presacral neurectomy, uterosacral nerve ablation or ligation, uterine suspension)

IX. **Psychosocial aspects.** Endometriosis can have a significant effect on quality of life and reproductive capacity. The Endometriosis Association is an international organization that provides support and education for women with endometriosis.

X. **Endometriosis and infertility**
   A. The **success rate** of surgery is related to the severity of endometriosis. A 60% pregnancy success rate is seen in patients with moderate disease, and a 35% rate is achieved in severe disease. The highest pregnancy rate occurs within the first year after surgery. Therefore, many physicians avoid postoperative medical therapy, which suppresses ovulation, in patients who desire pregnancy.
   B. Patients with endometriosis who remain infertile despite conservative surgery or hormonal therapy or both are candidates for assisted reproductive technologies using in vitro fertilization.

35. AMENORRHEA

Julie Huh and Joseph Whelan

I. **Definition and epidemiology.** Amenorrhea is the absence of spontaneous menses during the reproductive years. It is physiologic during lactation and pregnancy.

   A. **Primary amenorrhea** refers to the absence of menarche by age 16. It occurs in fewer than 0.1–2.5% of reproductive-age women.

   B. **Secondary amenorrhea** refers to the absence of menses for 3 cycle lengths in the setting of oligomenorrhea, or for 6 months after establishing regular menses. The incidence is variable, but in the general population it ranges between 1% and 5%.

II. **Clinical evaluation.** Failure of menarche by age 16, regardless of presence or absence of secondary sexual characteristics, or absence of menses in a woman with previous periodic menses merits evaluation; however, an evaluation may be undertaken if there is no breast development by age 14, if sexual ambiguity or virilization is present, or if the patient or family or both are concerned.

   A. **History**

      1. Past medical and surgical history including pubertal milestones and abnormalities of growth and development; systemic diseases such as hypothyroidism, adrenal insufficiency, or growth hormone excess; and hemotherapy, radiation, or surgical procedures.

      2. Obstetric-gynecologic history including menstrual history, history of hemorrhage during delivery, dilation and curettage, infection, or hormonal contraception use.

      3. Drug use, including psychotropic drugs, oral contraceptives, antihypertensives, narcotics, chemotherapeutic agents, or cannabis.

      4. Family history of genetic or congenital illnesses.

      5. Review of systems including diet, exercise, weight changes, stress, symptoms of early pregnancy, galactorrhea, hirsutism, cyclic lower abdominal pain, hot flashes, vaginal dryness, virilizing symptoms.

   B. **Physical examination**

      1. Height and weight proportions.

      2. Signs of endocrinopathies. Thyroid disease (exophthalmos, thyromegaly, or thyroid nodule, macroglossia, heat or cold intolerance, hair thinning, deep tendon reflex changes), hyperprolactinemia (galactorrhea), Cushing syndrome (centripetal obesity, hypertension, proximal muscle weakness, abdominal striae, thinning of scalp hair, hirsutism).

      3. Secondary sexual characteristics. **Thelarche:** breast development, which occurs, on average, at 10.8 years of age and indicates estrogen exposure. **Adrenarche:** axillary and pubic hair development, which occurs, on average, at 11 years of age and indicates ovarian and adrenal androgen production and end-organ androgen response.

      4. Gynecologic examination. Speculum and bimanual examination to confirm the presence of cervix, endocervical canal, uterus, and adnexa. Decrease in breast size or vaginal dryness may indicate decreasing estrogen exposure (or increasing androgen exposure).

   C. **Initial workup** (Fig. 35-1). After pregnancy is excluded, the initial step in the workup is measurement of thyroid-stimulating hormone (TSH) and prolactin levels. Women with galactorrhea, regardless of their menstrual history, may also require radiographic evaluation. A **progestin challenge** is optional for assessing estrogenization of the endometrium. This test involves administering 100–200 mg of progesterone in oil intramuscularly or 10 mg of medroxyprogesterone acetate orally for 5–10 days to induce

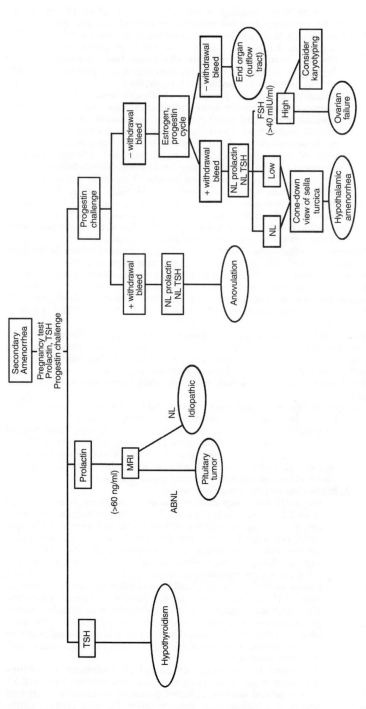

FIG. 35-1. Flow diagram for the evaluation of women with secondary amenorrhea. ABNL, abnormal level; FSH, follicle-stimulating hormone; LH, luteinizing hormone; NL, normal level; TSH, thyroid-stimulating hormone. (Adapted from Speroff L, Glass RH, Kase NG. Amenorrhea. In: *Clinical gynecologic endocrinology and infertility*, 6th ed. Baltimore: Lippincott Williams & Wilkins, 1999.)

uterine withdrawal bleeding. A withdrawal bleed within 10 days of the progestin challenge does not indicate the level of estrogen supply or the endometrium's histologic response to estrogen, nor does it rule out müllerian anomalies or uterine disease, such as Asherman syndrome.

1. **Positive result on progestin challenge test.** Bleeding within 10 days of the completion of the regimen indicates a positive test result, and the diagnosis of anovulation is established.

2. **Negative result on progestin challenge test.** Failure to induce uterine bleeding implies hypoestrogenemia, most likely due to a hypothalamic or pituitary disorder, or lack of communication from uterus to vaginal outflow tract. To clarify whether the outflow tract is inoperative or estrogen-influenced proliferation of the endometrium has not occurred, exogenous estrogen can be administered (1.25 mg conjugated estrogens or 2 mg estradiol, daily for 21 days). This is followed by the addition of medroxyprogesterone acetate 10 mg orally during the last 5 days to induce withdrawal bleeding. If bleeding occurs, the cause of inadequate estrogen production needs to be elucidated (i.e., ovarian cause or CNS cause). Serum gonadotropin levels should be assessed. If bleeding does not occur, a thorough evaluation of the müllerian system is warranted for anomalies or obstruction to outflow.

III. **Differential diagnosis** (Table 35-1). Although gonadal failure is the most frequent cause of primary amenorrhea, anorexia nervosa is the single most common cause of amenorrhea overall in teenagers. Uterovaginal agenesis is the second most common cause of primary amenorrhea. Of women with secondary amenorrhea who are not pregnant, 49–62% have hypothalamic disorders, 7–16% have pituitary disorders, 10% have ovarian disorders, and 7% have Asherman syndrome.

IV. **Classification into upper or lower genital tract causes, ovarian causes, and CNS causes.** Although it is traditional to categorize amenorrhea as primary or secondary, this distinction is less helpful than other categorizations, as some disorders cause both primary and secondary amenorrhea, and it should not necessarily be strictly relied on when evaluating an amenorrheic patient.

A. **Upper or lower genital tract causes and treatment**

1. Labial agglutination can be treated with estrogen cream.

2. Congenital defects of the vagina, imperforate hymen, fused vaginal septa. Symptoms may include cyclic, predictable abdominal pain. Treatment includes simple incision or excision. In cases of transverse vaginal septum, ultrasonography is helpful in determining the location and length of the septum before surgical repair is undertaken.

3. **Müllerian anomalies or agenesis**

a. **Mayer-Rokitansky-Küster-Hauser syndrome** affects a group of 46,XX patients. It is the second most frequent cause of primary amenorrhea, accounting for 15% of cases, and appears to be sporadic, not inherited. Affected patients have normal, functioning ovaries but either absent or rudimentary uterus, and lack a vagina. This syndrome is associated with an increased incidence of renal anomalies, including pelvic kidney or unilateral absence of a kidney, as well as skeletal, cardiac, and other congenital abnormalities. IVP can help determine the presence of renal anomalies. MRI or ultrasonography can distinguish this from complete androgen resistance by confirming the presence of ovaries. Treatment involves either nonsurgical dilatation of a blind-ending pouch or surgical construction of a neovagina with use of a skin graft (McIndoe procedure).

b. **Androgen insensitivity or complete androgen resistance** (testicular feminization syndrome). Affected patients have a 46,XY karyotype and have an X-linked dominant or recessive trait that results in a testosterone receptor defect. Patients produce mülle-

TABLE 35-1.   CLASSIFICATION OF AMENORRHEA

Upper and lower genital tract causes	Central nervous system causes
Labial agglutination/fusion	Pituitary causes
Imperforate hymen	Prolactinomas
Transverse vaginal septum	Craniopharyngiomas
Cervical agenesis, stenosis	Empty sella syndrome
Müllerian agenesis (Mayer-Rokitan-	Arterial aneurysm
sky-Küster-Hauser syndrome)	Sarcoidosis
Complete androgen resistance (testic-	Sheehan syndrome
ular feminization)	Hypothalamic correlations
Asherman syndrome (uterine scarring)	Chronic anovulation, estrogen present
Ovarian causes	Polycystic ovary syndrome
Gonadal agenesis	Thyroid dysfunction (hypothy-
Gonadal dysgenesis	roidism, hyperthyroidism)
Turner syndrome (45,XO)	Adrenal disease (Cushing dis-
Mosaicism	ease/syndrome, adult-onset
Pure gonadal dysgenesis	adrenal hyperplasia)
46,XX	Chronic anovulation, estrogen absent
46,XY (Swyer syndrome)	(hypogonadotropic hypogonadism)
Ovarian enzymatic deficiency	Tumors
17α-hydroxylase deficiency	Infection and other disorders
17,20-lyase deficiency	(Kallmann syndrome, tubercu-
Premature ovarian failure	losis, syphilis, sarcoidosis)
Idiopathic	Functional (stress, weight loss,
Autoimmune	malnutrition, psychological
Resistant ovary syndrome	factors, exercise)
Radiation or chemotherapy	
Mumps oophoritis	
Ovarian tumors	

rian duct inhibitory factor and have normal, functioning testes with a complete absence of internal female genitalia. Individuals have varying degrees of target tissue androgen unresponsiveness and, accordingly, range in appearance from completely normal females, without pubic or axillary hair, to normal phenotypic males whose only abnormality is infertility (mildest form). Phenotypically female patients have a blind vaginal pouch, abundant breast tissue, scant axillary and pubic hair, and normal external female genitalia. These patients usually have been raised as girls. After breast development and epiphyseal closure, the undescended gonads should be removed due to risk of gonadal neoplasia. Hence, gonadectomy can be deferred until secondary sexual development is complete (usually age 16–18).

4. **Uterine scarring.** Endometrial scarring or intrauterine adhesions (Asherman syndrome) may result from dilation and curettage, metroplasty, myomectomy, cesarean section, or tuberculosis or schistosomiasis. It can be confirmed using hysterosalpingography or hysteroscopy. Treatment involves directed hysteroscopic resection of scar tissue. After surgery, an intrauterine balloon catheter or pediatric Foley catheter can

be inserted for 7 days to prevent the walls of the uterine cavity from adhering. Pharmacologic doses of estrogen for 1–2 months (e.g., conjugated estrogen 2.5 mg/day for 3 weeks) and a progestin (e.g., medroxyprogesterone acetate 10 mg for 1 week, starting in the third week) are sometimes prescribed in the immediate postoperative interval in hopes of optimizing endometrial healing. Antibiotic coverage is advised while the balloon or Foley catheter is in place.

B. **Ovarian causes**
   1. **Gonadal dysgenesis** is the absence of germ cells, with ovaries replaced by fibrous streaks. Approximately half of patients with gonadal dysgenesis exhibit a mosaic karyotype or a structural abnormality of the X chromosome (e.g., deletion of long [*p*-] or short [*q*-] arm, ring chromosome, or isochromosome). In individuals with a Y chromosome, a 20% incidence of dysgerminoma and gonadoblastoma exists; therefore, gonadectomy is recommended for affected patients. Workup includes determination of karyotype.
      a. **Turner syndrome** (45,XO) is the most common karyotype found in cases of spontaneous abortion. Fewer than 0.3% of affected fetuses survive to term, for an incidence of 1 in 2000–3000 live births. The defect is usually not inherited. Affected individuals commonly may present with primary amenorrhea and somatic defects, including short stature, webbed neck, shield chest, short metacarpals, increased carrying angle of the arms, cardiovascular defects (coarctation of the aorta), and sexual infantilism.
      b. **Chromosomal mosaicism.** Individuals with the karyotypes XO/XY, XO/XYY, or XO/XY/XYY have clinical presentations that range from a syndrome similar to that of typical gonadal dysgenesis, to ambiguous genitalia, to phenotypic maleness. Individuals with the karyotypes X/XX, X/XXX, or X/XX/XXX have a low incidence of physical stigmata. Affected patients tend to be short and may undergo premature menopause; 20% produce enough estrogen to menstruate.
      c. **Pure gonadal dysgenesis** comprises the karyotypes 46,XY (**Swyer syndrome**) and 46,XX. The disorder may be inherited; however, in most cases the cause is unknown. The disorder may result from single gene defects or destruction of germinal tissue in utero by environmental or infectious agents. Patients present with primary amenorrhea, eunuchoid habitus, normal stature, and infantile internal and external female genitalia. One-third of patients have major cardiovascular or renal abnormalities. Some patients with 46,XX may have a few ovarian follicles, develop breasts, or menstruate for several years. Neurosensory deafness is common. Workup includes chromosomal karyotyping with gonadectomy if the Y chromosome is present, as the risk of developing gonadal neoplasm, sometimes at an early age, is as high as 25%. Approximately 10% of neoplasms occur before the age of 10, and most develop before age 30. Tumors include gonadoblastomas (50%), dysgerminomas (20%), gonadoblastoma with dysgerminomas (18%), and other histologic types (9%).
   2. **Premature ovarian failure** is cessation of ovarian function before age 40 and affects approximately 1% of women. In most cases, the cause is unknown; however, possibilities include destruction of follicles by infection (e.g., mumps oophoritis) or an autoimmune process. In 30–50% of cases, it is associated with autoimmune disorders of the adrenal, thyroid, or parathyroid glands and systemic lupus erythematosus. Radiation and chemotherapy, especially with alkylating agents, can injure ovaries and decrease the number of oocytes. A dose greater than 8 Gy directed to the ovary usually causes permanent failure, irrespective of age.
   3. In **resistant ovary syndrome** (resistance to follicle-stimulating hormone) primordial follicles arrest in development before the antral stage,

despite elevated gonadotropin levels, which results in sexual immaturity. Patients with resistant ovary syndrome can, on rare occasions, be treated successfully with high doses of gonadotropins.

4. **Ovarian tumors** may interrupt normal ovarian function and, therefore, should be considered in cases of amenorrhea with an enlarged adnexa.

5. **Diagnosis and treatment.** Ovarian failure should be suspected in all cases of primary amenorrhea with sexual infantilism and secondary amenorrhea with hot flashes and other signs of estrogen deficiency. Confirmation is made by documenting increased FSH levels in the menopausal range (higher than 40 IU/L) in repeated tests 4–6 weeks apart. For women younger than 30 years, a karyotype should be determined. The presence of a Y chromosome requires excision of the gonadal tissue to prevent malignant transformation, which occurs in 25% of patients. If indicated, 17α-hydroxyprogesterone levels (to rule out ovarian enzymatic deficiency), thyroid function indicators, or autoimmune antibody levels should be measured. Treatment involves estrogen and progesterone replacement. Patients with 17α-hydroxylase deficiency need glucocorticoids as well. Prophylactic oophoropexy may be helpful in women undergoing pelvic radiation therapy. Pretreatment with gonadotropin-releasing hormone (GnRH) analogs or other methods of ovulation suppression before chemotherapy may help maintain ovarian function.

C. **CNS causes**

1. **Pituitary disorders**

   a. Anatomic lesions include tumors, space-occupying lesions, and inflammatory lesions.

   b. **Hyperprolactinemia** due to prolactin-secreting adenomas, ingestion of drugs, or other disorders, interrupts gonadotropin secretion, probably by causing hypothalamic dysfunction. Ten percent of women with amenorrhea have elevated prolactin levels. Prolactin secretion is inhibited by dopamine and stimulated by serotonin and thyrotropin-releasing hormone. With elevated prolactin level, thyroid function should be evaluated. Primary hypothyroidism may cause elevated levels of thyrotropin-releasing hormone and, hence, prolactin. Women with persistent hyperprolactinemia, especially associated with amenorrhea or galactorrhea or both, should undergo radiographic evaluation. The prolactin level at which radiographic study is recommended is debatable. Some recommend evaluation with levels higher than 20–30 ng/mL, whereas others evaluate when levels exceed 50–100 ng/mL. MRI is superior to CT in clarity of definition of soft tissue, optic chiasm, and vasculature. If the patient desires to establish a pregnancy, administration of gonadotropins or pulsatile GnRH therapy may be considered. Treatment with a dopamine agonist (bromocriptine mesylate or cabergoline) may help normalize prolactin levels, especially in cases of microadenomas (tumors smaller than 10 mm diameter) and restore cyclical ovulation.

   c. **Sheehan syndrome,** partial or complete pituitary insufficiency, classically results from obstetric hemorrhage. Consequent hypogonadotropic hypogonadism results in amenorrhea, failure to lactate, or loss of genital and axillary hair. In severe cases, there is evidence of panhypopituitarism. Treatment involves replacement of appropriate hormones.

2. **Hypothalamic correlations**

   a. **Chronic anovulation, estrogen present** (see also Chap. 36)

      (1) **Polycystic ovary syndrome** or chronic hyperandrogenemic anovulation is due to inappropriate feedback signals to the hypothalamic-pituitary unit. It can cause infertility, hirsutism, obesity (two-thirds of patients), insulin resistance, menstrual disturbances (amenorrhea, oligomenorrhea, or dysfunctional uterine

bleeding), or a skin disorder (acanthosis nigricans). Ultrasonography may reveal multiple ovarian cysts; however, this finding is not uniformly present. The finding of a serum luteinizing hormone to FSH ratio of higher than 2:1 may help to confirm the diagnosis. Treatment involves administration of combination oral contraceptive pills or cyclical medroxyprogesterone acetate to cause cyclical uterine withdrawal bleeding if pregnancy is not desired. Ovulation-inducing drugs (e.g., clomiphene citrate) are options if pregnancy is desired. Metformin may also be added in patients who exhibit insulin resistance.

(2) **Thyroid dysfunction.** Both hypothyroidism and hyperthyroidism may cause amenorrhea. In hypothyroidism, high levels of thyrotropin-releasing hormone may potentiate prolactin secretion.

(3) **Cushing disease or syndrome.** In these disorders, androgen levels are not regulated by the usual negative feedback mechanisms and are consequently increased. This can result in hirsutism, increased muscle mass, frontal baldness, deepened voice, and hypertension.

b. **Chronic anovulation, estrogen absent (hypogonadotropic hypogonadism).** Hypogonadotropic hypogonadism may cause primary or secondary amenorrhea. Reversal of the primary cause is important.

(1) Anatomic lesions.

(2) Functional. Weight loss from extreme dieting or binging and purging (**anorexia nervosa** or **bulimia**) represents a common cause of secondary amenorrhea among young women. Patients are often white middle- to upper-class girls or women younger than 25 years. They may present with hypothermia, hypotension, bradycardia, hypercarotenemia, and constipation. Patients have normal to low gonadotropin levels, which is thought to result from diminished GnRH secretion. Exercise-induced amenorrhea may be caused by suppression of GnRH release by elevated levels of β-endorphin and catechol estrogens. Treatment for psychogenic causes requires psychiatric intervention. Cases of amenorrhea due to either psychogenic or behavioral factors (i.e., exercise-induced amenorrhea) require sex hormone replacement therapy to prevent bone loss until spontaneous menstrual cycling is reestablished.

(3) **Other disorders. Kallmann syndrome** is an isolated GnRH deficiency or inherited disorder (autosomal dominant) characterized by the absence of GnRH-secreting neurons originating from the olfactory bulb. Patients present with primary amenorrhea and absent to minimal sexual development. Associated findings include anosmia, color blindness, cleft lip, and sometimes congenital deafness. Treatment consists of continuous or cyclic sex hormone replacement therapy. Pulsatile GnRH agonist therapy or exogenous gonadotropin regimens may induce ovulation.

36. ABNORMAL UTERINE BLEEDING

Betty Chou and Nikos Vlahos

I. **Classification of abnormal uterine bleeding.** Normal menstrual bleeding is defined as cyclic menstruation every 21–35 days that lasts fewer than 8 days with 20–80 mL of blood loss. For practical purposes, any patient who complains of a change in her previously established menstrual pattern may be considered to have abnormal uterine bleeding.

A. **Definitions**
1. Polymenorrhea is uterine bleeding at intervals of fewer than 21 days.
2. Oligomenorrhea is uterine bleeding at intervals of more than 35 days.
3. Hypermenorrhea (menorrhagia) is excessive bleeding at regular intervals.
4. Metrorrhagia is bleeding at irregular intervals.
5. Menometrorrhagia is heavy, irregular bleeding.
6. Intermenstrual bleeding is bleeding between regular menses.

B. **Differential diagnosis.** The causes of abnormal uterine bleeding may be categorized as either **organic** or **nonorganic.** Organic causes can be further classified as reproductive tract disease, systemic disease, trauma, and pharmacologic alterations. The diagnosis of nonorganic cause, or **dysfunctional uterine bleeding,** is assumed when an organic cause cannot be found (Table 36-1).

II. **Evaluation.** To determine the cause of a patient's abnormal uterine bleeding, a complete workup must be performed, including history, physical examination, laboratory evaluation, possible imaging studies, and possible tissue sampling (Table 36-2).

A. **History.** The history must include a qualification of the abnormal bleeding, specifically determining the onset, duration, frequency, amount, and pattern of the bleeding. In addition, the degree of associated pain, vaginal discharge, fever, nausea, and vomiting should be clarified. Other sources of the bleeding, such as from the GI or urinary tract, should be ruled out. For women of childbearing age, sexual and contraceptive history should be explored to help determine likelihood of pregnancy. Menopausal symptoms should be explored in appropriate patients. Any change in the patient's diet, weight, and exercise pattern is relevant. The patient's age, parity, hormonal contraception or hormone replacement history, past medical history, gynecologic and obstetric history, and medication regimen are pertinent to the evaluation. Family history of diseases, including gynecologic cancer or bleeding disorders, should be discussed.

B. **Physical examination.** The patient should first be evaluated to ensure that she is hemodynamically stable. If the patient does not require immediate resuscitative intervention, attention should be directed to the abdomen and pelvis. Examination of the abdomen can determine if the patient has an acute or surgical abdomen that requires urgent surgical intervention. Inspection of the vaginal vault can demonstrate the degree of current bleeding, source of the bleeding, discharge suggestive of infection, or evidence of trauma, lesions, polyps, tissue, or masses. A bimanual examination should be performed to establish the status of the internal os, presence of cervical motion tenderness, presence of any palpable masses or lesions, size and contour of uterus and adnexa, and presence of any tenderness on manipulation of any of the pelvic organs. Finally, more specific physical findings can be associated with abnormal uterine bleeding caused by systemic diseases (see sec. **III.C**).

C. **Laboratory studies.** To establish the acuteness and severity of the abnormal vaginal bleeding, the patient's hemoglobin level or hematocrit or both

TABLE 36-1. DIFFERENTIAL DIAGNOSIS OF ABNORMAL UTERINE BLEEDING

Organic causes	Reproductive tract disorders
	Complications of pregnancy (ectopic pregnancy, miscarriage)
	Benign disease—fibroids, polyps, infections, endometrial hyperplasia
	Malignancy—endometrial, cervical cancer
	Trauma or foreign body
	Systemic diseases
	Coagulation disorders
	Endocrinopathies—hypothyroidism, hyperprolactinemia
	Liver failure
	Obesity
	Iatrogenic/pharmacologic causes
	Psychotropic medications
	Hormonal contraception/replacement
Nonorganic	Dysfunctional uterine bleeding
	Anovulation (more common)
	Ovulation

should be determined. Any patient of childbearing age must be assumed to be pregnant until proven otherwise; therefore, a urine level of human chorionic gonadotropin, β-subunit (β-hCG) must be obtained. Other laboratory tests that may be of interest include a Pap smear (if the patient is not actively bleeding) to evaluate for cervical dysplasia; WBC to look for other evidence of infection; platelet count, prothrombin time, and partial thromboplastin time to rule out a coagulation disorder; liver function tests to assess for hepatic disease; and thyroid function tests to investigate the possibility of thyroid disorders. A perimenopausal patient may need hormonal assays to evaluate her current hormonal state (follicle-stimulating hormone, estradiol).

TABLE 36-2. COMPLETE EVALUATION

Hemodynamic stabilization	Vital signs, orthostatics, general appearance
History	Duration, frequency, severity of bleeding
	Associated pain, discharge, abdominal symptoms
	Contraceptive history, medical history, obstetric-gynecologic history, medications
Physical examination	Vital signs, abdominal examination, pelvic examination
Laboratory tests	β-hCG level, CBC, PT/aPTT, LFTs, TFTs, prolactin level
Imaging studies	Ultrasonography, CT scan, SHG
Tissue sampling	D & C, endometrial biopsy, hysteroscopically directed biopsy

aPTT, activated partial thromboplastin time; β-hCG, human chorionic gonadotropin, β-subunit; D & C, dilation and curettage; LFTs, liver function tests; PT, prothrombin time; SHG, sonohysterography; TFTs, thyroid function tests.

D. **Imaging studies.** Depending on the differential diagnosis, various imaging studies may be necessary.

1. **Ultrasonography.** Ultrasonography is useful to evaluate for the presence of benign reproductive tract conditions such as fibroids, possible polyps, intrauterine pregnancy, and ectopic pregnancy. In the workup for possible malignant processes, sonography can be used to search for a thickened endometrial stripe and masses within the uterus, adnexa, or cervix.

2. **Sonohysterography (SHG).** SHG involves the instillation of a sterile solution (usually crystalloid) into the uterine canal during ultrasonography. SHG is the most sensitive noninvasive method of diagnosis for endometrial polyps and submucous myomata; its sensitivity approaches that of hysteroscopy.

3. **CT scanning.** CT imaging is used primarily in patients in whom the suspicion for malignancy is high. The CT scan can be used to help evaluate the location and extent of the disease.

E. **Tissue sampling.** Assessment of the endometrium is almost never needed for patients younger than 30 years (unless for endometrial dating). Endometrial sampling may be indicated in patients aged 30–40 years with risk factors for carcinoma. In premenopausal patients older than 40 years, the endometrium should be assessed if abnormal bleeding occurs. Postmenopausal bleeding must be assumed to be due to a malignancy until proven otherwise by tissue sampling.

1. **Office biopsy.** Office sampling using a Novak curette or a Pipelle or Vabra aspirator is simple, safe, and cost effective. Complications are extremely rare.

2. **Office hysteroscopy and biopsy.** Hysteroscopy can be used to visualize the endometrial cavity directly to look for lesions or pathology and to perform a directed biopsy. Complications are rare (less than 1%).

3. **Dilation and curettage (D & C).** D & C is a simple procedure. Performing the procedure, however, incurs the cost of an expensive operating room and carries the inherent risks of anesthesia.

III. **Diagnosis and treatment**

A. **Benign reproductive tract disease**

1. **Complications of pregnancy.** Any patient of childbearing age must be assumed to be pregnant until proven otherwise.

a. **Diagnosis.** A positive result on a urine β-hCG test is the definitive indicator of pregnancy. If findings of the urine β-hCG test are positive, a careful pelvic examination must be performed and an ultrasonographic study obtained to determine if the patient has an ectopic pregnancy or a threatened, inevitable, incomplete, or missed abortion. A quantitative serum β-hCG test may be helpful.

b. **Treatment.** Any patient who is hemodynamically unstable, bleeding heavily, or septic requires surgical intervention, such as a D & C for an early intrauterine pregnancy or abdominal surgery for an ectopic pregnancy.

2. **Leiomyomata. (fibroids)** are the most common uterine neoplasm. These benign smooth muscle tumors are found in 20–30% of patients older than 30 years and are uncommon in younger patients. The most common bleeding pattern associated with leiomyomata is hypermenorrhea. (See Chap. 33 for diagnosis and treatment.)

3. **Polyps.** Endometrial polyps are generally benign lesions that are found in fewer than 2% of premenopausal patients who undergo D & C. Benign cervical polyps are found in up to 4% of patients undergoing routine speculum examination. Although cervical polyps are often asymptomatic, associated symptoms most commonly include intermenstrual bleeding and postcoital spotting.

a. **Diagnosis.** Polyps can be diagnosed by a sonogram, hysterosalpingogram, or hysteroscopy.

b. **Treatment.** Polyps can be treated by simple polypectomy. Hypermenorrhea associated with endometrial polyps may respond to hormonal therapy.

4. **Infection.** Abnormal bleeding is not a common presenting symptom of either endometritis or cervicitis. If present, bleeding associated with endometritis is most commonly intermenstrual, and bleeding associated with cervicitis is postcoital.

   a. **Diagnosis.** Endometritis is diagnosed by fundal tenderness and fever. Any recent history of instrumentation of the uterus adds to the suspicion of endometritis. Cervicitis is diagnosed by clinical examination and results of cervical cultures.

   b. **Treatment.** Endometritis and cervicitis should be treated with antibiotics. (See Chap. 24.)

5. **Typical endometrial hyperplasia**

   a. **Diagnosis.** An endometrial tissue sample, either from an endometrial biopsy or a D & C, is required to make the diagnosis of typical endometrial hyperplasia.

   b. **Treatment.** In the absence of attempts at conception, these patients should probably be maintained on a regimen of cyclic monthly progestin withdrawal or oral contraceptive pills to prevent recurrence. An endometrial biopsy should be repeated if abnormal bleeding persists during treatment or recurs after therapy. Treatment should be continued for 4–6 months, at which time an endometrial biopsy should be performed to confirm regression of the hyperplasia.

6. **Atypical endometrial hyperplasia**

   a. **Diagnosis.** Diagnosis of atypical hyperplasia requires an endometrial tissue sample.

   b. **Treatment.** Treatment is always required, because in approximately 25% of cases, atypical hyperplasia progresses to carcinoma. Hysterectomy is an acceptable first-line treatment. As many as 25% of uteri removed in the treatment of atypical hyperplasia harbor a focus of well-differentiated carcinoma. For patients who wish to retain their fertility, progestational therapy is an acceptable approach. Continuous regimens of megestrol acetate (20–40 mg twice daily) may achieve an adequate response. Preliminary data suggest that even lower dosages may be effective. Treatment is continued for 6 months, with endometrial biopsies performed at 3 and 6 months. Dosing is increased if regression is not observed. Progesterone withdrawal regimens are not consistently effective and should not be used in the treatment of atypical hyperplasia; they may, however, be useful in preventing recurrence. (See Chap. 44.)

B. **Malignant reproductive tract disease**

1. **Endometrial cancer.** Endometrial carcinoma is rare in patients younger than 40 years and uncommon in the perimenopausal years. Postmenopausal bleeding, however, should be assumed to represent endometrial cancer until proven otherwise. (See Chap. 44.)

   a. **Diagnosis.** In a postmenopausal woman not receiving HRT, the presence of a thickened endometrial stripe (larger than 5 mm) on ultrasonography can be suggestive, but an endometrial tissue sample taken by D & C or endometrial biopsy is required for diagnosis.

   b. **Treatment.** Total abdominal hysterectomy with bilateral salpingo-oophorectomy and staging is the standard therapy. The need for postoperative radiation therapy is dependent on the stage and risk of recurrence.

2. **Cervical cancer.** Cervical carcinoma is a disease of both the relatively young and the old. Although it is rarely the cause of abnormal bleeding, it must be considered in the differential diagnosis. Almost all cervical lesions that cause abnormal bleeding are visible on examination. The

most common bleeding patterns associated with cervical carcinoma are intermenstrual and postcoital bleeding. (See Chap. 43 for additional discussion of diagnosis and treatment.)

a. **Diagnosis.** Patients are screened for cervical cancer with routine Pap smears. Abnormal smears can be followed by colposcopy. Lesions warrant biopsy.

b. **Treatment.** Depending on the stage of the cervical cancer, the patient may require surgical resection, chemotherapy, radiation, or a combination of these.

3. **Ovarian cancer.** Estrogen-producing ovarian tumors, such as a granulosa-theca cell tumor, can produce endometrial hyperplasia and abnormal uterine bleeding. (See Chap. 45.)

a. **Diagnosis.** Diagnosis usually involves a sonographic finding or a tissue diagnosis after resection.

b. **Treatment.** Ovarian cancer is treated by resection with or without adjuvant therapy.

C. **Systemic disease or disorder**

1. **Disorders of coagulation.** Coagulopathies may lead to abnormal uterine bleeding, often by exacerbating another underlying mild abnormality such as fibroids. Coagulopathies, however, are a relatively rare cause of abnormal uterine bleeding. **von Willebrand's disease** is the most common inherited bleeding disorder in women (occurring in up to 1 in 1000 patients). Other entities such as idiopathic thrombocytopenic purpura, hypersplenism, and hematologic malignancy (e.g., leukemia) may also be associated with abnormal uterine bleeding.

a. **Diagnosis.** Menorrhagia during adolescence should be attributed to a coagulation disorder until proven otherwise. Blood tests to evaluate the platelet count, prothrombin time, and partial thromboplastin time are indicated. Bleeding from multiple sites (nose, gingiva, intravenous sites, GI and genitourinary tracts) can be suggestive of a coagulopathy.

b. **Treatment.** Therapy usually involves treating the underlying cause and may require administration of blood products.

2. **Endocrinopathies** that cause anovulation. Anovulation can create an environment of unopposed estrogen. In the absence of progestin, the endometrium eventually breaks down, which may or may not lead to the formation of hyperplasia. **Hypothyroidism** and **hyperprolactinemia** are common disorders that can lead to anovulation.

a. **Diagnosis.** Signs and symptoms of hypothyroidism (fatigue, weight gain, cold intolerance, goiter, myxedema, delayed reflexes) and hyperprolactinemia (galactorrhea or visual changes from mass effect) should be reviewed and examined. Laboratory studies are diagnostic; therefore, thyroid function tests (measurement of levels of thyroid-stimulating hormone and free thyroxine) and measurement of prolactin level are indicated.

b. **Treatment.** Thyroid replacement therapy may be necessary for hypothyroidism. Bromocriptine mesylate or surgical resection of any macroadenoma of the pituitary, or both, may help relieve symptoms of hyperprolactinemia. Oral contraceptive pills (OCPs) or progestin may help eliminate the bleeding resulting from anovulation.

3. **Liver failure.** Decreased metabolism of estrogen and decreased clotting factor synthesis may lead to endometrial glandular and stromal breakdown, which may or may not produce endometrial hyperplasia. Anovulation may also ensue. Menometrorrhagia is common.

a. **Diagnosis.** Liver function tests are necessary to make the diagnosis. Physical examination findings of jaundice, ascites, hepatosplenomegaly, palmar erythema, pruritus, and spider hemangiomata are suggestive of liver failure.

b. **Treatment.** If possible, the underlying cause of the liver disease should be treated. If the patient is coagulopathic and is hemorrhaging from her disorder, administration of fresh frozen plasma may be indicated. Progesterone therapy may also be beneficial.

D. **Pharmacologic alterations.** Various medications may cause abnormal uterine bleeding. Any medication that acts on the hypothalamic-pituitary axis can lead to anovulation and abnormal bleeding.

1. **Psychotropic medications.** Certain medications used in the treatment of psychiatric patients can affect the hypothalamic-pituitary axis and interfere with ovulation. **Antidepressants** are among the commonly used medications associated with anovulation. The **antipsychotics** can also interfere with the normal menstrual cycle.

2. **Hormonal manipulation**
   a. **Levonorgestrel implants.** Sixty percent to 80% of patients experience irregular bleeding during the first year of levonorgestrel implant (Norplant) use.
   b. **Medroxyprogesterone acetate.** Approximately 30% of patients taking medroxyprogesterone (Depo-Provera) experience irregular bleeding during the first year. After the first year, 75% of patients on medroxyprogesterone are amenorrheic.
   c. **Combination oral contraceptive preparations.** Intermenstrual (breakthrough) bleeding is experienced by 10–30% of patients during the first month of OCP use, and by 1–10% during the subsequent 2 months. With long-term use, abnormal bleeding may result from endometrial atrophy. Abnormal bleeding for longer than 6 months requires further evaluation.
   d. **Progestational agents.** High doses of progesterone often are used in the treatment of abnormal uterine bleeding and endometrial hyperplasia. Prolonged use of these agents may result in endometrial atrophy, which itself often can cause abnormal uterine bleeding.

3. **Anticoagulants.** If the dosage of anticoagulants is too high, the patient can experience abnormal uterine bleeding.

4. Other drugs that may cause abnormal uterine bleeding include digitalis, phenytoin, and corticosteroids.

E. **Intrauterine devices.** Inert and copper-containing intrauterine devices can frequently cause heavy and irregular bleeding secondary to local inflammation and increased endometrial fibrinolytic activity. Such bleeding is often treated successfully with nonsteroidal anti-inflammatory agents.

F. **Dysfunctional uterine bleeding (DUB).** DUB is defined as abnormal uterine bleeding without a demonstrable organic cause and is found in approximately one-third of all patients evaluated. Treatment is directed toward stabilizing the endometrium and balancing the hormonal alterations. Medical therapy can include nonsteroidal anti-inflammatory agents, antifibrinolytic agents, high-dose estrogens, progestins, OCPs, danazol, and gonadotropin-releasing hormone agonists.

1. **Anovulation.** The predominant cause of DUB is anovulation. By definition, this anovulation is not secondary to a demonstrable organic cause. Anovulation is multifactorial and related to alterations of the hypothalamic-pituitary-ovarian axis. Anovulation associated with **polycystic ovary disease** and other forms of hyperandrogenism lacks a discrete organic cause, and associated bleeding abnormalities may be considered to be DUB. **Morbid obesity** can also cause DUB. Peripheral conversion of androstenedione to estrone occurs in adipose tissue. Elevated estrogen levels may lead to anovulation, which causes unopposed estrogen exposure and DUB.

2. **Ovulation.** Occasionally, DUB may be associated with ovulatory cycles. A persistent corpus luteum that does not regress in 12–14 days may result in DUB.

IV. **Acute vaginal hemorrhage.** Occasionally, patients experience severe vaginal bleeding. These patients usually present to the emergency department. Under such circumstances, endometrial sampling is inappropriate.

A. **History and physical examination.** An abbreviated history and physical examination is performed. Particular attention is paid to menstrual history and reproductive tract disease, as pregnancy and leiomyomata are by far the most common offenders. It is also necessary to look for vaginal tears from coitus or trauma and rectal bleeding, which are other common causes of acute hemorrhage.

B. **Laboratory studies.** A pregnancy test should be performed, and CBC, prothrombin time, and activated partial thromboplastin time should be obtained.

C. **Treatment.** Intravenous fluid resuscitation should be initiated immediately. If anemia is severe or symptomatic and bleeding persists, blood transfusion should be initiated.

1. **Endometrial atrophy.** Patients on chronic megestrol acetate therapy occasionally present with vaginal hemorrhage. Patients bleeding from endometrial atrophy may be treated with conjugated equine estrogens (Premarin), 25 mg intravenously every 2–4 hours (up to four doses). Antiemetics also should be administered to alleviate nausea associated with high-dose estrogen therapy. Patients may continue to take oral Premarin or OCPs. After 2 weeks of Premarin therapy, progestin should be added. An OCP taper also may be used as the primary therapy.

2. **Endometrial hyperplasia.** Often, morbidly obese patients present with signs and symptoms of endometrial hyperplasia. An OCP taper or high-dose continuous progestin therapy should be initiated. Megestrol 20 mg can be given twice each day and should be continued for at least 1 month. An endometrial sample should be obtained after the bleeding is controlled.

3. **Unclear etiology or suspected myoma.** An OCP taper usually controls the bleeding. No data suggest a superiority of any available formulation or taper regimen. A common approach is to administer four tablets/day for 4 days, three tablets/day for 4 days, two tablets/day for 4 days, then one tablet/day for a total of 2 months (omitting placebo pills). Patients are then continued on OCP therapy with normal monthly withdrawal for at least 4 months. Intravenous Premarin is an acceptable alternative for patients who cannot tolerate oral medication. Bleeding usually is controlled within 48 hours.

4. **Pregnancy.** Acute vaginal hemorrhage associated with previable pregnancy usually is caused by incomplete abortion. Such hemorrhage in first or second trimester pregnancies is best treated with suction curettage or evacuation. Antimicrobial prophylaxis (e.g., doxycycline 100 mg before the procedure) is warranted. If any signs of infection are present, broad-spectrum coverage with intravenous cefotetan disodium and doxycycline or triple antibiotics should be initiated.

5. **Bleeding requiring surgical intervention.** Surgical intervention is indicated if blood loss cannot be replaced with transfusion or if bleeding shows no signs of abating after 48 hours. D & C should be performed, although it may provide only temporary attenuation and should be followed by hormonal therapy. The patient should provide informed consent for hypogastric artery ligation and hysterectomy, which are the next lines of therapy should D & C fail. If available, hypogastric/uterine artery embolization may be considered as an alternative to ligation.

37. HYPERANDROGENISM

Kerry L. Swenson and Howard A. Zacur

I. **Hyperandrogenism** is characterized by the laboratory finding of an abnormally elevated serum concentration of androgens or the physical findings of androgen excess, or both. Physical characteristics of hyperandrogenism are as follows.

   A. **Hair distribution**

   1. **Normal.** During gestation, all hair follicles of the developing fetus produce fine, unpigmented hair known as **lanugo**. The total number of hair follicles is predetermined late in the second trimester of pregnancy. With age, some of these hair follicles on particular areas of the body produce thick, darkly pigmented hair in response to androgen exposure. This thick, dark hair is called terminal hair. The remaining hair follicles produce villus hair, which is finer than terminal hair and not as darkly pigmented. Hair follicles on the lower arms and legs do not respond to androgen stimulation and continue to produce villus hair.

   2. **Hirsutism** refers to the growth of dark terminal hair on the face, chest, back, lower abdomen, and upper thighs caused by overactivity of circulating androgen hormones. Androgens stimulate hair growth, increase the diameter of the hair shaft, and deepen the pigmentation of the hair. In contrast, estrogens slow hair growth and decrease hair diameter and pigmentation. Hirsutism is often associated with amenorrhea, anovulation, and hyperinsulinemia.

   3. **Hypertrichosis.** Excessive growth of villus hair is referred to as hypertrichosis. This condition may be caused by genetic factors or exposure to drugs such as phenytoin (Dilantin), or may be associated with an underlying malignancy. Hypertrichosis should not be mistaken for hirsutism.

   4. **Male pattern baldness.** Recession of frontal hair, as well as loss of hair in the temporal regions of the scalp and the crown of the head, is commonly seen in men as they age and occurs in response to androgens. The fact that excessive androgen activity stimulates hair growth on some parts of the body while causing hair loss from others remains unexplained.

   B. **Acne.** Infections of the pilosebaceous glands adjacent to hair follicles result in the formation of dermal abscesses, called **acne**. These skin lesions may exist on the surface of the skin or within the dermis. Lesions within the dermis are known as pustular acne. Because of the ability of androgens to stimulate secretions from pilosebaceous glands, it has long been believed that development of severe cases of acne is a manifestation of excessive androgenic hormone activity. Pustular acne involving the face and back is thought to result from excessive androgen stimulation.

   C. **Oily skin.** Release of secretions from pilosebaceous glands in response to androgen stimulation may result in excessive skin oiliness.

   D. **Voice changes.** In response to excessive androgen exposure, vocal cords undergo an irreversible thickening. This results in lowering of the tone of the voice.

   E. **Male body habitus.** Hypertrophy of major muscle groups, such as arm and leg muscles, occurs in response to androgen exposure. Not only do muscle cells become larger in response to androgen exposure, but their number increases as well. Hypertrophy of major muscle groups results in the development of what is commonly described as a male body habitus.

   F. **Enlargement of the clitoris.** Enlargement of the clitoris may occur in response to excessive androgen exposure. This is a dose-dependent event and is irreversible.

G. **Virilization** is a more severe state of excess androgenic activity than hirsutism. It refers to a constellation of symptoms including deepening of the voice, male body habitus, male pattern baldness, clitoromegaly, and reduction of breast size. Virilization is very rare and may be associated with adrenal tumors and hyperplasia or ovarian tumors such as theca lutein cysts, luteomas and arrhenoblastomas.

H. **Hyperinsulinemia.** Hyperandrogenism has been associated with hyperinsulinemia and insulin resistance. Insulin resistance is defined as a reduced glucose response to a given amount of insulin. Acanthosis nigricans is a gray-brown velvety discoloration of the skin and is a reliable indicator of insulin resistance and hyperinsulinemia. It is often seen in obese patients with hirsutism and is usually found in the groin, neck, axilla and vulva.

II. **Androgens.** Androgenic hormones include those that stimulate terminal hair growth and cause voice and muscle changes, hair loss, clitoral enlargement, and reduction in breast size. The most common androgens are testosterone and androstenedione. Dehydroepiandrosterone sulfate (DHEAS) is an androgen precursor.

A. **Testosterone** is the most potent androgenic hormone. In women, testosterone is secreted in equal amounts from the adrenal glands and from ovaries, and these sources account for 50% of the total testosterone found in the circulation. The remaining 50% is produced by peripheral conversion of androstenedione, which is also secreted by the adrenal glands and ovaries. Normal circulating concentrations of testosterone in women range from 20 to 80 ng/dL. This range is far lower than the concentrations found in men, which range from 300 to 800 ng/dL. Approximately 80% of testosterone is bound to sex hormone–binding globulin (SHBG). In women, approximately 19% of the remaining testosterone is loosely bound to albumin, which leaves approximately 1% in the free and active form.

B. **Androstenedione** is produced in equal amounts by the adrenal glands and the ovaries, and most of the androstenedione secreted is converted to testosterone. Androstenedione is a less potent androgen than testosterone but can produce significant androgenic biological effects when present in excess amounts. Normal serum concentration of androstenedione in women ranges from 60 to 300 ng/dL.

C. **Dehydroepiandrosterone (DHEA)** and its sulfate (DHEAS) are androgen precursors produced almost exclusively by the adrenal glands. DHEA is metabolized quickly. As a consequence, measurement of its serum concentration does not reflect adrenal gland activity. DHEAS has a much longer half-life than DHEA, and measurement of its serum level is used to assess adrenal function. Levels of DHEAS in women vary widely, with a normal range of 38 to 338 μg/dL.

D. **Dihydrotestosterone (DHT).** Testosterone is converted to DHT by 5α-reductase, an enzyme found in many androgen-sensitive tissues such as skin. DHT is a very potent androgen and is primarily responsible for androgenic effects on hair follicles. Hirsutism in women with normal androgen levels may indicate increased activity of 5α-reductase.

E. **Sex hormone–binding globulins (SHBGs).** Because androgenicity is determined mainly by unbound testosterone, the circulating concentration of SHBG influences the hormonal state. Testosterone and insulin both decrease SHBG levels, whereas estrogen and thyroid hormone increase its levels. Symptoms of hyperandrogenism may be seen in a patient with a normal total testosterone level if the level of SHBGs is decreased enough to significantly increase the free testosterone concentration.

III. **Diagnosis of hyperandrogenism**

A. **History and physical examination.** Hyperandrogenism may be diagnosed if biological signs of androgen excess are present. These signs include excessive sexual hair growth, male pattern baldness, deepening of the voice, enlargement of the clitoris, reduction in breast size, and male muscular development. A careful breast examination should be performed to look for galactorrhea. Symptoms of a thyroid disorder should be investigated. Signs of hyperinsulinemia such as presence of acanthosis nigricans, should be sought.

B. **Laboratory evaluation.** Measurements of serum or plasma androgen levels may be obtained to diagnose hyperandrogenism. Testosterone and androstenedione levels are commonly measured. DHEAS levels should be determined to assess adrenal gland androgen production. Levels higher than 700 ng/dL are considered markers for abnormal adrenal function. Levels of 17α-hydroxyprogesterone (17-OHP) should be determined. Levels of prolactin should be checked and thyroid function tests performed as well. The role of 17-OHP in the development of hyperandrogenism is described later in this chapter in the section on adrenal hyperplasia. Hyperprolactinemia and thyroid disorders may produce hyperandrogenism directly by affecting androgen production and indirectly by creating an anovulatory state. Because hyperandrogenism and hyperinsulinemia are often associated, a comprehensive workup includes assessment of insulin function. Diabetes mellitus may be excluded by determining that the fasting glucose level is lower than 116 mg/dL. Impaired glucose tolerance is indicated by a fasting glucose level of between 116 and 126 mg/dL. Diabetes is diagnosed by a fasting glucose level exceeding 126 mg/dL. A fasting glucose to insulin ratio of less than 4.5 is consistent with insulin resistance.

IV. **Causes of hyperandrogenism.** Five major causes of hyperandrogenism have been identified: hyperandrogenemic chronic anovulation syndrome, late-onset adrenal hyperplasia, tumors of the ovary or adrenal glands, Cushing syndrome, and idiopathic or drug-induced processes.

A. **Hyperandrogenemic chronic anovulation syndrome.** In 1935 Stein and Leventhal described seven women who were amenorrheic, obese, and hirsute and who had cystic ovaries. From this initial description, the term **Stein-Leventhal syndrome** was used to identify other similarly affected women. Because of the cystic changes found within the ovaries of affected patients, the terms **polycystic ovary syndrome** (PCOS), and **polycystic ovary disease** (PCOD) were also used to describe these patients. Orderly follicular development, which ultimately leads to the emergence at monthly intervals of a dominant follicle that releases an oocyte, does not occur routinely in patients with PCOD. Although follicle development occasionally proceeds to ovulation in affected patients, development of the follicle to only its initial growth stage is common. As a consequence, the ovarian cortex becomes populated with numerous small follicles, or "cysts," in these patients. This effect may be induced in the ovaries of unaffected women who are exposed to persistently elevated androgen levels. The hyperandrogenemic state is believed to be a cause of incomplete follicular development. Because of these observations, the term **hyperandrogenemic chronic anovulation syndrome** is preferred to other terms to describe these patients. In 1990, a National Institutes of Health consensus conference on PCOS was held. At this meeting, use of the term *hyperandrogenemic chronic anovulation* was recommended in lieu of PCOS or PCOD. Evidence of hyperandrogenism demonstrated either by hirsutism or measurement of elevated levels of androgens coupled with a history of six or fewer vaginal bleeding episodes per year were recommended as criteria for the diagnosis of PCOS. It was also suggested that this diagnosis be made by exclusion.

1. **Symptoms.** Patients with hyperandrogenemic chronic anovulation syndrome present with hirsutism, oligomenorrhea, amenorrhea, obesity, infertility, and pelvic pain. All or only some of these symptoms may be present. Virilization is not a common finding in affected patients. Hyperinsulinemia and insulin resistance are often associated with this syndrome.

2. **Pathogenesis.** The cause of hyperandrogenemic chronic anovulation syndrome remains unknown. Abnormalities of the hypothalamic-pituitary

axis and the ovarian or adrenal steroidogenic pathway have been suggested as possible explanations for this condition.

a. At the level of the hypothalamic-pituitary axis, an increase in the frequency and amplitude of luteinizing hormone (LH) pulses has been recorded in affected patients. An increase in the ratio of LH to follicle-stimulating hormone from 1 to greater than 2 is observed in patients with hyperandrogenemic chronic anovulation syndrome. Disordered regulation of hypothalamic-pituitary secretion of gonadotropin-releasing hormone is believed to be the cause of this increase in LH secretion.

b. Increased secretion of androgens from the ovaries and adrenal glands in patients with hyperandrogenemic chronic anovulation syndrome also has been observed. This increased secretion may result from stimulation of thecal cells by the elevated level of LH to produce androgens. In patients with insulin resistance, insulin may stimulate androgen secretion from the adrenals or ovaries.

c. Increased secretion of androgen from the adrenal glands has been suggested as a cause of hyperandrogenemic chronic anovulation syndrome. The mild elevation of DHEAS levels frequently seen in these patients has been cited as supporting evidence for this theory. Unfortunately, studies designed to detect adrenal gland enzyme deficiencies or excesses that could cause excessive secretion of androgens in patients with hyperandrogenemic chronic anovulation have identified such disorders in only a small number of patients.

d. Consequences of anovulation. Ovulation for many women with hyperandrogenemic chronic anovulation syndrome may occur infrequently. Nevertheless, ovaries in these patients may continue to secrete low levels of estrogen. Over time this may cause menorrhagia and, in some cases, endometrial hyperplasia or even endometrial cancer.

e. Hyperinsulinemia and insulin resistance. Increased resistance to insulin is often observed in patients with hyperandrogenemic chronic anovulation whether or not they are obese. Insulin may cause or contribute to the hyperandrogenic state by activating insulin receptors within the ovary, augmenting androgen secretion, or by acting on insulin-like growth factor receptors. Furthermore, insulin decreases production of SHBG by the liver, which ultimately increases the level of free and active testosterone.

B. **Late-onset adrenal hyperplasia.** The most common adrenal enzyme defect is 21-hydroxylase (21-OH) deficiency. Deficiencies of 11β-hydroxylase and 3β-hydroxysteroid dehydrogenase are rarely seen. The 21-OH converts progesterone to deoxycorticosterone, or 17-OHP to deoxycortisol. A deficiency in the activity of this enzyme causes a decrease in cortisol production, which results in increased pituitary secretion of adrenocorticotropic hormone (ACTH). Increased stimulation of the adrenal gland by ACTH may result in the production of increased amounts of the deoxycortisol precursor 17-OHP. Androstenedione is produced from 17-OHP by the enzyme 17α-hydroxylase-17,20-desmolase. Androstenedione is in turn converted to testosterone by 17-ketosteroid reductase. Increased levels of 17-OHP result in increased secretion of androstenediol and testosterone from the adrenal gland. Elevated basal levels of 17-OHP and increased release of 17-OHP by the adrenal gland in response to ACTH stimulation are seen in patients with late-onset adrenal hyperplasia. In an anovulatory woman, basal levels of 17-OHP should be measured in the morning and should be less than 200 ng/dL. Levels exceeding 200 ng/dL require ACTH-stimulation testing. Patients with late-onset hyperplasia have 17-OHP levels higher than 1200 ng/dL in response to a 250-mg dose of ACTH after 1 hour. Only 3–5% of hyperandrogenemic patients can be shown to have a partial deficiency in 21-

OH. This percentage is approximately the same as the expected prevalence of partial 21-OH deficiency in the general population.

C. **Androgen-producing ovarian or adrenal tumors.** Tumors of the ovary or adrenal gland that secrete androgens are quite rare. The presence of an androgen-producing tumor is suspected on the basis of clinical findings. Palpation of an adnexal mass in a patient with symptoms of hyperandrogenism or rapid onset of virilization even in the presence of normal testosterone levels should prompt a workup for a pelvic tumor. Testosterone levels exceeding 200 ng/dL warrant concern about the presence of an ovarian or adrenal androgen-producing tumor. A concentration of DHEAS exceeding 1000 μg/dL suggests the possibility of an adrenal androgen-producing tumor.

D. **Cushing syndrome.** Patients with Cushing syndrome usually are identified easily by specific physical findings such as moon facies, increased nuchal fat (buffalo hump), abdominal striae, facial erythema, and truncal obesity. This syndrome may result from excess levels of ACTH from a pituitary adenoma (Cushing disease), ectopic ACTH production, adrenal overproduction of cortisol, an ovarian tumor, or, rarely, ectopic production of corticotropin-releasing hormone. Increased 24-hour urinary excretion of free cortisol and inability to suppress fasting serum or plasma cortisol levels to less than 5 μg/dL 12 hours after oral administration of 1 mg of dexamethasone are laboratory tests used to confirm the diagnosis of Cushing syndrome. Further studies including a high-dose dexamethasone suppression test and radiographic imaging are required to determine the cause of the disorder.

E. **Idiopathic and drug-induced hirsutism.** Idiopathic hirsutism is diagnosed in individuals who are hirsute but who do not demonstrate abnormal findings on the standard laboratory tests ordered to identify known causes of hirsutism. Although estimates vary depending on the study cited, it is calculated that perhaps 5–15% of all hirsute patients may have idiopathic hirsutism.

1. Because the presence of hirsutism is a biological manifestation of hyperandrogenism, the inability to identify a specific androgen that is elevated in patients with idiopathic hirsutism may simply reflect a lack of knowledge about the androgen responsible for the condition.

2. An alternative explanation is based on the hypothesis that patients with idiopathic hirsutism demonstrate increased skin sensitivity to androgens. It has been suggested that patients with idiopathic hirsutism convert testosterone to DHT in greater quantities than normal due to increased activity of 5α-reductase.

3. Occasionally drug ingestion may be responsible for hirsutism. Danazol, a 17 α-ethinyl derivative of testosterone used for treatment of endometriosis, and methyltestosterone, used in hormone replacement therapy, are two examples of drugs that may cause iatrogenic hirsutism.

V. **Treatment** of the patient with hirsutism or hyperandrogenism depends on what the cause is and whether or not pregnancy is desired.

A. Treatment of patients with hyperandrogenemic chronic anovulation syndrome depends on their desire to conceive.

1. **If pregnancy is not desired,** therapy is directed toward stopping the development of new hair growth, removing existing excessive hair growth, and regulating the menstrual cycle. Hirsutism is slow to respond to hormone suppression, and results may not be seen for up to 6 months. In addition, previously established hair patterns do not change with androgen suppression. Mechanical methods of hair removal such as shaving, waxing, depilatories, and electrolysis should also be considered.

a. **Oral contraceptive preparations (OCPs)** diminish circulating gonadotropin levels and increase SHBG levels. Lowering of gonadotropin levels results in decreased ovarian androgen secretion, which produces lower circulating levels of androgens. Increasing SHBG levels result in less free testosterone available for conversion to DHT in the hair follicle. Progestins also decrease activity of 5α-reductase. Lowered total and free androgen levels in women treated with OCPs cause a reduction in the formation of new androgen-dependent hair growth and androgen-stimulated acne. All low-dose OCP preparations are believed to have similar results. However, one particular combination OCP (ethinyl estradiol and norgestimate) has received Food and Drug Administration approval to be prescribed specifically for the treatment of acne. If therapy with OCPs is disappointing, addition of an antiandrogen such as spironolactone or finasteride is recommended.

b. **Medroxyprogesterone acetate.** If combination OCPs are contraindicated or not desired, medroxyprogesterone acetate given as 10 mg for 10–12 days every month or every other month may be used to produce regular withdrawal bleeding to reduce the risk of menorrhagia or endometrial hyperplasia or both. Patients should be cautioned that, unless contraception is used, pregnancy is possible with cyclical progestin therapy.

c. **Spironolactone** therapy is often initiated if OCP use is not an option for treatment of hirsutism or if results from OCP therapy are not optimal. An aldosterone antagonist, spironolactone is a steroid compound originally dispensed as an antihypertensive agent. Its activity as an antiandrogen was detected after men receiving the compound developed gynecomastia. It is now known that spironolactone inhibits the binding of DHT to its receptor and directly inhibits 5α-reductase. Spironolactone also decreases androgen synthesis by inhibiting 17α-hydroxylase and 17,20-lyase. After 6 months of therapy at 100–200 mg/day, reduction in the diameter of terminal hair and cessation of new terminal hair growth are observed. Doses may be tapered down to a maintenance dose of 25–50 mg/day. Because of potential adverse effects on the development of the external genitalia of male fetuses, spironolactone should be used together with contraception in sexually active women. Side effects include diuresis, fatigue, dysfunctional uterine bleeding, hyperkalemia, and breast enlargement.

d. **Flutamide** is a nonsteroidal antiandrogen that blocks the binding of androgen to its receptor. It was developed initially for the treatment of prostate disease. When administered in a dosage of 250 mg/day, decreased terminal hair diameter and cessation of new hair growth are observed. Side effects include dry skin and a rare but severe hepatotoxicity. Liver function should be monitored. During pregnancy, flutamide may have a detrimental effect on male fetal development. Therefore, concurrent therapy with OCPs or other contraception is encouraged.

e. **Finasteride.** An inhibitor of type II 5α-reductase, finasteride was developed initially as a treatment for prostate hypertrophy and cancer. By inhibiting 5α-reductase, the drug decreases DHT activity at the hair follicle. Two types of 5α-reductase enzyme activity exist, type I and type II. Although finasteride treatment prevents new hair growth and decreases the terminal hair shaft diameter, it does not appear to completely inhibit type I 5α-reductase, which is present in skin. Finasteride is orally dosed at 5 mg daily. As of yet, no major side effects have been associated with this drug. There is potential risk during pregnancy as DHT participates in the development of male external genitalia. Adequate contraception should be used. Finasteride is also available in a lower-dose preparation, 1 mg (Propecia), and has been approved for the treatment of hair loss in men.

    f. **Surgery.** Older women who have no desire for fertility and who do not desire continued hormonal therapy may be considered for bilateral oophorectomy with or without hysterectomy.

  2. **If pregnancy is desired** by individuals with hyperandrogenemic chronic anovulation syndrome, assistance with ovulation induction frequently is required. This assistance may be provided by the oral medication clomiphene citrate or by systemic administration of gonadotropins. This is further discussed in Chapter 31.

    a. **Clomiphene citrate** may act by blocking the binding of estrogen to its receptor in the hypothalamus. Clomiphene citrate usually is administered orally in dosages of 50–100 mg/day for 5 days on a monthly basis. Monitoring the patient using a basal body temperature chart, pelvic ultrasonography, or measurement of serum progesterone 14 days after the last clomiphene citrate tablet is taken can document ovulation. For the patient resistant to clomiphene citrate, many studies have shown that the use of the hypoglycemic agent metformin hydrochloride (500 mg three times daily), either alone or in combination with clomiphene citrate, may result in ovulation. Metformin hydrochloride decreases hepatic production of glucose, which may lower insulin resistance. Although clomiphene citrate is approved by the Food and Drug Administration as an ovulation-inducing drug, metformin hydrochloride is not yet approved for this purpose. Metformin should be considered for use in ovulation induction only in the well-informed patient who has not been able to ovulate using clomiphene citrate alone.

    b. **Gonadotropins.** Direct stimulation of the ovary to induce ovulation is achieved by injecting gonadotropins intramuscularly or subcuticularly.

B. **Late-onset adrenal hyperplasia**

  1. Individuals diagnosed with late-onset adrenal hyperplasia may be treated by administration of glucocorticoid agents to restore ovulation. This treatment also reduces circulating androgen levels. Glucocorticoid administration is therefore appropriate therapy for infertility or hirsutism in individuals with late-onset adrenal hyperplasia. In patients with 21-OH deficiency, prednisone, 5 mg before bedtime, is used to suppress endogenous ACTH.

  2. Alternatively, the same hormone therapy indicated for individuals with hyperandrogenemic chronic anovulation may be used in individuals with late-onset adrenal hyperplasia. OCPs or antiandrogens may be used successfully to treat hirsutism, alone or in combination with dexamethasone. Ovulation-inducing drugs may also be used to treat infertility.

C. Androgen-producing ovarian or adrenal tumors usually are treated surgically. Depending on the type of tumor, additional treatment with chemotherapy or radiation therapy may be required.

D. Cushing syndrome. Surgery of the pituitary or adrenal gland may be required to treat Cushing's disease or adrenal hyperplasia causing Cushing's syndrome.

E. Idiopathic hirsutism. The same medications used to treat hirsute patients with hyperandrogenemic chronic anovulation may be used to treat patients with idiopathic hirsutism.

38. FEMALE SEXUAL FUNCTION AND DYSFUNCTION

Karen Hoover and Andrew Goldstein

I. **Introduction.** Female sexual dysfunction is a broad diagnosis. More than a century ago Freud dubbed female sexuality "the dark continent of the soul." Now 100 years later, the etiology of female sexual dysfunction is still considered complex and is poorly understood. The cause is almost always multifactorial. Anatomic, physiologic, psychological, and interpersonal factors all play a role in sexual dysfunction and make the diagnosis and treatment difficult and complicated. Compared to male sexual dysfunction, clinical and basic research and the treatment of female sexual dysfunction has lagged until only recently. Much of our understanding and treatment of women's problems has been extrapolated from male sexual dysfunction studies. Although the anatomy and physiology of male and female sexuality partially parallel each other, there are significant differences between men and women with regard to their sexuality and sexual function. The success of sildenafil citrate (Viagra) in the treatment of male erectile dysfunction has fueled public interest in female sexual dysfunction. Current treatment choices are minimal, but there is the hope that with improved understanding will come more options.

II. **Epidemiology.** Sexual dysfunction is prevalent, affecting 43% of all women, compared to 31% of all men. The best data to date has come from the National Health and Social Life Survey of 1992. This study surveyed 1749 women and 1410 men aged 18–59 years. The completion rate was greater than 79%. Among the findings are that problems are less prevalent in women who are married, are more educated, and have higher incomes. Women are more likely to report problems in all categories if they suffer from stress or emotional problems. The survey also revealed that female sexual dysfunction is associated with a decreased sense of physical and emotional satisfaction and with a decreased sense of overall well-being. The problem affects the woman's quality of life and has a negative impact on her relationship with her partner.

III. **Female sexual anatomy and physiology.** Knowledge of female pelvic anatomy is essential in the diagnosis, treatment, and especially the prevention of female sexual dysfunction. This is especially true for obstetricians and gynecologists, as we perform surgeries such as hysterectomy, oophorectomy, and episiotomy that can injure nerves or decrease hormones essential for normal sexual function.

The labia minora are especially important structures in sexual function. They are composed of spongy tissue containing blood vessels and glands. The medial side of the labia minora is continuous with the vaginal mucosa and bears sensory nerve endings. Anteriorly the labia minora fuse to form the prepuce of the clitoris, and posteriorly they join to form the frenulum. The labial formation is innervated by the perineal and posterior branches of the pudendal nerve. The blood supply arises from both the inferior perineal and posterior labial branches of the internal pudendal artery and from superficial branches of the femoral artery.

The vestibular bulbs are bilateral structures beneath the skin of the labia. They consist of erectile tissue that lies on the superficial aspect of the vaginal wall, adjacent to the clitoris and urethra. The greater vestibular glands are deep to the vestibular bulbs and secrete lubricating mucus during arousal. In addition to the vestibular bulbs, the clitoris is also part of the erectile tissue of the female pelvis. The clitoris consists of three parts: the glans, corpus, and crura. The glans is the visible portion of the clitoris. The corpus extends from the glans but is beneath the dermis. The crura are bilateral and are posterolateral to the corpus, and their distal segments attach to the ischiopubic rami under the pubis. The clitoris is suspended to the anterior abdominal wall by a suspensory ligament. The crura are the corpora cavernosa and consist of a trabecula of vascular smooth muscle, lacunar sinusoids, and collagen layer surrounded by the tunica albuginea. The clitoris is highly innervated and sensitive. Both the sacral and hypogastric plexi provide sympathetic and parasympathetic fibers to the clitoris. Somatic sensory innervation of the clitoris arises in the skin and consists of pacinian corpuscles, Meissner's corpuscles, Merkel tactile discs, and free nerve endings. These sensory fibers ascend via the dorsal nerve of the clitoris to the pudendal nerve and then to the sacral spinal cord. (The pudendal nerve also provides somatic sensory innervation to the proximal two-thirds of the vagina.) The clitoral blood supply is from the internal pudendal artery, which becomes the common clitoral artery after it passes through Alcock's canal. The common clitoral artery gives rise to the dorsal clitoral artery and the clitoral cavernosum arteries.

The pelvic floor muscles support the abdominal and pelvic organs and play an important role in sexual function, as well as helping to maintain urinary and fecal continence (see Fig. 22-9 in Chap. 22, Anatomy of the Female Pelvis). The pelvic diaphragm, which is composed of the levator ani muscles, the urogenital diaphragm, and the perineal membrane, is especially important for pelvic support. The perineal membrane has three components—the ischiocavernosus, bulbocavernosus, and superficial transverse perineal muscles—and is adjacent to the clitoris and vestibular bulbs. These muscles are involved in the orgasmic response and undergo involuntary rhythmic contractions during orgasm. When voluntarily contracted, they can also intensify orgasmic sensation for both the woman and her partner. The levator ani muscle consists of the pubococcygeus and iliococcygeus muscles. These muscles modulate the orgasmic motor responses and, when relaxed, provide vaginal receptivity. Vaginismus is the involuntary spasm of the muscles of the pelvic floor that is triggered by vaginal penetration and causes dyspareunia, which leads to sexual dysfunction. Conversely, pelvic floor laxity and hypotonia can lead to decreased sensation, anorgasmia, and incontinence during intercourse. Autonomic innervation of the clitoris, perineum, and vagina arises from the sacral and hypogastric plexi. The fibers coalesce bilaterally at the bases of the broad ligament beside the cervix to form the uterovaginal plexus. This plexus then travels to the perineum through the uterosacral and cardinal ligaments. These ligaments are always severed during a total abdominal hysterectomy (TAH), which disrupts the neural pathway essential for normal sexual response.

The physiologic female sexual response is mediated by a complex interplay between vasocongestive and neuromuscular events. The result is increased vaginal wall engorgement and lumen diameter, increased vaginal lubrication, and increased clitoral length and diameter. During arousal, blood flow to the vestibular bulbs of the labia minora leads to a two- to threefold increase in labial diameter and to eversion of the labia with resulting exposure of the inner surface. Engorgement of the vagina and clitoris occurs by relaxation of smooth muscle along with increased pelvic blood flow to the pudendal arterial bed. Blood flow also increases to the clitoral cavernosal arteries with excitement, which causes increased intracavernosus pressure. This results in tumescence and extrusion of the glans clitoris during arousal but does not cause rigidity. Unlike the penis, the clitoris does not have a subalbugineal venous plexus between the erectile tissue and the tunica albugineal layer. This venous plexus exists in men and during arousal it becomes engorged and expands against the tunica albuginea, preventing venous outflow, and this leads to penile rigidity. Vaginal blood flow increases during excitement, and the blood vessels of the middle muscularis become infiltrated. The elastin and collagen mesh surrounding the vagina expand and provide support. The increased vaginal blood flow leads to increased capillary pressure, and a transudate forms in the subepithelial vascular bed. The transudate is passively transported through the intraepithelial spaces to the vaginal mucosa and coalesces to form a lubricating vaginal film. Additional lubrication comes from cervical secretions and possibly from Bartholin's gland secretions.

Increased sensation during sexual activity results from stimulation of somatic sensory nerve fibers in the female sexual organs, especially in the clitoris, labia minora, and vagina. CNS regulation of arousal arises in the medial preoptic area, anterior hypothalamic region, and limbic-hippocampal structures. These pathways are further regulated by higher brain centers that are responsible for the emotional, intellectual, and psychological aspects of behavior. The arousal centers transmit their signals peripherally via parasympathetic and sympathetic nerve fibers. The specific role of peripheral neurotransmitters and hormones in the regulation of sexual arousal and function are being studied. As a result, the sexual response in the genitalia, vagina, and clitoris is becoming better understood. In these target tissues, nitric oxide (NO) and vasoactive intestinal peptide are the proposed neurotransmitters that mediate smooth muscle relaxation during the female sexual response.

IV. **Classification of dysfunction**

    A. The current **classification systems** of sexual dysfunction are the *Diagnostic and Statistical Manual of Mental Disorders, Fourth Edition*, the *International Classification of Diseases, 10th Revision,* and the American Foundation of Urologic Diseases classification. These systems are based on a three-phase model of the female sexual response. Masters and Johnson devised the first model of the female sexual response in 1966, which identified excitement, plateau, orgasm, and resolution occurring as successive phases. In 1974 Kaplan proposed a model that is a revision of the Masters and Johnson model, which specifies the three phases of desire, arousal, and orgasm. Although the Kaplan model is probably oversimplified, it does provide a framework for identifying and standardizing different areas of female sexual dysfunction. A more realistic model of female sexual response has been diagrammed by Basson (Fig. 38-1). This model takes into account the psychosocial aspects of female sexual response, which are left out of the Kaplan model.

    B. **American Foundation of Urologic Diseases classification**

        1. **The American Foundation of Urologic Diseases Consensus Panel** devised the most recent classification system for sexual dysfunc-

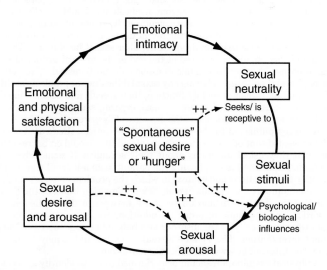

FIG. 38-1. Basson's model of female sexual response.

tion in October 1998. This international multidisciplinary panel convened to establish a classification system that would guide research and treatment of female sexual dysfunction. The classification attempts to integrate both physiologic and psychogenic causes of dysfunction to provide diagnostic criteria and a framework for identifying research gaps. Each of the following diagnoses is subtyped as lifelong versus acquired, as generalized versus situational, and by origin.

a. **Hypoactive sexual desire** disorder is the persistent or recurrent deficiency or absence of sexual fantasies and thoughts, or the absence of desire for or receptivity to sexual activity.

b. **Sexual aversion disorder** is the persistent or recurrent phobic aversion to and avoidance of sexual contact with a partner.

c. **Sexual arousal disorder** is the persistent or recurrent inability to attain or maintain sufficient sexual excitement. It may be expressed as a lack of subjective excitement or as a lack of genital or other somatic responses.

d. **Orgasmic disorder** is the persistent or recurrent difficulty in, delay in, or absence of attaining orgasm after sufficient sexual stimulation and arousal.

e. **Sexual pain disorders** include dyspareunia, vaginismus, and noncoital sexual stimulation.

   (1) **Dyspareunia** is the persistent or recurrent occurrence of genital pain associated with sexual intercourse.

   (2) **Vaginismus** is the persistent or recurrent involuntary spasm of the musculature of the lower third of the vagina that interferes with vaginal penetration.

   (3) **Noncoital sexual pain** disorder is persistent or recurrent genital pain induced by noncoital sexual stimulation.

2. These diagnoses are applied only if the problem causes personal distress to the patient. Also, the assignment of one of these diagnoses requires that the problem be persistent or recurrent.

V. **Diagnosis.** Evaluation of sexual dysfunction begins with a detailed medical history, review of systems, and physical examination. First, a thorough medical history can reveal systemic conditions such as hypertension, diabetes mellitus, depression, and multiple sclerosis that might predispose a patient to sexual dysfunction. Second, a list of current medications should be elicited from the patient, as certain drugs may have a significantly adverse effect on libido or sexual function. Last, a social history can reveal dependence on cigarettes, alcohol, or substances of abuse that can dramatically alter sexual functioning. The patient's sexual history should be explored at the end of the medical history after rapport has been established. Two simple questions should be asked: "Are you sexually active?" and then "Are you having any sexual difficulties or problems at this time?" If questioning reveals sexual dysfunction, then specific and detailed inquiries can be made regarding sexual desire, arousal, orgasm, satisfaction, sexual thoughts and fantasies, masturbation, and the presence of dyspareunia.

A survey published in the *Journal of the American Medical Association* in 1999 revealed that 68% of patients were afraid they would embarrass their physician if they asked questions about their sexuality. If sexual dysfunction is identified from the history, having the patient keep a journal can be helpful to identify the situations and context in which the problem arises. A validated sexual questionnaire such as the Female Sexual Function Index or the Female Sexual Distress Scale can help differentiate between a desire disorder, arousal disorder, and orgasmic disorder. In addition, these questionnaires can help quantify the severity of the disorder and help follow the success of any subsequent intervention. The Female Sexual Function Index may be downloaded from the Internet at www.FSFIquestionnaire.com.

A physical examination should be performed to try to identify gynecologic and nongynecologic causes of sexual dysfunction. Specifically, the vulva should be examined for anomalies, lesions, ulcerations, vulvar dystrophies, condyloma, atrophy, and areas of tenderness. The pelvic floor muscles should be evaluated for vaginismus or the inability to contract. The bulbocavernosus reflex and "anal wink" should be elicited to test genital and perineal sensation. A bimanual examination is especially important in patients who experience dyspareunia. Of note, dyspareunia is the sexual dysfunction complaint most likely to have an organic cause, such as vaginitis, uterine leiomyoma, adnexal masses, pelvic inflammatory disease, endometriosis, or adhesive disease. Laboratory values of serum follicle-stimulating hormone, luteinizing hormone, estradiol, free and total testosterone, dehydroepiandrosterone (DHEA), thyroid-stimulating hormone, and prolactin should be obtained for all women with sexual dysfunction.

VI. **Etiology.** The cause of female sexual dysfunction is almost always multifactorial and complex. The cause of a problem can be hormonal, vascular, neurologic, pharmacologic, or psychogenic, but it is more likely to be due to more than one factor.

Estrogens, androgens, oxytocin, and dopaminergic agonists are believed to promote the female sexual response, whereas progesterone, prolactin, and serotonin are thought to play an inhibitory role. Serum estradiol levels below 50 pg/mL are highly correlated with complaints of sexual dysfunction. Specifically, estrogen deficiency is associated with decreased desire, decreased sexual response, decreased genital sensation, decreased orgasm, and increased dyspareunia. Declining estrogen levels cause decreased vaginal NO levels and increased fibrosis of the vagina. Administration of estrogen reverses the process, restoring normal vaginal NO levels and decreasing the rate of mucosal cell apoptosis. Estrogen prevents thinning and drying of the vaginal wall by maintaining the epithelium and muscularis, and by increasing lubrication. Adequate estrogen is also essential in maintaining touch receptor zones along the distribution of the pudendal nerve, which preserves sensory function that is essential for arousal and orgasm. Estrogen may also prevent atherosclerosis of the iliohypogastric arterial system and thereby preserve vaginal, clitoral, and urethral blood flow. In addition, estrogen itself acts as a vasodilator.

The most common cause of a low estrogen state is menopause, either natural or surgical. A state that mimics menopause may be induced by gonadotropin-releasing hormone agonists, which are used to treat endometriosis or uterine leiomyomata. Medroxyprogesterone acetate (Depo-Provera), levonorgestrel (Norplant), or progestin-only birth control pills can cause a low estrogen state and possibly sexual dysfunction. Lactation is also associated with a hypoestrogenic state, and this is partially responsible for postpartum sexual dissatisfaction and dyspareunia in breast-feeding mothers. It is important to note that the perimenopausal woman with a normal follicle-stimulating hormone level may have decreased serum levels of estradiol.

The exact physiologic and biochemical role of androgens in female sexual response is under investigation and is controversial. It is generally accepted, however, that there is an androgen deficiency syndrome with symptoms that include decreased sexual desire, decreased genital sensation, decreased libido, decreased orgasm, and a general sense of diminished well-being. Data show that androgens are important in maintaining the structural and metabolic integrity of female genital tissues, so critical in sexual arousal. Also, studies have shown that testosterone replacement improves sexual desire, arousal, and orgasm. Approximately 5 years after menopause, androstenedione, the primary ovarian androgen, decreases 75%, and DHEA sulfate, the principal adrenal androgen, declines 50%. More significantly, there is a reduction of circulating free testosterone because it is bound to increased sex hormone–binding globulin-binding sites made available by decreased estrogen production. Oophorectomy can greatly diminish serum androgens and has been associated with sexual dysfunction even with adequate estrogen replacement therapy.

Hypertension, hypercholesterolemia, diabetes mellitus, and smoking all contribute to vascular injury of the small vessels of the vagina and clitoris. Subsequent decreased blood flow to the vagina and clitoris during arousal leads to a blunted sexual response. In addition, poorly controlled diabetes can cause a peripheral neuropathy that can affect the nerves innervating the vagina and clitoris. This peripheral neuropathy can progress to decreased sensation in the vagina and clitoris, anorgasmia, or, in rare instances, vaginal or clitoral pain.

Injury to nerves and vessels of the vagina and clitoris can occur during pelvic surgery. The most common of these surgeries is hysterectomy. Approximately 600,000 hysterectomies are performed annually in the United States, most for benign disease. The hysterectomy usually performed, a total abdominal hysterectomy (TAH), removes the uterus and cervix and traumatizes the uterovaginal plexus in the uterosacral and cardinal ligaments. These nerves provide autonomic innervation to the vagina, clitoris, and labia. Postoperatively, arousal and genital sensation is often abnormal. Most studies indicate that sexual satisfaction improves after hysterectomy, but there are inherent confounding variables in these studies. For example, a woman undergoing hysterectomy for menorrhagia or pelvic pain may suffer from low sexual satisfaction before her hysterectomy, because of the disease process itself. Surgery alleviates these overwhelming symptoms, and the patient is more receptive to sexual activity. Ironically, although frequency of intercourse increases after hysterectomy, the patient may have an irreversibly diminished quality of sexual satisfaction. Data derived from nonrandomized clinical studies suggest that there is better preservation of sexual function (increased orgasm, decreased pain) with supracervical hysterectomy (SCH) than with TAH. This is because the nerves of the uterovaginal plexus are not injured during SCH. Munro at the University of California at Los Angeles wrote that more than 95% of hysterectomies performed before 1940 were SCHs. The trend shifted to TAH to prevent cervical cancer. This rationale, however, is undermined by our current ability to detect and cure preinvasive cervical cancer.

Many commonly prescribed drugs can affect desire, arousal, and orgasm. Antidepressant medications, especially selective serotonin reuptake inhibitors (SSRIs), have been shown to cause sexual dysfunction (including decreased desire and arousal, and anorgasmia) in up to 60% of patients. Most authors postulate that this sexual dysfunction is the result of an increased serotonin effect and a decreased dopaminergic effect in the CNS. Sildenafil citrate has proven efficacious in alleviating SSRI-induced sexual dysfunction. Bupropion hydrochloride, a non-SSRI antidepressant with dopaminergic activity, may be substituted for SSRIs or may be added to SSRI regimens with resulting improvement in sexual dysfunction. Oral contraceptives pills (OCP) are the most prevalent form of birth control for women younger than 35 years. Four randomized controlled studies have examined the effect of OCPs on sexual function. Three of these studies show a modest population-dependent decrease in sexual desire in OCP users. Also, the relatively high discontinuation rate of OCP use within the first 4 months after initiation may be partly due to decreased sexual function. OCPs increase serum levels of sex hormone–binding globulin, which binds to free serum testosterone and decreases the amount of circulating free testosterone. The decrease in testosterone leads to decreased sexual desire.

In a woman, issues such as poor body image, low self-esteem, and inability to communicate with her partner are as important as organic disease in the etiology of her sexual dysfunction. In addition, psychological disorders such as depression, anxiety, and obsessive-compulsive disorder are frequently associated with female sexual dysfunction. This results from both the symptoms and manifestations of the illnesses, and the side effects of medications used to treat them. Finally, prior sexual experiences, especially negative experiences such as sexual abuse, can have a profound lifelong negative impact on sexual function. Frequently, vaginismus is a complaint with a psychogenic cause, especially in a patient with a history of sexual abuse. Evaluation of the psychosocial aspects of sexual dysfunction should be performed by a qualified sex therapist or by a psychologist experienced in the treatment of sexual dysfunction.

VII. **Treatment.** Female sexual dysfunction may be due to concurrent causes. Synergism may be achieved by using more than one treatment modality. The evaluation and treatment of female sexual dysfunction is optimized by a collaborative effort between a physician and sex therapist using a biopsychosocial model. In addition to a thorough medical evaluation, the patient should undergo evaluation by a psychologist or sex therapist who is familiar with female sexual dysfunction. The patient's partner or spouse may need to be included in this evaluation. After the physiologic and psychological causes of dysfunction are identified, a treatment regimen can be initiated. In the majority of cases, both pharmacologic therapy and sexual counseling are necessary.

Estrogen replacement therapy at standard dosages is an integral component of treating sexual dysfunction in naturally or surgically menopausal women. In postmenopausal women, estrogen replacement restores clitoral and vaginal vibration and sensation to levels close to those of premenopausal women. All routes of estrogen administration (oral, transdermal, or topical) provide relief of complaints due to vaginal atrophy, such as dryness, pain, and burning during intercourse. In women who have not undergone hysterectomy, addition of a progestin is necessary to avoid increasing the risk of endometrial carcinoma. Unfortunately, the added progestin has an inhibitory effect on the patient's sexual function.

Androgen replacement therapy can improve libido, arousal, number of orgasms, and subjective enjoyment of sex in women who have low serum levels of androgens. Androgen replacement increases sexual desire, sexual arousal, clitoral sensitivity, and vaginal lubrication. Currently, androgen replacement therapy can be orally administered in the form of DHEA, methyltestosterone, fluoxymesterone, or testosterone undecenoate. Testosterone can also be administered intramuscularly or topically with transdermal patches. A transdermal patch designed specifically to replace physiologic amounts of testosterone in women is under development. One benefit of oral DHEA and topical testosterone is that serum levels can be followed to prevent supraphysiologic replacement. Careful monitoring of these blood levels can prevent the side effects of androgen replacement, including hoarseness, acne, hirsutism, clitoromegaly, hepatotoxicity, alopecia, and undesirable lipoprotein alterations. Extended supraphysiologic replacement can lead to male pattern baldness, worsening hirsutism, and permanent clitoromegaly. Before androgen replacement therapy is initiated, baseline liver function tests and a fasting blood lipid profile should be obtained. Women must be advised of the potential side effects and be counseled to recognize them early. Finally, in women who are of reproductive age, adequate birth control is essential, as exogenous androgens can masculinize a female fetus.

The amino acid L-arginine is a precursor of NO that mediates relaxation of vascular and nonvascular smooth muscle in the genitalia. In small studies, the use of L-arginine in combination with yohimbine, an alpha$_2$-antagonist, increased genital sexual arousal in postmenopausal women with an arousal disorder.

Apomorphine is a dopamine agonist that improves erection responses in men with erectile dysfunction due to both psychogenic and organic causes. Efficacy in treating sexual dysfunction in women is being studied.

Bupropion, an antidepressant of the aminoketone class that has dopaminergic properties, has been successful in treating SSRI-induced sexual dysfunction. In addition, in a small single-blind placebo-controlled trial, bupropion was shown to improve sexual desire in women with hypoactive sexual desire disorder.

A vacuum clitoral therapy device, the Eros-CTD, is a device approved by the U.S. Food and Drug Administration for the treatment of female sexual arousal disorder and female orgasmic disorder. The treatment increases clitoral engorgement when a gentle vacuum is applied to the clitoris. In small studies, use of the Eros-CTD resulted in increased sensation, lubrication, and ability to achieve orgasm in women with arousal or orgasmic disorders.

39. MENOPAUSE AND HORMONE REPLACEMENT THERAPY

Karen Hoover and Edward E. Wallach

I. **Definition.** Menopause is the permanent cessation of menses as a result of ovarian follicle inactivity. It is dated by the last menstrual period that is followed by 12 months of amenorrhea. Menopause can occur naturally as part of the climacteric, the transition period from reproductive capacity to nonreproductive state. The average age of menopause is 50 years, with a range of 43 to 57 years. It can also be induced by oophorectomy or by iatrogenic ablation of ovarian function. Perimenopause is the period before menopause and 1 year after menopause. Reduction in ovarian function during the climacteric is associated with the cessation of ovulation and a marked decline in estradiol production and a modest decline in androgen production.

When any doubt exists about the diagnosis of menopause, other causes of secondary amenorrhea must be ruled out. Laboratory studies should include a serum pregnancy test and measurement of prolactin and follicle-stimulating hormone (FSH) levels. The best time to measure serum FSH level is during days 2–4 of a normal menstrual period. Ideally, FSH is measured twice, with samples drawn 2 weeks apart, to avoid a midcycle FSH peak. An elevation in FSH level to 15–20 mIU/mL is associated with early ovarian failure. For perimenopausal women on oral contraceptives, FSH level may be measured late in the pill-free week. When the serum FSH level is persistently elevated during the pill-free week, the patient can be switched to hormone replacement therapy (HRT).

II. **Hormone replacement therapy** with estrogen has been demonstrated to protect against development of osteoporosis and vaginal atrophy, and may protect against Alzheimer's disease, macular degeneration, and colon cancer. Before initiation of HRT, workup should include breast examination, mammography if the patient is older than 50 years or if otherwise indicated, pelvic examination, Pap smear, endometrial sampling if indicated by abnormal bleeding, and BP and weight measurement.

Possible routes of HRT include oral, transdermal, and transvaginal (Table 39-1). Although estrogen may be administered intramuscularly or subcutaneously, these routes are not used in clinical practice. The oral route is the most common mode of administration, although oral dosing results in plasma level fluctuations. Transdermal estrogen patches deliver estrogen at a relatively constant rate of 50–100 µg/dL. This is comparable to premenopausal endogenous estrogen production of 60–600 µg/dL. Thus, estradiol levels comparable to those in the follicular phase of the menstrual cycle are achieved by transdermal administration. The transdermal route also maintains the 1:1 ratio of estradiol to estrone that approximates the natural, premenopausal ratio. In contrast, oral administration of estrogen results in an estradiol to estrone ratio of less than 1.

Transvaginal delivery of estrogen achieves a fairly constant plasma level. The magnitude of the plasma level depends on the type of estrogen, the dose delivered, and the drug vehicle. Plasma levels are typically 25–75% of the levels obtained by oral dosing of the same quantity of steroid. Both transdermal and transvaginal estrogen administration avoid the first-pass liver metabolism effect, which prevents an effect on synthesis of clotting factors and decreases the effect on lipid metabolism. Estring is a plastic ring embedded with small amounts of estrogen that provides local estrogen with minimal systemic absorption. Vagifem is a vaginal tablet that provides only local estrogen exposure.

Estrogen must be given along with a progestin to a patient with an intact uterus to prevent endometrial hyperplasia or carcinoma. The progestin is administered either continuously with daily dosing or cyclically with daily dosing only during the last half of each cycle.

TABLE 39-1. HORMONE REPLACEMENT THERAPY

Drug	Dosage
Oral estrogens	
Ethinyl estradiol (Estinyl)	0.02–0.05 mg daily
Conjugated equine estrogen (Premarin, C.E.S., Congest)	0.3–1.25 mg daily
Synthetic conjugated estrogen (Cenestin)	0.625–1.25 mg daily
Micronized estradiol (Estrace, Gynodiol)	1–2 mg daily
Esterified estrogens (Estratab, Menest)	0.3–1.25 mg daily
Estropipate (Ogen, Ortho-Est)	0.625–5.0 mg daily
Oral progestins	
Micronized progesterone (Prometrium)	200 mg h.s. for 12 d or 100 mg daily
Medroxyprogesterone acetate (Provera, Cycrin, Amen, Curretab)	10 mg daily for last 12 d or 2.5–5.0 mg daily
Norethindrone acetate (Aygestin, Norlutate)	2.5–10.0 mg for last 12 d
Oral estrogen/progestin combinations	
Continuous	
Conjugated estrogens/medroxyprogesterone acetate (Prempro)	0.625/2.5 mg daily or 0.625/5 mg daily
Estradiol/norethindrone (Activella)	1.0/0.5 mg daily
Estinyl estradiol/norethindrone (FemHRT)	5 µg/1 mg daily
Cyclical	
Estradiol/norgestimate (Ortho-Prefest)	1 mg estradiol for 15 d, and then 1 mg estradiol/0.99 mg norgestimate for 15 d
Conjugated estrogens/medroxyprogesterone acetate (Premphase)	0.625 conjugated estrogens for 14 d, then 0.625 conjugated estrogens/5 mg medroxyprogesterone for 14 d
Transdermal estradiol (Alora, Climara, Esclim, Estraderm, FemPatch, Vivelle, Vivelle-Dot)	Variable dosing
Transdermal estrogen/progestin combinations (CombiPatch)	0.05/0.14 mg or 0.05/0.25 mg weekly
Vaginal estrogen creams (Premarin, Estrace, Ogen, Ortho Dienestrol	Variable dosing
Vaginal estradiol ring (Estring)	Replace every 90 d
Vaginal estradiol tablets (Vagifem)	25 µg daily for 2 wks, then twice weekly

III. **Vasomotor symptoms.** Seventy-five percent of menopausal women experience hot flashes. Eighty percent of those who have hot flashes endure them for longer than 1 year and 50% for longer than 5 years. Vasomotor instability causes the hot flash, characterized by a sudden reddening of the skin over the head, neck, and chest, accompanied by a feeling of intense body heat and concluding with profuse perspiration. Estrogen administration is currently the most effective treatment for hot flashes. Its effect is not immediate; the full benefit may not be realized until several months after beginning therapy. For women who cannot take estrogen because it is medically contraindicated or produces unacceptable side

TABLE 39-2. RISK FACTORS FOR OSTEOPOROSIS

Modifiable risk factors
  Cigarette smoking
  Low body weight: <127 lb for average height
  Estrogen deficiency due to:
    Menopause
    Early menopause: <45 years old
    Prolonged premenopausal amenorrhea: >1 year
  Lifelong low calcium intake: <400 mg/day
  Excessive alcohol intake
  Impaired vision
  Inadequate physical activity
  Poor health and frailty
Nonmodifiable risk factors
  Personal history of fracture as an adult
  History of a fracture in a first-degree relative
  White race
  Advanced age
  Dementia
  Poor health and frailty

---

effects, alternative therapies exist. Medroxyprogesterone acetate, 150 mg per month intramuscularly, has been shown to be 90% effective in the treatment of hot flashes. Clonidine (0.05–0.15 mg/day), propranolol hydrochloride (60 mg/day), and belladonna alkaloids (Bellergal) also have been shown to be useful in the treatment of hot flashes.

IV. **Osteoporosis** is a condition of decreased bone mass and bone microarchitectural deterioration with resulting skeletal fractures. It results from a dominance of osteoclastic activity. Estrogen deficiency causes an increased rate of skeletal remodeling, with an increase in resorption that is greater than the increase in bone formation. The spine, hip, and wrist are very common sites of fractures associated with osteoporosis.

A. **Treatment and prevention** of osteoporosis can avoid the occurrence of painful, debilitating fractures in postmenopausal women. Identification and modification of risk factors for development of this disease constitute the first step in management. Known risk factors account for 30% of osteoporosis incidence (Table 39-2). Guidelines for prevention and treatment can be found in Table 39-3.

B. **Diagnosis** is by determination of bone mineral density (BMD). The four most widely used methods for assessing bone density are single-photon absorptiometry, dual-photon absorptiometry, dual-energy x-ray absorptiometry, and quantitative CT. BMD should be measured in any postmenopausal patient who presents with a fracture. Other candidates for BMD determination are all women older than 65 years, postmenopausal women under age 65 with one or more risk factors, and women in whom decreased BMD would influence the decision to initiate HRT. BMD is best measured at the hip and is predictive of hip fracture and fracture at other sites. T-values are assigned and are scored as standard deviations above or below the mean BMD of a young woman of approximately 25 years. Normal bone T-scores are above –1.0; osteopenia T-scores are between –1.0 and –2.5; osteoporosis

TABLE 39-3. NATIONAL OSTEOPOROSIS FOUNDATION GUIDELINES FOR PREVENTION AND TREATMENT OF OSTEOPOROSIS

Calcium, 1200 mg/day

Vitamin D, 400–800 IU/day

Regular weight-bearing, muscle-strengthening exercise

Smoking cessation

Moderate alcohol consumption

Treatment for all women with a vertebral or hip fracture

Preventive treatment for women with

    T-score below –2.0

    T-score below –1.5 with risk factors

Estrogen replacement as first-line therapy

T-scores are at or below –2.5. For each reduction in bone mass of one standard deviation, the risk of fracture doubles.

A prospective study found that patients on HRT had increased spine and hip BMD, whereas women receiving placebo had a decrease in BMD. Although retrospective studies reveal decreased incidence of spine and hip fractures in patients on HRT, no large prospective study has demonstrated that estrogen prevents fractures. However, a 12-month study of 75 women with osteoporosis who used transdermal estrogen found that HRT patients had fewer vertebral fractures than did patients in the placebo group.

V. **Alternative therapies** may be advised for a patient with contraindications to estrogen use.

  A. **Alendronate sodium** is a bisphosphonate approved for prevention and treatment of osteoporosis. Bisphosphonates are a class of drugs analogous to the physiologically occurring inorganic pyrophosphates and are inhibitors of bone resorption. The U.S. Food and Drug Administration (FDA) has approved alendronate 5 mg daily for prevention of osteoporosis and 10 mg daily for treatment. A formulation with a once-weekly dose of 70 mg has been released. Treatment with oral alendronate not only prevents bone loss but progressively increases the bone mass of the spine, hip, and total body. It also reduces the risk of vertebral fractures, the progression of vertebral deformities, and height loss in postmenopausal women with osteoporosis.

  B. **Risedronate sodium,** also an oral bisphosphonate, has been recently approved by the FDA for the same indications as alendronate. Recommended dosing is 5 mg daily for prevention and treatment of osteoporosis. A 2-year prospective study of postmenopausal women with normal lumbar spine BMD values found that patients receiving 5 mg daily had an increase in spine and femoral trochanter BMD, whereas patients in the placebo group experienced decreases in BMD at both sites. The benefits of treatment are sustained: 1 year after cessation of therapy, lumbar spine BMD was 2.3% lower than baseline in patients given risedronate but 5.6% lower in patients receiving placebo.

  C. **Side effects** of alendronate and risedronate include heartburn, esophageal irritation, esophagitis, abdominal pain, and diarrhea. Oral calcium supplementation may interfere with the absorption of bisphosphonates. The patient should take each dose after an overnight fast while sitting in the upright position and should follow by drinking a glass of water. The patient must remain upright and not eat for 30 minutes after administration. Long-term side effects are unknown.

  D. **Raloxifene hydrochloride** is a selective estrogen receptor modulator. It has estrogen-like effects on bone and the cardiovascular system, but antiestrogen effects on the breast and uterus. Raloxifene has received FDA approval for the prevention and treatment of osteoporosis. A daily dose of 60 mg is recommended. A study involving postmenopausal women both with and without osteoporosis found that patients treated with raloxifene daily for 2 years had statistically significant increases in lumbar spine and hip BMD compared to patients receiving placebo, who had decreased BMD. Side effects include hot flashes and leg cramps. There is an increased risk of thromboembolic events with raloxifene use. However, a trial involving postmenopausal women with osteoporosis found a decreased risk of breast cancer in these patients.

E. **Calcitonin,** a peptide hormone, inhibits bone resorption by decreasing osteoclast activity. It may also have an analgesic effect. Because calcitonin is degraded when taken orally, parenteral administration is required. A nasal form of salmon calcitonin, Miacalcin 200 IU daily, has been used effectively in the treatment of postmenopausal osteoporosis. It can also be administered in a 100-IU dose subcutaneously or intramuscularly every other day. Calcitonin, in both injectable and nasal spray preparations, is also effective in preventing early postmenopausal bone loss. Side effects of calcitonin therapy include nausea and flushing. Rhinitis and epistaxis may occur with intranasal dosing. There are no long-term adverse effects.

VI. **Heart disease.** Firm recommendations regarding HRT and primary prevention of heart disease require the results of ongoing clinical trials. One in two women will die from cardiovascular disease (CVD) or stroke. In contrast, one in nine women develop breast cancer. Epidemiologic studies have demonstrated that women using HRT have a 40–50% lower risk of death from CVD than those not on HRT.

Clinical research to date. One study demonstrated that long-term use of estrogen in a postmenopausal woman was associated with reduced overall mortality risk. This risk reduction occurred primarily through a reduction in cardiovascular-related deaths. In one report, the use of estrogen was associated with a decrease in serum levels of low-density lipoprotein cholesterol and an increase in high-density lipoprotein cholesterol. These effects occur with both oral and vaginal administration of ethinyl estradiol, and with oral, but not vaginal, use of conjugated estrogens. The transdermal patch has not been shown to have the same beneficial effect on lipid levels as other routes of delivery.

The **Heart and Estrogen/Progestin Replacement Study (HERS)** studied the effect of estrogen on prevention of recurrent CVD events. Postmenopausal women with CVD and an intact uterus received 0.625 mg conjugated equine estrogen along with 2.5 mg medroxyprogesterone acetate or placebo. There was no significant difference between the HRT group and the placebo group in CVD events after 4 years of follow-up. However, the HRT group had a higher risk of a second CVD event during the first year of therapy than did the placebo group. The relative risk showed a trend downward with each successive year. During the first year of treatment, HRT patients had a 14% decrease in low-density lipoprotein cholesterol and an 8% increase in high-density lipoprotein cholesterol, but a 10% increase in triglycerides. Progesterone was found to attenuate the estrogen effect on lipid profile. HRT patients had an increased incidence of thromboembolic events and pulmonary emboli. The American Heart Association recently concluded that there are insufficient data to support initiation of HRT for the sole purpose of primary prevention of CVD. Furthermore, initiation and continuation should be predicated on established noncoronary benefits and risks, possible coronary benefits and risks, and patient preference. The American Heart Association also recommends that HRT not be initiated for the secondary prevention of CVD.

VII. **Other benefits of HRT.** The vagina, urethra, and bladder trigone have high estrogen receptor concentrations. The loss of estrogen that accompanies menopause thus leads to urogenital atrophy. The atrophic vulva loses most of its collagen, adipose tissue, and water-retaining ability, and becomes flattened and thin. Sebaceous glands remain intact, but secretions decrease. Vaginal shortening and narrowing occur, and the vaginal walls become thin, lose elasticity, and become pale in color. The atrophic vagina secretes less, which causes vaginal dryness. Dyspareunia is the most common complaint related to vaginal atrophy. The treatment of urogenital atrophy is an indication for HRT, and the mainstay of therapy is systemic or local estrogen.

The effect of estrogen deficiency on the urethra and bladder is associated with urethral syndrome, which is characterized by recurrent episodes of urinary frequency and urgency with dysuria. Estrogen therapy relieves urgency, urge incontinence, and dysuria, and may protect against recurrent lower urinary tract infections. Estrogen therapy does not, however, improve stress incontinence.

VIII. **Side effects and contraindications of HRT** include pregnancy, estrogen-dependent neoplasms, distant or recent history of breast cancer, undiagnosed vaginal bleeding, acute vascular thrombosis or emboli, and severe liver disease. Side effects include breast tenderness, uterine bleeding, and bloating. Many women suffer the effects of estrogen deficiency after treatment for endometrial cancer. Women traditionally have not been offered HRT after being diagnosed and treated for endometrial cancer, because of the theoretical risk that dormant cancer cells may be activated by HRT. Many experts believe that, for women with a history of endometrial cancer, the proven risks of long-term estrogen deficiency far outweigh the presumed risk of cancer recurrence, and reports suggest that HRT can be prescribed safely after appropriate treatment for endometrial cancer.

Long-term risks of HRT are especially a concern of patients. The most controversial issue is the association between breast cancer and HRT. Some studies have demonstrated an increased risk of breast cancer in women taking HRT, but others have not. The reanalysis of 51 studies by the Collaborative Group on Hormonal Factors in Breast Cancer demonstrated an increased risk of 6 cases per 1000 with 10 years of continuous HRT. The effect was reduced with discontinuation of therapy, and almost disappeared 5 years after discontinuation. Data from the Iowa Women's Health Study, however, revealed that HRT exposure was associated with a higher risk of developing invasive breast cancer with a favorable prognosis than with developing ductal carcinoma in situ or invasive ductal or lobular carcinoma. Another study examined the risk of breast cancer in women with a previous histologic diagnosis of benign breast disease and found that estrogen replacement therapy does not significantly increase the risk of invasive breast disease. This study concludes that estrogen replacement therapy is not contraindicated in these patients. Recently published results from the Breast Cancer Detection Project indicate a small but statistically significant increased risk of breast cancer in estrogen-progestin users compared to users of estrogen alone.

The increased risk of endometrial cancer in women with an intact uterus taking unopposed estrogen is well established. The two- to threefold greater risk of developing endometrial cancer is eliminated by the addition of at least 12 days of progestin therapy each month.

There are other demonstrated risks of HRT. Oral HRT raises serum triglyceride levels. The Nurses Health Study found a relative risk ratio of 1.5–2.0 for development of gallbladder disease in HRT users. During the initial year of HRT, there is a slightly increased risk of excess cases of deep venous thrombosis of approximately 1:5000, as demonstrated in two studies. Another study found 1:20,000 excess cases of pulmonary embolism.

IX. **Management of perimenopause.** Because of the changing hormonal milieu, complaints of irregular bleeding are very common during the climacteric. If episodes of bleeding occur more often than every 21 days, last longer than 8 days, are very heavy, or occur after a 6-month interval of amenorrhea, particularly if such bleeding occurs in an irregular pattern, an evaluation must be undertaken to rule out neoplasm.

Oral contraceptive pills (OCPs) are recommended for estrogen supplementation in the perimenopausal woman. Benefits of this therapy, in addition to relief of vasomotor symptoms, are contraception, decreased risk of endometrial and ovarian cancers, establishment of regular menses, and increased bone density. An OCP with 20 μg of ethinyl estradiol and 150 μg of desogestrel has the same efficacy and side effects as OCPs with 30 or 35 μg of estrogen, yet carry virtually no increased risk of coagulation pathology. The transition from OCPs to HRT is recommended when the FSH level is higher than 20 IU/mL on day 6 or 7 of the pill-free week. A blood sample can be obtained annually starting at age 50 years to determine the serum FSH level; however, because of variability in FSH levels in perimenopausal women, the measurement is not always accurate. An alternative is to allow the patient to continue to take low-dose OCPs into her midfifties and to change to HRT empirically. As with a menopausal woman, the perimenopausal patient should receive calcium and vitamin D supplementation, maintain a healthy diet, engage in regular exercise, and avoid smoking.

Section Five. GYNECOLOGIC ONCOLOGY

40. BENIGN VULVAR LESIONS

Carolyn J. Alexander, Cornelia Liu Trimble, and Edward Trimble

I. **Infections.** Many benign lesions of the vulva are infectious. A number of these infections can involve squamous epithelium elsewhere. The vulva and perineum have estrogen and progesterone receptors and thus are subject to stronger hormonal influences than skin elsewhere. Furthermore, as the vulva and perineum are often sequestered by clothing, they are prone to chronic dampness from perspiration.

A. **Bacterial infections.** Common bacterial infections include those that cause folliculitis (*Staphylococcus*), furuncles (*Staphylococcus*), and Bartholin's gland abscesses (polymicrobial). Treatment strategies should focus on hygiene measures, with sitz baths and antibiotic treatment if necessary.

B. **Sexually transmitted diseases (STDs).** When an STD is suspected, assessment for other STDs should be considered and a Pap smear should be taken.

1. **Syphilis**

a. The primary lesion is a painless, indurated papule that can be 2 cm in diameter. This lesion progresses to a shallow ulcer with raised edges, which resolves in 2–8 weeks. Inguinal lymph nodes may be shotty. The chancres may be multiple and, on the vulva, may be superinfected. The diagnosis can be made by dark-field microscopic examination.

b. Vulvar manifestations of secondary syphilis include soft, nontender papules that may be larger than the primary lesions.

c. The pathognomonic lesions of tertiary syphilis are condylomata lata, which are large, raised gray-white lesions with a moist appearance.

d. For treatment, see Chap. 24, Infections of the Genital Tract.

2. **Chancroid** may present as a tender, nonindurated vulvar ulcer with a friable purulent erythematous base. The incubation period ranges from 3 to 10 days. These lesions typically are quite painful. Bilateral inguinal adenopathy is common. Because the causative organism, *Haemophilus ducreyi*, is difficult to culture, biopsy and Gram staining are often necessary for diagnosis. For treatment options, refer to Chap. 24, Infections of the Genital Tract.

3. **Granuloma inguinale** is a contagious, chronic STD caused by *Calymmatobacterium granulomatis*. The lesions are painless papules or ulcers with rolled borders and a friable base that are granulomatous and locally destructive. Histologic or cytologic demonstration of the Donovan body, which is highlighted with Wright or Giemsa staining, is diagnostic. Although the acute lesion responds to tetracycline, surgery may be indicated in later, chronic stages to remove areas of chronic infection and distortion.

4. **Lymphogranuloma venereum** is a chronic STD more frequently seen in men than in women that is caused by three serotypes of *Chlamydia trachomatis*, L1, L2, and L3. Phase one is erosion of the skin, forming a primary lesion that may present as a papule, a shallow ulcer, or a small, herpetiform lesion. This arises after an incubation period of 3–12 days. Phase two involves inguinal lymphadenopathy; a **bubo** is an enlarged inguinal lymph node. This generally occurs 10–30 days after initial infection but may occur 4–6 months later. Phase three involves fibrosis and destruction. Chronic, untreated infection can lead to proctocolitis and bowel strictures, progressive vulvar induration and fibrosis, and, in some cases, stenosis of the urethra and vagina. The diagnosis is based on posi-

tive serologic test results, isolation of the organism, or histologic identification of the bacterium. Effective antibiotics include tetracycline, sulfadiazine, chloramphenicol, erythromycin, and rifampin. If surgery is indicated for repair of strictures or fistulas, patients should receive antibiotics for several months before the operation. For treatment options, refer to Chap. 24, Infections of the Genital Tract.

5. **Gonorrhea** often presents as an acute inflammatory reaction in the region of the urethra, or at Bartholin's or Skene's glands. Diagnosis is made by culture.

C. **Viral infections**

1. **Herpes simplex virus (HSV)** infection is the most common cause of vulvar ulcers.

   HSV type 1 is typically associated with oral infections, although it can produce genital lesions. HSV type 2 is more often the cause of lesions of the lower genital tract. The infection is highly contagious. It may be preceded by malaise, fever, or a prodromal tingling sensation at the site of the eventual lesion. Recurrent ulcers are often in the same location. They are frequently painful. Of note, viral shedding may persist for several weeks after the ulcers have resolved, although this is much more likely with a primary infection. Recurrences are usually milder than primary lesions. Treatment for both the initial lesions and recurrences consists of acyclovir, 200 mg, five times a day for 10 days.

   According to the American College of Obstetricians and Gynecologists, women with primary HSV infection at any time during pregnancy should be treated with antiviral therapy. Cesarean delivery should be performed on women with first-episode HSV infection who have active genital lesions at delivery and on pregnant women with prodromal symptoms at delivery. Expectant management of patients with preterm labor or preterm premature rupture of membranes and active HSV infection may be warranted.

2. **Condyloma acuminatum,** or venereal warts, are caused by the human papillomavirus (HPV) infection. HPV types 6 and 11 are the most common types producing exophytic lesions on the lower genital tract. These lesions are frequently multifocal, papillary, verrucous, or papular. Malignant transformation is uncommon. The exophytic lesions may be pruritic and may become superinfected. Although they may regress spontaneously during pregnancy or other immunocompromised states, they may instead flourish.

   a. Approximately 1% of all sexually active adults (aged 15–49) either have or have had genital warts. The highest rates occur in sexually active women younger than 25 years.

   b. Treatment consists of the following (please refer to Chap. 24, Infections of the Genital Tract, for dosing details):
      (1) Trichloroacetic acid 80–90%, or
      (2) Imiquimod (Aldara) 5% cream, or
      (3) Podophyllin 0.5% solution or gel, or
      (4) Cryotherapy, or
      (5) Systemic and intralesional interferon

   c. A Pap smear of the cervix should be obtained. Only a very small percentage of those infected with HPV actually develop genital warts. Infection with HPV (types 16, 18, 31, 33) typically does not manifest as exophytic lesions but rather as vulvar intraepithelial neoplasia and is covered in more detail in the section on squamous carcinomas.

3. **Molluscum contagiosum virus** is a poxvirus that is spread by close contact. The lesions are multiple, small, umbilicated papules filled with white, waxy material. Most patients are entirely asymptomatic. Although the diagnosis is most often made clinically, histologic demonstration of intracytoplasmic molluscum bodies is pathognomonic. Therapy consists of curettage and excision of the lesions under local anesthesia.

II. **Inflammatory lesions**
   A. In **Crohn's disease,** cutaneous ulcerations occur in areas where there is close apposition of skin, such as the vulva and submammary areas. Vulvar ulcers may precede GI symptoms by months or even years. Crohn's disease ulcers are typically multiple, linear, and deep and can cause a granulation tissue response. They may become secondarily infected or result in draining fistulas, or both. Lymphadenopathy is rare.
   B. **Behçet's syndrome** is a triad of relapsing oral ulcers, genital ulcers, and ocular inflammation. Other findings include acne, cutaneous nodules, thrombophlebitis, and colitis. Uveitis is less frequent than genital ulcerations, which are small and deep and may result in fenestration of the labia. They tend to resolve spontaneously, but systemic corticosteroids are the most widely used and effective treatment. Sitz baths and careful hygiene of the area is recommended.
   C. **Hidradenitis suppurativa** is an apocrine gland disorder causing deep, painful, subcutaneous nodules that progress and produce confluent masses, which may ulcerate the epidermis and result in draining sinuses and extensive scarring. Total excision of the involved areas is necessary for advanced cases.
   D. **Vulvar vestibulitis** is associated with exquisite tenderness of the minor vestibular glands and erythema of the vestibule. The only histologic finding is that of chronic inflammation, and there is no evidence of allergic reaction. No specific organisms have been identified. Treatment is ill defined. Antibiotics, corticoids, retinoids, chloracetic acid, 5-fluorouracil, and laser therapy have all proven ineffective. Spontaneous remissions may occur in as many as 50% of patients. Vestibulectomy, particularly complete resection of the vulvar skin, improves symptoms in some patients, but there are substantial risks of scarring, introital narrowing, and dyspareunia.
   E. **Dermatologic causes** of vulvar lesions include pemphigoid, familial benign pemphigus, keratosis follicularis, and psoriasis.

III. **Benign neoplastic lesions**
   A. **Acrochordons,** or skin tags, are frequently pedunculated but may be sessile and have a rubbery consistency. These do not need to be removed unless they are symptomatic. On histologic examination, they are fibroepithelial polyps.
   B. **Seborrheic keratoses** are flat, raised pigmented lesions common elsewhere on the body. Although these lesions are benign, all pigmented vulvar lesions should be evaluated carefully. Both melanoma and squamous carcinoma of the vulva may be similar in appearance.
   C. **Lipomas** are benign tumors composed of adipose tissue. They are soft and sometimes pedunculated.
   D. **Ectopic tissue** can cause symptoms on the vulva.
      1. **Papillary hidradenomas** occur on the milk line and present as firm, encapsulated nodules that can measure up to 2 cm in greatest dimension. These nodules are asymptomatic and occur predominantly in postpubertal white women. The most frequent location is on the labia majora or in the interlabial folds.
      2. **Endometriotic foci** on the vulva are relatively uncommon. They may occur in a site of previous surgery, such as an episiotomy site. These lesions appear bluish red and undergo cyclic enlargement.
   E. **Other benign lesions** that may occur on the vulva include granular cell tumors, syringomas, hemangiomas, and pyogenic granulomas. These are all rare lesions.

IV. **Benign pigmented and hypopigmented lesions**
   A. **Hyperpigmented lesions**
      1. **Lentigo simplex** is the most common hyperpigmented lesion of the vulva. These lesions are isolated areas of epidermis within which is a population of functioning melanocytes. They vary in epidermal pigmentation and biopsy specimens are usually taken, although they are benign.

2. **Nevi** of the intradermal, junctional, and compound varieties are common on the external genitalia. These lesions should be excised carefully, as the differential diagnosis includes melanoma and squamous carcinoma. Nevi are either pigmented or white (hypopigmented or amelanotic).

3. Both seborrheic keratoses and vulvar intraepithelial lesions may be pigmented.

B. **Hypopigmented conditions**

1. **Vitiligo** is an inherited disorder in which the melanocytes are lost from areas of skin, frequently the vulva.

2. **Leukoderma** (postinflammatory depigmentation) occurs in areas of previous ulcerations, especially after herpetic and syphilitic infections.

V. **Benign cystic tumors**

A. **Bartholin cyst.** Bartholin's glands produce a clear, mucoid secretion that provide continuous lubrication for the vestibular surface. These glands are lined by transitional epithelium and are prone to obstruction, which results in cyst formation. This cyst may become superinfected, which manifests as an abscess. These lesions are usually polymicrobial in origin, although approximately 10% may be caused by *Neisseria gonorrhoeae*. Of note, attempts at incision and evacuation are therapeutic only when the lesion has become fluctuant. The incision should be made proximal to the hymeneal ring, and a Word catheter may be inserted. To bring a firm lesion to fluctuance, sitz baths are recommended. Recurrences are common. Surgical marsupialization may be required. In postmenopausal women, surgical excision is recommended because of the risk of Bartholin adenocarcinoma, which tends to be in the tissue adjacent to the cyst wall.

B. **Keratinous cysts** are epithelial inclusion cysts that are frequently seen on the labia majora and contain a white to pale yellow cheesy material without hair. Histologically, giant cells are seen adjacent to the cyst wall with a stratified squamous epithelial lining. These are not premalignant.

C. **Mucous cysts** are found within the vestibule. They are lined by mucus-secreting simple columnar epithelium without myoepithelial cells. Squamous metaplasia may be present within the cyst lining.

D. **Cysts of the canal of Nuck** are peritoneal-lined cysts found in the superior aspect of the labia majora. They are believed to arise from inclusions of the peritoneum at the insertion of the round ligament to the labia majora. These cysts can become substantially large and must be distinguished from an inguinal hernia.

VI. **Nonneoplastic epithelial disorders**

A. **Lichen sclerosus** is characterized by itching and the presence of low, flat-topped white maculopapules on the vulva and perineum. These can grow together to form well-defined plaques. Often, the labia minora may disappear from atrophy. Most commonly postmenopausal white women are affected. Multiple punch biopsies should be performed to confirm the diagnosis. Topical testosterone appears to be the most successful agent to decrease pruritus, edema, and scarring associated with lichen sclerosus. Lichen sclerosus is sometimes associated with vulvar squamous cell carcinoma, but it is not considered a premalignant lesion.

B. In **squamous hyperplasia,** there are variable increases in the thickness of the horny layer of skin (hyperkeratosis), as well as in the basal layer (acanthosis). An isolated, heaped-up lesion consistent with squamous hyperplasia is called a **keratoacanthoma.** These may be red or white, well-delineated or poorly defined. Commonly, women between the ages of 30 and 60 are affected. Evaluation should include colposcopy and full-thickness biopsy. There is no proven association between hyperplasia and squamous carcinoma. Topical corticosteroids are the treatment of choice for squamous hyperplasia of the vulva. Chronic candidiasis can be differentiated by silver staining for fungus or periodic acid–Schiff staining for the organisms.

41. VULVAR AND VAGINAL CANCERS

Robert DeBernardo, Cornelia Liu Trimble, and Edward Trimble

I. **Vulvar neoplasms.** It is estimated that 3–5% of all primary malignancies of the female genital tract develop on the vulva. Squamous cell carcinoma is the most common type of histopathology found in vulvar cancer, followed by melanoma, basal cell carcinoma, and sarcoma. Paget's disease of the vulva may herald an underlying adenocarcinoma in 20% of patients. These lesions frequently present as pruritus and are often misdiagnosed by health care providers.

   A. **Squamous cell carcinomas** of the vulva comprise over 85% of cases and can be divided into two distinct categories based on etiology: those that are associated with the human papillomavirus (HPV) and those that are not.

      1. **Vulvar carcinoma associated with HPV.** The risk factors are similar to those for cervical carcinoma, including early age at first intercourse, multiple lifetime sexual partners, immunosuppression, and cigarette smoking. Vulvar carcinoma associated with HPV occurs at a younger age than do those cancers not associated with the virus. Like squamous cell cancers of the cervix, this type of vulvar carcinoma is associated with an intraepithelial precursor lesion, vulvar intraepithelial neoplasia (VIN). HPV types most commonly found in these lesions are type 16 and, to lesser extent, types 18 and 31. Because VIN tends to be multifocal, colposcopic examination and directed biopsy of the entire lower genital tract, including the cervix, vagina, and vulva, is warranted.

         a. **Pathologic features.** Like cervical dysplasia, vulvar dysplasia may involve only the deeper layers of the epidermis and rete pegs (VIN 1). As cellular atypia progresses, lack of maturation of the nucleus and cytoplasm is seen in cell layers closer to the surface (VIN 2). Full-thickness atypia is called VIN 3. Grossly, VIN 3 lesions are slightly elevated, rough, and delineated. They may be white, red, or brown.

         b. **Assessment.** Initial evaluation should include vulvar colposcopy and full-thickness biopsy. After the diagnosis of VIN has been confirmed, the lesion should be removed with a wide local excision. Occasionally, laser ablation is used for a lesion close to the urethra or clitoris. The rate of progression from VIN to invasive vulvar cancer is low, with slow progression occurring over years to decades.

      2. **Vulvar carcinoma not associated with HPV** tends to occur in older women as unifocal lesions. Affected patients often give a history of pruritus. No known precursor lesion develops, although either lichen sclerosus or squamous hyperplasia often is found near these cancers.

      3. **Treatment.** Accurate surgical staging predicts prognosis and directs treatment in squamous cell cancer of the vulva. In addition, the International Federation of Gynecology and Obstetrics (FIGO) staging system (Table 41-1) allows for uniform reporting of data. Treatment of early-stage vulvar carcinomas initially may be surgical. For these lesions, the primary surgery is generally tailored to the lesion. A common procedure, which is more conservative than a traditional radical vulvectomy, has been termed a **radical local excision,** or **partial vulvectomy.** The lateral clear margins should be 1–2 cm, and the deep margin should extend to the urogenital diaphragm. Inguinal lymph node dissection is reserved for lesions with invasion of 3 mm or deeper, those in which lymphovascular invasion is identified, or those accompanied by clinically palpable nodes. Inguinal node dissection is unilateral for lateralized lesions and bilateral for central lesions. Adjuvant pelvic

TABLE 41-1. INTERNATIONAL FEDERATION OF GYNECOLOGY AND OBSTETRICS (FIGO) STAGING SYSTEM FOR SQUAMOUS CELL CANCER OF THE VULVA

Stage	Description
0	Carcinoma in situ.
I	Tumor confined to vulva or perineum; lesion <2 cm. No palpable nodes.
II	Tumor confined to vulva or perineum; lesion >2 cm. No palpable nodes.
III	Tumor of any size extending to lower urethra, vagina, or anus, and/or unilateral nodal metastasis.
IVA	Tumor invading upper urethra, bladder, rectal mucosa, or pelvic bone, with or without regional nodal metastasis.
IVB	Distant metastasis to any site, including pelvic lymph nodes.

radiation therapy is indicated for patients with more than two affected inguinal lymph nodes. Larger or more advanced stage lesions, particularly those close to the urethra, vagina, or rectum, are treated initially with primary chemoradiation, which generally enables more conservative surgery that preserves function and body image.

B. **Verrucous carcinoma** is a variant of squamous carcinoma that occurs in postmenopausal women. The tumors of verrucous carcinoma are large, fungating masses that may be mistakenly diagnosed as condyloma acuminata resistant to treatment. Because the histologic appearance of verrucous carcinoma so closely resembles that of normal squamous epithelium, a sufficiently deep biopsy must be obtained for diagnosis. It is helpful to include a good clinical history with the pathology specimen. Although lymph node metastasis is exceedingly rare, tumor recurrence is common. Treatment consists of radical local excision. Radiation is *contraindicated* because it may induce increased aggression in malignant activity.

C. **Melanomas** constitute the second most common primary malignancy of the vulva, with a peak frequency in the sixth to seventh decades of life. The lesions of melanomas are typically raised, with irregular pigmentation and irregular borders. The lesions are found with approximately equal frequency on the labia majora and on mucosal surfaces. Prognosis depends primarily on tumor thickness and on the presence or absence of lymph node involvement. Radical local excision is recommended for the primary lesion. The role of regional lymphadenectomy is not well defined.

D. **Basal cell carcinomas,** despite being the most common type of carcinoma of the skin, constitute only 2–3% of all vulvar carcinomas. They occur most commonly in postmenopausal white women. Most patients complain of pruritus. Grossly, these lesions appear as a whitish nodule or plaque. The prognosis is good, despite a roughly 20% risk of local recurrence. Metastases to the inguinal lymph nodes are rare; wide local excision is usually sufficient treatment.

E. **Sarcomas** of the vulva are rare but can arise in any connective tissue component of the vulva.

1. **Leiomyosarcomas** are the most common of the vulvar sarcomas. These lesions develop most frequently in the labium majus or in the region of Bartholin's glands. Standard treatment includes radical local excision. An effective chemotherapeutic agent has not yet been developed for this disease.

2. **Rhabdomyosarcoma** is the most common soft tissue tumor of childhood. In 20% of cases, the pelvis or genitourinary system is involved. In such cases, the vagina is more frequently affected than the vulva. Combination chemotherapy generally is used as primary treatment, followed by conservative surgery.

3. **Malignant fibrous histiocytoma,** although uncommon, is the second most common vulvar sarcoma in adults. The tumor involves deep soft tissue and skeletal muscle. The patient usually presents with a solitary mass that grows relatively rapidly. Although first-line therapy consists of radical local excision, radiation therapy has been reported to decrease the rate of local recurrence.

4. **Alveolar soft part sarcoma** most frequently involves the soft tissue of extremities in young adults. Very rarely, alveolar soft part sarcoma can involve the vulva. Standard therapy consists of radical local excision.

5. **Dermatofibrosarcoma protuberans** is a low-grade sarcoma that can in rare cases occur in the vulva. This lesion may appear initially as an indurated plaque on which multiple firm reddish or bluish nodules may appear. Although the lesion may recur locally, systemic metastases are uncommon. Standard therapy consists of radical local excision.

F. **Paget's disease** of the vulva is rare. Most affected patients are in their seventh or eighth decade of life and experience local irritation and pruritus. The lesion has slightly raised edges and is red, with islands of white epithelium. The lesions are sharply demarcated and often have foci of excoriation and induration. Unlike in Paget's disease of the breast, in the majority of cases, no underlying adenocarcinoma is present. An adenocarcinoma of the underlying sweat glands is found in 15–20% of patients who have intraepithelial Paget's disease.

1. **If the disease is limited to the epithelium,** its clinical course may be both prolonged and indolent. Wide local excision is the mainstay of treatment. Although grossly wide surgical margins are indicated, the use of frozen-section evaluation of margins at the time of operation is a subject of controversy. Although recurrence is common when the surgical margins show positive findings, the histologic analysis on permanent section is more accurate than that possible on frozen section.

2. **If an underlying adenocarcinoma is identified,** the patient should undergo radical excision and inguinal lymphadenectomy. The prognosis in patients with lymph node involvement is poor.

II. **Vaginal neoplasms** are one of the least common types of malignancy of the female genital tract. The majority of vaginal neoplasms are squamous cell lesions, although other cell types can occur. It is thought that most vaginal squamous cell lesions are associated with HPV infection. Patients with malignant squamous lesions of the cervix and vulva are at increased risk of having vaginal lesions as well. Careful examination and colposcopy of the vagina should be performed on patients in whom a vulvar or cervical cancer is diagnosed. The spectrum of squamous lesions parallels that of squamous lesions in the cervix or vulva and ranges from vaginal intraepithelial lesions (VAINs, classified as VAIN 1, 2, or 3, depending on the thickness of the atypia) to invasive vaginal carcinoma. VAINs may be treated with local excision, laser ablation, or topical 5-fluorouracil cream. Early-stage vaginal cancer may be treated with local excision, brachytherapy, or both, whereas advanced-stage vaginal cancer is treated best with chemoradiation therapy.

A. **Clear cell carcinomas** of the vagina are uncommon. However, in women exposed to diethylstilbestrol (DES) in utero, particularly before 18 weeks' gestation, careful surveillance of the vagina and cervix is prudent. DES was used until 1972 to treat pregnant women thought to be at risk for miscarriage. Although most patients with DES-related clear cell carcinoma of the vagina are diagnosed between the ages of 18 and 24 years, the oldest reported patient with a clear cell primary cancer of the vagina was 42 years old at the time of diagnosis.

1. **Diagnosis.** The most frequent location of clear cell adenocarcinoma is the upper one-third of the vagina. Many clear cell adenocarcinomas occur on the anterior surface and may present as a submucosal nodule. Therefore, it is necessary to rotate the speculum 90 degrees to visualize the anterior vaginal wall in addition to performing a careful bimanual

examination. Many patients present with abnormal bleeding or vaginal discharge. The most important prognostic factor is stage at diagnosis.

2. **Treatment.** Small tumors limited to the vagina may be treated with partial vaginal excision and brachytherapy. Larger tumors or tumors close to the cervix may require partial vaginectomy, radical hysterectomy, and pelvic lymph node dissection. Patients with late-stage disease are treated with radiation.

B. **Sarcoma botryoides** occurs most often in children younger than 5 years. In this group, sarcoma botryoides is the most common vaginal neoplasm. As the age of the patient increases, the most frequent site of occurrence moves distally. The most common presenting symptom is vaginal bleeding. The lesion manifests as one or more polypoid excrescences that are pinkish red and translucent. Conservative surgery after neoadjuvant chemoradiation is the current standard of treatment.

42. CERVICAL INTRAEPITHELIAL NEOPLASIA

Julie Huh, Robert Bristow, and Cornelia Liu Trimble

I. **Epidemiology and risk factors.** Each year, an estimated 500,000 cases of cervical cancer are newly diagnosed. Worldwide, it is the second leading cause of cancer death in women. In the United States, despite federally mandated screening programs, it remains the sixth most commonly diagnosed malignancy in women. Cervical cancer is thought to be caused by a sexually transmitted disease, human papillomavirus (HPV) infection of the cervix. HPV infection is common among women, and some studies suggest that more than 70% of women will have had an infection by the end of their sexual experience. Infection with a high-risk type of HPV is a requisite for development of preinvasive and invasive squamous neoplasia of the cervix. Other risk factors include multiple sexual partners, intercourse at an early age, poor personal hygiene, immunocompromise, other sexually transmitted diseases (such as herpes simplex virus type 2), and cigarette smoking.

II. **Pathophysiology.** Nearly all cervical intraepithelial neoplasia (CIN) lesions arise in the transformation zone, which is the area of glandular epithelium that undergoes a process of squamous metaplasia. Maximal metaplasia occurs during fetal development, adolescence, and first pregnancy. Cells actively undergoing metaplasia are vulnerable to carcinogens, which may explain the epidemiologic association between early age of first coitus and cervical cancer.

III. **Terminology and definitions**
   A. The concept of **cervical intraepithelial neoplasia** stems from the hypothesis that cervical dysplasia represents a continuum of a single disease process. The three grades of precursor lesions recognized are CIN I (mild dysplasia, involving the lower one-third of the epithelium), CIN II (moderate dysplasia, involving up to two-thirds of the epithelium), and CIN III (severe dysplasia, involving the upper third of the epithelium, or carcinoma in situ). The microscopic features of dysplasia include disordered maturation, nuclear hyperchromatism, increased nuclear to cytoplasmic ratio, pleomorphism, mitoses, and dyskeratosis.
   B. **The Bethesda system** divides cervical lesions into the following categories: atypical squamous cells of undetermined significance (ASCUS), low-grade squamous intraepithelial lesion (LSIL), high-grade squamous intraepithelial lesion (HSIL), and atypical glandular cells of undetermined significance (AGUS). The category of LSIL consolidates HPV cellular changes with those of CIN I. HSIL includes CIN II and CIN III.
   C. **Specimen adequacy.** A cytologic specimen reported as "unsatisfactory for evaluation" requires a repeat Pap smear. If a specimen is reported to be "satisfactory but limited by . . . ," the test may or may not be repeated, depending on the clinical situation. Specifically, an inadequate transformation zone component on Pap smear in a low-risk patient may require only routine follow-up smear. In a high-risk patient, the physician should consider repeating the endocervical portion of the Pap test.

IV. **Molecular evidence.** Infection with low-risk HPV can cause genital condyloma acuminatum and other manifestations of HPV infection that rarely progress to cervical carcinoma. Viral production occurs in low-grade lesions and is restricted to basal cells. Infection with high-risk HPV can lead to the development of cervical intraepithelial neoplasm and invasive carcinoma in approximately 1% of infected women. In most high-grade lesions, as well as in carcinomas, viral DNA is integrated into the host genome and no intact viral production is seen. The viral oncoproteins E6 and E7 inactivate the cell cycle regulators p53 and retinoblastoma (Rb), respectively, providing the initial events in progression to malignancy.

A. **The HPV screening** methods available include DNA dot blot hybridization systems and the more sensitive polymerase chain reaction testing. A great majority of patients diagnosed with LSIL have positive test results for HPV DNA. In the Atypical Squamous Cells of Undetermined Significance/ Low-Grade Squamous Intraepithelial Lesions Triage Study Group (ALTS trial), HPV DNA was detected by Hybrid Capture II assay in over 80% of women with LSIL. Hence, the high percentage of HPV DNA positivity in LSIL cases may limit the usefulness of HPV DNA testing for triage of LSIL. Others, however, have reported that testing may be useful for triage of women with Pap smears showing ASCUS.

B. **HPV typing.** The high-risk HPV subtypes 16, 18, 31, 33, and 51 have been recovered from more than 95% of cervical cancers. HPV-16, alone, is found in over 70% of high-grade lesions. The finding of high-risk HPV and a positive Pap smear result more likely indicates a squamous intraepithelial lesion (SIL) rather than a benign process. The finding of a low-risk HPV type, which rarely is found in cancers in nonimmunosuppressed women, suggests that the lesion is not likely to progress. The future contribution of HPV testing to the management of cervical dysplasia is uncertain; however, it may help identify high-risk HPV in cytologic reports describing the findings as ASCUS.

C. **HPV viral load.** The risk of carcinoma in situ has been shown to increase with consistently high viral loads of HPV-16. The amount of HPV DNA may predict the risk of developing cervical cancer before any cytologic alterations are visible and long before the appearance of tumors. Some authors suggest that HPV quantitative testing, particularly for HPV-16, might help distinguish between infections that have a high or low risk of progressing into cervical cancer.

D. **HPV vaccines.** In animal papillomavirus models, vaccination against viral capsid proteins provides protection against infection. This involves virus type–specific neutralizing antibodies. Prophylactic vaccines produced using recombinant DNA technology are in phase I/II clinical trials for HPV-6 and HPV-11, and for HPV-16. Therapeutic vaccines targeted at the HPV-16 E7 antigen are currently being evaluated in phase I/II clinical trials.

V. **Progression of cervical intraepithelial neoplasia.** CIN I and CIN II/III are thought to represent distinct processes, with CIN I being the morphologic manifestation of a self-limited sexually transmitted HPV infection and CIN II/ III being a cervical cancer precursor. Approximately 60% of CIN I lesions regress spontaneously. Ten percent of CIN I lesions progress to CIN III, and 1% may ultimately progress to invasive cancer. Persistent positive test results for oncogenic HPV types may indicate a significant risk for the development of HSIL and cancer.

VI. **The Pap smear test and other diagnostic tools**

A. **Cytologic analysis**

1. **Screening** for cervical cancer. Women who are sexually active or have reached the age of 18 should undergo an annual Pap smear and pelvic examination. After three or more consecutive satisfactory smear findings, the test may be performed less frequently, at the discretion of the physician. The false-negative rate ranges between 15% and 30% and usually results from inadequate sampling, poor processing, or laboratory error.

2. **Technique.** To sample the ectocervix, a wooden spatula is placed against the external os and rotated 360 degrees. To sample the endocervix, a cytobrush is inserted into the external os and rotated. The sample obtained by the spatula and cytobrush is spread on a glass slide and immediately placed in a fixative, usually 95% ethanol. Another method is the use of a liquid-based Pap smear (thin preparation), which was developed to improve the preservation and presentation of cells for cervical cytologic analysis. This method may be more sensitive in detecting

SILs than the conventional technique. The specificity of both methods, however, may be equivalent. In addition, the residual fluid that remains after processing a liquid specimen may be used for HPV DNA testing.

3. **Atypical findings.** Infection, inflammatory or reparative changes, and the effects of irradiation can result in atypical smear results suggestive, but not diagnostic, of CIN. In these cases, smears should be repeated in 3–6 months. If there is evidence of a specific infectious agent causing atypical inflammation, antibiotic or antifungal therapy may be appropriate.

4. **Positive findings.** Patients with Pap smear findings suggesting HSIL require colposcopy.

B. **Colposcopy** allows examination of the cervix at magnifications ranging from 6- to 40-fold. Use of a green filter better defines vascular architecture by absorbing red light and making blood vessels appear black and more prominent. Colposcopy does not evaluate disease in the endocervical canal.

1. **Technique.** Acetic acid (3.0% or 5.0%) is applied to the cervix. This removes mucus and dehydrates cells. The more protein in the cell, the whiter it becomes. Dysplastic cells contain large nuclei with abnormally large amounts of chromatin (protein). The application of acetic acid coagulates these intracellular proteins and makes them opaque and white. Hence, cells with an increased nucleus to cytoplasm ratio appear opaque on colposcopic examination.

2. **Abnormal or unsatisfactory results.** Abnormal features that may represent CIN include epithelium that whitens with the application of acetic acid (acetowhitening), mosaicism, and punctation. Several processes, including inflammation, can cause acetowhite changes. Typically, intraepithelial lesions are characterized by discrete, sharp margins. Classification of examination results as "unsatisfactory" indicates that the transformation zone was not completely visualized or the full extent of the lesion was not visualized. Biopsy should be performed on abnormal areas.

3. **Endocervical curettage (ECC)** helps evaluate the endocervical canal for the presence of dysplasia.

VII. **Low-grade squamous intraepithelial lesions**

A. **Principles for evaluation.** Most Pap smear findings suggestive of LSIL represent lesions that regress spontaneously. A few women with results in this category, however, have a lesion that progresses. Between 20% and 30% of women with smear results indicating mild dysplasia actually have a high-grade lesion present. Such women usually are identified by continued cytologic surveillance. The clinical challenge is to distinguish the patients who have LSIL that will persist unchanged or regress spontaneously.

B. **Strategies for evaluation and management.** In more than 75% of immunocompetent women with a diagnosis of LSIL, the condition resolves without intervention in 9 months. Thus, LSILs may be followed conservatively, depending on the degree of patient compliance.

1. **Reliable or low-risk patients.** Observation with repeat Pap smear every 4–6 months for 1 year is recommended for reliable or low-risk patients. After three consecutive negative findings on Pap smears that are satisfactory for evaluation, routine screening protocol is resumed. If LSIL persists, colposcopy, ECC, directed biopsy, or some combination of these, is recommended.

2. **Unreliable or high-risk patients.** Colposcopy is recommended to identify the 20–30% of high-risk patients who may have an underlying HSIL. If directed biopsy confirms HSIL, these patients require the appropriate treatment (refer to sec. **X** on HSIL management). If colposcopy confirms LSIL, these patients may be followed every 6–9 months with repeat cytologic examination. If LSIL persists, they may require repeat colposcopy and appropriate treatment. Excision or ablation should be considered for patients who are not likely to return for follow-up. Carbon dioxide laser or cryotherapy is used for ablation. The

loop electrosurgical excision procedure is both diagnostic and therapeutic, and is the preferred method of treatment, with a cure rate of approximately 96%. Before an ablative procedure is performed, biopsy samples should be obtained to evaluate the extent of the lesion and rule out higher-grade disease. Ablative or destructive procedures are not always curative. In addition, the healing process may draw the transformation zone proximally into the endocervical canal, which makes subsequent surveillance and diagnosis more difficult.

VIII. **Atypical squamous cells of undetermined significance.** The term **atypia** is reserved for abnormalities that do not qualify as a SIL or reactive change.

    A. **Incidence.** Variation exists in the criteria used by different laboratories to designate ASCUS. This cytologic diagnosis is expected in no more than 5% of routine Pap smears. In high-risk populations with a higher prevalence of SILs, a correspondingly higher prevalence of ASCUS is to be expected. It has been useful to qualify ASCUS by adding the statement "favor reactive" or "favor dysplasia." Less than 5% of women with ASCUS classified as "favor reactive" are eventually confirmed histologically to have HSIL; however, women with ASCUS designated "favor dysplasia" have biopsy-confirmed HSIL or invasive cancer in 8–10% of cases.

    B. **Management**

        1. **Unqualified results.** Pap smear results may be followed without colposcopy in reliable patients. A smear should be repeated every 4–6 months for 2 years until there have been three consecutive (and adequate) smears with negative findings, at which point the patient can be monitored routinely. If a second ASCUS result is obtained during the 2-year period, colposcopy should be considered. The diagnosis of unqualified ASCUS with severe inflammation should be reevaluated after 2–3 months.

        2. **ASCUS in high-risk patients** requires colposcopy and directed biopsy as indicated.

        3. **Infections.** If chlamydiosis, gonorrhea, or vaginitis (due to *Candida* or *Trichomonas*) is identified, antibiotic or antifungal treatment is appropriate.

        4. **Postmenopausal patients** not on hormone replacement therapy have atrophic cells that may resemble parabasal cells with a high nucleus to cytoplasm ratio, suggestive of dysplasia. Use of topical estrogen may be helpful in resolving the cellular atypia. If ASCUS remains, colposcopy is recommended.

        5. **Results favoring dysplasia.** If the diagnosis of ASCUS favors dysplasia, the patient, particularly a patient at high risk, should undergo colposcopy. Some studies indicate that HPV DNA testing in women with ASCUS on cytologic examination may be helpful in identifying patients with underlying HSIL.

IX. **Atypical glandular cells of undetermined significance**

    A. The classification of **AGUS** was proposed in 1988 by the Bethesda system and refers to suspected glandular lesions that cannot be definitely classified as reactive or neoplastic. Histologic correlation ranges from benign glandular conditions such as reactive atypia or an endometrial polyp, to preinvasive disease and frank malignancy. AGUS may be found in 0.5–2.5% of Pap smears. Atypical cells may arise from the endocervix, ectocervix, or any glandular epithelial source within the pelvis. AGUS can be associated with a significant percentage of underlying disease, especially HSIL. Risk factors are unknown, although menopausal status and vaginal bleeding as the presenting complaint have been associated with clinically significant lesions.

    B. **Evaluation and management.** Glandular lesions of the cervix are diagnostically and therapeutically more challenging because of their rarity, relative absence of colposcopic findings, irregular shedding, small size, endocervical location, and broader differential diagnosis. There is no formal recommendation by the American College of Obstetricians and Gynecologists regarding standard management in cases with this cytologic diagnosis. The American Society for Colposcopy and Cervical Pathology published guidelines for the management of AGUS identified on Pap smears as follows:

1. AGUS on Pap smear: cervical and vaginal colposcopy and ECC.
2. Unqualified AGUS on Pap smear, with negative colposcopic and ECC findings: repeat Pap smear every 4–6 months, until four normal smear results are obtained.
3. AGUS categorized as favoring neoplasia on Pap smear, with negative colposcopic and ECC findings: cervical conization.
4. Unqualified AGUS on Pap smear, with positive ECC findings: cervical conization.
5. Endometrial biopsy, hysteroscopy, or endometrial curettage if cells appear to be of endometrial origin. Endometrial biopsy is generally recommended in older women (i.e., 50 years or older, or 35 years or older if there are risk factors for endometrial cancer such as polycystic ovarian syndrome).

X. **High-grade squamous intraepithelial lesions: evaluation and treatment.** All patients with HSIL on Pap smear require colposcopy and directed biopsy. After biopsy to confirm the presence of a high-grade lesion and the distribution of the lesion, excisional or ablative therapy aimed at removal or destruction of the entire lesion and the transformation zone is performed.

XI. **Local therapy** is appropriate for patients with a preinvasive lesion that has been confirmed cytologically and histologically, and completely visualized colposcopically, and for which invasion has been ruled out. Current therapeutic options all involve tissue resection or destruction. Tissue destruction must extend to a depth of 6–7 mm, as this is the depth of the endocervical gland. There is a 90% success rate after first treatment. Persistent disease, which occurs in 5–10% of cases, is usually diagnosed within the first 12 months after treatment. The sequelae of tissue resection and ablation include cervical stenosis or incompetence, increased risk of preterm delivery, infertility, and migration of the transformation zone proximally. Sexual abstinence for 4 weeks allows healing of the transformation zone. Patients return in 6–8 weeks and are followed with Pap smears every 3–4 months until three consecutive negative Pap smear results have been obtained, at which point the patient may be monitored with annual Pap smears.

A. **Ablation**

1. **Cryotherapy.** A nitrous oxide or carbon dioxide cryoprobe is used. Application of the probe to the cervix produces an ice ball that must extend 5 mm beyond the edge of the lesion. Results are best when a double-freeze technique is used: 3 minutes of freezing, 5 minutes of thawing, 3 minutes of refreezing. Complications include uterine spasm producing a low pelvic ache and, occasionally, a feeling of faintness. A success rate of over 90%, depending on the lesion size, grade, and presence of endocervical gland involvement, has been reported. A profuse watery discharge may persist up to 3 weeks.

2. **Carbon dioxide laser.** Tissue is vaporized by conversion of cellular water to steam. The treatment can usually be undertaken satisfactorily in an outpatient setting using local anesthesia. A burning sensation is commonly reported by patients during the procedure.

B. **Cone biopsy**

1. **Loop electrosurgical excision procedure or large loop excision of the transformation zone** can be both diagnostic and therapeutic.

   a. **Indications** include cytologic or colposcopic evidence of HSIL (CIN II or III); unsatisfactory colposcopy results in the presence of a Pap smear showing HSIL, persistent LSIL, or LSIL in high-risk, noncompliant patients, and the necessity of ruling out invasive cancer in AGUS.

b. **Technique.** The procedure can usually be performed in an office setting. The cervix is examined colposcopically and local anesthesia is injected circumferentially around the cervix (i.e., at 2, 4, 8, and 10 o'clock positions). The electrosurgical generator is set at cut/blend to 25–50 W. (The patient should be grounded.) A tungsten wire loop is drawn across the area of cervical dysplasia, excising a dish-shaped specimen. Frequently, a second pass is performed to excise a portion of the endocervical canal. Coagulation with the ball electrode, set at 60 W, is used for hemostasis. In addition, ferric subsulfate may be applied. Patients with CIN extending to the margin of resection have a recurrence risk of approximately 30% and should be followed with close cytologic surveillance and colposcopy rather than re-treated immediately. If the limits of the lesion and the transformation zone are not entirely visible, cervical conization should be performed. Bleeding (2–5% of patients) and discomfort are common short-term sequelae. The success rate is higher than 90%.

2. **Cold knife or carbon dioxide laser beam conization.** The morbidity is proportional to the size and depth of the cone. Adverse effects include cervical stenosis, cervical incompetence, decreased fertility caused by excision of the gland-bearing part of the endocervix that produces mucus at ovulation, and immediate or delayed hemorrhage requiring hospital admission and possible blood transfusion. **Indications** include

a. HSIL (CIN II or III) with a lesion that extends beyond the view into the endocervical canal (i.e., unsatisfactory colposcopy).

b. Cytologic or colposcopic suggestion of microinvasive or invasive disease.

c. Pap smear showing HSIL with normal findings on colposcopic examination or an abnormal ECC result.

d. Pap smear suggesting adenocarcinoma in situ.

XII. **Human immunodeficiency virus (HIV) infection and intraepithelial lesions.** Women infected with HIV are at increased risk for cervical SILs, although little is known about the causes of this association. Ellerbrock et al. (*JAMA*, 283/1031, 2000) concluded that 1 in 5 HIV-infected women, versus 1 in 20 uninfected women, with no evidence of cervical disease will develop biopsy-confirmed SILs within 3 years. This is probably dependent on the degree of immunocompromise, with patients having CD4 counts below 200 at the highest risk.

XIII. **Pregnancy and intraepithelial lesions.** Cervical cancer is the most common malignancy in pregnancy. The epidemiologic risk factors are similar to those in the nonpregnant state. Nearly 86% of all cervical abnormalities that occur during pregnancy are classified as LSILs.

The evaluation of women with abnormal Pap smears in pregnancy can be done with a combination of cytologic study, colposcopy, and careful use of colposcopically directed biopsy. ECC is contraindicated in pregnancy due to the risk of bleeding and premature rupture of membranes.

Colposcopy should be performed on all patients with an abnormal cytologic result. It is up to the physician to determine if colposcopically directed biopsy is necessary, especially in the case of LSIL on Pap smear. Of note, even if the colposcopic impression is consistent with LSIL, as many as 10% of such lesions show histologic evidence of HSIL. Biopsy-confirmed LSIL lesions can be followed through pregnancy without risk of progression to invasive cancer. Cervical cytologic analysis should be performed during each trimester and 8–12 weeks postpartum. The diagnosis of HSIL requires close cytologic and colposcopic surveillance, every 8–12 weeks (Fig. 42-1). All patients should be reevaluated with colposcopy 8–12 weeks postpartum.

Conization is recommended for pregnant patients with cytologic evidence of invasive cancer that is not confirmed by colposcopy. The optimal time for a cone

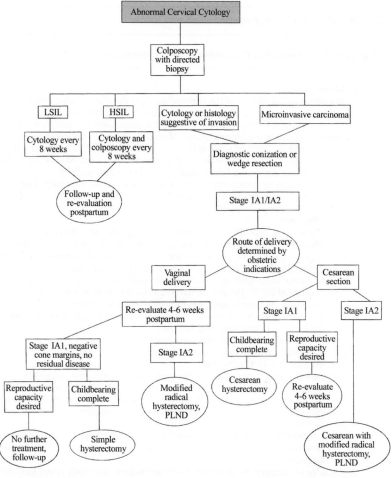

FIG. 42-1. Management of abnormal cervical lesions identified by cytologic examination during pregnancy. HSIL, high-grade squamous intraepithelial lesion; LSIL, low-grade squamous intraepithelial lesion; PLND, pelvic lymph node dissection. (Adapted from Bristow RE, Montz FJ. Cervical cancer in pregnancy. In: Trimble EL, Trimble CL, *Cancer obstetrics and gynecology*. Philadelphia: Lippincott Williams & Wilkins, 1999:157–175.)

biopsy is between 14 and 20 weeks' gestational age. It should not be attempted if delivery is expected within 4 weeks, because of the risk of cervical laceration and excessive bleeding from the conization bed. Bleeding and pregnancy loss can occur in as many as 32% of patients undergoing cone biopsy, especially during the first trimester.

43. CERVICAL CANCER

Robert Bristow, Nicholas C. Lambrou, and Frederick J. Montz

I. **Epidemiology**
   A. **Incidence.** Carcinoma of the uterine cervix is the second most common cancer among women worldwide, occurring most commonly in Africa, Asia, and South America. Cervical cancer is the third most common malignant gynecologic neoplasm in the United States. Mortality and incidence rates for cervical cancer have declined in most developed countries, which is attributed to the introduction of screening with the Pap smear (see Chap. 34). In the United States, where screening for cervical cancer is readily available, most women who are found to have cervical cancer are not screened regularly. The mean age for diagnosis of cervical cancer is 52.2 years, and the distribution of cases is bimodal, with peaks at 35–39 years and 60–64 years.
   B. **Risk factors**
      1. **Race.** The rate of cervical cancer among African-Americans remains about twice as high as that among whites at all ages. The incidence is approximately two times higher for Hispanic Americans, and even higher for Native Americans. Asian groups experience rates similar to or lower than that of whites. These differences are at least partially accounted for by the strong inverse association between cervical cancer incidence and socioeconomic factors. When socioeconomic differences are controlled for, the excess risk of cervical cancer among African-Americans is substantially reduced from over 70% to less than 30%. Racial differences are also apparent in survival; 57% of all African-Americans with cervical cancer survive 5 years, compared with 69% of all whites with the disease.
      2. **Sexual and reproductive history.** First intercourse before the age of 16 is associated with a twofold increased risk of cervical cancer compared with women with first intercourse after the age of 20. Cervical cancer risk is also directly proportional to the number of lifetime sexual partners.
      3. **Cigarette smoking** has emerged as an important etiologic factor in cervical carcinoma. The increased risk for smokers is approximately twofold.
      4. Use of **barrier methods of contraception,** especially those that combine both mechanical and chemical protection, have been shown to lower the risk of cervical cancer.
      5. **Male partner contribution.** The sexual histories (e.g., history of venereal infections, early sexual experiences, and nonmonogamous behavior) of the male partners of women with cervical cancer may be etiologically important.
      6. **Immunosuppression.** Cell-mediated immunity appears to be a factor in the development of cervical cancer. Immunocompromised women may be at higher risk of developing the disease and may demonstrate more rapid progression from preinvasive to invasive lesions. Patients testing positive for human immunodeficiency virus infection appear to present with invasive cervical cancer earlier than patients testing negative for the virus, and with more advanced disease at the time of diagnosis when CD4 cell counts are reduced (below 200/mm^3).
   C. **Etiology.** Evidence supports a significant role for **human papillomavirus (HPV) infection** in the etiology of cervical neoplasia. These DNA tumor viruses colonize mucosal or cutaneous epithelium and induce hyperprolifer-

ation, which results in the formation of warts at the site of infection. Based on differences in DNA sequencing, more than 70 different types of HPV have been identified, more than 20 of which are known to infect the anogenital tract. HPV types 16, 18, 31, 45, 51–53, and 56 are associated with invasive carcinoma. HPV DNA (predominantly of types 16, 18, and 31) has been isolated from 80–100% of cervical carcinomas.

II. **Detection and prevention.** Cervical neoplasia is presumed to be a continuum from dysplasia to carcinoma in situ to invasive carcinoma. For this reason, screening for cervical cancer with the use of exfoliative cytologic study (Pap smear examination) can have significant effects on the incidence, morbidity, and mortality of invasive disease by facilitating the eradication of precursor lesions. A single negative Pap smear result may decrease the risk of developing cervical cancer by 45%, and nine negative smear findings during a lifetime decrease the risk by as much as 99%.

III. **Clinical presentation**

A. **Presenting symptoms.** The most common symptom of cervical cancer is abnormal vaginal bleeding or discharge. Abnormal bleeding may take the form of postcoital spotting, intermenstrual bleeding, or heavy menstrual bleeding (menorrhagia). Serosanguineous or yellowish vaginal discharge, at times foul smelling, may occur with particularly advanced and necrotic carcinomas. Pelvic pain may result from locally advanced disease or tumor necrosis. Extension to the pelvic side wall may cause sciatic pain or back pain associated with hydronephrosis. Metastatic involvement of the iliac and para-aortic lymph nodes can extend into the lumbosacral nerve roots and also present as lumbosacral back pain. Bladder or rectal invasion by advanced-stage disease may produce urinary or rectal symptoms (e.g., hematuria, hematochezia).

B. **Physical findings.** Cervical carcinoma most commonly appears as an exophytic cervical mass that characteristically bleeds on contact. With endophytic tumors, the neoplasm develops entirely within the endocervical canal, and the external cervix may appear normal. In these cases, bimanual examination may reveal a firm, indurated, often barrel-shaped cervix. Cervical cancer may also take the form of a small, shallow, ulcerative crater.

C. **Spread of disease** (Fig. 43-1)

1. **Direct extension**

a. **Paracervical and parametrial extension.** The lateral spread of cervical cancer occurs through the cardinal ligament, and significant involvement of the medial portion of this ligament may result in ureteral obstruction. Tumor cells commonly spread through parametrial lymphatic vessels to expand and replace parametrial lymph nodes. These individual tumor masses enlarge and become confluent, eventually replacing the normal parametrial tissue. Less commonly, the central tumor mass reaches the pelvic side wall by direct contiguous extension of the tumor from the cervix through the cardinal ligament.

b. **Vaginal extension.** The upper vagina is frequently involved (50% of cases) when the primary tumor has extended beyond the confines of the cervix. Anterior extension through the vesicovaginal septum is most common, and often the dissection plane between the bladder and underlying cervical tumor is obliterated, which makes surgical therapy difficult or impossible. A deep posterior cul-de-sac can represent an anatomic barrier to direct tumor spread from the cervix and vagina to the rectum posteriorly.

c. **Bladder and rectal involvement.** Anterior and posterior spread of cervical cancer to the bladder and rectum is uncommon in the absence of lateral parametrial disease.

2. **Lymphatic spread** of cervical carcinoma follows an orderly and reasonably predictable pattern. The most commonly involved, in descending order of incidence, are the obturator, external iliac, and hypogastric

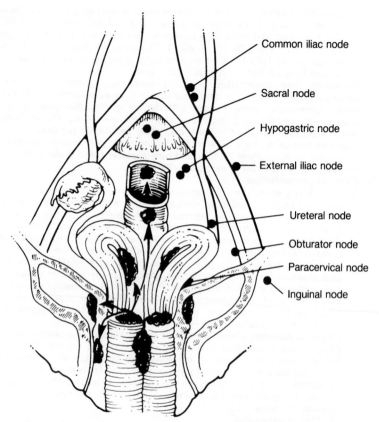

FIG. 43-1. Possible sites of direct extension of cervical cancer to adjoining organs or metastases to regional lymph nodes. The uterus, cervix, and vagina are depicted bisected and opened to reveal the possible sites of tumor implantation. (From Scott JR, DiSaia PJ, Hammond CB, et al. *Danforth's obstetrics and gynecology*, 7th ed. Philadelphia: Lippincott–Raven Publishers, 1997:909, with permission.)

lymph node groups (Fig. 43-1). The parametrial, inferior gluteal, and presacral lymph nodes are less frequently involved. Secondary nodal involvement (common iliac, para-aortic) rarely occurs in the absence of primary nodal disease. The percentage of involved lymph nodes increases directly with primary tumor volume. In patients with clinically advanced or recurrent disease, metastatic disease may be detected in the scalene nodes.

IV. **Staging**
   A. **Clinical staging**
      1. **System of the International Federation of Gynecology and Obstetrics.** In 1995, the International Federation of Gynecology and Obstetrics (FIGO) revised the clinical staging of cervical carcinoma (Table 43-1 and Fig. 43-2). The most notable changes were for stage IA1 (microinvasive carcinoma), which is now defined as stromal invasion no greater than 3.0 mm in depth and no wider than 7.0 mm. This new definition reflects data indicating that patients with less than 3.0 mm of

TABLE 43-1. STAGING FOR CARCINOMA OF THE CERVIX UTERI (INTERNATIONAL FEDERATION OF GYNECOLOGY AND OBSTETRICS, 1995)

Stage	Description	Comments
0	Carcinoma in situ, intraepithelial carcinoma.	
I	The carcinoma is strictly confined to the cervix.	
IA	Invasive cancer identified only microscopically. All gross lesions, even with superficial invasion, are stage IB cancers. Invasion is limited to measured stromal invasion with maximum depth of 5 mm and width of 7 mm.*	The diagnosis of both stage IA1 and IA2 cases should be based on microscopic examination of removed tissue, preferably a cone, which must include the entire lesion. The lower limit of stage IA2 should be measurable macroscopically (even if dots need to be placed on the slide before measurement), and the upper limit of stage IA2 is given by measurement of the two largest dimensions in any given section. The depth of invasion should not be more than 5 mm
IA1	Measured invasion of stroma no greater than 3 mm in depth and no wider than 7 mm.	taken from the base of the epithelium, either surface or glandular, from which it originates. The second dimension, the horizontal spread, must not exceed 7 mm. Vascular space involvement, either venous or lymphatic, should not alter the staging but should be specifically recorded, as it may affect treatment decisions in the future.
IA2	Measured invasion of stroma greater than 3 mm and no greater than 5 mm in depth, and no wider than 7 mm.	Lesions of larger size should be classified as stage IB.
IB	Clinical lesions confined to the cervix or preclinical lesions higher than stage IA.	As a rule, it is impossible to estimate clinically whether a cancer of the cervix has extended to the corpus or not. Extension to the corpus should therefore be disregarded.
IB1	Clinical lesions no larger than 4 cm.	
IB2	Clinical lesions larger than 4 cm.	
II	The carcinoma extends beyond the cervix but has not extended to the pelvic wall. The carcinoma involves the vagina but not as far as the lower one-third.	A patient with a growth fixed to the pelvic wall by a short and indurated but not nodular parametrium should be assigned to stage IIB. It is impossible, at clinical examination, to decide whether a smooth and indurated parametrium is truly cancerous or only inflammatory. Therefore, the case should be placed in stage III only if the parametrium is nodular on the pelvic wall or if the growth itself extends to the pelvic wall.
IIA	No obvious parametrial involvement.	
IIB	Obvious parametrial involvement.	

(continued)

TABLE 43-1. (*Continued*)

Stage	Description	Comments
III	The carcinoma has extended to the pelvic wall. On rectal examination, there is no cancer-free space between the tumor and the pelvic wall. The tumor involves the lower one-third of the vagina. All cases with a hydronephrosis or nonfunctioning kidney are included unless these are known to be due to other causes.	The presence of hydronephrosis or nonfunctioning kidney due to stenosis of the ureter by cancer permits a case to be allotted to stage III even if, according to the other findings, the case should be assigned to stage I or stage II.
IIIA	No extension to the pelvic wall.	
IIIB	Extension to the pelvic wall and/or hydronephrosis or nonfunctioning kidney.	
IV	The carcinoma has extended beyond the true pelvis or has clinically involved the mucosa of the bladder or rectum. A bullous edema as such does not permit a case to be allotted to stage IV.	The presence of bullous edema, as such, should not permit a case to be assigned to stage IV. Ridges and furrows in the bladder wall should be interpreted as signs of submucous involvement of the bladder if they remain fixed to the growth during palpation (i.e., examination from the vagina or the rectum during cystoscopy). A finding of malignant cells in cytologic washings from the urinary bladder requires further examination and biopsy of the wall of the bladder.
IVA	Spread of the growth to adjacent organs.	
IVB	Spread to distant organs.	

From Shingleton HM, Orr JW. *Cervical cancer*. Philadelphia: JB Lippincott Co, 1995, with permission.

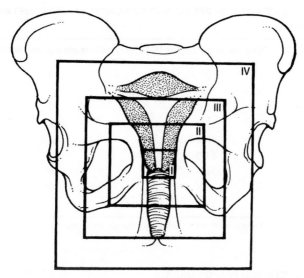

FIG. 43-2. Clinical stages of carcinoma of the cervix. In stage I, only the cervix is involved. In stage II, the parametrium or upper two-thirds of the vagina is involved. In stage III, the malignancy extends to the pelvic side walls or involves the lower one-third of the vagina. In stage IV, areas beyond the true pelvis are involved. (From Scott JR, DiSaia PJ, Hammond CB, et al. *Danforth's obstetrics and gynecology*, 7th ed. Philadelphia: Lippincott–Raven Publishers, 1997:909, with permission.)

       invasion are at very low risk of metastatic disease and may be treated more conservatively (Table 43-2).

       FIGO's clinical staging system for cervical carcinoma is based on clinical evaluation (inspection, palpation, colposcopy); radiographic examination of the chest, kidneys, and skeleton; and endocervical curettage and biopsies as needed. Lymphangiograms, arteriograms, CT scan findings, MRI, and laparoscopy and laparotomy findings should not be used for clinical staging (Table 43-3). Routine laboratory studies should include a CBC, electrolyte and chemistry panel, and urinalysis.

    2. **Evaluation of disease extent.** The clinical stage is determined by inspection and palpation of the cervix, vagina, and pelvis and by examination of extrapelvic areas, specifically the abdomen and supraclavicular lymph nodes. It is important to palpate the entire vagina to determine whether disease is limited to the cervix (IB), extends to the upper two-thirds of the vagina (IIA), or also involves the lower one-third of the vagina (IIIA). Tumor extension into the parametrial tissue (IIB) or to the pelvic side wall (IIIB) is best appreciated on rectovaginal examination. Examination under anesthesia is preferred. When there is doubt concerning the stage to which a tumor should be assigned, the earlier stage is chosen. Once a clinical stage has been determined and treatment has begun, subsequent findings on either extended clinical staging or surgical exploration should not alter the assigned stage.

  B. **Surgical staging.** The 1995 FIGO staging classification for cervical cancer is based on pretherapy clinical findings. Only the subclassifications of stage I (IA1, IA2) require pathologic assessment. Discrepancies between clinical staging and surgicopathologic findings range from 17.3% to 38.5% in patients with clinical stage I disease to 42.9–89.5% in patients with stage III

TABLE 43-2. INCIDENCE OF PELVIC AND PARA-AORTIC NODAL METASTASIS BY STAGE

Stage	Positive pelvic nodes (%)	Positive para-aortic nodes (%)
IA1	0	0
IA2		
(1–3 mm)	0.6	0
(3–5 mm)	4.8	<1
IB	15.9	2.2
IIA	24.5	11
IIB	31.4	19
III	44.8	30
IVA	55	40

Adapted from Berek JS, Hacker NF, eds. *Practical gynecologic oncology*, 2nd ed. Baltimore: Williams & Wilkins, 1994.

TABLE 43-3. STAGING PROCEDURES

Physical examination[a]	Palpation of lymph nodes
	Examination of vagina
	Bimanual rectovaginal examination (under anesthesia recommended)
Radiologic studies[a]	IVP
	Barium enema
	Chest
	Skeletal radiograph
Procedures[a]	Biopsy
	Conization
	Hysteroscopy
	Colposcopy
	Endocervical curettage
	Cystoscopy
	Proctoscopy
Optional studies[b]	CT scan
	Lymphangiography
	Ultrasonography
	MRI
	Radionucleotide scanning
	Laparoscopy

[a]Allowed by International Federation of Gynecology and Obstetrics (FIGO).
[b]Information that is not allowed by FIGO to change the clinical stage.
Adapted from Berek JS, Hacker NF, eds. *Practical gynecologic oncology*, 2nd ed. Baltimore: Williams & Wilkins, 1994.

disease. Specifically, CT scans have only a 35% sensitivity in predicting nodal disease. Positron emission tomography and MRI may prove more useful. This has led some to emphasize surgical staging in women with locally advanced cervical carcinoma to identify occult tumor spread and allow treatment of metastatic disease beyond the traditional pelvic radiation field. There is also evidence suggesting a benefit to debulking macroscopically positive lymph nodes. The use of transperitoneal surgical staging procedures followed by abdominopelvic irradiation is associated with appreciable complications, particularly enteric morbidity. To avoid entering the peritoneal cavity, an extraperitoneal surgical approach relying on a paraumbilical or paramedian incision can be used and allows accurate assessment of disease status. Depending on physician training and preference, laparoscopy offers another method of surgical staging and may allow for earlier treatment with radiation therapy.

V. **Tumor characteristics.** Prognostic variables directly related to surgicopathologic tumor characteristics and their effect on survival include FIGO stage, tumor histologic subtype, histologic grade, and lymph node status. In addition, tumor volume and depth of invasion have also been shown to have a significant impact on survival (Table 43-4).

  A. **Stage.** Clinical stage of disease at the time of presentation is the most important determinant of subsequent survival regardless of treatment modality. Five-year survival declines as FIGO stage at diagnosis increases from stage IA (97%) to stage IV (12.4%). Significant declines in survival are seen for every stage compared with stage IA.

  B. **Histologic subtype.** There are conflicting data on the influence of histologic subtype on tumor behavior, prognosis, and survival.

  C. **Histologic grade.** Significant decreases in 5-year survival rates are associated with histologic grades of moderately differentiated (63.7%) and poorly differentiated (51.4%) compared with well-differentiated tumors (74.5%).

  D. **Lymph node involvement.** Among surgically treated patients, survival is directly related to the number and location of lymph node metastases. For all stages of disease, when both pelvic and para-aortic lymph nodes are negative, 5-year survival is 75.2%. Survival decreases to 45.6% with positive pelvic nodes, whereas involvement of para-aortic nodes lowers 5-year survival to 15.4%. With the use of extended radiation fields and adjuvant chemotherapy, 5-year survival for patients with pelvic and para-aortic nodal disease may increase to higher than 50%. Patients with bilateral pelvic lymph node involvement have a worse prognosis than those with unilateral disease. The recurrence rate is 35% for patients with one positive node, 59% for those with two or three positive nodes, and 69% for those with more than three positive nodes.

  E. **Tumor volume.** Lesion size is an important predictor of survival, independent of other factors. Greater tumor volume is associated with higher rates of parametrial involvement and decreased survival. For stages IB through IIB, 5-year survival decreases from 84.9% to 69.6% when the parametria are involved with tumor.

  F. **Depth of invasion.** Survival is also strongly correlated with depth of tumor invasion into the stroma, with 3-year survival rates of 86–94% for depths less than 10 mm, 71–75% for 11–20 mm, and 60% for 21 mm of invasion.

VI. **Pathology**

  A. **Microinvasive carcinoma (MICA).** MICA is a lesion not apparent clinically that is diagnosed by histologic examination of a cone biopsy or hysterectomy specimen that includes the entire lesion. Involvement of the cone margins by invasive carcinoma or even a high-grade intraepithelial lesion precludes a diagnosis of MICA, because deeper invasion may exist higher in the endocervix. Histologically, MICA is characterized by the presence of irregularly shaped tongues of epithelium projecting from the base of an

TABLE 43-4. PROGNOSTIC VARIABLES: TUMOR CHARACTERISTICS

Characteristic	5-year survival (%)
Stage[a]	
IA	97.0
IB	78.9
IIA	54.9
IIB	51.6
IIIA	40.5
IIIB	27.0
IV	12.4
Histologic findings[a]	
Squamous	67.2
Adenocarcinoma	67.7
Adenosquamous	54.9
Grade[a]	
Well-differentiated	74.5
Moderately differentiated	63.7
Poorly differentiated	51.4
Lymph node status[a]	
Negative	75.2
Positive pelvic	45.6
Positive para-aortic	15.4
Tumor volume[b]	
<2 cm	90
>2 cm	60
>4 cm	40
Depth of invasion[c,d]	
<10 mm	86–94
11–20 mm	71–75
>20 mm	60

[a]From Kosary CL. FIGO stage, histology, histologic grade, age and race as prognostic factors in determining survival for cancers of the female gynecological system: an analysis of 1973–87 SEER cases of cancers of the endometrium, cervix, ovary, vulva, and vagina. *Semin Surg Oncol* 1994;10:31–46, with permission.

[b]From Hatch KD. Cervical cancer. In: Berek JS, Hacker NF, eds. *Practical gynecologic oncology,* 2nd ed. Baltimore: Williams & Wilkins, 1994.

[c]From Delgado G, Bundy BN, Fowler WC Jr, et al. A prospective surgical pathological study of stage I squamous carcinoma of the cervix: a Gynecologic Oncology Group study. *Gynecol Oncol* 1989;35:314–320, with permission.

[d]Three-year survival.

intraepithelial lesion into the stroma. The FIGO staging system for cervical carcinoma separates microscopic lesions into stage IA1 (measured invasion of stroma 3.0 mm or less in depth and no wider than 7.0 mm) and stage IA2 (stromal invasion of 3.1–5.0 mm and width of less than 7.0 mm). Lymph vascular involvement does not alter the classification. The Society of Gynecologic Oncologists has defined MICA as neoplastic epithelium that invades the stroma in one or more places to a depth of 3.0 mm or less below the basement membrane of epithelium and in which lymph or blood vascular involvement is not demonstrated. Lesions fulfilling the Society of Gynecologic Oncologists criteria of MICA have virtually no potential for either metastases or recurrence because lymph vascular involvement is associated with a higher incidence of pelvic node metastases. Therefore, this definition appears to be the most useful for guiding clinical management.

B. **Invasive squamous cell carcinoma.** Squamous cell carcinoma is the most common histologic type of cervical cancer, comprising 75–90% of cases in most series.

1. **Grade.** Histologic differentiation of cervical carcinomas includes three grades. Grade 1 tumors are **well differentiated** with mature squamous cells, often forming keratinized pearls of epithelial cells. Mitotic activity is low. **Moderately well-differentiated** carcinomas (grade 2) have higher mitotic activity and less cellular maturation accompanied by more nuclear pleomorphism. Grade 3 tumors are composed of **poorly differentiated** smaller cells with less cytoplasm and often bizarre nuclei. Mitotic activity is high.

2. **Subclassification.** Squamous cell carcinomas are also subclassified according to cell type (or degree of differentiation). The most commonly used descriptive evaluation divides squamous cell carcinomas into **large cell keratinizing, large cell nonkeratinizing,** and **small cell** types. Small cell squamous carcinomas should not be confused with small cell anaplastic carcinomas, which resemble oat cell carcinoma of the lung and are generally associated with reduced survival rates.

3. **Variants of squamous cell carcinomas. Verrucous carcinoma** is a distinct type of extremely well differentiated squamous cell carcinoma that microscopically appears exophytic, with an undulating hyperkeratotic surface composed of rounded papillary projections that lack central fibrovascular cores. The lack of fibrovascular cores is particularly useful in discriminating these tumors from giant condylomata acuminata, which display prominent fibrovascular cores. **Papillary squamous cell carcinoma** is a rare variant of squamous carcinoma. The cells have the appearance of a high-grade squamous intraepithelial lesion with hyperchromatic nuclei and scant cytoplasm, resembling transitional cell carcinoma of the urinary bladder.

C. **Adenocarcinoma.** Grossly, cervical adenocarcinoma may appear as a polypoid or papillary exophytic mass. Conversely, diffuse cervical enlargement may be the only indication that an endophytic lesion is present. In approximately 15% of adenocarcinomas, the lesion is located entirely within the endocervical canal and escapes visual inspection. Histopathologically, cervical adenocarcinomas may exhibit a variety of glandular patterns composed of diverse cell types.

1. **Mucinous adenocarcinoma** is the most common type. Three histologic variants of mucinous adenocarcinoma may occur alone or in combination. Endocervical tumors tend to be well or moderately differentiated, and mucin production may be plentiful. Less common intestinal-type lesions and signet-ring–type lesions may occur.

2. **Endometrioid carcinoma,** accounting for up to 30% of cervical adenocarcinomas, is composed of cells resembling those of typical adenocarcinomas of the uterine corpus. Endometrioid carcinomas should be distinguished from endometrial adenocarcinoma extending to the endocervix, if possible.

3. **Clear cell carcinoma** accounts for approximately 4% of adenocarcinomas of the cervix. The gross appearance of these tumors varies from nodular, reddish lesions to small, punctate ulcers. Histologically, tumor cells are characterized by abundant, clear cytoplasm. Diethylstilbestrol

exposure is a risk factor, and clear cell carcinomas that develop in the absence of exposure occur most commonly in postmenopausal women.

4. **Minimal deviation adenocarcinoma,** or adenoma malignum, is reported to represent 1% of cervical adenocarcinomas. It is a well-differentiated tumor, characterized by cytologically bland but architecturally atypical glands that vary in size, shape, and depth of stromal penetration.

D. **Other malignant epithelial tumors**

1. **Adenosquamous carcinoma.** Primary cervical carcinoma with both malignant-appearing glandular and squamous elements is referred to as adenosquamous carcinoma. This entity should not be confused with adenocarcinoma and its histologically benign squamous differentiation. The clinical behavior of these tumors is controversial, with some studies suggesting lower survival rates and others higher survival rates than with the more common squamous tumors.

2. **Glassy cell carcinoma** represents approximately 1% of cervical cancers and is characterized by large cells with a distinctive "ground-glass" or granular cytoplasm. The prognosis and clinical course of these tumors are similar to those of other poorly differentiated carcinomas.

VII. **Treatment**

A. **General management by stage.** Surgery and radiation therapy are the two therapeutic modalities most commonly used to treat invasive cervical carcinoma. In general, primary surgical management is limited to disease of stages I and IIA. There are several advantages to surgical therapy that make it an attractive option, particularly for younger women. Surgery allows for a thorough pelvic and abdominal exploration, which can identify patients with a disparity between the clinical and surgicopathologic stages. These patients can be offered an individualized treatment plan based on their disease status. Surgery also permits conservation of the ovaries with their transposition out of subsequent radiation treatment fields. Radical hysterectomy results in vaginal shortening; however, with sexual activity, gradual lengthening will occur. Fistula formation (urinary or bowel) and incisional complications related to surgical treatment tend to occur early in the postoperative period and are usually amenable to surgical repair. Other indications for the selection of radical surgery over radiation include concomitant inflammatory bowel disease, previous radiation for other disease, and the presence of a simultaneous adnexal neoplasm.

Radiation therapy, on the other hand, can be used for all stages of disease and for most patients, regardless of age, body habitus, or coexistent medical conditions. Radiation therapy has evolved to include concurrent chemotherapy as a radiosensitizer, which results in improved disease-free progression and overall survival compared with radiation alone. Preservation of sexual function is significantly related to the mode of primary therapy. Pelvic irradiation produces persistent vaginal fibrosis and atrophy, with loss of both vaginal length and caliber. In addition, ovarian function is lost in virtually all patients undergoing tolerance-dose radiation therapy to the pelvis. Fistulous complications associated with radiation therapy tend to occur late and are more difficult to repair because of radiation fibrosis, vasculitis, and poorly vascularized tissues.

1. **Stage IA1.** The 5-year survival rate of these patients approaches 100% with primary surgical therapy. In the absence of lymph vascular space invasion, the incidence of pelvic lymph node metastases is 0.3%. Extrafascial hysterectomy is adequate treatment of this group of patients. Conization may be used selectively if preservation of fertility is desired, provided that the surgical margins are free of disease. Lymph vascular involvement increases the risk of pelvic node metastases to 2.6%. Pelvic lymphadenectomy and extrafascial hysterectomy should be performed in these cases. If enlarged pelvic nodes are encountered, the procedure can be converted to a modified radical hysterectomy (class II

hysterectomy; see later). In medically inoperable patients, stage IA carcinoma can be effectively treated with radiation.

2. **Stage IA2.** Microinvasive carcinoma with stromal invasion of 3.1–5.0 mm is associated with positive pelvic lymph nodes in 3.9–8.2% of cases. The preferred treatment of these lesions is modified radical (class II) hysterectomy with pelvic lymphadenectomy. In patients desiring preservation of fertility, radical trachelectomy with laparoscopic or extraperitoneal lymphadenectomy has been performed with success.

3. **Stages IB1, IB2, IIA.** Radical surgery (class III hysterectomy; see later) and adequate irradiation are equally effective in treating stages IB and IIA carcinoma of the cervix. Five-year survival rates of 85% for stage IB and 70% for IIA have been reported for both primary surgical and radiation treatment.

   Management of patients with bulky stage I disease (IB2) should be individualized. Most of the available survival data for cervical cancer were published before the FIGO subclassification of stage IB (IB1 and IB2). Expansion of the upper endocervix and lower uterine segment can distort cervical anatomy and lead to suboptimal placement of intracavitary radiation sources. Consequently, the central failure rate is 17.5% in patients with cervical lesions larger than 6 cm treated with irradiation alone. One approach is to combine external irradiation (4000 cGy) with a single intracavitary implant followed in 6 weeks by extrafascial hysterectomy. Although many clinicians confine the use of radical hysterectomy to patients with small IB tumors (less than 3–4 cm) or IIA lesions, there is evidence that acceptable survival rates can be obtained for patients with bulkier disease confined to the cervix with primary surgical treatment. Five-year survival ranges from 73.6% to 82.0% after radical hysterectomy and bilateral pelvic lymphadenectomy for cervical lesions larger than 4 cm. Survival decreases to 66% at 5 years for lesions larger than 6 cm.

4. **Stages IIB, III, IVA, IVB.** Radiation therapy is the treatment of choice for patients with stage IIB and more advanced disease. Radiation therapy for invasive cervical cancer is given as a combination of external and intracavitary therapy. The average total dose required to control disease within the treated area in 90% of cases ranges from 5000 cGy for lesions smaller than 2 cm to more than 8000 cGy for tumors exceeding 6 cm (Table 43-5). Long-term survival rates with irradiation therapy alone are approximately 70% for stage I disease, 60% for stage II disease, 45% for stage III disease, and 18% for stage IV disease. With the routine use of chemoradiation since the published reports of five

TABLE 43-5. SQUAMOUS CELL CARCINOMA OF THE CERVIX, DOSE-TUMOR VOLUME RELATION: AVERAGE DOSE OF RADIATION REQUIRED TO OBTAIN 90% CONTROL IN TREATED AREA

Tumor volume (cm)	Dose (cGy)
<2	5000
2	6000
2–4	7000
4–6	7500–8900
6	8000–10,000

From Shingleton HM, Orr JW. *Cancer of the cervix: diagnosis and treatment.* New York: Churchill Livingstone, 1995:160, with permission.

TABLE 43-6. TYPES OF ABDOMINAL HYSTERECTOMY

Type of surgery	Intrafascial	Extrafascial class I	Modified radical class II	Radical class III
Cervical fascia	Partially removed	Completely removed	Completely removed	Completely removed
Vaginal cuff	None removed	Small rim removed	Proximal 1–2 cm removed	Upper one-third to one-half removed
Bladder	Partially mobilized	Partially mobilized	Mobilized	Mobilized
Rectum	Not mobilized	Rectovaginal septum partially mobilized	Mobilized	Mobilized
Ureters	Not mobilized	Not mobilized	Unroofed in ureteral tunnel	Completely dissected to bladder entry
Cardinal ligaments	Resected medial to ureters	Resected medial to ureters	Resected at level of ureter	Resected at pelvic side wall
Uterosacral ligaments	Resected at level of cervix	Resected at level of cervix	Partially resected	Resected at postpelvic insertion
Uterus	Removed	Removed	Removed	Removed
Cervix	Partially removed	Completely removed	Completely removed	Completely removed

From Perez CA. Uterine cervix. In: Perez CA, Brady LW, eds. *Principles and practice of radiation oncology,* 2nd ed. Philadelphia: JB Lippincott Co, 1992, with permission.

randomized trials that all support the benefit of chemoradiation over radiation alone, long-term survival and disease-free progression are expected to increase for all stages of disease. Patients with stage IVB disease are usually treated with chemotherapy alone or chemotherapy in combination with local irradiation. These patients have a uniformly poor prognosis regardless of treatment modality.

B. **Surgical management**
  1. **Types of hysterectomy.** There are five distinct variations or classes of hysterectomy used in the treatment of cervical cancer (Table 43-6).
     a. **Class I** hysterectomy refers to the standard **extrafascial total abdominal hysterectomy.** This procedure ensures complete removal of the cervix with minimal disruption to surrounding structures (bladder, ureters).
     b. **Class II** hysterectomy is also referred to as a **modified radical hysterectomy.** This procedure involves dissection of the ureters from the parametrial and paracervical tissues down to the ureterovesical junction. This permits removal of all parametrial tissue medial to the ureters as well as the medial half of the uterosacral ligament and proximal 1–2 cm of vagina. This operation may be performed with pelvic lymphadenectomy.
     c. In **class III** hysterectomy or **radical abdominal hysterectomy,** the ureters are completely dissected from within the paracervical tunnel, and the bladder and rectum are extensively mobilized.

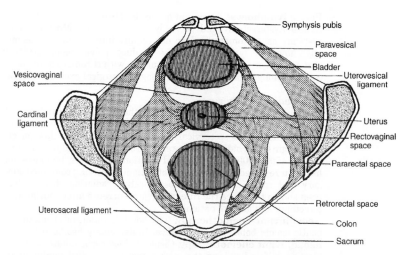

FIG. 43-3. The pelvic ligaments and spaces. (From Dunnihoo DR. *Fundamentals of gynecology and obstetrics*, 2nd ed. Philadelphia: JB Lippincott Co, 1992:28, with permission.)

Establishment of the paravesical and pararectal spaces facilitates the removal of all the parametrial tissue out to the pelvic side wall, complete resection of the uterosacral ligaments, and excision of the upper one-third to one-half of the vagina (Fig. 43-3). Bilateral pelvic lymphadenectomy may be performed either before or after radical hysterectomy, at the discretion of the surgeon.

    d. **Class IV and class V.** A class IV or **extended radical hysterectomy** includes removal of the superior vesical artery, periureteral tissue, and up to three-fourths of the vagina. In a class V or **partial exenteration operation,** the distal ureters and portion of the bladder are resected. Class IV and class V procedures are rarely performed today, because patients with disease extensive enough to require these operations can be more adequately treated using primary radiation therapy.

2. **Complications of radical abdominal hysterectomy**

    a. **Acute complications.** Modern surgical techniques and anesthesia have reduced the operative mortality rate to 0.6%. Febrile morbidity is common and is reported to occur in 25–33% of patients after radical hysterectomy. The major causes include pulmonary atelectasis, urinary tract infections, wound infections or hematomas, and pelvic cellulitis. Potentially lethal pulmonary embolism occurs in 1–2% of patients. Ureterovaginal and vesicovaginal fistulas occur in 2% and 0.9% of patients, respectively.

    b. **Bladder dysfunction** is the most commonly observed subacute and chronic complication after radical hysterectomy and results from partial denervation of the detrusor muscle during excision of the paracervical and paravaginal tissue. In the early postoperative period, patients experience a loss of bladder sensation and inability to initiate voiding. Various degrees of long-term urinary dysfunction are seen, ranging from a hypertonic low-compliance bladder to a hypotonic bladder subject to overdistension. Extensive paravaginal dissection may also result in a denervated, atonic urethra with resultant stress urinary incontinence.

c. **Pelvic lymphocyst** formation occurs in 2.0–6.7% of patients after radical hysterectomy and pelvic lymphadenectomy. Most lymphocysts are asymptomatic and do not require intervention. Occasionally, however, lymphocysts may produce pelvic pain, ureteral obstruction, or partial venous obstruction with thrombosis. In these cases, prolonged percutaneous drainage or surgical excision may be indicated.

3. **Surgical adjuvant therapy**
   a. **Postoperative adjuvant radiation** therapy has been advocated for patients with microscopic parametrial invasion, pelvic lymph node metastases, deep cervical invasion, and positive or close surgical margins. Morbidity is acceptable, provided the total dose is limited to 4500–5000 cGy in divided fractions. However, lymphedema has been reported in up to 23.4% of patients receiving combined surgery and radiation therapy. Postoperative radiation therapy has been shown to reduce the rate of pelvic recurrence after radical hysterectomy in high-risk patients.
   b. **Neoadjuvant chemotherapy.** The administration of chemotherapeutic agents before or after radical hysterectomy has been termed **neoadjuvant chemotherapy.** Cisplatin, bleomycin sulfate, and vinblastine sulfate has been the most extensively studied combination. Preoperative chemotherapy offers the advantage of increasing the operability of initially large, unresectable tumors. Complete clinical response rates range from 17% to 44%, with overall response rates of 80–90%. In addition to increasing surgical resectability, preoperative chemotherapy also decreases the number of positive pelvic lymph nodes and improves 2- and 3-year survival rates compared with historical controls. Chemotherapy after radical hysterectomy has also been advocated when histopathologic analysis reveals nodal metastases, lymph vascular space invasion, positive surgical margins, parametrial extension, or poorly differentiated histology; however, the long-term survival benefits of this approach are yet to be established.

C. **Radiation therapy.** External-beam irradiation is usually delivered from a linear accelerator. Thin patients can be treated with two opposing anteroposterior ports. Larger patients require the addition of two lateral ports to achieve optimal dose distribution within the pelvis. Once external therapy has been completed, brachytherapy can be delivered using a variety of intracavitary techniques, including intrauterine tandem and vaginal colpostats, vaginal cylinders, or interstitial needle implants.

1. **Dose.** Microscopic or occult tumor deposits from epithelial cancers require 4000–5000 cGy for local control. Clinically obvious tumor requires in excess of 6000 cGy.
   a. Two reference points are commonly used to describe the dose prescription for cervical cancer.
      (1) Point A is 2 cm lateral and 2 cm superior to the external cervical os.
      (2) Point B is 3 cm lateral to point A and corresponds to the pelvic side wall.
   b. The summated dose to point A (from intracavitary and external radiation therapy) believed to be adequate for central control is usually between 7500 and 8500 cGy.
   c. The prescribed dose to point B is 4500–6500 cGy, depending on the bulk of parametrial and side wall disease.
2. **Treatment volume** describes the tumor volume receiving the prescribed tumor dose, plus or minus 5%. The treatment volume is designed to encompass the primary tumor in the pelvis and its possible adjacent extensions, as well as the appropriate first- and second-echelon draining lymph nodes. The pelvis is usually treated to within acceptable tolerance of normal tissues.

3. **The borders** of the treatment field are as follows.
   a. The **inferior border** usually lies at the inferior aspect of the obturator foramina and encompasses the obturator nodes. If vaginal extension has occurred, the border is moved inferiorly to 2 cm below visible and palpable tumor.
   b. The **superior border** is usually between L4 and L5 or in the mid-vertebral level of L5. The reason to treat up to this level is to provide some dose to the common iliac nodes, although in most cases it is unclear whether additional therapeutic benefit results from taking the field up to the L5 level, as opposed to the L5 and S1 junction.
   c. The **lateral borders** are at least 1 cm (usually 2 cm) lateral to the margins of the bony pelvis, noted on a flat plate. Appropriate shielding along the common iliac nodes decreases the volume of normal tissue irradiated.
4. **Complications** of radiation therapy can be divided into acute (those occurring during or immediately after therapy) and chronic (those that occur months to years after completing therapy).
   a. **Acute complications of radiation therapy** include the following.
      (1) **Uterine perforation** may occur at the time of intracavitary therapy and, if unrecognized, may cause significant blood loss, radiation damage, and peritonitis. Ultrasonography or CT scanning can be used to locate the uterine tandem if perforation is suspected. Laparoscopy can also be used if perforation cannot be excluded by noninvasive studies. Appropriate management consists of removal of the implant and administration of broad-spectrum antibiotics if signs of infection are evident.
      (2) **Proctosigmoiditis** occurs in up to 8% of patients undergoing radiation therapy for cervical cancer, usually in those receiving more than 5000 cGy of external-beam radiation. Symptoms of proctosigmoiditis include abdominal pain, diarrhea, and nausea. Management consists of the use of antispasmodics, a low-gluten and low-lactose diet, and steroid enemas. Severe cases may require hyperalimentation and diverting colostomy.
      (3) **Acute hemorrhagic cystitis** occurs in approximately 3% of patients receiving radiation therapy for cervical cancer. Symptoms can usually be controlled with bladder irrigation, antispasmodics, and antibiotics as necessary.
   b. **Chronic complications of radiation therapy** include the following.
      (1) **Vaginal stenosis** has been reported in up to 70% of patients receiving radiation therapy for cervical cancer. The severity of stenosis can be minimized by continued sexual activity, use of vaginal dilators, and application of conjugated estrogen vaginal cream.
      (2) **Rectovaginal and vesicovaginal fistulas** each complicate approximately 1% of cases of cervical cancer treated with irradiation. Proctosigmoidoscopy or cytoscopy should be used to visualize the fistula site, and biopsy specimens should be taken from the edge of the fistula to rule out recurrent tumor. Diversion of the fecal stream (colostomy) or urinary stream (percutaneous nephrostomy) is usually required to allow adequate healing (3–6 months) before surgical repair. Bulbocavernosus or omental flaps can be used to provide a new vascular supply to the irradiated operative site.
      (3) **Small bowel obstruction** occurs in approximately 2% of patients undergoing definitive radiation therapy for cervical cancer and is more common in patients who have vascular disease or who have undergone previous abdominal surgery. The most common site of small bowel obstruction is the terminal ileum, which is relatively fixed within the radiation field by the cecum. Mild or partial small bowel obstruction can be treated conservatively with

nasogastric suction, blood and electrolyte replacement, and total parenteral nutrition. Complete small bowel obstruction or cases recalcitrant to conservative therapy require surgical treatment.

D. **Chemotherapy**

1. **Single-agent chemotherapy** is used to treat patients with extrapelvic metastases as well as those with recurrent tumor who have been previously treated with surgery or irradiation and are not candidates for exenteration. Cisplatin has been the most extensively studied agent and has demonstrated the most consistent clinical response rates. Although there is some variation among different studies, single-agent cisplatin therapy results in a complete response in 24% of cases, with an additional 16% of patients demonstrating a partial response. In most series, however, responses to cisplatin are short-lived (3–6 months). Ifosfamide, an alkylating agent similar to cyclophosphamide, has produced overall response rates as high as 29% in cervical cancer patients; however, such efficacy has not been confirmed by all investigators. Other agents demonstrating at least partial activity against cervical cancer include carboplatin, doxorubicin hydrochloride, vinblastine sulfate, vincristine sulfate, 5-fluorouracil, methotrexate sodium, and hexamethyl melamine.

2. The most active **combination chemotherapy** regimens used to treat cervical cancer all contain cisplatin. The agents most commonly used in combination with cisplatin are bleomycin, 5-fluorouracil, mitomycin C, methotrexate, cyclophosphamide, and doxorubicin. National Cancer Institute Gynecologic Oncology Group trials are currently under way comparing the efficacy of various chemotherapeutic combinations. The results of these trials are pending.

3. **Chemoradiation.** The use of chemoradiation has become widely recognized as providing survival benefit over radiation alone in the treatment of cervical cancer. The use of combined chemotherapy and radiation therapy is based on the theory of synergistic cell kill—the therapeutic effect of two treatment modalities used in combination is greater than if the effects of the two modalities individually were simply added together. When combined with radiation, weekly cisplatin administration reduces the 2-year risk of progression by 43% (2-year survival = 70%) for stage IIB through stage IVA cervical cancer. Similarly, for patients with bulky IB disease, the relative risk of progression of disease and death is 50% lower when patients are treated with weekly doses of cisplatin 40 mg/m^2 concurrent with radiation therapy than when they are treated with radiation alone. When used in this scenario, cisplatin appears to act as a radiosensitizer, yielding a large reduction in the rate of local recurrence and a more modest reduction in the rate of distant metastases.

E. **Posttreatment surveillance.** Among patients with recurrent cervical cancer, recurrence is detected within 1 year in 50% of cases and within 2 years in more than 80%. Pelvic examination and evaluation of lymph nodes, including supraclavicular nodes, should be performed every 3 months for 2 years and then every 6 months for an additional 3 years. Because over 70% of women with pelvic recurrence have abnormal cervical/vaginal cytologic findings, appropriate cytologic smears should be obtained at the time of each routine examination. An annual chest radiograph is indicated to detect pulmonary metastases. If a palpable pelvic mass is detected or symptoms suggest urinary obstruction, a CT scan of the abdomen and pelvis with intravenous contrast should be obtained to rule out recurrent tumor and delineate ureteral involvement. CT-guided fine-needle aspiration biopsy can then be performed to confirm recurrent disease.

F. **Treatment of recurrent cervical cancer.** Cervical cancer detected within the first 6 months after therapy is often termed **persistent cancer,** whereas that diagnosed later is usually referred to as **recurrent disease.**

TABLE 43-7. PREOPERATIVE CONTRAINDICATIONS TO EXENTERATION IN PATIENTS WITH RECURRENT CERVICAL CANCER

Absolute
  Extrapelvic disease
  Triad of unilateral leg edema, sciatica, and ureteral obstruction
  Tumor-related pelvic side wall fixation
  Bilateral ureteral obstruction (if secondary to recurrence)
  Severe, life-limiting medical illness
  Psychosis or the inability of the patient to care for herself
  Religious or other beliefs that prohibit the patient from accepting transfusion
  Inability of physician or consultants to manage any or all intraoperative and postoperative complications
  Inadequate hospital facilities
Relative
  Age older than 75 years
  Large tumor volume (>4 cm)
  Unilateral ureteral obstruction
  Metastasis to the distal vagina

Adapted from Shingleton HM, Orr JW. *Cancer of the cervix: diagnosis and treatment.* New York: Churchill Livingstone, 1995:265.

Appropriate treatment of recurrent cervical cancer is dictated by the site of recurrence and the modality of primary therapy. Generally, patients in whom recurrent cervical cancer develops after primary surgery should be considered for radiation therapy. Conversely, surgical treatment should be considered for those patients with recurrent disease who initially received irradiation. Patients who have had suboptimal or incomplete primary irradiation may be candidates for additional radiation therapy; however, the risk of urinary or enteric fistula formation is usually prohibitive. Distantly metastatic recurrent tumor is not amenable to therapy modality alone and is an indication for palliative chemotherapy, radiation therapy, or both.

Only patients with recurrent tumor confined to the central pelvis are candidates for surgical intervention. Total hysterectomy is inadequate treatment for patients who have centrally recurrent cervical cancer. Approximately 15% of patients with recurrent cervical cancer have a small-volume central pelvic recurrence. These patients can be treated with radical hysterectomy, which results in 5-year survival rates approaching 30–50%; however, the inability to accurately assess tumor volume may be associated with failure in situations in which a more radical procedure might have resulted in cure. In addition, radical hysterectomy after tolerance doses of radiation therapy is associated with a 20–50% rate of ureteral stricture, urinary fistula, and other serious complications. Therefore, pelvic exenteration is usually the procedure of choice for centrally recurrent cervical cancer.

   1. **Preoperative considerations.** A thorough investigation should be undertaken to rule out extrapelvic metastases. Abdominopelvic CT scan can identify enlarged para-aortic lymph nodes and liver metastases. Physical examination includes palpation of inguinal and supraclavicular lymph nodes. Fine-needle aspiration biopsy of suspicious areas should be performed, with CT guidance if necessary. Other contraindications are shown in Table 43-7. Pelvic side wall involvement may be difficult to

differentiate from radiation fibrosis on physical examination. Although many lesions may seem to be clinically nonresectable during examination, the philosophy of most gynecologic oncologists is that the operating room is the court of last resort; in the absence of documented extracervical disease, most women should be considered surgical candidates. In most series, approximately 25% of patients with recurrent cervical cancer are deemed satisfactory candidates for exenterative surgery. Thorough preoperative psychological and nutritional preparation is essential to optimize outcome.

2. **Operative approaches**

   a. **Anterior exenteration** is indicated for the treatment of recurrent cervical cancer limited to the cervix, anterior vagina, and bladder, or a combination. The procedure combines radical cystectomy with radical hysterectomy and vaginectomy. Negative findings on proctoscopic examination do not exclude tumor involvement of the rectal serosa or muscularis; consequently, the decision to limit the procedure to anterior resection must be based on intraoperative findings.

   b. **Posterior exenteration** combines abdominal perineal resection of the rectum with radical hysterectomy and vaginectomy and is indicated for lesions confined to the posterior fornix and rectovaginal septum. Using surgical stapling devices, low-rectal reanastomosis can be accomplished in approximately 70% of cases.

   c. **Total pelvic exenteration** is most often required for recurrent cervical cancer. The procedure involves the en bloc excision of the bladder, uterus, rectum, and vagina. A continent urinary diversion can be created using a segment of ascending colon and terminal ileum, with a buttressed ileocecal valve providing the continence mechanism (Indiana pouch, Miami pouch). Reconstruction of the pelvic floor can be accomplished with the use of an omental pedicle flap. A neovagina can be created by a variety of techniques, including gracilis or bulbocavernosus myocutaneous flaps. Vaginal reconstruction using a transverse or vertical rectus abdominus musculocutaneous flap or an omental J flap with split-thickness skin graft also gives excellent functional results and may reduce postoperative morbidity.

3. **Survival.** With modern surgical techniques and ICU support, perioperative mortality has not exceeded 7% in recent series. With proper patient selection and surgical judgment, 5-year survival rates after pelvic exenteration range from 45% to 61% in recent large series.

VIII. **Special problems**

A. **Cervical cancer in pregnancy.** Depending on the patient's socioeconomic status and the hospital's referral base, cervical cancer occurs in 0.02–0.90% of all pregnancies (1 in 110 to 1 in 5000). Conversely, 0.1–7.6% of all cervical cancer patients are pregnant at the time of diagnosis. Cervical cancer coincident with pregnancy requires complex diagnostic and therapeutic decisions that may jeopardize both mother and fetus.

   1. **Diagnosis.** Cervical cytologic screening should be part of routine antenatal care. Directed biopsy should be performed when high-grade intraepithelial lesions or microinvasion is suspected. Cervical conization is generally performed in pregnancy only for diagnostic, rather than therapeutic, purposes. Conization is indicated in any patient whose cytologic smear or biopsy results suggests invasive carcinoma when a diagnosis of invasive disease may result in a treatment or delivery modification. Conization should be performed only in the second trimester because of the increased risk of perioperative hemorrhage and spontaneous pregnancy loss (as high as 33%) associated with first trimester procedures.

   2. **Pretreatment evaluation.** Pregnant women with cervical cancer should undergo the same pretreatment metastatic evaluation as non-

pregnant women. It should be noted that urinary tract dilatation normally associated with pregnancy may mimic obstructive uropathy. Because the bimanual examination may be difficult in pregnancy, MRI may be useful to delineate extracervical disease while minimizing fetal radiation exposure.

3. **Treatment.** Traditionally, vaginal delivery of pregnant cervical cancer patients has been avoided because of the theoretical potential for dissemination of tumor cells during cervical dilatation. However, overall survival after vaginal delivery (52.9%) is not significantly different from that after abdominal delivery (46.1%). Although these data are not adjusted for gestational age and tumor volume, the risk of tumor dissemination is probably only theoretical. Hemorrhage remains a significant risk of vaginal delivery in patients with large cervical carcinomas, and in these cases abdominal delivery is advisable.

   a. **MICA.** In patients with stages IA1 and IA2 disease, there appears to be no harm in delaying definitive therapy until after fetal maturity has been attained. Patients with less than 3 mm of invasion and no lymph vascular space involvement may be followed to term and delivered vaginally. If delivery is by cesarean section, extrafascial hysterectomy can be performed at the time of delivery or after a delay of 4–6 weeks if further childbearing is not desired. Patients with 3–5 mm of invasion or lymph vascular invasion can also be safely followed until fetal maturity has been reached. In these cases, however, surgical treatment should include a modified radical hysterectomy with pelvic lymph node dissection performed either at the time of cesarean delivery or 4–6 weeks postpartum. Radiation therapy is associated with survival rates comparable to those after surgical treatment.

   b. **Stages IB1, IB2, and IIA.** In patients with large-volume cervical cancer, a delay in therapy in excess of 6 weeks may be detrimental to the mother's chance of survival. If the diagnosis is made after 20 weeks' gestation, consideration may be given to postponing therapy until fetal viability, as neonatal intensive care allows salvage rates of approximately 80% for infants born at 28 weeks. Standard treatment consists of classic cesarean delivery followed by radical hysterectomy and pelvic and para-aortic lymph node dissection; however, this procedure is associated with longer operative time and greater blood loss than in nonpregnant patients. Radiation therapy results in equivalent survival rates and may be preferable for patients who are poor surgical candidates.

   c. **Advanced-stage disease.** Radiation therapy is indicated for patients with stage IIB to IV disease and for poor surgical candidates with smaller-volume disease. When advanced carcinoma is diagnosed in the second trimester, consideration may be given to delaying therapy until fetal viability. If the fetus is viable, it should be delivered by classic cesarean section and radiation treatment begun postoperatively. When radiation therapy is used during the first trimester, the fetus should be left in situ, as spontaneous abortion will occur in 70% of cases before the administration of 4000 cGy. Pyometra occurs in infrequent cases.

4. **Prognosis.** Five-year survival is not significantly different for patients with stage I and stage II disease whether they are diagnosed during the first, second, or third trimester. Pregnancy has no known adverse effects on the ultimate survival of patients with cervical cancer. Diagnosis at a late gestational age or postpartum, however, is associated with more advanced clinical stage and correspondingly poor long-term survival rates.

B. **Preservation of fertility.** For patients desiring the preservation of fertility, radical trachelectomy with either laparoscopic or extraperitoneal lymph node dissection offers an alternative to radical hysterectomy for patients with stage IA2 through IB disease. Published series observe a 2-year disease-free survival rate of 95% and successful pregnancy rates of 33–100%. Late miscarriages occur in up to 25% of cases; however, placement of a cerclage at the time of operation may reduce the risk of both spontaneous loss and pre-term delivery.

C. **Incidental cervical carcinoma found at simple hysterectomy.** Occasionally, invasive cervical carcinoma is incidentally discovered in the surgical specimen after simple extrafascial hysterectomy has been performed. Unless disease is limited to stage IA1, microinvasive carcinoma (less than 3 mm) without lymph vascular involvement, simple hysterectomy is inadequate treatment, as the parametrial soft tissue, vaginal cuff, and pelvic lymph nodes may still harbor residual tumor. Additional treatment is dictated by the patient's age, the volume of disease, and the status of the surgical margins of resection.

1. **Surgery.** Although it may be technically difficult to perform an adequate radical resection after previous simple hysterectomy, reoperation should be considered in selected clinical situations, particularly for young patients in whom ovarian preservation is desired. Radical post–simple hysterectomy surgery for invasive cervical cancer generally includes radical parametrectomy, resection of the cardinal ligaments, excision of the vaginal stump, and pelvic lymphadenectomy. Use of postoperative adjuvant radiation therapy is dictated by surgical and pathologic findings. Survival after successful reoperation for patients with stage I disease is comparable to that for patients treated primarily with radical hysterectomy.

2. **Radiation therapy.** Cervical carcinoma at the margins of resection after simple hysterectomy and the presence of gross residual tumor are absolute indications for radiation therapy. These patients have a much less favorable prognosis than patients without residual tumor and patients with comparable disease who have been appropriately staged and treated with radiation alone. Survival after radiation therapy correlates with the volume of disease, the status of the surgical margins, and the delay between the performance of the simple hysterectomy and initiation of radiation treatments.

D. **Small cell carcinomas** of the uterine cervix are similar to small cell "neuroendocrine" tumors of the lung and other anatomic locations. These tumors are clinically aggressive, demonstrating a marked propensity to metastasize locally and to distant sites. At the time of diagnosis, disease is often widely disseminated, with bone, brain, and liver being the most common sites. Because of the high metastatic potential of small cell carcinomas, local therapy alone (surgery, radiation, or both) rarely results in long-term survival. Multiagent chemotherapy, in combination with external-beam and intracavitary radiation therapy, is the standard therapeutic approach. The two most commonly used chemotherapeutic regimes are vincristine, doxorubicin, and cyclophosphamide (Cytoxan), and etoposide and cisplatin.

E. **Bilateral ureteral obstruction and uremia** can occur secondary to lateral extension of cervical cancer within the pelvis. Women with ureteral obstruction resulting from untreated cervical cancer or recurrent disease after primary surgical therapy are candidates for radiation therapy. When there is no evidence of distant metastatic disease, urinary stents may be placed percutaneously and radiation therapy instituted with curative intent. If the ureteral obstruction precludes stent placement, urinary diversion may be accomplished by way of percutaneous nephrostomy tubes. In patients previously treated with maximum-dose radiation therapy, bilateral ureteral obstruction is due to radiation fibrosis in only 5% of cases; recurrent carcinoma is the cause of obstruction in the vast majority of patients. The management of patients with recurrent disease is more complex. Additional radiation therapy leads to troublesome fistula formation and bowel complications. Distant metastatic disease precludes exenterative surgery and limits the therapeutic options for these patients. Some have suggested that these patients should not undergo urinary diversion, as uremia may be a more preferable method of expiration than hemorrhage or progressive cachexia with severe pelvic pain. Nevertheless, ureteral stent placement or urinary diversion with percutaneous nephrostomy tubes is effective in alleviating bilateral obstruction.

F. **Cervical hemorrhage.** Profuse vaginal bleeding from large cervical malignancies is a challenging therapeutic situation. Generally, conservative measures to control cervical hemorrhage are preferable to emergency laparotomy and vascular (hypogastric artery) ligation. Attention must first be directed toward the stabilization of the patient with appropriate intravenous fluid and blood product replacement. Immediate control of cervical hemorrhage can usually be accomplished with a vaginal pack soaked in Monsel's solution (ferric subsulfate). Topical acetone (dimethyl ketone) applied with a vaginal pack placed firmly against the bleeding tumor bed has also been used successfully to control vaginal hemorrhage from cervical malignancy. Definitive control of cervical hemorrhage can be accomplished with external radiation therapy of 180–200 cGy/day if the patient has not previously received tolerance doses of pelvic irradiation. Alternatively, arteriography can be used to identify the bleeding vessel(s) and Gelfoam or steel coil embolization can then be performed. Vascular embolization has the disadvantage of producing a hypoxic local tumor environment and potentially compromising the efficacy of subsequent radiation therapy.

44. CANCER OF THE UTERINE CORPUS

Ginger J. Gardner and Frederick J. Montz

ENDOMETRIAL CANCER

I. **Epidemiology**
   A. **Incidence and mortality.** Endometrial cancer is the most common gynecologic malignancy and the fourth most common cancer in American women, with an estimated 36,100 cases occurring in 2000. Worldwide, endometrial cancer is the eighth most common malignancy, with an age-adjusted incidence four to five times lower in non-European countries or North America.

   The typical endometrial cancer patient is a postmenopausal white woman who presents with vaginal bleeding and is noted to have disease confined to the uterus. This stereotype illustrates the fact that endometrial cancer is more frequent in white than in African-American women. Similarly, three-fourths of endometrial cancer patients are postmenopausal at the time of diagnosis; 5% are younger than 40 years. Approximately 70% of affected women present with early-stage disease; the remainder present with advanced disease or with an especially aggressive variant. The overall 5-year survival rate for endometrial cancer in the United States is 83%, and approximately 6500 American women die of endometrial cancer yearly.

   B. **Risk factors and etiology.** In the majority of instances, endometrial cancer is a hormone-mediated process. Unopposed estrogenic stimulation of the endometrium is the final common pathway for most of the known risk factors (Table 44-1). Elevated estrogen levels may be a result of increased endogenous synthesis (i.e., granulosa cell tumors), decreased estrogen metabolism (i.e., hepatic disease), or an inappropriate hormone replacement regimen.

   Postmenopausal patients who are obese and nulliparous have a fivefold increased risk of developing endometrial cancer compared to patients without these risk factors. Diabetes is an independent risk factor in obese women. Hypertension and coronary artery disease are found in approximately 25% of patients with endometrial cancer, although they are not found to be independent risk factors after controlling for patient age and weight. African-American women have a lower overall incidence of endometrial cancer than white women. African-American women diagnosed with endometrial cancer have a higher mortality rate than patients from other ethnic groups. This may be due to the increased percentage of cases with high-risk cell types and advanced-stage disease, treatment differences, or sociodemographic factors.

II. **Disease prevention.** The primary method of disease prevention for endometrial cancer is to minimize risk factors and ensure appropriate detection and treatment of precursor lesions.

   A. **Avoidance of unopposed estrogens.** Hormone replacement therapy must contain adequate progesterone to counterbalance the estrogenic stimulation to the uterus.

   B. **Maintenance of ideal body weight**

   C. **Oral contraceptive use** decreases the risk of endometrial cancer. A 0.5% reduced risk of developing endometrial cancer for up to 10 years was demonstrated in women who had taken oral contraceptives for at least 12 months.

   D. **Abnormal bleeding and other symptoms should be promptly evaluated** by endometrial sampling. A patient who presents with abnormal vaginal bleeding has approximately a 20% chance of an underlying endometrial

TABLE 44-1. RISK FACTORS FOR ENDOMETRIAL CANCER

Unopposed or inadequately opposed estrogen therapy, tamoxifen therapy	Family history of breast, ovarian, or colon cancer, Lynch syndrome type II, hereditary nonpolyposis colorectal cancer
Obesity	Personal history of breast or colon cancer
Nulliparity	Hepatic failure
Early menarche or late menopause	Granulosa cell tumors of the ovary
Chronic anovulation	Polycystic ovary syndrome

hyperplasia or malignancy. Prompt evaluation is therefore necessary. (See sec. **III**, Diagnosis.)

E. **Appropriate treatment of a precursor lesion: endometrial hyperplasia.** Endometrial hyperplasia is associated with both the presence of and an increased risk of progression to endometrial cancer. The risk that endometrial hyperplasia will progress to endometrial cancer depends on the architectural complexity of the lesion and, to a greater extent, the presence of atypical cytologic findings.

1. **Simple hyperplasia and complex hyperplasia** can be treated with progestational agents and follow-up endometrial sampling.
2. **Hyperplasia with atypia** should be considered a premalignant lesion, especially when it occurs in postmenopausal patients. There is approximately a 2% risk of progression to carcinoma in patients without cytologic findings of atypia compared to a 23% risk in patients with cytologic findings of atypia. Simple extrafascial hysterectomy provides definitive therapy for atypical hyperplasia. Progestational agents can reverse many of these lesions, but progestin therapy must be continued as long as risk factors persist. This treatment strategy also requires serial endometrial biopsies to confirm therapeutic success. High progestin dosages may be required. Consequently, hormonal therapy is generally reserved for poor surgical candidates or for compliant patients who have a reasonable desire for future fertility.

III. **Diagnosis**

A. **Screening.** There are few uniform findings on physical examination or radiography associated with endometrial cancer. This fact underscores the necessity to promptly evaluate the endometrial lining of each patient who presents with symptoms. The frequent diagnosis of precursor and early-stage lesions in patients presenting with symptoms renders general population screening for endometrial cancer a low-yield activity and therefore not cost effective. A high-risk population that benefits from asymptomatic screening may exist. Although such a group could theoretically be identified by risk factor assessment, there are no definitive data to support any screening in an asymptomatic patient population.

B. **Symptoms.** At least 90% of patients with endometrial cancer present with symptoms. The following are the most frequently presenting symptoms.

1. **Abnormal vaginal bleeding,** including any postmenopausal bleeding (other than regular withdrawal bleeding on cyclic hormone replacement therapy), or any abnormal bleeding pattern in an at-risk premenopausal patient
2. **Abnormal vaginal discharge**
3. **Pelvic heaviness, crampiness, or pain**
4. **Reported abnormal Pap smear.** Glandular cells or endometrial cells on cervical cytologic examination should prompt further evaluation if cytologic atypia is present, the patient is postmenopausal, or the cells are shed out of cycle.

C. **Diagnostic techniques.** When a patient presents with symptoms, several diagnostic options are available.
   1. **Endometrial biopsy** (using a Pipelle or Curvette device) has demonstrated high sensitivity and specificity in detecting endometrial cancer and is generally well tolerated as an office procedure. The false-negative rate is less than 10%.
   2. **Endovaginal ultrasonography** is a useful evaluation tool for patients for whom an office endometrial biopsy is not feasible or is declined. Studies have demonstrated that no cases of endometrial neoplasia are present in postmenopausal women with an endometrial stripe of less than 5 mm; conversely, an endometrial stripe of more than 10 mm is associated with a 10–20% incidence of endometrial hyperplasia or malignancy. Therefore, patients with an endometrial stripe larger than 5 mm should undergo sampling.
   3. **Hysteroscopy** enables direct inspection of the uterine cavity and lining. Recent data, however, have demonstrated that hysteroscopic procedures lead to an increased incidence of malignant cells in peritoneal cytologic specimens at the time of surgical staging. The impact of this association on patient prognosis has not been defined.
   4. **Dilation and curettage** provides the most thorough screen for endometrial neoplasia. When symptoms persist or there is diagnostic uncertainty after endometrial biopsy or ultrasonography, an assessment should be made by dilation and curettage.
D. **Histologic analysis.** Endometrial malignancies are most commonly adenocarcinomas. The major histologic subtypes of endometrial cancer as classified by the World Health Organization in 1994 are described in the following subsections. Histologic review allows the tumors to be further subdivided into grades 1, 2, and 3, based on the degree of differentiation, percentage of solid growth, and amount of nuclear atypia.
   1. **Endometrioid** is the most common type of endometrial cancer, comprising 80% of endometrial cancers, the majority of which are well-differentiated (grade 1) lesions. It is the degree of architectural distortion and cytologic atypia that distinguishes endometrioid carcinoma from its precursor lesion, complex atypical hyperplasia. This distinction is subtle and is best determined by an experienced gynecologic pathologist.
   2. **Uterine papillary serous carcinoma (UPSC)** comprises up to 10% of endometrial malignancies. UPSC generally occurs in older parous women who are close to their ideal body weight. UPSC has a histologic appearance and clinical course similar to those of serous ovarian carcinoma and is considered to be highly aggressive. A papillary pattern is not unique to this type of endometrial cancer, as other cell types can develop papillary projections. Therefore, some authors suggest referring to UPSC simply as serous endometrial carcinoma. Clinically, UPSC has the propensity for intra-abdominal spread, even in cases with minimal or no myometrial invasion. Up to 30–50% of patients in whom intrauterine UPSC is confined to an endometrial polyp have extrauterine disease identified by thorough surgical staging. In those instances in which complete surgical staging demonstrates disease confined to the endometrial lining, the prognosis is more optimistic than previously thought. The prognosis and treatment scheme for UPSC is dependent on stage and underscores the importance of thorough surgical staging.
   3. **Clear cell carcinoma** comprise 2–3% of endometrial cancers. These tumors are histologically similar to those arising in the vagina, cervix, and ovary. An association between clear cell cancer of the endometrium and exposure to diethylstilbestrol has not been demonstrated. These tumors tend to be deeply invasive.
   4. **Pure squamous cell carcinoma** of the endometrium is extremely rare (0.1% of endometrial cancers). There is a strong association with cervical stenosis, pyometra, and chronic inflammation. Microscopically, squamous

TABLE 44-2. SURGICAL STAGING OF ENDOMETRIAL CANCER

Stage I	Confined to uterine corpus
IA	Limited to endometrium
IB	Invades <50% of the myometrium
IC	Invades >50% of the myometrium
Stage II	Involves uterine corpus and cervix
IIA	Limited to endocervix
IIB	Invades cervical stroma
Stage III	Regional tumor spread to the pelvis
IIIA	Invades serosa and/or adnexa and/or malignant cells found in peritoneal cytologic examination
IIIB	Vaginal metastases
IIIC	Metastases to pelvic and/or para-aortic lymph nodes
Stage IV	Advanced pelvic disease or distant metastases
IVA	Invades bladder and/or bowel mucosa
IVB	Distant metastases (upper abdomen, inguinal lymph nodes, supraclavicular lymph nodes, lungs, liver, bones, brain)

Each stage of disease is evaluated for the degree of cellular differentiation and assigned a grade. The grading system is based primarily on architectural findings, which are described by the percentage of solid tumor growth.

Grade 1	5% or less of a solid growth pattern
Grade 2	6–50% of a solid growth pattern
Grade 3	>50% of a solid growth pattern

Notable nuclear atypia raises the grade of the tumor by one level according to the 1988 grading system of the International Federation of Gynecology and Obstetrics.

carcinomas of the endometrium can be difficult to differentiate from squamous lesions of the cervix in a curettage specimen.
5. **Undifferentiated carcinomas** have a prevalence of 1–2% and, by definition, fail to show evidence of either glandular or squamous differentiation. These lesions are typically described as either large or small cell tumors. They behave similar to grade 3 endometrioid tumors.
6. **Mixed types** contain two or more pure types of tumor and comprise 10% of all endometrial cancers.
7. **Miscellaneous epithelial tumors.** Especially rare neoplasms of the uterus include glassy cell carcinoma, argyrophilic cell carcinoma, yolk sac tumor, and metastatic lesions. Choriocarcinomas, which may be endometrial in locale, are described separately in Chap. 46, Gestational Trophoblastic Disease.
IV. **Staging and prognosis**
   A. **Clinical staging.** Because clinical staging tends to underestimate the extent of disease, criteria for surgical staging were adopted in 1988 by the International Federation of Gynecology and Obstetrics (FIGO) (Table 44-2). *All patients are now surgically staged.* Comorbidities may limit the patient's capacity to tolerate a complete surgical staging procedure. In these cases, a stage is assigned based on the available surgical pathology and serves as a basis to discuss the appropriate adjuvant treatment options.

B. **Surgical staging** includes hysterectomy and bilateral salpingo-oophorectomy (BSO). A laparotomy or a vaginal approach with laparoscopic assistance is used. Peritoneal washings are collected and sent for cytologic evaluation. At a minimum, when extrauterine disease is grossly evident or when the patient is considered to be at risk for occult extrauterine disease, pelvic and para-aortic lymph node sampling is performed. Risk of occult extrauterine disease is determined by considering the grade and cell type of the lesion, the volume of the intrauterine malignancy, and the depth and extent of invasion (i.e., cervical involvement). Patients meeting any of the following criteria are at increased risk of nodal involvement: tumor size larger than 2 cm, more than 50% myometrial invasion, cervical involvement, nonendometrioid cell type, histologic grade 2 or 3, or palpably enlarged lymph nodes. Lymph node sampling, with its additional small although real surgical risk, is warranted in these patients. Similarly, patients with a well-differentiated, superficial endometrioid lesion do not benefit from routine lymph node sampling. For clear cell or serous tumors, an omentectomy is performed at the time of lymph node sampling because of the propensity for these subtypes of endometrial cancer to spread to the upper abdomen. After removal from the operative field, the uterus should be bivalved and rapid histologic sampling performed if the findings would modify the extent of the operative procedure.

C. **Prognostic factors. FIGO stage** is the most important prognostic indicator. Five-year survival rates are as follows: stage I, 86%; stage II, 66%; stage III, 44%; and stage IV, 16%. In addition, within a given stage of disease, a variety of clinical and histologic factors serve as additional prognostic variables:

1. **Depth of myometrial invasion**
2. **Malignancy of peritoneal washings**
3. **Histologic grade**
4. **Histologic type**
5. **DNA ploidy**
6. **Lymphatic space invasion**
7. **Tumor bulk**
8. **Estrogen and progesterone receptors,** when present, are independently favorable prognostic factors.
9. **Patient age.** Young patients tend to fare better than older patients.

V. **Types of endometrial carcinoma.** Epidemiologic and clinical data suggest that there may be two different forms of endometrial cancer (Table 44-3). Type I, representing well and moderately differentiated endometrioid carcinoma, is thought to result from an estrogen-dependent process that progresses from hyperplasia through cellular atypia to cancer. This type arises

TABLE 44-3. CHARACTERISTICS OF TYPES OF ENDOMETRIAL CARCINOMA

	Type I	Type II
Unopposed estrogen	Present	Absent
Hyperplasia	Present	Absent
Menopausal status	Pre- and perimenopausal	Postmenopausal
Racial predominance	White	African-American
Grade	Low	High
Myometrial invasion	Minimal	Deep
Histologic subtypes	Endometrioid	Serous, clear cell
Behavior	Stable	Aggressive

in younger, perimenopausal women with obesity, hyperlipidemia, and signs of hyperestrogenism. It is highly sensitive to progestins and carries a favorable prognosis (85% 5-year survival). Type II appears to arise de novo and is thought to be caused by one or more carcinogens. It can occur in patients with a genetic predisposition or prior pelvic radiation. Type II is a non–estrogen-dependent type and arises in women with few overt signs of hyperestrogenism. Type II endometrial cancer tends to be poorly differentiated with decreased sensitivity to progestins and has an overall poor prognosis (58% 5-year survival).

VI. **Clinical management**
   A. **Pretreatment evaluation** focuses on two primary issues:
      1. **Extent of disease.** Anticipating the degree of disease spread is important to plan the appropriate therapeutic intervention and informatively counsel the patient.
      2. **Operative risk of the patient.** Endometrial cancer is typically a disease of women in their fifties to seventies who have comorbidities that need to be appropriately managed before surgery.

         In a patient with endometrial cancer, the history should be taken and a physical examination performed; CBC, serum creatinine level, electrolyte levels, and blood glucose level should be measured; liver function tests and urinalysis should be carried out; and ECG, chest radiograph, endometrial biopsy, and endocervical curettage should be performed. Proctoscopy, barium enema, CT scan, or MRI should be reserved for clinical situations in which advanced disease is suspected, when a precise diagnosis is unclear, or when the findings could modify the recommended therapy.

   B. **Treatment of stage I and stage IIA disease.** The core of endometrial cancer treatment is surgical and includes a class I extrafascial hysterectomy with BSO. This alone is curative for most cases of localized disease. Lymph node sampling and omentectomy are performed in women at risk of occult extrauterine disease (see earlier). Patients with known cervical involvement should receive a class II radical hysterectomy, as this treatment improves 5-year survival compared to a class I simple hysterectomy.

      The final pathologic results determine whether or not a patient would benefit from adjuvant treatment. Patients determined to be at high risk of recurrence are offered postoperative pelvic radiation. Adjuvant radiation therapy for stage I or II disease has been shown to decrease local recurrence but has not been shown to improve overall survival. On the Kelly Gynecologic Oncology Service (KGOS), patients with negative lymph nodes but more than 50% myometrial invasion, grade 3 histology, nonendometrioid cell types, endocervical involvement (if a class II radical hysterectomy was not performed), or extensive lymph vascular space invasion are offered pelvic irradiation (typically, 5000 cGy external-beam radiation in fractionated doses). Some centers offer vaginal cuff radiation to patients with low- or intermediate-risk disease, although this is not routinely recommended on our service unless the patient had high-volume cervical disease.

      Poor surgical candidates with endometrial cancer are considered for primary radiation treatment. Historically, endometrial cancer was treated initially with radiation; however, this approach risks underestimation of disease spread and has an associated 15% decrease in cure rate compared to optimal surgical management.

   C. **Treatment of stage IIB disease.** The KGOS protocol for stage IIB disease includes a class II radical hysterectomy, BSO, and bilateral pelvic and para-aortic lymph node sampling. Radiation treatment is given postoperatively based on the risk for recurrence as described earlier for stage I and IIA disease.

   D. **Treatment of stage III disease.** In addition to surgical staging, tumor debulking should be performed (as for ovarian cancer). Surgical debulking has a proven survival advantage. Adjuvant treatment for stage III disease is controversial, and trials are ongoing. Off trial, patients with gross extrauterine disease but no positive nodes receive four cycles of doxorubicin hydrochloride (Adriamycin) and cisplatin if the tumor is endometrioid or carboplatin and paclitaxel (Taxol) if serous. Chemotherapy is followed by pelvic radiation. For intraperitoneal disease in which the lymph nodes are also positive, we offer radiation first, irradiating to the "next level up" for a clear port, and then give chemotherapy. If nodes only are positive (no intraperitoneal disease is identified), the current standard of care includes radiation only.

Patients with metastases to the vagina undergo partial vaginectomy at time of surgical staging. Patients with inoperable disease, including cases in which tumor extends to the pelvic side wall, receive a combination of intracavitary and external-beam radiation.

E. **Treatment of stage IV disease.** As with stage III disease, patients should first undergo surgical staging and tumor debulking. Adjuvant treatment is then provided on an individualized basis as described for stage III disease.

F. **Follow-up.** Most patients are evaluated at 3- to 6-month intervals for 2 years. The patient is assessed for the development of recurrent disease or for the development of a second primary tumor, especially breast cancer. After 2 years, the patient may be seen every 6 months to 1 year. Routine CT scans and chest radiographic studies do not effectively detect preclinical recurrences and should be reserved for the symptomatic patient.

There is currently no consensus on the use of hormone replacement therapy in patients after treatment for endometrial carcinoma. The use may be individualized, with the potential cardiovascular and skeletal benefits of hormone replacement therapy weighed against the theoretical risk of stimulating cancerous growth. The Gynecologic Oncology Group of the National Cancer Institute has a prospective randomized trial under way investigating this question.

VII. **Recurrent disease.** The overall survival rate of patients with recurrent endometrial cancer is less than 30%. Patients with recurrence have a better prognosis if their recurrence is a small, localized lesion that develops 3 years or more after the primary diagnosis and in a field that has not been previously irradiated. Treatment of recurrent disease is based on the location of the disease and the type of previous therapy. Surgery may be appropriate for selected patients with recurrent localized disease. Radiation therapy may be offered to patients who have not previously received it or to control symptoms at distant sites, such as bone or brain. Other patients should be treated with systemic chemotherapy or progestins.

UTERINE SARCOMAS

I. **Epidemiology.** Sarcomas of the uterus are a heterogeneous group of tumors that contain malignant mesodermal elements. These tumors comprise 3–5% of uterine malignancies and generally have a poor prognosis. The most common uterine sarcomas are carcinosarcomas (50%), followed by leiomyosarcomas (30%), and endometrial stromal sarcomas (15%).

A. **Carcinosarcoma (CS).** The median patient age at the time of diagnosis is 62 years. The risk factors for CS are similar to those for adenocarcinoma of the endometrium: nulliparity, obesity, and diabetes. Some evidence suggests, however, that CS is three times more common in African-American women than in white women, and up to 10% of patients with CS have a history of radiation therapy.

B. **Leiomyosarcoma (LMS).** Patients with LMS have an average age at diagnosis of 53 years. No clear risk factors have been identified, although 20% of patients with LMS are nulliparous.

C. **Endometrial stromal sarcoma (ESS)** is usually found in postmenopausal women, although younger women and girls may also be affected. No reliable risk factors have been identified.

TABLE 44-4. HOMOLOGOUS VERSUS HETEROLOGOUS SARCOMAS

	Homologous	Heterologous
Pure	Endometrial stromal sarcoma (endolymphatic stromal myosis)	Rhabdomyosarcoma
	Leiomyosarcoma	Chondrosarcoma
	Angiosarcoma	Osteosarcoma
	Fibrosarcoma	Liposarcoma
Mixed	Carcinosarcoma	Mixed mesodermal sarcoma
	Malignant mixed müllerian tumors, also called mixed mesodermal sarcoma, include both the homologous and heterologous mixed tumors.	

II. **Histologic characteristics.** Uterine sarcomas are traditionally categorized into pure and mixed sarcomas. Pure sarcomas contain only malignant mesodermal elements such as those arising from smooth muscle, endometrial stroma, blood vessels, or lymphatics. Mixed sarcomas contain not only sarcomatous elements, but also malignant epithelial elements. Pure and mixed sarcomas can be described as homologous (containing only elements native to the uterus) or heterologous (containing extrauterine tissue such as striated muscle) (Table 44-4). The presence of heterologous elements does not affect prognosis.

LMS must be distinguished histologically from other smooth muscle tumors, which include intravenous leiomyomatosis and disseminated peritoneal leiomyomatosis. In contrast to LMS, these tumors tend to be estrogen responsive and are often treated with progestins or with hysterectomy and oophorectomy. LMS also must be distinguished from leiomyomas of uncertain malignant potential, also called cellular myomas, which have fewer mitoses per high-power field and no cytologic atypia. Leiomyomas of uncertain malignant potential are treated by hysterectomy or myomectomy alone.

Endometrial stromal tumors are divided into endometrial stromal nodules, and the two malignant forms: low-grade ESS, and high-grade ESS. Endometrial stromal nodules are benign and have fewer than five mitoses per high-power field, pushing boundaries, minimal cytologic atypia, and no evidence of lymph vascular space invasion. Endometrial stromal nodules can be treated with hysterectomy or even localized resection. The low-grade sarcomas have a similar histologic appearance to endometrial stromal nodules, except that low-grade ESS demonstrates growth into lymphatic and vascular spaces, and high-grade ESS has greater cytologic atypia.

III. **Staging.** No official staging system exists for uterine sarcomas. By convention, the 1988 FIGO surgical staging system for adenocarcinoma of the endometrium is used.

IV. **Diagnosis**

A. **Carcinosarcoma.** Patients with CS most frequently present with postmenopausal bleeding. Many patients also have pelvic pain or an abnormal vaginal discharge. Half of affected women are found to have a polypoid mass, which often protrudes through the cervical os. Biopsy results usually confirm the diagnosis.

B. **Leiomyosarcoma.** Patients with LMS most frequently present with pain, pelvic pressure, or abnormal bleeding. LMS typically arises de novo, rather than from a preexistent leiomyoma. The symptoms and physical examination findings of patients with LMS are virtually indistinguishable from those of patients with benign myomas. The diagnosis of LMS is therefore usually made after hysterectomy. Only 0.7% of patients undergoing surgery for leiomyomata are found to have LMS. Patients may present with symptoms of distant metastasis such as cough, back pain, or ascites. Some postmenopausal patients with LMS present with a rapidly enlarging solitary fibroid. Evidence suggests that color-flow Doppler ultrasonographic studies may aid in the preoperative diagnosis of LMS, but the validity of this technique and its applicability to the general population remain to be demonstrated.

C. **Endometrial stromal sarcoma.** Patients with ESS usually present with abnormal uterine bleeding or pelvic pain. Although ESS can be entirely an intramural lesion, most such tumors involve the endometrial lining, so that the diagnosis can be made by endometrial biopsy.

V. **Management**

A. **Surgical exploration.** Surgery is the only proven effective treatment option to date for uterine sarcomas. Patients should be managed by exploratory laparotomy, total abdominal hysterectomy, BSO, peritoneal washings, and a complete tumor resection. Surgical staging, including omentectomy and lymph node sampling, offers prognostic information but has not been shown to affect survival. Surgical staging may influence postoperative decisions regarding the appropriate follow-up and adjuvant therapy.

B. **Adjuvant therapy**

1. **Carcinosarcoma.** For patients with stage I or II CS, the most effective adjuvant therapy remains controversial. A recent Gynecologic Oncology Group trial randomly assigned patients with optimally debulked CS to either whole abdominal and pelvic radiation therapy or to treatment with ifosfamide and cisplatin. Initial analysis suggests that adjuvant chemotherapy is warranted in these patients. On the KGOS, patients with advanced disease are treated with chemotherapy. If they have had subtotal resection, consideration is given to local radiotherapy.

2. **Leiomyosarcoma.** LMS tends to be resistant to both radiation and hormonal therapy. In women with grossly evident recurrent disease, treatment with doxorubicin and ifosfamide has shown a moderate (25%) response.

3. **Endometrial stromal sarcoma.** The clinical behavior of low-grade ESS is difficult to anticipate, and adjuvant treatment with either progestins or pelvic irradiation is warranted. Pelvic radiation is recommended for patients with stage I ESS. Patients with more advanced disease should receive progestins or tamoxifen citrate if their tumors are hormone receptor positive and doxorubicin-based chemotherapy if their tumors are hormone receptor negative.

VI. **Prognosis.** Stage appears to be the most important prognostic factor for uterine sarcomas. The 5-year survival rate is 50% for patients with stage I disease and only 20% when extrauterine disease is identified.

45. OVARIAN CANCER

Raquel Dardik, Linda Duska, and Robert Bristow

I. **Epithelial ovarian cancer** accounts for approximately 90% of all cases of ovarian cancer. The tumors are derived from the coelomic epithelium.
   A. **Epidemiology.** Ovarian cancer is the fifth most common malignancy in American women. In the United States, it is the leading cause of death from gynecologic cancer. Ovarian cancer is the seventh most common malignancy worldwide.
      1. **Incidence and mortality.** Ovarian cancer currently has the highest fatality to case ratio of all the gynecologic malignancies. In 2000, approximately 23,100 new cases of ovarian cancer were diagnosed, and 14,000 women died from their disease. For women in the United States, lifetime risk of developing the disease is approximately 1 in 70, or 1.4%. The occurrence of epithelial ovarian cancer is unusual in women younger than 40 years and peaks in women aged 60–64 years (Fig. 45-1). Although the overall incidence of ovarian carcinoma decreases in women older than 64 years, the age-adjusted incidence continues to rise. The incidence of ovarian cancer shows wide geographic variation, with the highest incidence rates (11.5–15.3 per 100,000 women) in Scandinavian countries, Israel, and North America, and the lowest rates (3.3–7.8 per 100,000 women) in developing countries and Japan. The incidence of ovarian cancer has remained stable over the last three decades in high-risk (developed) countries, whereas increasing incidence has been reported in low-risk (developing) countries (Fig. 45-2).
      2. **Risk factors.** The causes of ovarian cancer are poorly understood, but several factors have been associated with an increased or decreased risk of the disease.
         a. **Individual risk factors.** Age over 40 years, white race, nulliparity, infertility, history of endometrial or breast cancer, and family history of ovarian cancer consistently have been found to increase the risk of invasive epithelial cancer. Higher parity, use of oral contraceptive pills (OCPs), history of breast feeding, tubal ligation, and hysterectomy have been associated with a decreased risk of ovarian cancer. The relationship of a number of additional factors to the risk of ovarian cancer has not been well elucidated; these factors include age at menarche, age at menopause, use of fertility drugs, use of estrogen replacement therapy, talc use, dietary factors, lactose intolerance, and history of mumps and other infectious diseases.
         b. **Family history.** Patients with a family history of ovarian, breast, endometrial, or colon cancer are at increased risk of developing ovarian carcinoma. Although the lifetime risk of developing ovarian cancer in American women is estimated to be 1.4%, the risk increases to 5% in women with one first-degree relative with the disease and further to 7% when two first-degree relatives have ovarian cancer. Hereditary familial ovarian cancer accounts for approximately 5% of all newly diagnosed cases. Of these women, a large proportion have a mutation in the *BRCA1* or *BRCA2* gene. A subset of women with two first-degree relatives with ovarian cancer have one of the three distinct autosomal dominant syndromes that have been termed **familial ovarian cancer:** site-specific ovary, breast-ovary, and Lynch type II syndromes. (Lynch syndrome type II is a hereditary condition characterized by nonpolyposis colorectal cancers and associated endometrial and ovarian cancer.) These syndromes can

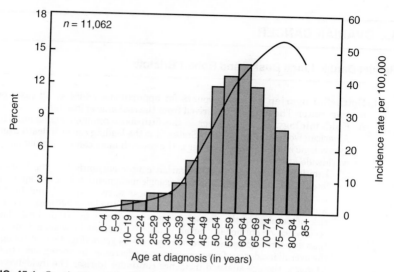

FIG. 45-1. Ovarian cancer incidence rates by age, 1973–1982. (From Yancik R, Ries LG, Yates JW. Ovarian cancer in the elderly: an analysis of Surveillance, Epidemiology, and End Results program data. *Am J Obstet Gynecol* 1986;154:639–647, with permission.)

involve the breast, ovary, colon, and endometrium. For a woman who has two or more affected first-degree relatives and whose family carries familial ovarian cancer, the risk of developing the disease has been estimated to be 40–50%. Hereditary ovarian cancer syndromes are rare, accounting for less than 1% of all reported ovarian cancer cases. The recent identification of the breast and ovarian cancer susceptibility genes (*BRCA1* and *BRCA2*) is an important advance in the field of genetic epidemiology. These genes have been linked to familial breast cancer and are linked to the breast-ovary and site-specific ovarian cancer syndromes. Women who are positive for *BRCA1* or *BRCA2* may have as much as a 50% risk of developing ovarian carcinoma. Furthermore, these women develop the disease at an earlier age than those women without the BRCA genes. Several genes for Lynch II syndrome have also been identified. Screening tests for these genes are available.

c. **Environmental factors** may play a role in ovarian cancer. An association between diet and ovarian cancer was suggested on the basis of the geographic variation of ovarian cancer incidence and mortality. Some have suggested that diets high in animal fat increase the risk of ovarian cancer. Decreased risk has been associated with higher total intake of vegetables, vitamin A, and vitamin C. An association between talc use and ovarian cancer has been proposed; the epidemiologic data, however, remain inconclusive.

d. **Reproductive factors** play an important role in ovarian cancer risk. Increasing parity decreases the relative risk of developing ovarian cancer. Conversely, nulliparity has been associated with an increased risk of ovarian cancer. The use of OCPs also has been associated with a decreased relative risk. Increasing duration of OCP use has been associated with decreasing risk, and evidence suggests that the protective effect of OCP use persists for 10 or more years after discontinuation of use. Women with a history of breast feeding have

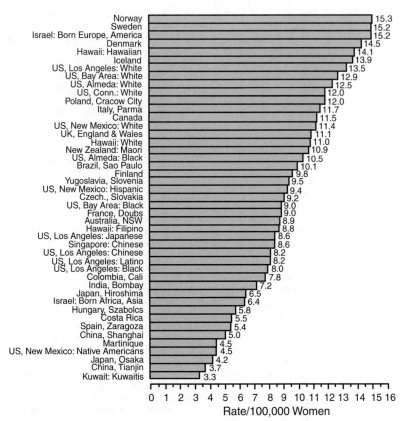

FIG. 45-2. Age-adjusted incidence rates of ovarian cancer in selected populations, 1978–1982. Rates adjusted to the world standard population. (From Tortolero-Luna G, Mitchell MF, Rhodes-Morris HE. Epidemiology and screening of ovarian cancer. *Obstet Gynecol Clin North Am* 1994;21:3, with data from Muir C, Waterhouse J, Mack T, et al. *Cancer incidence in five continents.* Lyon, France: International Agency for Research on Cancer, 1987:892–893, with permission.)

been reported to have a lower risk of ovarian cancer than nulliparous women and parous women who have not breast fed. Women with infertility have an elevated risk of ovarian cancer, independent of nulliparity. Although fertility drugs have been implicated in the development of ovarian cancer, their association has not been clearly separated from the risk that nulliparity and infertility confer. Tubal ligation or hysterectomy with ovarian preservation both lower the risk of ovarian cancer.

3. **Etiology.** The etiology of ovarian cancer is multifactorial. Three main hypotheses have been proposed to explain the pathogenesis: the incessant ovulation, gonadotropin, and pelvic contamination theories. The first two theories have received the most support from epidemiologic data. The possibility that a combination of these hypothetical causes occurs during the complex process of carcinogenesis has also been suggested, and future results from studies should help to clarify the issue.

a. **The incessant ovulation hypothesis** postulates that repeated minor trauma to the epithelial surface of the ovary, caused by uninterrupted ovulatory cycles, increases the likelihood of ovarian cancer. The protective effects of ovulation suppression by parity, OCP use, and lactation support this hypothesis. The differences in protective effect provided by pregnancy and OCP use, however, undermine this hypothesis.

b. **The gonadotropin hypothesis** postulates that exposure of the ovary to continuously high circulating levels of pituitary gonadotropin increases the risk of malignancy. This theory is supported by the protective effects of parity and OCP use and the increased risk observed with fertility drugs. This theory is undermined by the fact that premenopausal women develop ovarian carcinoma. In addition, the protective effect of lactation, which increases follicle-stimulating hormone, is inconsistent with the gonadotropin hypothesis. The lack of association of ovarian cancer with late age at menopause also is inconsistent with both the incessant ovulation hypothesis and the gonadotropin hypothesis.

c. **The pelvic contamination theory** suggests that carcinogens may come into contact with the ovary after passing through the genital tract. Although the protection afforded by tubal ligation and hysterectomy supports this hypothesis, the significant role of other reproductive factors is not explained by the pelvic contamination theory.

B. **Detection and prevention**

1. **Criteria for effective screening tools.** Early ovarian cancer is a silent and often asymptomatic disease. An effective screening test must have sufficient specificity, sensitivity, and positive predictive value for the disease it is used to detect. To be used to screen large populations of women, the screening test must also be cost effective. A sufficiently high positive predictive value is difficult to achieve for a disease with as low an incidence as ovarian cancer (compared with breast cancer, which occurs in 1 of 9 women, ovarian cancer occurs in 1 of 70). Currently, no available screening test has sufficient positive predictive value for early-stage ovarian cancer.

2. **Routine yearly pelvic examination** is currently in use for the general population as a screening tool. The rectovaginal pelvic examination, however, does not have sufficient sensitivity to diagnose early disease.

3. **Cancer antigen 125 (CA-125),** first described in the 1980s, is an antigen expressed by 80% of nonmucinous epithelial ovarian cancers. A level higher than 35 U/mL is considered abnormal. In premenopausal women, however, CA-125 levels may also be elevated in a number of benign conditions, including pelvic inflammatory disease, endometriosis, pregnancy, and hemorrhagic ovarian cysts. In addition, approximately 50% of women with early ovarian cancer have a normal CA-125 level. Other markers for ovarian cancer, such as carbohydrate antigen 19-1 (CA 19-9), CA-15-3, OVX1, *Her-2/neu,* and human chorionic gonadotropin (hCG) fragments, have been investigated. However, an appropriately sensitive and specific combination has not been identified.

4. **Transvaginal ultrasonography** also has been considered as a screening tool, in combination with color Doppler imaging. However, transvaginal ultrasonography has a poor positive predictive value when used to screen the general population. If the use of ultrasonography as a screening tool is limited to high-risk populations (postmenopausal patients or women with a significant family history), then 17 surgeries are required to find 1 case of stage I cancer. Multimodal screening using CA-125 measurement with sonography has been evaluated and found not to be efficacious as a general screening tool.

5. **Current recommendations for screening** include a comprehensive family history and annual rectovaginal pelvic examination for women with no significant family history of ovarian cancer. Women with two or

more first-degree relatives with ovarian cancer have a 3% chance of having a familial ovarian cancer syndrome, which carries a 40% lifetime risk of ovarian cancer; these women should be examined and counseled by a gynecologic oncologist. Women with a familial ovarian cancer syndrome should undergo annual rectovaginal pelvic examination, CA-125 determination, and transvaginal ultrasonography. Most authors agree that, after women at high risk of ovarian cancer complete their childbearing, they should consider a prophylactic oophorectomy. Participation in clinical trials for screening should be encouraged. *BRCA1/BRCA2* testing helps to identify patients at highest risk of hereditary ovarian cancer.

6. **Prevention**
   a. If a woman is undergoing pelvic surgery for other reasons, **prophylactic removal of the ovaries** may be considered to eliminate her risk of future ovarian cancer almost entirely (although the risk of peritoneal cancer still exists after removal of both ovaries). The associated risks of premature menopause, with its potential for bone loss and heart disease, must be weighed against the risk of developing ovarian cancer, as discontinuation of hormone replacement therapy is common.
   b. Because their use has been shown to be protective, a number of authors suggest encouraging the use of OCPs. High-risk groups may be the most appropriate candidates for **OCP prophylaxis.**
   c. **Investigational methods.** No chemoprophylactic agents are currently available for ovarian cancer. Research on numerous agents, however, including retinoids, may improve our armamentarium against ovarian cancer.

C. **Pathology of epithelial ovarian cancer.** Epithelial tumors are thought to arise from the surface epithelium of the ovary, which is closely related to the coelomic epithelium lining the peritoneal cavity. The tumors are classified by cell type and behavior as benign, atypically proliferating, or malignant. Atypically proliferating tumors are associated with a small risk of recurrence, may have invasive implants, and may decrease survival. Malignant tumors recur, metastasize, and decrease survival.

1. **Serous tumors.** The serous histologic subtype is the most common, accounting for 46% of all epithelial ovarian tumors. The mean age of patients at diagnosis is 56 years. The epithelium resembles the normal lining of the fallopian tube. Seventeen percent of serous tumors are atypically proliferating, and 33% are malignant. Thirty-three percent of atypically proliferating tumors are bilateral, and carcinomas are bilateral in 33–67% of cases.

2. **Mucinous tumors** are lined by cells that resemble the cells of the endocervical glands. Eighty percent of all ovarian mucinous tumors are benign; malignant mucinous ovarian tumors are quite rare. Less than 5% of mucinous tumors are malignant, and 16% are atypically proliferating tumors. The mean age of patients diagnosed with malignant tumors is 52 years. Mucinous tumors can become quite large, filling the abdominal cavity. Malignant tumors are commonly bilateral, although atypically proliferating mucinous tumors are bilateral in only 8% of cases.

3. **Endometrioid tumors** account for 6–8% of epithelial tumors, and most are malignant. Twenty percent may be atypically proliferating. The mean age of patients diagnosed with malignant tumors is 57 years. A significant proportion of cases have been associated with adenocarcinoma of the endometrium, and 10% of cases are associated with endometriosis.

4. **Clear cell carcinomas** account for 3% of ovarian cancers. These tumors are the ovarian neoplasms most commonly associated with paraneoplastic syndromes, including hypercalcemia and hyperpyrexia. Histologically, hobnail-shaped cells are characteristic of the clear cell

carcinomas. The mean age at diagnosis is 53 years. Bilaterality occurs in 13% of cases. Clear cell carcinomas also have been associated with endometrial cancer and endometriosis.

5. **Malignant Brenner tumors** are very rare and are defined as a benign Brenner tumor associated with an invasive component of another type of carcinoma.

D. **Pattern of metastasis.** Ovarian cancer can spread by direct extension, by exfoliation of cells into the peritoneal cavity (transcoelomic spread), via the bloodstream, or via the lymphatic system. The most common pathway of spread is believed to be transcoelomic. Cells from the tumor are shed into the peritoneal cavity and circulate, following the path of the peritoneal fluid up the paracolic gutters, along the intestinal mesenteries, and up to the diaphragm. Commonly, the omentum also is involved. Essentially all peritoneal surfaces are at risk. Lymphatic spread to the pelvic and para-aortic lymph nodes can occur. Hematogenous spread to the liver or lungs can occur in advanced disease.

E. **Clinical evaluation**

1. **Presentation.** Approximately 60% of patients diagnosed with epithelial ovarian cancer have advanced (stage III or greater) disease. Although some women with early disease experience symptoms, including pelvic pain or pressure, and urinary frequency, the majority of women are asymptomatic. When symptoms develop they are vague, and include abdominal bloating, early satiety, weight loss, constipation, anorexia, and irregular menstrual bleeding. On physical examination, a pelvic mass is an important sign of disease (Fig. 45-3). Some authors have suggested that a palpable ovary in a postmenopausal patient should be evaluated further, although this suggestion is controversial. In more advanced stages of disease, abdominal distention may develop, and chest examination may reveal evidence of pleural effusion.

2. **Evaluation of pelvic mass** varies depending on the patient's age, significant medical and family history, and the sonographic characteristics of the mass. After the decision to proceed to surgical evaluation is made, the preoperative evaluation should include a full history and physical examination, including a pelvic examination and a Pap smear. Additional tests such as a CBC, electrolyte levels and liver function tests, an ECG and chest radiograph, pulmonary function tests, arterial blood gas measurement, and echocardiogram should be performed on the basis of a patient's risk factors and underlying medical status. Consideration should be given to the possibility of metastatic disease. A barium enema or colonoscopy should be performed to rule out primary bowel disease, and in postmenopausal women a mammogram to evaluate for metastatic disease should be considered. Surgery should be preceded by a thorough preparation of the bowel. All patients undergoing surgery must have available a gynecologist capable of performing an adequate staging procedure.

F. **Staging.** Ovarian cancer is surgically staged. The assigned stage of disease is based on surgical and pathologic findings (Table 45-1). The importance of complete surgical staging in developing a proper treatment plan and prognosis cannot be overemphasized. In a cooperative national study in which 100 patients with apparent stage I and II disease underwent additional surgical staging, 28% of stage I disease and 43% of stage II disease was changed to a higher stage. Thus, with complete surgical staging approximately 31% of cases of apparent stage I or II disease were upstaged; in 75% of cases, disease was upstaged to stage III. The surgical staging procedure involves exploring the abdomen and pelvis through a vertical incision; taking washings from the pelvis, gutters, and diaphragm; taking multiple biopsy specimens from peritoneal sites, including pelvic side walls, surfaces of the rectum and bladder, cul-de-sac, lateral abdominal gutters, and diaphragm; removing the infracolic omentum; and sampling the pelvic and para-aortic

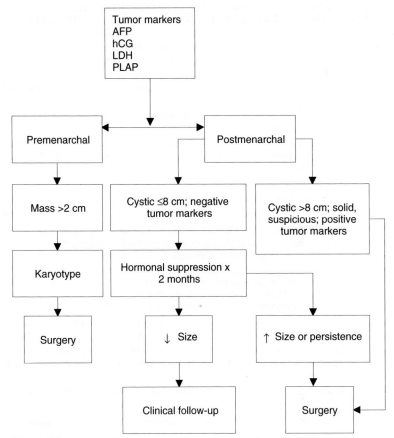

FIG. 45-3. Evaluation of a pelvic mass in young female patients. ↑, increased; ↓, decreased; AFP, alpha-fetoprotein; hCG, human chorionic gonadotropin; LDH, lactate dehydrogenase; PLAP, placental alkaline phosphatase. (From Berek JS, Hacker NF, eds. *Practical gynecologic oncology,* 2nd ed. Baltimore: Williams & Wilkins, 1994:381, with permission.)

      lymph nodes. In addition, a bilateral salpingo-oophorectomy is performed. Often a hysterectomy is performed in an attempt to remove existing disease, although it is not necessary for adequate staging.

  G. **Prognostic factors.** The overall 5-year survival rate of patients with ovarian cancer is 30%, but individual prognoses vary depending on stage, grade, histology of the tumor, and amount of residual disease remaining after initial debulking surgery.

    1. **Stage.** The 5-year survival rate of patients with epithelial ovarian cancer correlates directly with tumor stage. Patients with stage I disease have a 90% 5-year survival rate. This rate assumes that the patient has been surgically staged thoroughly and that microscopic disease in the abdomen has not been missed. Patients with stage II disease have a 5-year survival rate of 50–65%. Patients with stage III or IV disease have 5-year survival rates of 15–20% and less than 5%, respectively.

TABLE 45-1. STAGING OF PRIMARY CARCINOMA OF THE OVARY (INTERNATIONAL FEDERATION OF GYNECOLOGY AND OBSTETRICS, 1985)

Stage	Tumor characteristics
I	Growth limited to the ovaries.
IA	Growth limited to one ovary; no ascites; no tumor on the external surface; capsule intact.
IB	Growth limited to both ovaries; no ascites; no tumor on the external surfaces; capsule intact.
IC	Tumor either stage IA or IB but with tumor on surface of one or both ovaries; or with capsule ruptured; or with ascites present containing malignant cells; or with positive peritoneal washings.
II	Growth involving one or both ovaries with pelvic extension.
IIA	Extension or metastases to the uterus or tubes.
IIB	Extension to other pelvic tissues.
IIC	Tumor either stage IIA or IIB, but with tumor on surface of one or both ovaries; or with capsule ruptured; or with ascites present containing malignant cells; or with positive peritoneal washings.
III	Tumor involving one or both ovaries with peritoneal implants outside the pelvis and/or positive retroperitoneal or inguinal nodes. Superficial liver metastasis equals stage III. Tumor is limited to the true pelvis but with histologically proven malignant extension to small bowel or omentum.
IIIA	Tumor grossly limited to the true pelvis with negative nodes but with histologically confirmed microscopic seeding of abdominal peritoneal surfaces.
IIIB	Tumor of one or both ovaries with histologically confirmed implants of abdominal peritoneal surfaces, none exceeding 2 cm in diameter; nodes are negative.
IIIC	Abdominal implants >2 cm in diameter or positive retroperitoneal or inguinal nodes.
IV	Growth involving one or both ovaries, with distant metastases. If pleural effusion is present, cytologic findings must be positive to allot a case to stage IV. Parenchymal liver metastasis equals stage IV.

Adapted from Hoskins WJ, McGuire WP, Brady MF, et al. The effect of diameter if largest residual disease on survival after primary cytoreductive surgery in patients with suboptimal residual epithelial ovarian carcinoma. *Am J Obstet Gynecol* 1994;170:974–980, with permission.

2. **Grade and histologic type.** Histologic type historically has not been thought to be important in terms of prognosis. Some studies, however, have indicated that clear cell carcinomas are associated with a worse prognosis than other histologic cell types. Histologic grade is clearly a prognostic factor. The overall 5-year survival for patients with grade 1 epithelial malignancies is 40%, compared with 20% for those with grade 2 cancers and 5–10% for those with grade 3 cancers.
3. **Cytoreduction.** Debulking, also called *cytoreduction*, is defined as removal of as much tumor as possible during the initial operation. Optimal debulking implies that tumor nodules of no larger than 1 cm in diameter are left behind. Microscopic residual disease is the goal, how-

ever. Aggressive attempts at cytoreduction have been shown to improve long-term survival.

4. **Biological factors.** Tumor ploidy has been demonstrated to be an independent prognostic variable, with one study showing a median survival of 5 years for patients with diploid tumors, versus a median survival of 1 year for those with aneuploid tumors. Some studies have shown a correlation between proliferation fraction measured by flow cytometry and prognosis.

H. **Treatment** of epithelial ovarian cancer depends on the stage and grade of the disease, type of disease (primary or recurrent), prior treatment, and the patient's performance status.

1. **Atypically proliferating tumors** show a different behavior pattern than their malignant counterparts. Approximately 15% of all epithelial ovarian malignancies are atypically proliferating tumors. These tumors most commonly are of serous or mucinous histology. Unlike their malignant counterparts, atypically proliferating tumors are often found in younger patients, with mean patient age at diagnosis of approximately 40 years (compared with 61 years for malignant tumors). The majority of affected patients present with early-stage disease, although 20% show intra-abdominal spread, and should be treated with surgical staging and debulking as for epithelial malignant tumors. Mucinous atypically proliferating tumors may be associated with a concurrent appendiceal primary tumor, and affected patients also should undergo appendectomy. Because of the indolent growth of atypically proliferating tumors, controversy exists about the need for subsequent chemotherapy or radiation therapy. If disease recurs, it recurs an average of 10 years after initial diagnosis, and resection can be performed again at the time of recurrence. Most patients die with the disease rather than of the disease. In addition, early-stage disease in women who want to maintain fertility may be treated with unilateral salpingo-oophorectomy, or even with unilateral cystectomy, with good results. Patients who present with stage I disease have a 99% 5-year survival rate.

2. **Early-stage malignant disease** (stages I and II) may be divided into favorable and unfavorable categories. Patients with stage IA or IB disease and with grade 1 tumors are considered to have a favorable prognosis, with a 5-year survival of 94–96%. Patients with moderately or poorly differentiated tumors of any stage, stage IC disease, or stage II disease are considered to have an unfavorable prognosis. Patients with an unfavorable disease designation have a relapse rate of at least 20%.

   a. **Surgical therapy.** Initial surgical therapy is necessary for establishing a histologic diagnosis and appropriate staging. A full staging procedure is particularly important for patients with disease that appears to be confined to the pelvis. In approximately one-third of such patients, disease is upstaged by the results of a complete surgical evaluation. After a full staging procedure, approximately 40% of patients with epithelial ovarian cancer are found to have stage I or II disease. Patients with apparent stage I disease may wish to preserve the uterus and one ovary for future childbearing. If the tumor is localized and has favorable histologic characteristics (i.e., grade 1 tumor), such an option may be considered after appropriate counseling of the patient by a gynecologic oncologist. The remainder of the surgical staging should be performed, however, to ensure that the disease is indeed confined to the pelvis. After the procedure, the woman should be followed closely with pelvic examinations and CA-125 measurements. Total abdominal hysterectomy and bilateral salpingo-oophorectomy should be performed after childbearing is completed.

   b. **Chemotherapy.** For patients with early-stage disease and favorable prognostic factors, no chemotherapy is indicated. Patients with unfavorable prognostic factors should receive postoperative chemotherapy. Chemotherapy consists of multiagent treatment with a platinum-based regimen. The secondary agent usually is paclitaxel (Taxol). The appropriate chemotherapy regimen for patients with early-stage disease still is being evaluated in clinical trials.

  c. **Radiation.** Patients with early-stage disease have been treated with whole abdominal radiation or intraperitoneal radiocolloids (phosphorus 32). This treatment results in increased disease-free periods, but overall 5-year survival rates are identical with those after surgical therapy. Radiation therapy is very infrequently used today, however.

3. **Advanced disease** always requires an effort at optimal surgical debulking and a course of chemotherapy after initial surgery to improve patients' chances for survival.

  a. **Primary cytoreductive surgery,** or debulking, is the most important treatment of advanced disease. No universal agreement on the precise definition of optimal debulking has been reached. Different authors use different definitions of optimal in their measures of residual disease; these values range from 1–2 cm. The measurement of residual disease does not include the total volume of tumor cells left behind but merely the diameter of the largest residual nodule. For example, a patient with one unresected nodule measuring 2.5 cm has not undergone optimal debulking, whereas debulking is considered to be optimal in a patient with miliary studding of the entire peritoneal cavity with residual tumor implants. Although surgery has traditionally been performed before chemotherapy is begun, neoadjuvant chemotherapy followed by cytoreductive surgery is an appropriate alternative for patients whose performance status prohibits initial surgery. In addition, for patients in whom suboptimal debulking is likely, neoadjuvant chemotherapy has been used before surgery to attempt to increase the likelihood of optimal cytoreduction.

  b. **Combination chemotherapy** most often is used as postoperative treatment for advanced epithelial ovarian cancer. Combination chemotherapy with six courses of cisplatin or carboplatin plus paclitaxel is the treatment of choice for patients with advanced disease. A cycle is given every 3–4 weeks, with monitoring of tumor status by physical examination, measurement of CA-125 levels, and imaging studies if appropriate.

    (1) **Cisplatin** acts by binding to DNA and producing cross-links and DNA adducts. Important side effects include severe nausea and vomiting, dose-related nephrotoxicity, ototoxicity, peripheral neuropathy, and myelosuppression.

    (2) The mechanism of action of **carboplatin** is the same as that of cisplatin; the side effects, however, differ greatly. The most important side effect of carboplatin is thrombocytopenia. Leukopenia and anemia also occur but are less severe. Neurotoxicity and nephrotoxicity are less severe with carboplatin than with cisplatin. Other important side effects include alopecia and mucositis.

    (3) **Paclitaxel** acts as a mitotic spindle poison. Some patients exhibit hypersensitivity to paclitaxel. Other important side effects include myelosuppression, neuropathy, mucositis, diarrhea, alopecia, nausea, and vomiting.

  c. **Whole abdominal radiation** may be used as an alternative to chemotherapy, although it is not widely employed as a first-line treatment in the United States. Radiotherapy is most effective in patients who have no macroscopic residual disease after primary debulking. Acute side effects include fatigue, nausea, and vomiting. Long-term side effects are more severe and include bowel damage resulting in obstruction, which sometimes requires surgical therapy.

d. **New therapies.** Disappointingly low long-term survival rates in patients with advanced epithelial ovarian cancer have stimulated continued innovation in treatment approach. Experimental first-line postoperative treatments include concomitant chemotherapy and radiation therapy and dose-intensity strategies using autologous bone marrow transplant or peripheral stem cell support. Newer medications including vinorelbine tartrate (Navelbine) and doxorubicin hydrochloride (Doxil), which is a liposomal doxorubicin, are currently used for salvage therapy. Other new chemotherapeutic ideas for salvage include weekly single-agent regimens of paclitaxel or gemcitabine hydrochloride, as well as some new phase I drugs identified only by numbers. Alternative modalities, including biologic therapy using autologous tumor-infiltrating lymphocytes and monoclonal antibodies, are also under investigation.

e. **Second-look laparotomy** is performed in an experimental setting on patients with advanced epithelial ovarian cancer who have undergone primary debulking followed by a course of chemotherapy and who have no clinical evidence of disease. The technique is identical to that of the staging laparotomy and requires multiple peritoneal biopsies and washings if no gross disease is apparent. Laparoscopy can also be used to perform second looks, which decreases morbidity. Biopsy specimens from the peritoneal surfaces in the areas of previously documented tumor are most important to obtain because they are most likely to show a positive result. In 50% of patients, clinically occult disease appears on surgical exploration. For these patients, further treatment is indicated. Patients with persistent gross disease may be candidates for secondary cytoreduction. Of patients with negative findings on second-look laparotomy, 20–50% experience recurrence of disease. Consolidation treatment should be considered in these patients. Patients with negative findings on second-look laparotomy have a 5-year survival rate of 50%, compared with a rate of 5–35% for patients with a positive finding on second-look laparotomy. The use of second-look laparotomy (or laparoscopy) in the management of advanced epithelial ovarian cancer remains controversial. Second-look laparotomy has not been shown to affect patient survival and therefore should be performed only in the setting of a clinical trial, not as routine care for all patients.

f. **Second-look laparoscopy** may be performed as an alternative to second-look laparotomy. Visibility may be limited, however, by the presence of intra-abdominal adhesions. In addition, in laparoscopic procedures the operator is unable to perform a manual exploration of the entire bowel or the peritoneal cavity. Decreased patient morbidity and improved recovery time make laparoscopy an attractive option. The role of second-look laparoscopy is still being defined.

g. **Second-line chemotherapy.** Patients with persistent gross disease should be treated with second-line chemotherapy. However, response rates for second-line chemotherapy are only 10–30%. Depending on the initial chemotherapy, second-line chemotherapy may include platinum, paclitaxel, ifosfamide, or hexamethylmelamine. Regardless of the approach, chemotherapy in this setting is not curative.

h. **Appropriate follow-up for asymptomatic patients** after completion of primary surgery and a full course of chemotherapy should include routine history and physical examination, rectovaginal examination, and CA-125 testing. As discussed in sec. **I.H.3.e,** the role of second-look laparotomy is a subject of controversy. Patients should be seen every 3 months for the first 2 years. In patients whose CA-125 level was elevated preoperatively, CA-125 is a reliable marker of disease recurrence (although a negative CA-125 test result does not guarantee disease absence). The combination of thorough physical examination and CA-125 testing has been shown to detect recurrent disease in 90% of patients.

4. **Recurrent or persistent disease**
   a. **Secondary debulking.** Patients with recurrent or persistent disease may be candidates for further surgical therapy, or secondary cytoreduction. Surgery should be reserved for patients in whom therapy has a good chance of prolonging life or palliating symptoms; those with the longer disease-free intervals are the best candidates for secondary cytoreduction. The majority of patients with persistent or progressive disease after primary therapy do not benefit from secondary debulking, and at this time no effective salvage treatment is available for patients with recurrent or persistent disease.
   b. **Salvage chemotherapy.** Response rates for second-line chemotherapy are in the range of 10–30%. For women with recurrent disease resistant to platinum who have not received paclitaxel, it is the best salvage therapy currently available. Some interest has been shown in intraperitoneal chemotherapy; the complete response rate for intraperitoneal chemotherapy, however, is only 10–20%. Most commonly, intraperitoneal cisplatin is used. An intraperitoneal catheter must be surgically placed for intraperitoneal chemotherapy administration. Complications can occur with the catheter. In addition, patients with dense peritoneal adhesions are not candidates for intraperitoneal therapy because the drug cannot be distributed evenly. Newer approaches with weekly paclitaxel treatments are currently under way.
   c. **Whole abdominal radiation** was used in the past as a salvage therapy. It may be effective in patients with microscopic disease, but it is associated with high intestinal morbidity. Thirty percent of patients develop intestinal obstruction after whole abdominal radiation.
   d. **Hormone therapy** has been used as salvage treatment. Both megestrol acetate (Megace) and tamoxifen have been used in experimental protocols to treat recurrent disease. Response rates have been low: 15% and 45%, respectively.
   e. **Experimental protocols**
      (1) **Stem cell therapy.** Clinical trials are under way using high-dose chemotherapy regimens followed by autologous bone marrow transplant, although initial results have been disappointing.
      (2) **Immunotherapy.** Interferon has been found to have some activity in patients with minimal residual disease. Studies are being done with cytokines, tumor necrosis factor, and interleukin-2. Vaccine trials are under way, but results are not yet available.
      (3) **Genetic therapy.** Currently, experimental protocols are using adenovirus vectors administered intraperitoneally to correct deficits in tumor suppression oncogenes.
5. **Complications of advanced ovarian cancer**
   a. **Intestinal obstruction.** Many women with ovarian cancer develop intestinal obstruction, either at initial diagnosis or with recurrent disease. Obstruction may be related to mechanical blockage or carcinomatous ileus. Correction of intestinal obstruction at initial treatment is usually possible; obstruction associated with recurrent disease, however, is a more complex problem. Some of these obstructions may be treated conservatively with intravenous hydration, total parenteral nutrition, and gastric decompression. The decision to proceed with palliative surgery must be based on the physical condition of the patient and her expected survival. If patients are unable to undergo surgery or are judged to be poor operative candidates, placement of a percutaneous gastric tube may offer some relief.

      b. **Ascites.** Initial ascites on presentation with ovarian cancer is almost always improved by debulking surgery and several courses of chemotherapy. Persistent ascites is difficult to manage and is a very poor prognostic sign. Installation of bleomycin sulfate into the peritoneal cavity has been tried with limited success. Ascites is best managed by repeated paracenteses as needed and chemotherapy, if possible, for the patient's tumor.

I. **Survival**

    1. **Atypically proliferating tumors.** Overall survival of patients with atypically proliferating tumors is excellent. Unlike patients with epithelial malignancies, most patients with borderline tumors die with their disease rather than of their disease. Ten- and 20-year survival rates are 95% and 90%, respectively.

    2. **Early-stage malignant disease.** The 5-year survival rates for patients who are appropriately surgically staged with stage I or stage II disease are 80–100%, depending on the tumor grade.

    3. **Advanced disease.** The 5-year survival rate for patients with stage IIIA tumors is 30–40%. Patients with stage IIIB disease have a 5-year survival rate of 20%, and patients with stage IIIC and stage IV disease have a 5-year survival rate of 5%. Recall that approximately 60% of patients have at least stage III disease on presentation.

    4. **Recurrent disease.** Patients with no evidence of disease at second-look laparotomy have a 5-year survival rate of 50% (recall that most patients who undergo second-look laparotomy initially presented with stage III or higher disease). In contrast, patients with microscopic residual disease have a 5-year survival rate of 35%, and those with macroscopic residual disease have a 5-year survival of 5%.

    5. **Age.** Regardless of disease stage, patients younger than 50 years have a better 5-year survival than patients older than 50 years.

    6. **Performance status.** Patients whose Karnofsky index is low (less than 70) have a significantly shorter survival time than those with a Karnofsky index higher than 70.

J. **Peritoneal carcinoma.** The primary malignant transformation of the peritoneum is termed **primary peritoneal carcinoma** or **primary peritoneal papillary serous carcinoma,** and clinically and pathologically resembles serous carcinoma of the ovary. Primary peritoneal carcinoma therefore can appear to cause ovarian cancer in patients with a history of oophorectomy or with pathologically normal-appearing or minimally involved ovaries. Extensive upper abdominal disease is common, and clinical course, management, and prognosis are similar to those for epithelial ovarian cancer. Because this malignancy is ten times less common than ovarian cancer, there have been no large clinical trials on management of this disease. Although it is staged and treated in the same manner as ovarian carcinoma, no consensus exists on whether this malignancy behaves like its ovarian counterpart.

K. **Ovarian cancer in pregnancy** is very rare. Atypically proliferating tumors were present in 35% of these cases, epithelial cancers in 30%, dysgerminoma in 17%, granuloma cell tumor in 13%, and undifferentiated carcinoma in 5%. Seventy-four percent of patients were diagnosed with stage I disease. Early-stage disease can be treated with conservative surgery in the second trimester of pregnancy, usually with good maternal and fetal results. Late-stage and high-grade disease should be treated aggressively after appropriate counseling of the patient.

II. **Nonepithelial tumors of the ovary** are rare, compared with epithelial tumors, and account for 10–15% of cases of ovarian cancer.

A. **Germ cell tumors** (Fig. 45-4)

    1. **Epidemiology.** Twenty percent to 25% of all tumors of the ovary are of germ cell origin, but only 3% of these are malignant. Germ cell malignancies account for fewer than 5% of all cases of ovarian cancers in the

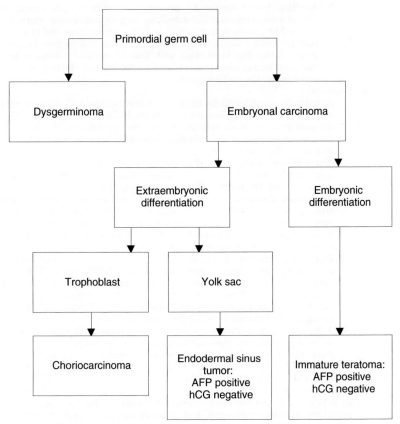

FIG. 45-4. Origin of malignant germ cell tumors and their markers. AFP, alpha-fetoprotein; hCG, human chorionic gonadotropin.

United States. In the first two decades of life, however, 70% of ovarian tumors are of germ cell origin and one-third are malignant. Germ cell tumors are quite rare after the third decade of life.

2. **Pathology.** Germ cell tumors are derived from the primordial germ cells of the ovary.

3. **Diagnosis.** Clinically, germ cell malignancies grow quickly and often are characterized by acute pelvic pain. The pain can be caused by distention of the ovarian capsule, hemorrhage, necrosis, or torsion. Adnexal masses that are 2 cm or larger in premenarchal girls or 8 cm or larger in premenopausal patients necessitate surgical exploration. Measurement of tumor marker levels may assist in the diagnosis of germ cell malignancies (Figs. 45-3 and 45-4).

4. **Preoperative workup** should include measurement of serum hCG and alpha-fetoprotein titers and lactate dehydrogenase levels, a CBC, and liver function tests. A chest radiographic study is important to rule out pulmonary metastases. A preoperative CT scan should be considered to assess for the presence or absence of liver metastases and retroperitoneal lymphadenopathy.

5. **Specific tumor types**
   a. **Dysgerminoma**
      (1) **Incidence.** Dysgerminoma is the most common germ cell tumor, comprising 30–40% of ovarian cancers of germ cell origin. In patients younger than 20 years, dysgerminoma accounts for 5–10% of ovarian cancers. Seventy-five percent of dysgerminomas occur in the second decade of life. Five percent of dysgerminomas occur in phenotypic female patients with gonadal dysgenesis. In these patients, the dysgerminoma may arise in a gonadoblastoma. More than 50% of gonadoblastomas left in situ in patients with gonadal dysgenesis have been reported to develop into malignancies.
      (2) **Diagnosis and presentation.** The diagnosis and presentation of dysgerminoma is typical of germ cell tumors in general.
      (3) **Treatment.** Primary treatment is surgical and should include proper surgical staging. A vertical midline incision should be used. Unilateral oophorectomy is performed. The remaining pelvic organs may be left in situ if maintenance of fertility is desired. A careful staging operation should be performed to rule out the presence of microscopic disease. Unilateral pelvic lymphadenectomy and para-aortic lymphadenectomy should be performed. A Tru-Cut biopsy of the contralateral ovary with frozen section should be performed, and the ovary should be removed only if disease is present. Dysgerminomas are very sensitive to radiation therapy; however, fertility is lost as a consequence of irradiation. Therefore, chemotherapy is the first-line treatment. Usually, combination therapy with three agents is used (one example is bleomycin, etoposide, and cisplatin, or BEP). Recurrent disease can be treated with radiation or chemotherapy.
      (4) **Prognosis and survival.** Seventy-five percent of patients with dysgerminomas present with stage I disease, and 85–90% of tumors are confined to one ovary. Ten percent to 15% of tumors are bilateral. The tumor spreads via the lymphatic system most commonly, although it also can spread via capsule rupture or via the bloodstream. For patients with stage IA disease, unilateral oophorectomy results in a 5-year disease-free survival rate of 95% or better. The survival rate for patients with advanced disease treated with surgery followed by combination chemotherapy is 85–90%.
   b. **Immature teratomas** contain tissues resembling those in an embryo.
      (1) **Incidence.** Pure immature teratoma accounts for 1% of ovarian malignancies but is the second most common ovarian germ cell tumor. In women younger than 20 years, immature teratomas comprises 10–20% of ovarian malignancies. Fifty percent of pure immature teratomas occur in female patients between the ages of 10 and 20 years.
      (2) **Diagnosis and presentation.** Test results for tumor markers are usually negative; some tumors may contain calcifications similar to those in mature teratomas.
      (3) **Treatment.** If the tumor appears to be confined to one ovary and the patient desires fertility, a unilateral oophorectomy and surgical staging is performed. A full staging operation, including total abdominal hysterectomy and bilateral salpingo-oophorectomy, should be performed in women who have completed childbearing. Biopsy of the contralateral ovary is unnecessary because immature teratoma is rarely bilateral. Chemotherapy should be used for any patient who has disease more advanced than stage I, grade 1. Combination platinum-based chemotherapy is the treatment of choice. (BEP is the combination of choice.)

(4) **Prognosis and survival.** Immature teratomas are graded from 1 to 3, based on the degree of differentiation of the most immature tissue present and the quantity of immature tissue. The most important prognostic factor is the grade of the tumor. Tumors with malignant squamous elements seem to have a poorer prognosis than tumors without malignant squamous elements. In addition, if the tumor is incompletely resected, survival drops from 94% at 5 years to 50%. The overall 5-year survival rate for patients with disease at all stages is 70–80%. The 5-year survival rate for grade 1 tumors is 82%, compared with 62% and 30% for grades 2 and 3, respectively.

c. **Endodermal sinus tumors** (yolk sac tumors) are derived from cells of the primitive yolk sac.

(1) **Incidence.** Endodermal sinus tumors are the third most frequently encountered malignant germ cell tumor of the ovary. Median age of presentation is 18 years. One-third of patients are premenarchal.

(2) **Diagnosis and presentation.** Abdominal and pelvic pain are the presenting symptoms in 75% of patients. Asymptomatic pelvic mass occurs in 10% of patients. Most endodermal sinus tumors secrete alpha-fetoprotein.

(3) **Treatment** consists of surgical exploration with unilateral salpingo-oophorectomy. Performing hysterectomy and contralateral salpingo-oophorectomy does not alter outcome. Gross metastatic disease should be resected and surgical staging performed, although most patients require subsequent chemotherapy. Cisplatin-based combination chemotherapy such as BEP is used for adjuvant therapy.

(4) **Prognosis and survival.** Most patients have early-stage disease at diagnosis. The 2-year survival rate is 60–70%.

d. **Embryonal carcinoma**

(1) **Incidence.** Embryonal carcinoma is extremely rare. Patients are very young, ranging in age from 4 to 28 years (median, 14 years). Embryonal tumors may secrete estrogen.

(2) **Presentation** is similar to that of endodermal sinus tumors. Because embryonal tumors may produce estrogen, patients may present with precocious pseudopuberty or irregular vaginal bleeding. Primary lesions tend to be large, and two-thirds of lesions are confined to the ovary. Embryonal lesions secrete alpha-fetoprotein and hCG.

(3) **Treatment** is unilateral oophorectomy, followed by combination platinum-based chemotherapy. Radiation is not useful.

e. **Choriocarcinoma**

(1) **Incidence.** Pure, nongestational choriocarcinoma of the ovary is extremely rare.

(2) **Diagnosis and presentation.** Almost all patients are premenarchal. The tumor often produces high levels of hCG. Isosexual precocious puberty is seen occasionally.

(3) **Treatment** is surgical excision, followed by combination chemotherapy.

(4) **Prognosis** is poor, because most patients have metastatic disease on presentation.

f. **Mixed germ cell tumors** contain characteristics of two or more of the germ cell tumors discussed earlier. The most common component is dysgerminoma. Lesions should be managed with combination chemotherapy. Prognosis depends on the size of the initial tumor and the relative amount of the most malignant component of the lesion.

B. **Sex cord stromal tumors** are derived from the sex cords and mesenchyme of the embryonic gonad and account for 5% of all ovarian tumors and 2% of cases of ovarian cancer.

1. **Granulosa cell tumor.** The granulosa cell tumor is the most common malignant sex cord stromal tumor. Granulosa cell tumors account for 2–3% of all ovarian malignancies. In the majority of cases, the tumor is estrogenic. Two forms exist: an adult form and a much rarer juvenile form. The tumor is bilateral in only 2% of cases. Histologically, the likely origin of these tumors is the normal granulosa cells of the coelomic epithelium.

   a. **Incidence.** Adult granulosa cell tumors occur in the perimenopausal years. Patients' mean age at presentation is 57 years. The highest incidence is in the immediate postmenopausal age group, women aged 51–60 years.

   b. **Diagnosis and presentation.** Patients may present with abdominal distention, pain, or a mass. Because most granulosa cell tumors produce estrogen, patients may present with a variety of menstrual irregularities. The incidence of concurrent endometrial hyperplasia is 50%, and the incidence of concurrent endometrial adenocarcinoma is at least 5%. The majority of affected patients present with stage I disease, mainly because the hormonal effects of the tumor cause symptoms early in the disease.

   c. **Treatment.** Surgery alone is usually sufficient treatment only for disease of stage IA or IB. For all other stages, chemotherapy is required. Radiation, chemotherapy, or both are used for recurrent disease. If the patient desires to maintain fertility, a unilateral salpingo-oophorectomy is adequate for treating stage IA tumors, and a staging operation also should be performed. If the patient has completed her childbearing, a total abdominal hysterectomy and bilateral salpingo-oophorectomy should be performed. If the uterus is left in situ, dilation and curettage should be performed to rule out endometrial hyperplasia or adenocarcinoma. Chemotherapy after surgery does not prevent recurrence of the disease.

   d. **Prognosis and survival.** Granulosa cell tumors have a propensity for late recurrence, with recurrence reported as many as 30 years after treatment for primary tumor. The 10-year survival rate is 90%, and the 20-year survival rate drops to 75%.

2. **Sertoli-Leydig cell tumor**

   a. **Incidence.** Sertoli-Leydig cell tumors account for only 0.2% of cases of ovarian cancer. Sertoli-Leydig cell tumors are diagnosed most commonly in the third and fourth decades of life. Seventy-five percent of Sertoli-Leydig cell lesions are present in women younger than 40 years. The tumors are most frequently low-grade malignancies.

   b. **Diagnosis and presentation.** Sertoli-Leydig cell tumors often produce androgens. Seventy percent to 85% of patients demonstrate clinical virilization.

   c. **Treatment.** In young patients, unilateral salpingo-oophorectomy may be performed to preserve fertility. In older patients, a total abdominal hysterectomy and bilateral salpingo-oophorectomy should be performed.

   d. **Prognosis and survival.** The 5-year survival rate is 70–90%.

C. **Sarcomas.** Malignant mixed-mesodermal tumors of the ovary are extremely rare. The lesions are very aggressive, and no effective treatment exists.

D. **Metastatic tumors** account for 5–8% of ovarian malignancies.

   1. **Metastatic gynecologic tumors** may involve the ovaries. Tubal carcinoma involves the ovaries by direct extension in 13% of cases. Cervical cancer very rarely spreads to the ovaries (less than 1% of cases). Endometrial cancer may metastasize to the ovaries; more often, however, synchronous endometrioid adenocarcinoma is the primary lesion that involves the ovary and the endometrium.

TABLE 45-2. SURGICAL STAGING OF FALLOPIAN TUBE CANCER

Stage	Characteristics
I	Carcinoma confined to fallopian tube(s)
IA	Unilateral disease; no ascites
IB	Bilateral disease; no ascites
IC	Either IA or IB with ascites and/or neoplastic cells in peritoneal washings
II	Carcinoma extending beyond fallopian tube(s) but confined to pelvis
IIA	Extension to uterus and/or ovary
IIB	Extension to other pelvic organs
IIC	Either IIA or IIB with ascites and/or neoplastic cells in peritoneal washings
III	Carcinoma extending beyond pelvis but confined to abdominal cavity
IIIA	Tumor microscopic only
IIIB	Tumor metastasis ≤2 cm
IIIC	Tumor metastasis >2 cm
IV	Carcinoma extending beyond abdominal cavity

Adapted from Podratz KC, Podczaski ES, Gaffey TA, et al. Primary carcinoma of the fallopian tube. *Am J Obstet Gynecol* 1986;154:1319.

2. **Metastatic breast cancer.** Among women who die of metastatic breast cancer, the ovaries are involved in 24% of cases. Most metastases to the ovaries from a primary breast cancer are bilateral.

3. **Gastrointestinal cancers** may metastasize to the ovary. Krukenberg's tumor accounts for 30–40% of metastatic tumors to the ovary. The metastasis is almost always bilateral and is characterized histologically by signet-ring cells, in which the nucleus is flattened against the cell wall by the accumulation of cytoplasmic mucin. One percent to 2% of women with intestinal cancer have ovarian metastases at the time of presentation. In postmenopausal women undergoing evaluation for an adnexal mass, metastatic colon cancer should be ruled out if possible, using colonoscopy.

4. **Metastatic carcinoid tumors** are very rare. If an ovarian carcinoid tumor is diagnosed, it is necessary to search for an intestinal primary cancer.

5. **Lymphomas** of the ovary are usually metastatic and bilateral. Burkitt's lymphoma may affect children or young adults. Rarely, ovarian lesions are the primary manifestation of disease in lymphoma patients.

III. **Fallopian tube cancers**

A. **Epidemiology.** Carcinoma of the fallopian tube is a very rare tumor, accounting for 0.3–1.0% of cases of genital tract cancer in women. Carcinoma of the fallopian tube is seen most often in the fifth and sixth decades of life, and affected patients present at a mean age of 55–60 years.

B. **Histology.** To confirm a diagnosis of fallopian tube cancer histologically, most of the tumor must be present in the fallopian tube, the mucosa of the tube must be involved, and a demonstrable transition from benign to malignant tubal epithelium must exist.

C. **Clinical presentation and diagnosis.** The classic triad of symptoms of fallopian tube carcinoma is watery vaginal discharge, hydrops tubae profluens, pelvic mass, and pelvic pain. Most patients, however, do not present with this triad. Vaginal discharge or bleeding is the most common presenting symptom. As in ovarian cancer, presentation may be nonspecific. Ascites may be present if the disease is advanced. Unlike ovarian cancer, fallopian tube carcinoma more often presents at an early stage.

D. **Natural history and patterns of spread.** Tubal cancers spread in a similar fashion to ovarian cancers. The main route of spread is transcoelomic.

E. **Staging.** The ovarian cancer staging system has been adapted for the fallopian tube. Twenty percent to 25% of patients have stage I disease on presentation, 20–25% have stage II, 40–50% have stage III, and 5–10% have stage IV (Table 45-2).

F. **Treatment** is similar to that of ovarian cancer, with surgical debulking the mainstay of treatment, followed by combination platinum-based chemotherapy. Chemotherapy for early-stage disease is the subject of controversy. In addition, the use of second-look laparotomy for primary fallopian tube carcinoma is controversial and should occur only in the setting of clinical trials.

G. **Prognosis and survival.** The overall 5-year survival rate for fallopian tube cancer is 40%. Prognosis is related to the stage of disease.

46. GESTATIONAL TROPHOBLASTIC DISEASE

Christine P. Nguyen and Robert Bristow

GESTATIONAL TROPHOBLASTIC DISEASE

I. **General features.** Gestational trophoblastic disease (GTD) is a group of neoplasms derived from placental trophoblastic tissue. GTD includes **hydatidiform mole, invasive mole, placental site trophoblastic tumor, and choriocarcinoma.**

   A. **Hydatidiform mole.** In the United States, hydatidiform moles are observed in approximately 1 in 600 therapeutic abortions and 1 in 1000–2000 pregnancies. Approximately 20% of patients with primary hydatidiform mole develop sequelae, that is, persistent GTD (invasive mole, choriocarcinoma, placental site trophoblastic tumor).

   B. **Invasive mole** is the most common sequela of hydatidiform mole, representing 70–90% of cases of persistent GTD. Up to 20% of invasive moles metastasize to extrauterine pelvic and distant sites (e.g., lungs).

   C. **Choriocarcinoma.** In the United States, choriocarcinoma occurs in 1 in 20,000–40,000 pregnancies. Approximately 50% of gestational choriocarcinomas develop after term pregnancies, 25% after molar gestations, and 25% after abortion or ectopic pregnancies.

   D. **Placental site trophoblastic tumor (PSTT)** is the most uncommon form of persistent GTD. PSTT accounts for approximately 1% of all cases of persistent GTD.

   E. The reported **incidence** of hydatidiform mole and choriocarcinoma varies widely throughout the world, with the highest rates found in Asia, Africa, and Latin America. Significantly lower rates are seen in North America, Europe, and Australia. Despite methodologic differences in studies calculating the incidence of GTD, it appears that developing countries do have a higher rate of GTD than Europe and North America. It has also been suggested that low socioeconomic conditions or dietary factors may contribute to the development of GTD.

   F. **Risk factors.** An increased risk of a complete hydatidiform mole is present at both extremes of reproductive age. Women older than 40 years have a 5.2-fold increased risk, whereas women younger than 20 years have a 1.5-fold increased risk. Persistent GTD also occurs more frequently in older patients. An obstetric history of spontaneous abortion is more common in patients with GTD than in women without such a history. A history of prior hydatidiform mole increases the risk of having a subsequent hydatidiform mole by 20-fold. With two prior hydatidiform molar pregnancies, the risk is increased 40-fold. Conversely, term pregnancies and live births have a protective effect. Nonwhite race is also a risk factor and is associated with an increased risk of 1.8- to 2.1-fold. An association has been reported between ABO blood group and choriocarcinoma, but not hydatidiform mole. Among patients with choriocarcinoma, blood group A is the most prevalent, and blood group O is the least prevalent.

II. **Placental anatomy and physiology.** Three distinctive types of trophoblastic cells have been recognized: cytotrophoblast, syncytiotrophoblast (ST), and intermediate trophoblast (IT). Each of these cell types is responsible for producing hormones specific to the placenta.

   A. **Morphology of normal trophoblast**

      1. **Cytotrophoblasts** are germinative, primitive trophoblastic cells that are polygonal to oval in shape, with a single nucleus and well-defined cell borders. Mitotic activity is evident.

TABLE 46-1. CLINICAL COMPARISON OF COMPLETE VERSUS INCOMPLETE HYDATIDIFORM MOLE

	Complete	Incomplete
Gestational age	8–16 wks	10–22 wks
Uterine size		
Large for gestational age	33%	10%
Small for gestational age	33%	65%
Diagnosis by ultrasonography	Common	Rare
Theca lutein cysts	25–35%	Rare
β human chorionic gonadotropin (mIU/mL)	>50,000	<50,000
Malignant potential	15–25%	<5%
Metastatic disease	17%	<1%

2. **Syncytiotrophoblasts** are highly differentiated cells that interface with the maternal circulation and produce most of the placental hormones. No mitotic activity is evident.

3. **Intermediate trophoblasts** show infiltrative growth into decidua, myometrium, and blood vessels dissecting the normal cells. IT characteristically invades the wall of large vascular channels until the wall is completely replaced. IT is the predominant cell of placental site trophoblastic tumors and exaggerated placental sites.

B. **Hormones** produced by the placenta include **human chorionic gonadotropin (hCG), human placental lactogen (hPL), estradiol, progesterone, and placental alkaline phosphatase (PLAP).** Most of these products are confined to the ST. The ST starts producing hCG at 12 days' gestation and maximizes its production by 8–10 weeks' gestation, after which the secretion steadily declines. By 40 weeks' gestation, hCG is present only focally in ST. Human placental lactogen also is localized in ST at 12 days' gestation and increases steadily thereafter. IT contains abundant hPL, which appears as early as 12 days after conception and peaks at 11–15 weeks of gestation. The hCG is present only focally in IT, appearing as early as 12 days' gestation and remaining until 6 weeks' gestation, at which time it disappears. Cytotrophoblast does not contain either hCG or hPL.

III. **Hydatidiform mole** is a noninvasive abnormal placental neoplasm characterized by enlarged, edematous, and vesicular chorionic villi accompanied by variable amounts of proliferative trophoblast. Hydatidiform mole is categorized as complete or partial based on gross characteristics, histologic findings, and karyotype (Table 46-1).

A. **Complete mole**

1. **Clinical features.** Complete moles typically present between 11 and 25 weeks' gestation, with an average gestational age of 16 weeks. Vaginal bleeding is the most common presenting symptom, occurring in 97% of cases, followed by excessive uterine enlargement, in 50% of cases. Severe vomiting (hyperemesis gravidarum) is seen in 25% of cases; pregnancy-induced hypertension in 25% of cases; and hyperthyroidism in 7% of cases. In approximately 33% of patients, the uterus is small for gestational date. Ovarian enlargement caused by multiple theca lutein cysts occurs in 25–35% of cases. Levels of hCG β-subunit (β-hCG) are typically above 50,000 mIU/mL, and ultrasonography often discloses a classic "snowstorm" appearance.

2. **Pathologic features.** Gross findings include massively enlarged, edematous villi that give the classic grape-like appearance to the placenta. Gross

characteristics include **lack of embryonic tissue.** Cases in which a fetus is present represent twin gestation, one of which is molar and the other a normal conceptus. Pathologic features include hydropic swelling in the majority of villi, accompanied by a variable degree of trophoblastic proliferation. Complete moles have widespread, diffuse immunostaining for hCG; moderately diffuse staining for hPL; and focal staining for PLAP.

3. **Chromosomal abnormalities.** Most complete moles are diploid, with a 46,XX karyotype; rare examples of triploid or tetraploid moles have been reported. In most cases, all of the chromosomal complements are paternally derived. In the diploid complete mole, the XX genotype results from duplication of a haploid sperm pronucleus in an empty ovum that has lost its maternal chromosomal haploid set. Three percent to 13% of complete moles have a 46,XY chromosome complement, presumably as a result of dispermy, in which an empty ovum is fertilized by two sperm pronuclei, one with an X and the other with a Y chromosome.

B. **Incomplete mole**

1. **Clinical features.** Incomplete, or partial, moles account for 25–74% of all molar pregnancies and occur between 9 and 34 weeks' gestation. Patients with partial moles may have signs and symptoms that are similar to those of patients with complete moles, but usually such symptoms are absent. Uterine size is generally small for gestational date; excessive uterine size is observed in only 4% of patients. Patients present with abnormal uterine bleeding in approximately 75% of cases. A clinical diagnosis of a missed or spontaneous abortion is made in 91% of cases of incomplete molar pregnancy. Serum hCG levels are in the normal or low range for gestational age. Preeclampsia occurs with lower incidence (2.5%) and presents much later with a partial mole than with complete moles, but can be equally severe.

2. **Pathologic features.** The partial mole has two populations of chorionic villi, one of normal size and the other grossly hydropic. On gross examination, the amount of tissue found is less than that found in a complete mole. Fetal tissue is nearly always present, although its discovery may require careful examination, because early fetal death is the rule (8–9 weeks' menstrual age). Partial moles show focal to moderate immunostaining for hCG and diffuse staining for hPL and PLAP.

3. **Chromosomal abnormalities.** Karyotypes of partial moles most frequently show triploidy (69 chromosomes), with two paternal sets and a maternal chromosome complement. The chromosomal complement is XXY in 70% of cases, XXX in 27% of cases, and XYY in 3% of cases. The abnormal conceptus in these cases arises from the fertilization of an egg with a haploid set of chromosomes either by two sperm, each with a set of haploid chromosomes, or by a single sperm with a diploid 46,XY complement.

IV. **Management of molar pregnancy**

A. **Workup.** The pathologic diagnosis of a hydatidiform mole is made from the findings of dilation and curettage (D & C) performed for an incomplete abortion or because of clinical suspicion of hydatidiform mole based on clinical findings (physical examination, β-hCG levels, ultrasonography). The following laboratory studies should be performed preoperatively:

1. Hematologic studies (CBC).

2. Prothrombin time, partial thromboplastin time.

3. Comprehensive panel of blood chemistry tests, including liver function tests.

4. Blood type and screen [any Rh-negative patient must be given Rh_0 (D) immune globulin (RhoGAM)].

5. Quantitative β-hCG level.

6. Chest radiograph.

B. **Treatment.** The primary treatment for hydatidiform mole is suction D & C.

1. The following steps should be taken before suction D & C:

a. Stabilization of medical complications (see sec. **IV.D**)

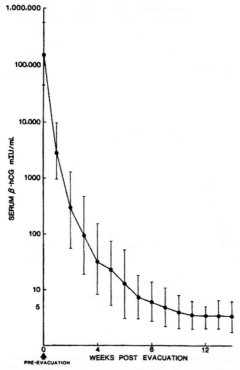

FIG. 46-1. Normal post–molar pregnancy curve for serum β human chorionic gonadotropin (β-hCG) levels by radioimmunoassay. Vertical bars indicate 95% confidence limits.

    b. Arrangement for full operating room support in a hospital setting
    c. Initiation of large-bore intravenous access, with possible central line monitoring
    d. Determination of active blood type and blood screen, with administration of Rh_0 (D) immune globulin to Rh-negative patients
    e. Initiation of oxytocin drip (during D & C)
    f. Induction of regional or general anesthesia
  2. Uterine evacuation is accomplished with the largest plastic cannula that can be safely introduced through the cervix. Intravenous oxytocin is begun after the cervix is dilated and suction initiated, and is continued for several hours postoperatively.
C. **Follow-up**
  1. After the surgical evacuation of a hydatidiform mole, all patients should be monitored as follows:
    a. Serum β-hCG level should be measured 48 hours after evacuation.
    b. Thereafter, β-hCG level should be determined weekly until results are normal for 3 consecutive weeks, then monthly until results are normal for 6–12 consecutive months.
    c. Pelvic examinations should be performed to monitor the involution of pelvic structures (e.g., ovaries, uterus) and to aid in early detection of metastasis.
    d. Repeat chest radiograph is indicated if the β-hCG titer plateaus or rises.
  2. Fig. 46-1 shows the normal post–molar pregnancy curve for serum β-hCG level. Fig. 46-2 outlines the follow-up management of molar pregnancy.

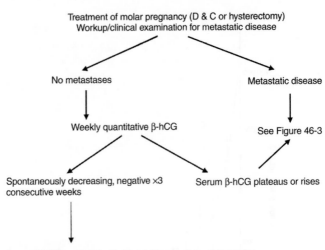

FIG. 46-2. Follow-up management of molar pregnancy. β-hCG, β human chorionic gonadotropin; D & C, dilation and curettage.

D. **Medical complications of hydatidiform mole**

1. **Common complications** include anemia, infection, hyperthyroidism, pregnancy-induced hypertension or preeclampsia, and theca lutein cysts. Anemia, defined as a hemoglobin level of less than 10 g/dL, is seen in 50% of patients with complete moles and results from excessive vaginal bleeding. Preeclampsia occurs in approximately 25% of cases and presents with the signs and symptoms of preeclampsia seen in nonmolar pregnancies (hypertension, proteinuria, edema). Seven percent of patients with complete moles present with hyperthyroidism, with clinical findings of tachycardia, hypertension, and tachypnea. Patients with hyperthyroidism should receive beta-sympathetic blockade before induction of anesthesia to prevent thyroid storm, which can be precipitated by surgery itself. Both hyperthyroidism and pregnancy-induced hypertension usually abate promptly after evacuation of the molar pregnancy and may not always require specific therapy. Theca lutein cysts (cysts larger than 6 cm) are observed in 50% of patients and result from β-hCG stimulation. These cysts may require 2–4 months to resolve completely. Any cyst larger than 6 cm that persists beyond this point necessitates surgical investigation.

2. **Pulmonary distress** is observed in 2% of patients. Frequently, it occurs at the time of evacuation of a mole in patients with marked uterine enlargement. Although the syndrome of trophoblastic embolization has been emphasized as an underlying cause for respiratory distress syndrome, many other potential causes for the syndrome have been identified in affected women, including high-output CHF caused by anemia or hyperthyroidism, preeclampsia, or iatrogenic fluid overload. Patients present with chest pain, shortness of breath, tachypnea, tachycardia, and hypoxemia. These signs and symptoms usually resolve within 72 hours of institution of supportive measures. In general, pulmonary complications should be treated aggressively with therapy directed by pulmonary artery catheter monitoring and with assisted ventilatory support as required.

E. **Contraception.** Effective contraception is recommended for the entire interval of β-hCG follow-up testing, namely, 6–12 months. It is important to prevent pregnancy, because a rising β-hCG titer due to a normal pregnancy cannot be distinguished from that of persistent GTD. If the patient does not desire surgical sterilization, either oral contraceptives or barrier methods may be chosen. An intrauterine device should not be inserted until the patient achieves normal gonadotropin levels, because of the risk of uterine perforation.

Patients who have had a partial or complete molar gestation have a 10- to 20-fold increased risk of a second mole in subsequent pregnancies. Therefore, all future pregnancies should be evaluated by ultrasonography early in their course. The magnitude of the risk of recurrent partial moles is not known, although recurrent partial mole has been documented.

PERSISTENT GESTATIONAL TROPHOBLASTIC DISEASE

I. **General features.** Persistent GTD includes *invasive mole, choriocarcinoma*, and *PSTT*. Twenty percent of evacuated complete moles are followed by persistent gestational trophoblastic disease.
   A. **A plateau or rise in β-hCG titers or the presence of metastasis** demonstrates persistent disease. Over 95% of malignant sequelae occur within approximately 6 months after evacuation of a hydatidiform mole. If β-hCG values rise or plateau over more than 2 weeks, immediate workup and treatment for persistent GTD is indicated.
   B. Important **clinical risk factors** identified in more than 60% of patients experiencing persistent GTD include large-for-date uterus, ovarian enlargement due to theca lutein cysts, recurrent molar pregnancy, uterine subinvolution, advanced maternal age, significantly elevated β-hCG level, and acute pulmonary compromise.
   C. **Metastatic disease** occurs in 17% of cases of complete mole. The risk of persistent GTD is considerably less for partial moles than for complete moles; approximately 5% of patients with partial hydatidiform mole develop persistent GTD.

II. **Specific features**
   A. **Invasive hydatidiform mole** is a disorder in which hydropic chorionic villi are present within the myometrium or its vascular spaces, or at distant sites. This lesion has been known as **chorioadenoma destruens, penetrating mole, malignant mole,** and **molar destruens.** Invasive mole accounts for 70–90% of cases of persistent GTD. Metastases occur in 20% of cases of invasive mole; metastases generally are found in the lungs, vagina, vulva, or broad ligament.
      1. **Gross findings.** In the uterus, invasive mole is an erosive, hemorrhagic lesion extending from the uterine cavity into the myometrium. Invasion can range from superficial penetration to extension through the wall, with uterine perforation and life-threatening hemorrhage. Molar vesicles are often grossly apparent.
      2. **Microscopic findings.** The diagnostic feature of invasive mole is the presence of molar villi and trophoblast within the myometrium or at an extrauterine site. Lesions at distant sites usually are composed of molar villi confined within blood vessels, without invasion into adjacent tissue.
   B. **Choriocarcinoma** is a pure epithelial neoplasm, comprising both neoplastic ST and cytotrophoblastic elements *without chorionic villi*. Choriocarcinoma may be associated with any form of gestation. The more abnormal the pregnancy, the more likely that choriocarcinoma may supervene. An incidence of 1 in 160,000 normal gestations, 1 in 15,386 abortions, 1 in 5333 ectopic pregnancies, and 1 in 40 molar pregnancies has been found. Early systemic hematogenous metastasis tends to develop in gestational choriocarcinoma.
      1. **Clinical features**
         a. **Pulmonary involvement.** At presentation, 80% of patients with metastatic disease show pulmonary involvement. Symptoms include

chest pain, persistent cough, hemoptysis, dyspnea, or asymptomatic chest lesions. The duration of these symptoms may be prolonged, or they may be acute. Patients may also experience pulmonary hypertension secondary to pulmonary arterial occlusion by trophoblastic emboli. Patients with extensive pulmonary involvement may have minimal gynecologic involvement.

b. **Vaginal metastases.** Approximately 30% of patients with extrauterine disease experience vaginal involvement. These patients can bleed profusely if biopsy is attempted. Because these lesions are highly vascular, they appear reddened or even violet.

c. **Hepatic metastases.** Ten percent of patients with metastatic disease have involvement of the liver. Hepatic disease is encountered almost exclusively in patients with delayed treatment and with extensive tumor burden. Lesions may be hemorrhagic and friable. Cases involving hepatic capsule leading to rupture and subsequent life-threatening hemorrhage have been reported.

d. **CNS disease** is seen in 10% of patients, mostly in those with advanced disease. These patients almost always have concurrent pulmonary or vaginal involvement, or both. These CNS lesions may undergo spontaneous hemorrhage leading to acute focal neurologic deficits.

2. **Histopathologic findings.** On gross examination, uterine choriocarcinoma generally is a dark red, hemorrhagic mass with a shaggy, irregular surface. Rarely, a lesion may lack significant hemorrhage and appear as a fleshy, tan-gray mass with necrosis. Metastases outside the uterus appear to be well circumscribed and hemorrhagic. Ill-defined infiltrative growth is unusual because of the rapid proliferation with hemorrhage and necrosis that typifies the neoplasm. On microscopic examination, choriocarcinoma is characterized by masses and sheets of trophoblastic cells *without chorionic villi* that invade surrounding tissue and permeate vascular spaces.

C. **Placental site trophoblastic tumor** is the rarest form of GTD and represents approximately 1% of cases of persistent GTD.

1. **Clinical features.** PSTTs exhibit the tendency to remain confined to the uterus and metastasize late in their course. Approximately 15% metastasize to extrauterine sites such as the lungs, liver, abdominal cavity, and brain. Because PSTTs are comprised predominantly of ITs, which produce small amounts of β-hCG, the baseline β-hCG level is typically low despite a large tumor burden. Because ITs secrete an abundant amount of human placental lactogen, however, serum hPL levels can be used to monitor disease progression or recurrence. *In contrast to other trophoblastic tumors, PSTTs are relatively insensitive to chemotherapy, thus surgical treatment is warranted.*

2. **Histopathologic findings.** The appearance of the lesion varies from a mass that is barely grossly visible to a diffuse nodular enlargement of the myometrium. Most tumors are well circumscribed, but they can be poorly defined. A PSTT may be polypoid, projecting into the uterine cavity, or may predominantly involve the myometrium. Invasion frequently extends to the uterine serosa and in rare instances extends to adnexal structures. The predominant cells of PSTT are ITs. Villi are only rarely present.

III. **Diagnosis**

A. **Clinical presentation.** Persistent disease is most often demonstrated by a plateau or rise in β-hCG titers. Patients may also present with recurrent vaginal bleeding after dilation and curettage for their molar pregnancies. Other presenting signs and symptoms are related to the anatomic sites involved with metastatic disease: chest pain, hemoptysis, or persistent cough with pulmonary involvement; vaginal hemorrhage from vaginal metastases; and focal neurologic deficits from cerebral hemorrhage. A diag-

TABLE 46-2. INTERNATIONAL FEDERATION OF GYNECOLOGY AND OBSTETRICS (FIGO) STAGING OF GESTATIONAL TROPHOBLASTIC DISEASE

Stage	Tumor characteristics
Stage I	Strictly confined to uterus
Stage II	Extension outside uterus but limited to pelvic structures
Stage III	Extension to lungs
Stage IV	All other metastatic sites

Each stage is further divided into A, B, or C as follows:

A = no risk factor

B = one risk factor present

C = two risk factors present

Risk factors affecting staging include: (1) β human chorionic gonadotropin level >100,000 mIU/mL, and (2) duration of disease >6 months from termination of the antecedent pregnancy.

nosis of persistent GTD is also made if there is histologic evidence of choriocarcinoma.

B. **Workup.** For all patients suspected of having persistent GTD, the following workup should be done to evaluate the extent of disease:
1. Complete history taking and physical examination
2. Measurement of serum β-hCG level, possibly serum hPL level
3. Tests of liver function, thyroid function, and renal function
4. CBC
5. Pelvic ultrasonography to evaluate for possible intrauterine pregnancy
6. Chest radiograph
7. CT of pelvis, abdomen, and brain
8. Stool guaiac test

C. **Differential diagnosis.** The diagnosis of persistent GTD is based on the quantitative pattern of serum β-hCG level, D & C findings, presence of metastatic disease, and histologic findings. Both invasive mole and choriocarcinoma after a hydatidiform mole are detected by a plateau or elevation in the β-hCG titer. It is often impossible to distinguish between these lesions clinically. These two entities can only be differentiated from pathologic specimens, either from biopsy or D & C. Obtaining a tissue diagnosis is not necessary, however, because the treatment for both invasive mole and choriocarcinoma is the same (see sec. **V.B**). PSTTs typically demonstrate low β-hCG levels; however, serum hPL level is often elevated and may be a more useful serologic marker.

IV. **Staging.** Anatomic staging for GTD has been adopted by the International Federation of Gynecology and Obstetrics (FIGO). Stage I is disease confined to the uterus. Stage II indicates extension outside the uterus but limited to pelvic structures. Stage III involves metastatic disease to the lungs. Stage IV includes metastases to all other sites, including head and liver. Each stage is further subdivided into the subcategories A, B, and C, depending on whether none, one, or two risk factors are present, respectively. The two risk factors affecting subcategory staging are (1) β-hCG level of more than 100,000 mIU/mL and (2) duration of disease longer than 6 months from termination of the antecedent pregnancy (Table 46-2). Other variables, in addition to anatomic site involvement, help to predict the likelihood of drug resistance. A prognostic scoring system endorsed by the World Health Organization guides the chemotherapy of patients with GTD (Table 46-3). When the prognostic score is

TABLE 46-3. WORLD HEALTH ORGANIZATION PROGNOSTIC SCORING INDEX

Score	0	1	2	4
Age	<39 yrs	>39 yrs	—	—
Antecedent pregnancy	Mole	Abortion	Term	—
Interval (mos) from antecedent pregnancy	<4	4–6	7–12	>12
Serum β human chorionic gonadotropin level (mIU/mL)	$<10^3$	10^3-10^4	10^4-10^5	$>10^5$
ABO blood group	—	A, O	B	—
Largest tumor size (cm)	—	3–5	>5	—
Metastases	Lung, pelvis	Spleen, kidney	Gastrointestinal tract, liver	Brain
Number of metastases	—	1–4	5–8	>8
Prior chemotherapy	—	—	One drug	Two or more drugs

8 or higher, the patient is considered high risk and should receive combination chemotherapy.

V. **Management.** Because persistent GTD is often diagnosed clinically, it is common not to have a histopathologic diagnosis before therapy is begun. Invasive mole and choriocarcinoma are treated in the same manner. Treatment modality depends on the presence of risk factors for treatment failure and on the extent of the disease (i.e., stage).

  A. **Risk factors**
    1. **Low risk**
      a. Short duration of disease (less than 4 months)
      b. Serum β-hCG level of 40,000 mIU/mL or less
      c. No brain or liver metastases
      d. No antecedent term pregnancy
      e. No prior chemotherapy
    2. **High risk**
      a. Long duration of disease (longer than 4 months)
      b. Serum β-hCG of more than 40,000 mIU/mL
      c. Brain or liver metastases
      d. Antecedent term pregnancy
      e. Prior chemotherapy
      f. World Health Organization score of 8 or higher
  B. **Treatment.** A summary of recommended treatment is presented in Fig. 46-3.
    1. **Nonmetastatic disease or low-risk metastatic disease**
      a. **Chemotherapy.** For patients with no extrauterine disease or metastatic disease with low-risk factors as mentioned earlier, single-agent chemotherapy with either methotrexate sodium or actinomycin D is the recommended primary therapy. The selected agent is administered on a predetermined schedule until a negative test result for serum β-hCG is obtained. An additional one to three cycles of consolidation chemotherapy are administered after a negative test result for serum β-hCG is obtained. If an inadequate response, defined as a plateau or rise in β-hCG titer, is observed after two courses of a chemotherapeutic agent, the patient is considered resistant to that agent, and the alternative chemotherapy

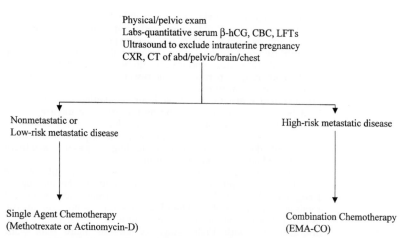

FIG. 46-3. Management of persistent gestational trophoblastic disease. β-hCG, β human chorionic gonadotropin; EMA-CO, etoposide, methotrexate, actinomycin D, cyclophosphamide (Cytoxan), and vincristine sulfate; LFT, liver function test; CXR, chest radiograph.

is promptly instituted (e.g., if methotrexate fails, actinomycin D is given). If both single agents fail, then a combination chemotherapy regimen is instituted. For patients who have completed childbearing, chemotherapy and a hysterectomy are recommended for best chances of cure.

b. **Prognosis.** Actinomycin D and methotrexate have comparable efficacy in treating nonmetastatic or low-risk metastatic GTN. Selection of chemotherapy should be based on the associated side-effect profiles and the convenience of administration schedules. For nonmetastatic disease, the overall remission rate is 75–90% with a single-agent regimen. The remission rate for low-risk metastatic disease is lower at 60%; however, for many of these patients salvage therapy with a second agent is successful. A resistant focus of disease occurs in 2–13% of cases, and is then treated with hysterectomy.

2. **High-risk metastatic disease**

a. **Chemotherapy.** For patients with high-risk metastatic disease, the recommended treatment is combination chemotherapy with etoposide, methotrexate, actinomycin D, cyclophosphamide (Cytoxan), and vincristine sulfate (EMA-CO). The chemotherapy is administered until three negative test results for β-hCG are achieved in three consecutive weeks or until intolerable side effects occur. After the normalization of β-hCG levels, an additional two courses should be given as consolidation therapy. For patients with complications of metastatic disease specific to the organ involved, the following interventions can be instituted.

(1) **Vaginal metastases.** These lesions can bleed profusely; bleeding can be controlled with packing for 24 hours. Prompt radiation treatment to the affected region may help to control further bleeding. Although infrequently used, radiographic embolization of the pelvic vessels may also be implemented in cases of life-threatening or recurrent hemorrhage.

(2) **Pulmonary metastases.** These lesions are usually treatable with chemotherapy. Occasionally, thoracotomy is required to

remove a persistent viable tumor nodule. It must be kept in mind that not all chest lesions clear radiographically, due to scarring and fibrosis from the injury and healing process.

(3) **Hepatic metastases.** If these lesions fail to respond to systemic chemotherapy, other options include hepatic arterial infusion of chemotherapy or partial hepatic resection to control bleeding or remove resistant tumor.

(4) **Cerebral metastases.** Whole-brain irradiation (approximately 3000 cGy) is initiated as soon as the extent of disease is confirmed. Radiation and chemotherapy reduce the risk of spontaneous cerebral hemorrhage. Craniotomy is infrequently performed for acute decompression or acute bleeding in cases in which there is hope of survival and cure is probable.

(5) **Hysterectomy** is indicated in cases with large intrauterine tumor burden, intrauterine infection, and uterine hemorrhage.

b. **Prognosis.** When EMA-CO is the primary treatment, the overall remission rate is 80–90%. When brain metastases are present, the overall remission rate is decreased to 50–60%. Higher failure rates are also seen with FIGO stage IV disease, more than eight metastases, and a history of prior chemotherapy. For patients refractory to or with recurrent disease after EMA-CO treatment, a combination regimen of etoposide, methotrexate, and actinomycin D followed by a repeat dose of etoposide and cisplatin on day 8 (EMA-CE) is administered as the second-line treatment. If EMA-CE fails, then salvage therapy such as experimental protocols and secondary surgical excision is considered.

C. **Follow-up.** The following schedule is recommended for all patients with persistent GTD. These patients require continued care because of the risk of late recurrence.

1. **Weekly measurement of β-hCG levels** until findings are negative for three consecutive weeks
2. **Thereafter, monthly measurement of β-hCG values** until findings are negative for 12 months (nonmetastatic or low-risk metastatic disease) or for 24 months (high-risk metastatic disease)
3. **Effective contraception** (oral contraceptive preparations, barrier methods) during the entire interval of hormonal follow-up
4. **Radiographic studies** as indicated (e.g., chest CT for pulmonary metastases, brain MRI for cerebral metastases)

47. CHEMOTHERAPY AND RADIATION THERAPY

Nicholas C. Lambrou and Edward Trimble

CHEMOTHERAPY

I. **Cell kinetic concepts**
   A. **Tumor growth.** The failure of the *regulated balance* between cell loss and cell proliferation differentiates tumorous tissues from normal tissues. Although cell proliferation occurs continuously in human tumors, it does not occur more rapidly than in normal tissues.
      1. **Gompertzian growth** is governed by the principle that, as a tumor's mass increases, the time required to double the tumor's volume also increases.
      2. **Doubling time** is the time it takes for the mass of a tumor to double its size. Considerable variation exists in doubling times of human tumors. Metastases generally have faster doubling times than primary lesions.
      3. **Clinically detectable** masses occur only after many tumor doublings (i.e., 30 doublings for a 1-cm mass). In late stages of tumor growth, a very few doublings in tumor mass have a dramatic impact on tumor size (e.g., a palpable tumor of 1 cm requires only three doublings to reach a size of 8 cm).
   B. **Cell cycle.** The principle of chemotherapy is to attain maximal therapeutic cytotoxic effects without extreme toxicity to normal tissues. Unfortunately, it is not always possible to obtain a therapeutic effect without temporarily or, in some instances, permanently altering the functions of other cells, tissues, organs, or systems. The kinetic behavior of individual tumor cells has been well described, and a classic cell cycle model has been developed (Fig. 47-1).
      1. **Growth fraction** is the number of cells in the tumor mass that are actively undergoing cell division.
      2. **Generation time** is the duration of the cycle from M phase to M phase. The largest variation in generation time among tumors occurs in the G_1 phase.
      3. **Cell cycle–specific drugs** depend on the proliferative capacity of the cell and on the phase of the cell cycle for their action. Effective agents act against tumors with relatively long S phases, high growth fractions, and rapid proliferation rates.
      4. **Cell cycle–nonspecific drugs** kill cells in all phases of the cell cycle, and their effectiveness is not very dependent on a tumor's proliferative capacity.
      5. **The log kill hypothesis** states that chemotherapeutic agents appear to work by first-order kinetics (they kill a constant fraction of cells rather than a constant number). One reason is because malignant cells are thought to have a less effective repair capacity than normal cells. Optimal dosing will achieve maximum tumor cell kill, with the next treatment cycle given when normal stem cells have had time to recover from the previous treatment cycle. This helps explain the need for intermittent courses of chemotherapy and also supports the rationale for multiple-drug therapy.
      6. **The Goldie-Coldman hypothesis** of drug resistance states that most mammalian cells start out with an intrinsic sensitivity to antineoplastic drugs but develop spontaneous resistance at variable rates by somatic mutation.
II. **Chemotherapy**
   A. **Primary therapy** is the use of chemotherapy as first-line treatment for a disease.

511

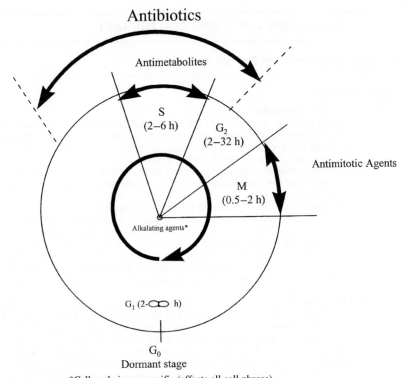

FIG. 47-1. Phases of the cell cycle, relative time intervals, and sites of action of the various classes of antineoplastic agents. (From Trimble EL, Trimble CL. *Cancer obstetrics and gynecology*. Philadelphia: Lippincott Williams & Wilkins, 1999:60, with permission.)

    B. **Adjuvant therapy** is the use of drugs to treat patients who are clinically disease free by surgical therapy but are known to be at high risk for the presence of micrometastases, and therefore recurrence.

    C. **Neoadjuvant therapy** is the use of drugs to treat patients before cytoreductive surgery.

    D. **Salvage therapy** is the use of drugs to treat patients with recurrent disease after first-line chemotherapy.

III. **Clinical trials**

    A. **Evaluation parameters. Complete response** is complete disappearance of all evidence of disease for at least 1 month. **Partial response** is the reduction of each measurable lesion by at least 50% for at least 1 month. **Stable disease** is maintenance for each lesion of criteria less than those required for either a partial response or increasing disease. **Increasing disease** is increase of a lesion by at least 50% or the appearance of a new lesion within 1 month.

    B. **Evaluation phases**

        1. **Phase I trials** determine the maximum tolerable dose, optimal schedule, and dose-limiting toxicity of the agent. These trials are usually conducted in a population of 15–30 patients. The drug is begun at a low

level and the dose is escalated after three patients have been treated safely at the given dose level. Phase I trials evaluating combinations of new and older agents also may be needed to define the optimal combination regimen.

2. **Phase II trials** determine the activity of each drug or drug combination against particular tumors. Multiple doses and schedules may be tested, and each requires a sufficient number of patients (15–40) to obtain an estimate of the response rate.

3. **Phase III trials** are randomized comparisons of the new agent alone or in combination with other active agents against the standard treatment for the tumor type in question.

4. **Phase IV trials** evaluate new agents as part of a treatment program, which may include surgery or radiation therapy or both, in a broad population of patients, generally in an effort to obtain additional information on side effects and cancer outcome.

IV. **Chemotherapeutic agents.** The agents commonly used for chemotherapy for cancers of the female reproductive system are listed in Table 47-1. Chemotherapy drugs are grouped according to their chemistry or mode of action.

A. **Alkylating agents** are cell cycle nonspecific. These agents contain an alkyl group that forms a covalent bond with the DNA helix, which prevents DNA duplication. They also attach to free guanine bases of DNA and prevent their action as templates for new DNA formation.

B. **Antimetabolites** are similar in chemical structure to metabolites required by both normal and tumorous cells for cell division to occur. These antimetabolites may be incorporated into new nuclear material or combined with enzymes to inhibit cell division.

C. **Vinca alkaloids** are derived from the periwinkle plant (*Vinca rosea*). They bind to tubules, which blocks microtubule formation and interferes with spindle formation. This leads to the arrest of metaphase and inhibits mitosis.

D. **Antitumor antibiotics** have many different modes of action, including increasing cell membrane permeability, inhibiting DNA and RNA synthesis, and blocking DNA replication.

E. **Miscellaneous agents** belonging to none of the above categories have different modes of action.

V. **Common side effects of chemotherapy**

A. **Local and dermal side effects** include alopecia (which is reversible after treatment stops), photosensitivity, phlebitis, tissue necrosis, and local infiltration or extravasation. Extravasation may be treated with topical steroids, local injection of hyaluronidase, or sodium thiosulfate, depending on the specific drug.

B. **Myelosuppression** can be the most dangerous and life-threatening side effect of chemotherapy and varies in severity according to the drug administered. Pancytopenia is the major dose-limiting toxicity associated with chemotherapy treatment. Generally, most agents can be readministered every 3–4 weeks if the patient has recovered from myelosuppressive effects. A nadir in white cell, red cell, or platelet count is usually observed 7–14 days after drug administration.

1. **Neutropenia.** Recombinant human granulocyte colony-stimulating factor (G-CSF) (Filgrastim, Neupogen) may be given for prevention or treatment of febrile neutropenia. G-CSF may be started after the onset of a febrile neutropenic episode and often is given prophylactically when the absolute neutrophil count is less than 500/mm³. In addition, G-CSF may be given during chemotherapy cycles for patients at risk of severe neutropenia. Recommended dosing is 5.0 μg/kg subcutaneously (SC) daily for 5–7 days beginning on day 2 or 3 after administration of chemotherapy. G-CSF use during the actual administration of chemotherapy is contraindicated.

TABLE 47-1. CHEMOTHERAPEUTIC AGENTS USED TO TREAT GYNECOLOGIC CANCER

	Route of administration	Toxicity	Diseases/sites treated
Alkylating agents			
Nitrogen mustard (Mustargen)	IV	Myelosuppression, nausea and vomiting	Ovary
Cyclophosphamide (Cytoxan)	IV/PO	Myelosuppression (WBCs affected more than platelets), hemorrhagic cystitis, bladder fibrosis, alopecia, hepatitis, amenorrhea	Ovary, breast, soft tissue sarcomas
Ifosfamide	IV	Myelosuppression, hemorrhagic cystitis, CNS dysfunction, renal toxicity	Ovary, cervix, uterine sarcomas, germ cell neoplasms of the ovary
Melphalan (Alkeran)	PO	Myelosuppression (platelets affected more than WBCs), nausea and vomiting, secondary malignancies (leukemia)	Ovary, breast
Chlorambucil (Leukeran)	PO	Myelosuppression, GI distress, hepatotoxicity, dermatitis	Ovary
Alkylating-like agents			
Cis-dichloro-diamino-platinum (cisplatin)	IV	Nephrotoxicity, nausea and vomiting, tinnitus and hearing loss, myelosuppression, peripheral neuropathy	Ovarian and germ cell carcinomas, cervix, vulva, endometrium
Carboplatin	IV	Less neuropathy, ototoxicity, and nephrotoxicity than cisplatin; more myelosuppression than cisplatin	Ovarian and germ cell carcinomas, endometrium
Hexamethylmelamine (Hexalen)	IV	Anorexia, nausea and vomiting, diarrhea, abdominal cramps, neurotoxicity	Ovary
Antitumor antibiotics			
Actinomycin D (dactinomycin)	IV	Nausea and vomiting, skin necrosis, mucosal ulceration, myelosuppression	Germ cell ovarian tumors, choriocarcinoma, soft tissue sarcomas
Bleomycin sulfate	IV, SC, IM, IP	Pulmonary toxicity, fever, anaphylactic reactions, dermatologic reactions	Germ cell ovarian tumors, cervix, vulva, malignant effusions
Mitomycin C (Mutamycin)	IV	Myelosuppression, nausea and vomiting, mucosal ulceration, nephrotoxicity	Breast, cervix, ovary

Drug	Route	Toxicity	Indication
Doxorubicin hydrochloride (Adriamycin)	IV	Myelosuppression, cardiac toxicity, alopecia, mucosal ulcerations, nausea and vomiting	Ovary, breast, endometrium
Liposomal doxorubicin hydrochloride (Doxil)	IV	Myelosuppression, skin and mucosal toxicity, hand-foot syndrome	Ovary, endometrium
Antimetabolites			
5-Fluorouracil (5-FU)	IV	Myelosuppression, nausea and vomiting, anorexia, alopecia	Breast, ovary, vulva, vagina
Methotrexate sodium (MTX)	IV, PO, IM	Myelosuppression, mucosal ulceration, hepatotoxicity	Choriocarcinoma, breast, ovary
Hydroxyurea (Hydrea)	PO, IV	Myelosuppression, nausea and vomiting, anorexia	Cervix
Gemcitabine hydrochloride	IV	Mild myelosuppression, flu-like syndrome	Ovary
Plant alkaloids			
Vincristine sulfate (Oncovin)	IV	Neurotoxicity, alopecia, myelosuppression, cranial nerve palsies	Ovarian germ cell, sarcomas, cervical cancer
Vinblastine sulfate (Velban)	IV	Myelosuppression, alopecia, nausea and vomiting, neurotoxicity	Choriocarcinoma, ovarian germ cell tumors
Epipodophyllotoxin (etoposide, VP-16)	IV	Myelosuppression, alopecia, hypotension	Ovarian germ cell, choriocarcinoma
Paclitaxel (Taxol)	IV	Myelosuppression, alopecia, allergic reactions, cardiac arrhythmias	Ovary, breast, endometrium
Docetaxel (Taxotere)	IV	Myelosuppression, hypersensitivity cutaneous reactions, alopecia	Ovary
Miscellaneous			
Topotecan hydrochloride	IV	Myelosuppression	Ovary
Dacarbazine (DTIC)	IV	Myelosuppression, nausea and vomiting, flu-like syndrome, hepatotoxicity	Uterine sarcomas, soft tissue sarcomas

2. **Anemia.** Erythropoietin [epoetin α (Epogen, Procrit)] may be used to treat anemia. Erythropoietin is administered SC at a dose of 150 U/kg (approximately 10,000 U three times per week or 15,000 U twice per week). Another option is to begin dosing with 30,000–40,000 U SC once per week. After 8 weeks of therapy, the dose may be increased (20,000 U three times per week or 30,000 units twice weekly) if a rise in hemoglobin level of more than 1 g/dL has not been achieved. Once the target is reached (hemoglobin level of 12 g/dL or hematocrit of 36–40%), the dose can be titrated down by 25%.

3. **Thrombocytopenia** usually is not treated with platelet transfusion until the platelet count drops below 15,000–20,000/mL unless clinical signs of spontaneous bleeding are evident. Thrombopoietin (oprelvekin, Neumega) may be given at a dosage of 50 μg/kg SC daily.

4. **Infections.** Infectious organisms associated with granulocytopenic defects include enteric Gram-negative bacteria, Gram-positive bacteria (*Staphylococcus epidermidis, Staphylococcus aureus,* and diphtheroid), viruses (herpes simplex and herpes zoster), and fungi (*Candida* and *Aspergillus* species). Infections generally are related to the severity and duration of the neutropenia and to alterations in the integrity of mucous membranes and skin. Fever in a neutropenic patient is sufficient evidence of occult infection to warrant antibiotic therapy after blood and urine culture specimens have been obtained. The administration of broad-spectrum antibiotics is generally recommended.

C. **Cardiac side effects**

1. **Daunorubicin citrate and doxorubicin hydrochloride** have significant cardiotoxic effects, including irreversible cardiomyopathies involving progressive CHF, pleural effusions, heart dilatation, and venous congestion. These side effects are generally cumulative; therefore, dosages of daunorubicin and doxorubicin are kept under the maximum. Commonly, multiple-gated acquisition (MUGA) scans are obtained before treatment with cardiotoxic agents to obtain a baseline ejection fraction and may be repeated as necessary.

2. **Paclitaxel (Taxol)** may cause asymptomatic and transient bradycardia (40–60 beats/minute), ventricular tachycardia, and atypical chest pain during infusion. These symptoms resolve with slowing of infusion.

D. **Pulmonary side effects. Bleomycin sulfate** may cause significant pulmonary fibrosis, and careful attention should be given to the lung examination in patients receiving this agent. Generally, this side effect is both dose and age related, but it can be idiopathic. Pulmonary function tests are performed to assess baseline pulmonary capacity before the first dose of bleomycin is administered and are repeated as needed.

E. **Hepatic side effects.** Transient elevations in transaminase and alkaline phosphatase levels may occur with chemotherapy. However, cholangitis, hepatic necrosis, and hepatic veno-occlusive disease, although rare, must be considered.

F. **Gastrointestinal side effects**

1. **Stomatitis and mucositis** may occur most commonly with antimetabolites such as methotrexate and with paclitaxel. Treatment is with either Larry's solution [three equal parts diphenhydramine hydrochloride elixir (Benadryl), magnesia and alumina oral suspension (Maalox), and viscous lidocaine] or nystatin, swish and swallow every 6 hours. Severe cases may require hospitalization for enteral or parenteral nutrition, intravenous hydration, and pain management.

2. **Nausea and vomiting** are two of the most common and most distressing side effects of chemotherapy. The severity and incidence of nausea and vomiting vary greatly, but the inability to effectively control these symptoms often can result in patient refusal of further potentially curative treatment. Three patterns of nausea and vomiting exist: *acute,*

TABLE 47-2. EMETOGENIC POTENTIAL OF COMMONLY USED CHEMOTHERAPEUTIC AGENTS

Very high (>90%)	High (60–90%)	Moderate (30–60%)	Low (<30%)
Cisplatin	Carboplatin	Etoposide	Bleomycin sulfate
Cyclophosphamide (high dose)	Cyclophosphamide	Ifosfamide	5-Fluorouracil
	Dactinomycin	Topotecan hydrochloride	Methotrexate sodium
			Paclitaxel
			Vincristine sulfate

delayed, and *anticipatory.* The incidence and severity of nausea and vomiting are related to the emetogenic potential of the drug, the dose, the route and time of day of administration, patient characteristics, and the combination of drugs used. Emetogenic potential of commonly used chemotherapeutic agents is listed in Table 47-2.

   a. **Diagnosis.** Symptoms of nausea and vomiting temporally related to the administration of chemotherapy are usually diagnostic of chemotherapy-induced emesis. Gastrointestinal obstruction must be ruled out, however, especially if abdominal distention or obstipation is present.

   b. **Treatment.** Ondansetron hydrochloride and granisetron hydrochloride, both serotonin S_3 receptor–blocking agents, have been shown to be particularly effective in reducing acute emesis associated with use of cisplatin and other highly emetogenic drugs. It is important to recognize that antiemetic medications are effective in the treatment of acute nausea and vomiting that result from the pattern of serotonin release, which is not a major factor in delayed emesis. Prevention is the key to management of delayed-onset nausea and vomiting. Patients are encouraged to take antiemetics as prescribed for 3–4 days after chemotherapy to prevent delayed emesis.

3. **Diarrhea** frequently accompanies stomatitis and, if temporally associated with the administration of chemotherapy, is most likely not infectious in origin. Patients are encouraged to increase their fluid intake to prevent postchemotherapy dehydration, with its risk of secondary side effects such as nephrotoxicity or electrolyte disturbances. If an infection is suspected, a stool specimen should be examined for the presence of WBCs, enteric pathogens (e.g., *Salmonella, Shigella*), ova and parasites, and *Clostridium difficile* toxin. In particular, if the patient has been on broad-spectrum antibiotics, *C. difficile* pseudomembranous colitis must be suspected. For diarrhea associated with *C. difficile* infection, therapy consists of oral metronidazole or intravenous vancomycin.

4. **Constipation** usually is seen in patients with neurogenic GI atony who are being treated with vinca alkaloids. In severe cases of constipation, ileus may ensue. Treatment includes hydration and administration of stool softeners (docusate sodium), laxatives (milk of magnesia), enemas, cathartics, and bulking agents.

G. **Acute allergic reactions** occasionally occur with the use of chemotherapeutic agents, most commonly etoposide. Acute pulmonary infiltrates have been known to occur with methotrexate and respond to steroid therapy. Bleomycin can cause anaphylaxis, skin reactions, fever, chills, and pulmonary fibrosis. Because of the high incidence of allergic reactions to bleomycin, patients are given a test dose of 2–4 U intramuscularly before the first dose of drug. Paclitaxel has been shown to cause hypersensitivity reactions in small numbers of patients within 2–3 minutes of infusion. The characteristic hypersensitivity reaction is bradycardia, diaphoresis, hypotension, cutaneous flushing, and abdominal pain. Premedications of diphenhydramine hydrochloride, dexamethasone, and ranitidine are given prophylactically.

H. **Hemorrhagic cystitis** may occur with cyclophosphamide and ifosfamide. Preventive measures include hydration and administration of diuretics, and treatment includes dosage reduction or discontinuation of the drug. **Mesna,** a uroprotector, is always administered simultaneously with ifosfamide to protect against bladder toxicity. Mesna acts to detoxify *acrolein*, the common metabolite of both cyclophosphamide and ifosfamide excreted by the kidneys.

I. **Neurotoxicity.** The vinca alkaloids in particular have been implicated in the development of peripheral, central, and visceral neuropathies. Neuropathies are cumulative side effects suggested by absent reflexes, constipation, and ileus. Rarely, cranial nerve abnormalities may be seen with neurotoxicity. Other agents, such as cisplatin and carboplatin, may cause a peripheral neuropathy characterized by paresthesias of the extremities. Cisplatin is thought to be more neurotoxic than carboplatin. Paclitaxel also has been shown to produce peripheral neuropathies, especially in heavily pretreated patients. Treatment of neurotoxicity involves discontinuation of the offending agent if neuropathies become debilitating.

J. **Nephrotoxicity.** Dose-related and cumulative renal insufficiency is the major dose-limiting toxic effect of cisplatin. Elevations may occur in BUN, serum creatinine, and serum uric acid levels within 2 weeks of treatment. Irreversible renal damage can occur. Prevention of nephrotoxicity with large amounts of intravenous hydration and diuretics is important during cisplatin treatment. Typically, 24-hour creatinine clearance is measured to establish baseline renal function before infusion of drug.

K. **Ototoxicity.** Tinnitus or high-frequency hearing loss may be observed in patients receiving cisplatin and may be more severe with repeated doses. It is unclear whether or not these effects are reversible. Audiograms may be obtained before treatment to acquire a baseline and throughout treatment to assess hearing loss.

RADIATION THERAPY

I. **Definitions and general concepts.** Destruction of tumor and normal cells by x-rays or gamma rays relies on the conversion in tissues of photon energy into kinetic energy of electrons and the subsequent chemical changes within molecules. Permanent cell damage occurs with the creation of oxygen free radicals and a multitude of other reactions resulting in DNA injury. The absorption of energy by tissue is measured in rads. One gray (Gy) = 100 rad and 1 centigray (cGy) = 1 rad. Current publications use centigray as the preferred unit. Tolerance doses of organs are listed in Table 47-3.

Clinical radiation sources can be divided into two basic types.

A. **Teletherapy** is external-beam radiation. Where available, linear accelerators have generally replaced cobalt units as sources of radiation. During external-beam radiation, the patient may be in either the prone or the supine position. The usual total dose of external-beam radiation to the pelvis ranges from 4000 to 5000 cGy, given in daily fractions of 180–200 cGy over 5 weeks.

B. **Brachytherapy.** In brachytherapy, the radiation device is placed either within or close to the target tumor volume (i.e., interstitial and intracavitary irradiation). The radiation applicators are called intrauterine tandems or colpostats.

1. **Intracavitary irradiation.** Intrauterine tandems are placed within the uterine cavity of a patient under anesthesia in an operating room.

TABLE 47-3. TOLERANCE DOSES (TD 5/5 TO TD 50/5) FOR WHOLE ORGAN IRRADIATION

Single dose (cGy)		Fractionated dose (cGy)	
Lymphatic system	200–500	Testes	200–1000
Bone marrow	200–1000	Ovary	600–1000
Ovary	200–600	Eye (lens)	600–1200
Testes	100–200	Lung	2000–3000
Eye (lens)	200–1000	Kidney	2000–3000
Lung	700–1000	Liver	3500–4000
Gastrointestinal system	500–1000	Skin	3000–4000
Colorectum	1000–2000	Thyroid	3000–4000
Kidney	1000–2000	Heart	4000–5000
Bone marrow	1500–2000	Lymphatic system	4000–5000
Heart	1800–2000	Bone marrow	4000–5000
Liver	1500–2000	Gastrointestinal system	5000–6000
Mucosa	500–2000	VCTS	5000–6000
VCTS	1000–2000	Spinal cord	5000–6000
Skin	1500–2000	Peripheral nerve	6500–7700
Peripheral nerve	1500–2000	Mucosa	6500–7700
Spinal cord	1500–2000	Brain	6000–7000
Brain	1500–2500	Bone and cartilage	>7000
Bone and cartilage	>3000	Muscle	>7000
Muscle	>3000		

VCTS, vasculoconnective tissue systems.
Adapted from Rubin P. The law and order of radiation sensitivity, absolute vs. relative. In: Vaeth JM, Meyer JL, eds. *Radiation tolerance of normal tissues,* vol. 23. Basel: Karger, 1989.

Their position is confirmed using radiographic studies. Vaginal ovoids or colpostats are designed for placement into the vaginal vault. Ovoids not only support the position of the tandem to keep it in place, they also may be loaded with radioactive sources. After the patient is transferred to her inpatient room, the hollow centers of the tandem and ovoids are then loaded with radioactive sources such as radium or cesium. Vaginal, endometrial, and cervical cancers may be treated by either high- or low-dose-rate intracavitary implants. It is becoming increasingly common in the United States and Europe to replace intracavitary brachytherapy treatments (usually cesium) with high-dose-rate intracavitary treatments (usually iridium 192). Among the advantages of high-dose-rate applications are that placement does not require anesthesia or operating room time and radiation exposure is 10–20 minutes for each outpatient visit (usually four to six visits are required), whereas use of low-dose-rate cesium implants requires hospitalization for 48–72 hours.

2. **Interstitial implants** are another form of brachytherapy. Various sources of radiation, such as iridium 192, iodine 125, and tantalum 182, may be configured as radioactive wires or seeds and placed directly within tissues. Hollow guide needles are inserted in a geometric pattern to deliver a relatively uniform dose of radiation to a target tumor vol-

ume. After the position of the guide needles is confirmed radiologically, they can be threaded with the radioactive sources (loaded) and the hollow guides removed.

3. The **inverse square law** states that the dose of radiation at a given point is inversely proportional to the square of the distance from the source of radiation. Therefore, in brachytherapy, the dose at a given distance from the source is determined largely by the inverse square law.

C. In **intracavitary radioisotope** therapy, radioactive isotopes are placed within a body cavity such as the abdomen and pelvis. To treat epithelial ovarian cancer, phosphorus 32 has been used, because its pattern of dissemination extends throughout the peritoneal cavity, theoretically irradiating all structures within the cavity. It has fallen out of favor, however, because it is toxic and has little proven benefit.

II. **Toxicity.** The severity of normal tissue reactions to radiation depends on total dose, dose fractionation, treatment volume, and energy of radiation.

A. **Skin toxicity.** Serious skin reactions are less frequent with megavoltage radiation than with regular-voltage radiation. Late subcutaneous fibrosis can develop, especially with doses higher than 6500 cGy. An acute skin reaction commonly becomes evident during the third week of therapy. The reaction is characterized by erythema, desquamation, and pruritus, and should resolve completely within 3 weeks of the end of treatment. Topical corticosteroids or moisturizing creams may be applied several times a day for symptomatic palliation and to promote healing. If the skin reaction worsens, it may be necessary to stop treatment and apply zinc oxide or silver sulfadiazine to the affected area until it improves enough to continue treatment. The perineum is at greater risk for skin breakdown than other areas because of its increased warmth and moisture, and lack of ventilation. The patient should be taught to keep the perineal area clean and dry in an effort to prevent skin breakdown.

B. **Hematologic toxicity.** The volume of marrow irradiated and the total radiation dose determine the severity of myelosuppression. In adults, 40% of active marrow is situated in the pelvis, 25% is in the vertebral column, and 20% is in the ribs and skull. Extensive radiation of these sites may cause significant myelosuppression. Blood transfusions or SC administration of erythropoietin may be required to support the patient's hematologic function during therapy.

C. **Gastrointestinal toxicity**

1. **Acute complications.** Nausea, vomiting, and diarrhea commonly occur 2–6 hours after abdominal or pelvic irradiation. The severity of the effect increases with the fraction size and treatment volume. Treatment involves supportive therapy with hydration and administration of antiemetics and antidiarrheals. Loperamide hydrochloride (Imodium) is generally used for first-line therapy, followed by diphenoxylate hydrochloride (Lomotil) if necessary. The usual dosage for both medications is one to two tablets after each loose stool, not to exceed eight doses per day. If the patient is having severe diarrhea, opiates may be used to decrease peristalsis. Opiate agents include opium tincture, 0.5–1.0 mL every 4 hours; paregoric elixir, 4 mL orally every 4 hours; or codeine, 15–30 mg orally every 4 hours. Occasionally, a reduction in fraction size or a break in treatment is necessary to control the acute GI effects. Finally, octreotide acetate (Sandostatin) may be given to reduce the volume of persistent high-output diarrhea. A recommended starting dosage of octreotide is 50–100 µg SC three times daily.

2. **Long-term complications.** Chronic diarrhea, obstruction caused by bowel adhesions, and fistula formation are serious complications of intestinal irradiation that occur in fewer than 1% of cases. Small bowel and rectovaginal fistulas can be caused by radiation effects on tissue or by recurrent disease. After recurrent disease is ruled out, the patient

may require a temporary or permanent colostomy to allow healing of the affected bowel. Fistulas often are associated with a foul odor, and good hygiene is important in eliminating the odor. Items that may assist with odor control are charcoal-impregnated dressings, skin cleansers, and air deodorizers.

D. **Genitourinary toxicity**
   1. **Cystitis** is characterized by inflammation of the bladder with associated symptoms of pain, urgency, hematuria, and urinary frequency. The bladder is relatively tolerant of radiation, but doses higher than 6000–7000 cGy over a 6- to 7-week period can result in cystitis. A diagnosis of radiation cystitis may be made after a normal urine culture result has been obtained. Hydration, frequent sitz baths, and possibly the use of antibiotics and antispasmodic agents may be necessary for treatment. **Hemorrhagic cystitis** may lead to symptomatic anemia that requires blood transfusions and hospitalization. Clot evacuation of the bladder with continuous bladder irrigation is often necessary. Bladder irrigation with 1% alum or 1% silver nitrate can alleviate bleeding. Persistent bleeding on continuous bladder irrigation or significant gross hematuria in the unstable patient requires immediate cystoscopic evaluation to localize and control the bleeding.
   2. **Vesicovaginal fistulas and ureteral strictures** are possible long-term complications of radiation therapy. Placement of nephrostomies, insertion of ureteral stents, and less commonly, surgical intervention may be necessary.

E. **Vulvovaginitis.** Pelvic irradiation often results in erythema, inflammation, mucosal atrophy, inelasticity, and ulceration of the vaginal tissue. Adhesions and stenosis of the vagina are not uncommon and result in painful intercourse and pain on pelvic examination. Treatment involves vaginal dilation, either by frequent sexual intercourse or by the use of a vaginal dilator. Vaginal dilation should be performed at least two to three times per week for up to 2 years. In addition, the use of estrogen creams is useful in promoting epithelial regeneration. Infections, including candidiasis, trichomoniasis, and bacterial vaginosis, may be associated with radiation-induced vaginitis.

F. **Fatigue.** During radiation therapy, many women report an overwhelming sense of exhaustion. The cause of this fatigue is unclear but most likely involves a combination of physiologic, psychological, and situational factors. Close monitoring of CBC findings is necessary to ensure that the patient is not anemic. It is often helpful for patients to rest immediately after treatment and to enlist family and friends to assist with daily activities and chores. Fatigue may continue for several months after completion of therapy.

48. TERMINAL AND PALLIATIVE CARE

Dana Virgo and Deborah Armstrong

I. **Palliative care.** The World Health Organization defines palliative care as the "active total care of patients whose disease is not responsive to curative treatment" but notes that curative care and palliative care are not mutually exclusive. The Canadian Palliative Care Association defines palliative care even more broadly as "the combination of active and compassionate therapies intended to comfort and support individuals and families who are living with a life-threatening illness." In other words, palliative care should focus on symptom relief and the psychosocial needs of patients and families regardless of prognosis. Palliative care should not be limited to patients without hope for cure; it functions as a useful aspect of curative care in that patients with improved quality of life better tolerate difficult treatment regimens. Palliative care should be considered a facet of total health care that increases in importance from diagnosis until death.

The issues surrounding the end of life—ranging from advance directives to pain control to depression and grieving—make many physicians and other health professionals uncomfortable. This discomfort commonly manifests itself as dissociation from dying patients and their families and failure on the part of the physician to address end-of-life issues. The SUPPORT trial, a recent 4-year study including over 9000 seriously ill patients, found that nearly half of patients who desired the withholding of cardiopulmonary resuscitation did not have "Do not resuscitate" orders written in their hospital charts. Despite the large number of patients who did not want resuscitation, nearly half of patients who died during the study were treated with mechanical ventilation within 3 days of death, and more than one-third spent at least 10 days in an ICU. The problem of the failure of end-of-life care to mesh with patients' and families' desires is due in part to the reluctance of health care providers to counsel patients on these sensitive issues. Studies have repeatedly found, however, that patients expect their physicians to bring up end-of-life issues. By educating ourselves about all aspects of this life stage, we can achieve the best possible care for terminally ill patients.

II. **Ethical and legal issues in palliative care.** Autonomy is defined as self-government. The principle of autonomy implies noninterference in decision making by others. In medicine, the importance of informed consent is derived from the weight given to patient autonomy. Another key term in palliative care, beneficence, is the obligation to do good. Its corollary is nonmaleficence: "First, do no harm." Medical decision making can be a tenuous balance between patient autonomy and beneficence, as patient decision making may not agree with physicians' assessment of the "best" treatment to optimize outcome and minimize harm. The principles of autonomy and informed consent are supported by modern American law, with certain limitations. Physician-assisted suicide, for example, remains illegal in 49 states.

The extremes of human life seem to carry the most potential for conflict between various ethical principles in medicine. The end of life, particularly, is a period in which patient and physician decisions may not agree, and in which both are subjected to occasionally contradictory, still-evolving laws.

A. **Euthanasia** is defined by *Merriam-Webster's New Collegiate Dictionary*, tenth edition, as "the act or practice of killing or permitting the death of hopelessly sick or injured individuals in a relatively painless way for reasons of mercy." Permitting death, however, is held by modern medical and ethical authorities to be quite distinct from the action of killing. Popularly, euthanasia is understood as the action of killing a sick individual. Euthanasia may be involuntary or voluntary.

1. **Involuntary euthanasia** is an intervention that ends a person's life without his or her consent. Despite the purported beneficent intent of such interventions, patient autonomy is popularly held to be much more important at the end of life. Involuntary euthanasia is illegal and an unpopular idea in the United States.

2. **Voluntary euthanasia** is an intervention ending a person's life at that person's request, with his or her informed consent. It assumes competency. Illegal in the United States, it nonetheless has been and continues to be practiced here. Estimates of the extent of its use vary greatly. Advocates of voluntary euthanasia see it as an extension of patient autonomy as well as physician beneficence, whereas some opponents define it as murder. Other opponents fear potential abuses of voluntary euthanasia.

B. **Assisted suicide** is the action of providing the means to commit suicide with the knowledge that the recipient plans to use the means to end his or her own life.

1. Assisted suicide is viewed by supporters as an extension of an individual's right to choose or refuse medical treatment. Opponents of the concept envision an extension of the "right to die" into a "duty to die," in which elderly, disabled, or dependent individuals will be coerced into suicide.

2. Physician-assisted suicide remains a subject of national debate. In June 1997, the U.S. Supreme Court handed down decisions in two cases challenging the legality of state bans on assisted suicide (*Washington v Glucksberg* and *Vacco v Quill*). In 9–0 votes, the Court found that there is no constitutional right to assisted suicide, and the matter of whether to ban or legalize assisted suicide was turned back to the states.

3. Oregon remains the only state to legalize physician-assisted suicide in certain circumstances.

C. **Withdrawal of medical treatment**

1. The constitutional right of an individual to request the withdrawal or withholding of medical treatment, even if doing so results in that person's death, was affirmed by the U.S. Supreme Court in 1990 in *Cruzan v Director of the Missouri Dept of Health*. This right was reaffirmed by the Court in 1997, in decisions that stressed the differences between this right and the right to physician-assisted suicide.

2. Most American legal, ethical, and medical authorities agree that no difference exists between withholding unwanted medical support and withdrawing unwanted life support after it has been started.

3. An individual's right to refuse treatment remains valid when he or she becomes incompetent. Written advance directives are authorized by all 50 states and the District of Columbia. Advance directives express the wishes of individuals in a legal document.

4. An exception in some instances to the right to refuse medical treatment has been in pregnancy. Thirty-six states have statutes explicitly forbidding the withdrawal or withholding of life support from a pregnant patient regardless of her choice.

5. An area of legal and ethical controversy exists regarding the administration of medical treatment contrary to the instructions in an advance directive. Several recent court decisions have found nonconsensual medical treatment to be legal battery.

D. **Medical futility**

1. The other side of the patient autonomy debate is the right of patients to request treatments considered futile or inappropriate by the medical community.

2. This issue assumes another dimension when considered in light of the high cost of some of these treatments. There is no legal or societal con-

sensus for situations in which patients and families disagree with physicians' recommendations to stop treatment. Overall, the medical community agrees that patient autonomy should dictate the continuance of treatment in these situations.

E. **Advance care planning** is the process of discussing end-of-life care with one's physician and family. It involves the explicit formulation and recording of the patient's wishes.

1. Multiple studies have shown that patients believe that their physicians should initiate discussion of advance care planning.

2. Advance care planning is best discussed with the patient and family by health care providers who know them well. Frequently, sensitive issues are neglected before hospitalization, so that resident physicians and hospitalists who have never met the patient are left facing an urgent need for decision making in an acute setting.

3. In December 1991, the federal Patient Self-Determination Act went into effect. The act requires health care institutions participating in the Medicaid and Medicare programs to inform all adult patients of their rights "to make decisions concerning medical care, including the right to accept or refuse medical or surgical treatment and the right to formulate an advance directive." Institutions are legally required to provide this information to patients on admission for care. The institution must note in the chart the existence of the advance directive and must respect the directive to the fullest extent possible under state law. Despite passage of the act and increasing attention to issues surrounding the end of life, only approximately 20% of hospitalized patients nationwide have advance directives.

4. An advance directive is oral or written instructions about future medical care in the event the individual is unable to communicate.

5. Health care power of attorney is a legal document in which a patient appoints someone to make decisions if he or she is unable to do so; also known as a health care proxy, durable power of attorney for health care decisions, or appointment of a health care agent.

6. A living will is a written form of advance directive in which a patient describes his or her wishes regarding administration of medical treatment if the patient is unable to communicate.

7. Situations in which patients' surrogate decision makers may disagree with previously formulated advance directives are common. Legally and ethically, it is clear that a surrogate decision maker must follow the advance directive formulated by a competent patient.

III. **Management of symptoms.** A major tenet of palliative care is patient comfort. Relief of distressing symptoms is key to patient endurance of difficult treatment regimens. When patient comfort is optimized, the patient is able to maintain a greater quality of life and often thereby life is prolonged.

A. **Pain**

1. Adequate relief of pain in the dying patient is crucial for promoting a peaceful death. Unfortunately, this goal is not achieved for the majority of patients. The SUPPORT trial found that half of conscious patients who died in the hospital reported experiencing moderate to severe pain the majority of the time.

2. Health professionals and patients frequently hold misconceptions about pain relief measures that impede their effectiveness. Fears of oversedation and addiction to narcotics often limit the administration of appropriate levels of pain relief agents.

3. Considerations in selecting pain medication include the type of pain, effectiveness of medications, route of administration, duration of relief, and patient preferences.

4. Common pain syndromes include bony pain due to metastases; abdominal (visceral) pain; and neuropathic pain (peripheral neuropathies; acute herpes zoster and postherpetic neuralgia).

5. When adequacy of pain relief is being assessed, regimens should be in place for a minimum of 24 hours. Patients should receive additional boluses of pain medications as necessary while adjusting to new regimens.
6. Pain relief tends to more effective when medications are given on a scheduled basis, rather than as necessary.
7. Severity of pain may be assessed by asking the patient to rate pain on a scale of 0 to 10, or using a visual analog scale.
8. The World Health Organization recommends a stepwise approach to pain relief depending on the severity of the pain. Mild pain may be treated initially with nonopioid analgesics. Moderate pain can be initially treated with weaker opioids (such as codeine and oxycodone and severe pain with stronger opioids (morphine sulfate and hydromorphone hydrochloride) supplemented by nonopioid coanalgesics. Adjuvant analgesics may be used throughout. (See Tables 48-1 through 48-3.)
9. Regimens for relief of mild to moderate pain tend to rely initially on oral medications, with intramuscular medications, infusions, and transdermal medications playing more important roles when oral formulations are inadequate. Both constant infusions of narcotics (i.e., morphine or fentanyl patient-controlled analgesia) and transdermal fentanyl patches provide constant levels of narcotics, which promotes more even relief of pain. These long-acting formulations should be supplemented with periodic oral or intravenous boluses for breakthrough pain. Fig. 48-1 depicts a protocol for starting patients on patient-controlled analgesia.
10. The use of intramuscular injections is discouraged.
11. Familiarity with duration of relief is important. Not surprisingly, when narcotics are prescribed at intervals longer than the effective half-life of the drugs, pain returns before administration of the next dose.
12. The risk of addiction in the setting of terminal illness is minimal. Patients should be given adequate doses of narcotics on schedule.
13. Tolerance to narcotics will develop over time, and patients with stable disease often require increasing doses of narcotics to control their pain. It is important to distinguish physical tolerance from addiction.
14. Oversedation due to opioid analgesia is a common problem in the setting of severe pain. Approaches include eliminating contributing factors such as nonessential drugs; assessing the patient for possible metabolic disturbances; lowering opioid requirements by adding adjuvant analgesia; switching opioids; and administering psychostimulants. Reversing analgesia with naloxone hydrochloride is rarely indicated for oversedation.
15. Other common side effects of opioids include nausea, vomiting, pruritus, and constipation. Patients generally develop tolerance to most of these side effects, with the notable exception of constipation. All patients receiving opioids should be placed on a prophylactic bowel regimen.

B. **Fatigue**
1. Fatigue has been identified as the most prevalent symptom affecting cancer patients and has a greater impact on quality of life than pain.
2. Fatigue is usually multifactorial in origin, originating from metabolic and endocrine abnormalities (hypothyroidism, hypercalcemia), anemia, cachexia, insomnia, depression, medications (particularly narcotics and antiemetics), and lack of physical activity.
3. Interventions for fatigue include the following:
   a. Planning of the day to include periods of rest and activity
   b. Prioritization of activities
   c. Delegation of tasks to others

TABLE 48-1. COMPARATIVE DOSING RECOMMENDATIONS FOR OPIOID ANALGESICS

Opioid analgesic	Oral dosing	Parenteral/intramuscular dosing	Comments
Codeine	130 mg every 3–4 hrs	75 mg every 3–4 hrs	Do not give doses higher than 0.5 mg/kg due to increased toxicity. Usually effective for mild to moderate pain only.
Hydrocodone bitartrate (Anexsia, Lortab)	5–10 mg every 3–4 hrs	Not available	Often compounded with adjuvants, which limit dose.
Oxycodone hydrochloride (Percocet, Roxicodone)	5–10 mg every 3–4 hrs	Not available	See above.
Oxycodone hydrochloride, controlled release (OxyContin)	10 mg every 12 hrs	—	—
Morphine sulfate	30 mg every 3–4 hrs	10 mg every 3–4 hrs	Useful for initial dose titration and for break-through pain with long-acting opioids.
Morphine sulfate, controlled release (MS Contin, Oramorph)	30 mg every 8–12 hrs	Not available	Useful for basal pain around the clock.
Hydromorphone hydrochloride (Dilaudid)	7.5 mg every 3–4 hrs	1.5 mg every 3–4 hrs	Useful for initial dose titration and for break-through pain with long-acting opioids.
Fentanyl (Duragesic, Oralet)	Transmucosal lozenges (Actiq) available: 200–1600 µg, maximum 4 lozenges daily	0.1 mg every 1–2 hrs	Fentanyl patch used for basal pain (patches 25, 50, 75, 100 µg/hour).
Methadone hydrochloride (Dolophine)	15–20 mg every 6–8 hrs	7.5–10 mg every 6–8 hrs	Long, variable half-life complicates titration.
Levorphanol tartrate (Levo-Dromoran)	4 mg every 6–8 hrs	2 mg every 6–8 hrs	—

TABLE 48-2. NONOPIOID ANALGESICS

Class	Examples	Comments
Aspirin/nonsteroidal anti-inflammatory drugs	Aspirin, ibuprofen, cele-coxib, ketorolac tromethamine	Inhibit prostaglandin synthetase function. Musculoskeletal pain; bony pain due to metastases.
Tricyclic antidepressants and selective seroto-nin uptake inhibitors	Amitriptyline hydrochlo-ride, desipramine hydrochloride	Increase pain threshold through serotonergic augmentation. Neuropathic pain, especially if burning in nature. Treat pain-related insomnia and fatigue.
Corticosteroids	Dexamethasone	Spinal cord compression; brain tumors. Increase appetite, mood, sense of well-being.
Methylphenidate hydro-chloride (Ritalin)	—	Useful for analgesia-induced lethargy.
Anticonvulsants	Phenytoin, valproate sodium, gabapentin	Neuropathic pain, particularly if paroxysmal or shooting in nature.
Antihistamines	Hydroxyzine	Analgesic and antiemetic.
Muscle relaxants	Cyclobenzaprine hydro-chloride	Musculoskeletal pain.
Anticholinergics	Scopolamine	Visceral pain due to bowel obstruction. Bladder spasms.
Neuroleptics	Fluphenazine	Neuropathic pain.
Local anesthetics	Lidocaine	Neuropathic pain.
Other drugs for neuro-pathic pain	Baclofen, clonidine, calci-tonin, topical capsaicin	—
Other drugs for bony pain	Bisphosphonates, calci-tonin, radiopharma-ceuticals	—
Psychostimulants	Caffeine, methylpheni-date hydrochloride	Useful for analgesia-induced sedation.
Transcutaneous nerve stimulation	—	Localized pain (usually neuro-pathic).

Adapted from American Society of Anesthesiologists Task Force on Pain Management, Cancer Pain Section. Comprehensive evaluation and assessment of the patient with cancer pain. In Miller RD, ed. *Anesthesia*, 5th ed. Philadelphia: Churchill Livingstone, 2000:2843.

    d. Treatment of anemia with blood transfusions or erythropoietin
    e. Treatment of depression (see later)
    f. Provision of physical therapy during bed rest or other times of reduced physical activity
    g. Treatment of insomnia, including minimization of sleep disturbance
    h. Correction of metabolic and endocrine derangements

TABLE 48-3. COMPARATIVE DOSING RECOMMENDATIONS FOR
NONOPIOID ANALGESICS

Analgesic	Oral dosing	Parenteral/ intra-muscular dosing	Comments
Acetami-nophen (Tylenol)	650–975 mg every 4 hrs	Not available	No antiplatelet activity. Maximum daily dose, 4 g. Overdose associated with hepatotoxicity.
Aspirin	650–975 mg every 4 hrs	Not available	Maximum dose, 4 g/day. GI upset and prolonged bleeding time.
Ibuprofen (Advil, Motrin)	400 mg every 4–6 hrs	Not available	Maximum dose, 1.2 g/day. GI upset and bleeding.
Celecoxib (Celebrex)	100 mg every 12 hrs	Not available	Less risk of GI upset and bleeding than with other NSAIDs.
Ketoprofen (Orudis)	25 mg every 6–8 hrs	Not available	Maximum, 75 mg/day.
Naproxen (Naprosyn)	500 mg initial dose, then 250 mg every 6–8 hrs	Not available	Maximum dose, 1.25 g (first day), then 1 g/day.
Ketorolac tromethamine (Toradol)	10 mg every 6–8 hrs	30–60 mg initial dose, then 15–30 mg every 6 hrs	Use not to exceed 5 days.

NSAIDs, nonsteroidal anti-inflammatory drugs.

    C. **Anxiety**
       1. Nonpharmacologic management of anxiety
         a. Muscle relaxation
         b. Diaphragmatic breathing
         c. Biofeedback
         d. Self-hypnosis
         e. Meditation and prayer
         f. Counseling by social worker or psychiatrist
       2. Anxiolytics can be very beneficial.
         a. Benzodiazepines are commonly used (Table 48-4).
         b. Anxiolytics are also helpful for treatment of insomnia.
       3. Low doses of antipsychotic medications (i.e., thioridazine hydrochloride, 10 mg three times daily) may be useful in cases of severe anxiety that has not responded to therapeutic doses of benzodiazepines.
    D. **Depression**
       1. Depression is a normal part of the bereavement process for seriously ill patients. Like pain, depression should be addressed and treated.
       2. Nonpharmacologic considerations are important, including interaction with family and friends, an attempt to maintain activities of daily living, and attentiveness from caregivers and health care personnel. Many patients find counseling or spiritual guidance, or both, to be helpful.
       3. Antidepressants are a key adjunct to nonpharmacologic measures.
       4. Selective serotonin reuptake inhibitors (SSRIs) and secondary amines (a subset of the tricyclic antidepressants, or TCAs) are recom-

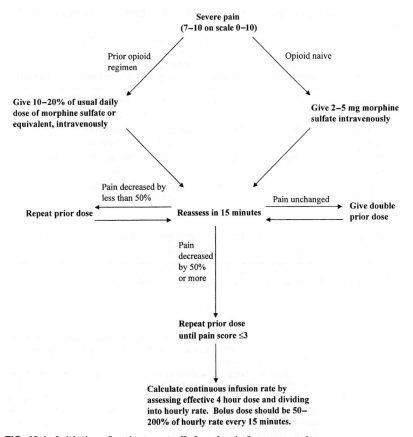

FIG. 48-1. Initiation of patient-controlled analgesia for severe pain.

mended first-line choices for treatment of depression. SSRIs and TCAs have been shown to be equally effective and well tolerated. Both groups of medications usually must be given for 6 to 8 weeks before benefits are seen.

    a. Fluoxetine hydrochloride (Prozac) usually is started at 20 mg/day; sertraline hydrochloride (Zoloft) at 50 mg/day. Most patients will have some response to these low starting dosages. Common side effects include mild nausea, insomnia, and transient worsening of anxiety.

    b. The SSRIs affect the cytochrome P-450 enzyme system and may interact with other medications, including warfarin sodium.

    c. Trazodone hydrochloride (Desyrel) is a less potent SSRI with more sedating effects. Because of the resulting sedation, it is often given in inadequate doses. Antidepressant benefit is not usually seen below 300 mg/day.

  5. Tricyclic antidepressants

    a. Secondary amines include desipramine hydrochloride and nortriptyline hydrochloride, which have a better side effect profile than the tertiary amines (amitriptyline hydrochloride, imipramine).

TABLE 48-4. BENZODIAZEPINES COMMONLY PRESCRIBED FOR TREATMENT OF ANXIETY

Drug	Dose equivalents	Route	Initial dosage (oral)	Absorption	Half-life
Lorazepam (Ativan)	1 mg	PO, IM, IV	0.5–2.0 mg tid	Intermediate	Intermediate
Oxazepam (Serax)	10 mg	PO	10–15 mg tid	Slow-intermediate	Intermediate
Alprazolam (Xanax)	0.5 mg	PO	0.25–1.0 mg tid	Intermediate	Intermediate
Chlordiazepoxide hydrochloride (Librium)	10 mg	PO, IM, IV	10–25 mg tid	Intermediate	Long
Diazepam (Valium)	5 mg	PO, IM, IV	2.5–10 mg tid	Fast	Long

Adapted from Lesko L. Psychologic issues. In: DeVita VT, et al. *Cancer: principles and practice of oncology,* 5th ed. Philadelphia: Lippincott-Raven Publishers, 1996:2884.

   b. The tertiary amines (amitriptyline, imipramine) have been more widely used but have more anticholinergic activity and cause more orthostatic hypotension.
   c. Most TCAs are begun at a dose of 50 mg and are increased in 25-mg increments as tolerated to 150–300 mg/day. Starting doses should be reduced by 50% in patients who are older or ill. Weekly increases in dosage are safest in ill patients, whereas healthy younger patients may tolerate dosage increases every few days. Giving the total daily dose at bedtime is most desirable.
   d. After 8 weeks of administration of a particular antidepressant, an adequate trial has been completed. If response is incomplete, blood levels may be monitored; otherwise, the patient should be switched to a different drug or referred to a psychiatrist.
E. **Delirium**
   1. Intermittent or persistent delirium is common in the final phases of terminal disease. Patients may experience inattentiveness, nonrecognition of family or friends, frank confusion, and so on.
   2. Early delirium may be mistaken for depression. Any abrupt behavioral changes should be thoroughly investigated.
   3. Causes are myriad and include metabolic derangements, infections, tumor metastases to the brain, use of analgesics or psychotropics, or a combination of factors. Unless death is imminent, all efforts should be made to reverse causes of delirium in the terminally ill patient.
      a. Electrolyte abnormalities should be corrected.
      b. Adequate caloric and fluid intake should be ensured.
      c. Infection should be ruled out.
      d. Withdrawal from alcohol or sedatives should be treated.
      e. Brain metastases should be diagnosed and treated palliatively.
      f. Analgesic or psychotropic regimens should be adjusted.
      g. Changes in other medications such as beta-blockers, H_2 blockers, and anticholinergics should be given attention.

4. Symptomatic treatment of delirium
   a. Frequent reassurance
   b. Avoidance of overstimulation
   c. Preservation of normal circadian rhythms
   d. Low-dose neuroleptics

F. **Dyspnea**
   1. Dyspnea is a common complaint in terminally ill patients. Some studies have found it to be the most common uncontrolled symptom in dying patients. It may be accompanied by anxiety and fear of suffocation.
   2. Causes of dyspnea may include extensive lung or pleural disease, ascites that causes pressure on the diaphragm, or chemotherapy- or radiation-induced lung injury, with pain and anxiety acting as strong contributors. Other medical problems, including chronic obstructive pulmonary disease, anemia, asthma, and heart failure, also are major contributors.
   3. Management of dyspnea
      a. Positioning of the patient upright in bed or on a chair.
      b. Administration of oxygen.
      c. Air circulation using fan or open window.
      d. Relaxation techniques.
      e. Reassurance.
      f. Low doses of opiates and sedatives, including morphine and lorazepam. Note that narcotics will decrease shortness of breath, but also decrease respiratory drive. It is acceptable, with the patient's consent, to titrate narcotic dosages upward for comfort, although this may hasten death.
      g. Nebulized beta-agonists or morphine. Morphine may be delivered in a nebulized form, which can be particularly useful in patients receiving large systemic doses of narcotics.
      h. Attention to the underlying cause of dyspnea, if appropriate. Patients with symptomatic pleural effusions may benefit from periodic therapeutic thoracentesis, for example.

G. **Nausea**
   1. Nausea may be caused by metabolic abnormalities, medications and chemotherapy, and psychological factors, as well as mechanical disorders such as constipation, ileus, or bowel obstruction. As with other symptom complexes, the cause is often multifactorial.
   2. Nonpharmacologic interventions
      a. Clear liquid diet should be given until symptoms resolve.
      b. Small, frequent portions of food are often tolerated better than large meals.
      c. For mild nausea, nibbling crackers and toast may be effective.
      d. Patients are advised to avoid lying down immediately after eating.
      e. Patients should avoid drinking liquids with food, which can increase the sensation of bloating.
      f. Ileus and bowel obstruction should be treated with GI rest and placement of a nasogastric tube as necessary. Terminally ill patients with carcinomatous ileus or other conditions in which bowel function is not expected to return expediently may benefit from placement of gastrostomy or jejunostomy tubes for bowel decompression, which are more comfortable than nasogastric tubes.
   3. Pharmacologic interventions
      a. Phenothiazines are effective against nausea due to narcotics. Prochlorperazine (5–10 mg orally or 25 mg per rectum every 4–6 hours) causes less sedation and hypotension than chlorpromazine. Cannabinoids can be even more useful than prochlorperazine, although restrictions on their administration precludes widespread use.
      b. Haloperidol (0.5–2.0 mg orally or subcutaneously every 6–8 hours) may be effective for nausea in an agitated patient.

    c. Gastroparesis may be treated with metoclopramide and cisapride.

    d. Corticosteroids (i.e., dexamethasone 8 mg every 8 hours) are also helpful, although the mechanism of their antiemetic action is unclear. Patients with advanced cancer may have adrenal insufficiency that leads to nausea and vomiting.

    e. Anticholinergics such as scopolamine can be useful for controlling secretions.

    f. For treatment of nausea due to chemotherapy, see Chap. 47. Benzodiazepines can be useful for controlling the anticipatory nausea and vomiting that develops in some patients receiving chemotherapy.

H. Anorexia

1. Anorexia is the second most common symptom in patients with advanced cancer, after fatigue. Anorexia and weight loss may be due to disease [particularly advanced cancer and acquired immunodeficiency syndrome (AIDS)], treatment, and psychological factors such as depression and anxiety.

2. Unpalatability of food is often the chief complaint. Patients understand the need to ingest food but cannot. Fatigue also plays an important role in that many patients are too tired to eat. It may be beneficial for treatment of anorexia to differentiate true anorexia, or food avoidance, from early satiety.

3. Patients with advanced cancer and AIDS, in particular, often have cachexia. Food intake is inadequate to keep up with the high energy demands of the illness.

4. Families become particularly concerned by anorexia, pressing the ill person to eat. It is important to realize, however, that anorexia is common and normal in progressive illness and especially in the final days of life.

5. Management of anorexia

    a. Educational and behavioral interventions

      (1) Consultation with a nutritionist may be beneficial.

      (2) Provision of small, frequent, high-calorie, appetizing meals may be helpful.

      (3) Social aspects of eating (sharing meals with family or friends) are often lost during illness and may be restored with some benefit.

      (4) Relaxation techniques and self-hypnosis may be useful when anxiety and other anticipatory phenomena contribute to poor intake.

    b. Medical interventions

      (1) The use of enteral tubes and parenteral nutrition is common in seriously ill patients. Numerous studies have discouraged the use of parenteral nutrition in terminally ill patients due to its high cost and potential complications, as well as lack of evidence of survival benefit. However, there has been little study of the impact of parenteral nutrition on quality of life and performance status in terminally ill patients. Parenteral nutrition may be beneficial in patients who are losing weight due to starvation as opposed to the cachexia syndrome, which does not respond to calorie replacement.

      (2) Medications

        (a) Steroids

        (b) Antidepressants

        (c) Cannabinoids function as antiemetics. Dronabinol, a synthetic cannabinoid marketed in the United States, has been shown to improve weight gain, reduce weight loss, and improve appetite. Smoked marijuana may be even more effective due to greater bioavailability and to the presence of active agents in crude marijuana that are absent in dronabinol and other synthetic cannabinoids. Crude marijuana remains illegal in the United States.

(d) Megestrol acetate (Megace) has been shown to increase appetite and weight gain in patients with cancer and AIDS. A dosage of 160–320 mg daily is typically given, although some studies have used much higher doses successfully (800–1600 mg daily).

I. **Constipation**
1. Constipation is a major problem in terminally ill patients, particularly those receiving narcotic pain medications. Other causes of constipation include lack of physical activity; lack of fluid or fiber intake, and use of other medications including anticholinergics. Hypercalcemia also may contribute.
2. A prophylactic approach to constipation is most effective.
3. Chronic constipation
   a. General recommendations include regular exercise, when possible. Increase in fluid intake (at least 1.5 L daily) can be helpful. Patients should attempt defecation daily for 10–15 minutes, approximately 30 minutes after breakfast. Patients with difficulty expelling stool may find that placing a 15-cm support under their feet to flex the hips while seated on the toilet may help.
   b. Dietary modifications include increasing dietary fiber to 20–30 g/day to increase stool bulk and water content.
      (1) Bran powder is inexpensive; 1–2 tbs twice daily mixed with fluids or sprinkled on food provides 10–20 g/day of fiber.
      (2) Fiber supplements, such as psyllium (Metamucil, 3–4 g) or methylcellulose (2 g), can be given 1–3 times daily. Adequate oral intake is required for such supplements to be effective.
   c. Pharmacologic therapy
      (1) Osmotic laxatives may be used to soften stools. These may be used long-term as dependency is not induced. They are typically titrated to a dose that results in soft to semiliquid stools.
      (2) Nonabsorbable sugars (lactulose, sorbitol 15–60 mL/day) are equally effective, but sorbitol is less expensive. Bothersome side effects include bloating, cramping, and flatulence due to malabsorbed sugars.
      (3) Saline laxatives (e.g., magnesium hydroxide, or milk of magnesia, 30–60 mL/day) may be administered. Hypermagnesemia may result from use in patients with impaired renal function.
      (4) Emollient laxatives (docusate sodium, 50–200 mg/day; mineral oil, 1–2 tbs/day) may be given orally to promote stool softening. Mineral oil should be avoided in patients with decreased neurologic function due to risk of aspiration.
      (5) Cisapride (a serotonin 5-hydroxytryptamine 4 agonist) increases colonic motility.
4. Acute constipation
   a. Cathartic laxatives stimulate fluid secretion and colonic contraction, resulting in a bowel movement within 6–12 hours after oral administration or 15–60 minutes after rectal administration. They may cause severe cramping and diarrhea. Chronic use may result in loss of normal colonic neuromuscular function. Specific cathartic laxatives include cascara (4–8 mL by mouth), bisacodyl (5–15 mg by mouth or 10-mg rectal suppository), and castor oil (15–45 mL by mouth).
   b. Osmotic laxatives produce evacuation in 30 minutes to 3 hours, generally with less discomfort than cathartic laxatives. Specific laxatives include magnesium citrate (18 g/10 oz); magnesium sulfate, or Epsom salts (10–30); sodium phosphate (15–30 g); and balanced polyethylene glycol lavage, or GoLYTELY.
   c. When acute constipation is particularly severe, it is best to start with enemas before giving laxatives.
      (1) Nonirritating: saline enemas (120–240 mL)

(2) Irritating: tap water enema (500–1000 mL)

(3) For hard or impacted stool: oil retention enema

d. Use of laxatives should be avoided in patients with large bowel obstruction or fecal impaction.

5. Fecal impaction

a. Fecal impaction may result in obstruction of fecal flow leading to a partial or complete large bowel obstruction. Presentation includes nausea, vomiting, abdominal pain, and distention. Patients may experience paradoxical diarrhea as liquid stool leaks around the impacted feces.

b. Initial treatment is aimed at relieving the impaction with enemas or digitally, with care taken not to injure the anal sphincter. Rarely, patients may require regional or general anesthesia. Myelosuppressed patients should not be digitally disimpacted. Once fecal impaction is relieved, long-term care follows as described earlier.

IV. **Psychosocial and spiritual considerations**

A. **Communication with patients and families**

1. Communication skills are not emphasized in medical training but may be learned by individual effort on the part of the caregiver.

2. Clear and empathetic communication of bad news is particularly difficult, and especially important. Bad news, whether it is a new diagnosis, treatment failure, or disease progression, necessitates a period of examination of patients' and families' goals. Discussion of practical matters, including changes in curative or palliative treatments, alterations in care, and any changes in advance directives, follows.

3. If the patient desires, family members or close friends should be included in discussions.

4. The physician should be clear when communicating with patients and families. The use of euphemisms should be avoided.

5. Patients should be given time to react to news. Typically, most information imparted after the delivery of bad news is not assimilated by the patient because it takes all the patient's mental energy to absorb the bad news alone. One should expect to repeat more information at a later date. Written information should be given to the patient.

6. Patient and family understanding should be checked during the discussion. The patient should be asked about his or her perception of the situation, which allows assessment of the level of understanding as well as the patient's fears and future needs.

7. When the discussion is finished, a specific date and time should be set for a follow-up appointment or discussion.

B. **Challenges of dying.** Patients with life-threatening illness face multiple psychosocial and spiritual as well as physical challenges. These include

1. Loss of ability to participate in employment or social activities because of symptoms, side effects, or concerns about infection

2. Guilt about the impact of illness on family and friends

3. Depression and anger (loss of a future)

4. Changes in body image, including loss of comfort with sexual intimacy

5. Discrimination or stigmatization by others

6. Role conflicts and meeting the demands of the role of the patient

7. Fear of the dying process and concerns about physical suffering, including pain and cachexia

C. **Hospice**

1. The first American hospice opened in New Haven, Connecticut, in 1974. In 1983, hospice services became part of the Medicare benefits program.

2. The National Hospice Organization defines hospice as comprehensive, medically directed, team-oriented care that aims to treat and comfort terminally ill individuals and their families either at home or in a homelike setting. Clinical goals include control of pain and other symptoms.

Psychological and spiritual suffering are prioritized as highly as physical suffering. Families are offered bereavement support.

3. Today, only about half of dying patients are referred to hospice services; those who do enter hospice programs often enter too late to benefit from the many support services offered.

4. Why are patients not offered hospice care, and why do patients refuse it when offered?

   a. To qualify for hospice care, Medicare patients must be certified by their physicians to have an expected survival of 6 months or less. This regulation has limited the use of hospice care by many patients who may benefit from its services.

   b. Denial of the patient's prognosis by the patient or the family is common. This denial is exacerbated by physicians' own tendencies toward denial, both of the patient's clinical reality and of their ability to prolong survival, control symptoms, and improve quality of life.

   c. Families and health care professionals perceive a need to continue to instill hope. Some patients may feel that hospice care amounts to abandonment by their health care team. Some patients and families feel that using hospice care amounts to "giving up."

   d. Patients may be candidates for research trials, which precludes hospice care.

   e. Financial disincentives to hospice care still exist for both families and physicians.

5. Hospice care may take place at home or in a hospital-based program. Most patients prefer to die at home; however, many patients and families do not feel prepared for the enormous burden of 24-hour care at home. These families may prefer an inpatient setting.

Section Six. APPENDIXES

Appendix A. DRUGS COMMONLY USED IN GYNECOLOGY AND OBSTETRICS

Janice Falls and Frank Witter

I. **Introduction.** Medications taken during pregnancy must be evaluated carefully to prevent the treatment of the illness from becoming more harmful to the woman and her fetus than the illness itself. It is imperative that those medications used during pregnancy be safe for the woman and her fetus. Today, teratogenic medications account for as many as 1–5% of all congenital anomalies.

Although growth and the CNS can be adversely affected later on in pregnancy, it is during the early stages of fetal development (embryogenesis) that the most deleterious effects of maternal drug ingestion can occur. This early developmental phase of embryogenesis is also a time during which the mother may not be aware of her pregnancy. It is therefore vital for the physician working with women of reproductive age to be cognizant of the fact that an undetected pregnancy may be present while treating other medical needs of the patient.

II. **Fetal development and teratogenesis.** If the human embryo is exposed to teratogenic substances during the first 2–3 weeks of life, the exposure will usually result in either abortion or no anomalies (known as the all-or-none effect). It is especially during the gestational ages of 3–8 weeks (or 31–71 days after the menstrual period in a regular 28- to 30-day menstrual cycle) that the embryonic organs are most susceptible to teratogenic effects. During the second half of pregnancy, medications can have less harmful, but still adverse, effects on the fetus. For example, tetracycline has been shown to discolor the fetus's teeth and alter bone growth after maternal ingestion during the latter half of pregnancy. It is important to note that, if a teratogenic substance is taken after vulnerable periods in fetal development, it cannot cause the same teratogenic effects as it would if ingested during the vulnerable time of embryonic/fetal development.

III. **Food and Drug Administration (FDA) pregnancy medication categories**

Category	Description
A	Controlled studies demonstrate no fetal risk in the first or later trimesters, and probability of fetal harm is remote.
B	Either animal studies alone show no fetal risk, or if fetal harm is demonstrated in animal studies, controlled human trials do not confirm adverse effect in the first trimester or later in the pregnancy.
C	Either adverse effects have been demonstrated in animal studies with no controlled human studies, or studies in humans or animals are not available.
D	Human studies reveal potential adverse effects to the fetus, but risks and benefits relative to the medical state of the mother may support drug's use.
X	Animal or human studies demonstrate fetal abnormalities or fetal risk; use is contraindicated during pregnancy or in women who may become pregnant.

It is important to note that paternal use of medications and their effects on sperm and subsequent teratogenicity is not well understood. To date, however, no documented teratogenicity has been associated with paternal medication exposure.

IV. **Dietary needs during pregnancy and lactation.** During pregnancy and lactation, it is recommended that the mother continue eating a well-balanced diet and not ingest too much or too little of vitamins and minerals. Negative fetal and neonatal effects can occur, for example, with consumption of too much vitamin A (CNS and cardiovascular anomalies, facial clefts) or too little vitamin D (decreased fetal growth, neonatal rickets, and defective tooth enamel).

The National Academy of Sciences recommended vitamin and mineral dietary allowances during pregnancy and lactation are as follows.

Vitamin/ mineral	Nonpregnant (age in yrs)			Pregnant	Lactating (up to 6 mos)
	15–18	19–24	25–50		
Vitamin A (μg)	800	800	800	800 (2700 IU)	1300
Vitamin B_1 (thiamin) (mg)	1.1	1.1	1.1	1.5	1.6
Vitamin B_2 (riboflavin) (mg)	1.3	1.3	1.3	1.6	1.8
Vitamin B_3 (niacin) (mg)	15	15	15	17	20
Vitamin B_6 (pyridoxine) (mg)	1.5	1.6	1.6	2.2	2.1
Vitamin B_{12} (μg)	2.0	2.0	2.0	2.2	2.6
Vitamin C (mg)	60	60	60	70	95
Vitamin D (μg)	10	5	5	10	10
Vitamin E (mg)	8	8	8	10	12
Folic acid (μg)	180	180	180	400	280
Calcium (mg)	1200	1200	800	1200	1200
Phosphorus (mg)	1200	1200	800	1200	1200
Magnesium (mg)	300	280	280	320	355
Iron (mg)	15	15	15	30	15
Zinc (mg)	12	12	12	15	19
Iodine (μg)	150	150	150	175	200
Selenium (μg)	50	55	55	65	75
Protein (g)	44	46	50	60	65

V. **Human teratogens.** Human teratogens include medications, as well as environmental chemicals (i.e., mercury, lead, chlorbiphenyls), and infectious agents (i.e., rubella virus, cytomegalovirus, *Toxoplasma gondii*, varicella virus). The only teratogenic category to be considered here is medications for human ingestion (whether prescribed or available without a prescription). Although the teratogenic potential of most substances is unknown, it seems appropriate to provide pregnant women with all of the facts available regarding the teratogenicity of any drug, chemical, or environmental agent to which they may be exposed.

Teratogen	Congenital malformation
Alcohol (4–5 drinks or 60–75 mL or more absolute alcohol daily)	Fetal alcohol syndrome (short palpebral fissures, maxillary hypoplasia, heart defects, mild to moderate mental retardation)
Aminopterin	Anencephaly, hydrocephaly, cleft lip and palate
Androgens	Masculinization of female genitalia (fused labia, clitoral hypertrophy)
Diethylstilbestrol	Malformations of the uterus, fallopian tubes, and upper vagina; vaginal cancer; malformed testes
Etretinate	Meningomyelocele, meningoencephalocele, facial dysmorphia, syndactylies, absent terminal phalanges
Isotretinoin	Small, malformed ears; mandibular hypoplasia; cleft palate; heart defects; hydrocephalus; microcephaly; limb reduction
Methotrexate sodium	Anencephaly, spina bifida, heart defects
Thalidomide	Limb defects, heart malformations
Vitamin A (more than 10,000 IU daily)	CNS and cardiovascular anomalies, microtia, facial clefts, neural tube defects
Warfarin sodium	Chondrodysplasia punctata (nasal hypoplasia, ophthalmologic abnormalities, bone stippling, mental retardation), microcephaly

VI. **Common medications used during pregnancy**

A. **Analgesics.** Aspirin has no teratogenic effects but does increase bleeding at the time of delivery, delays labor onset, and prolongs labor. Acetaminophen has no known teratogenicity. Prolonged use of other nonsteroidal antiinflammatory drug should be avoided in pregnancy due to an increased association with oligohydramnios. Indomethacin, if used for prolonged periods of time after 34 weeks' gestation, can cause constriction of the ductus arteriosus and neonatal pulmonary hypertension. In general, frequent use of narcotics should be avoided, as they can be become addictive to the patient and fetus, which results in withdrawal symptoms in the fetus or infant when either the patient stops use or the fetus is delivered.

Narcotic	FDA class	NSAID/analgesic	FDA class
Buprenorphine hydrochloride	C	Acetaminophen	B
Butorphanol tartrate	B[a]	Aspirin	C[b]
Codeine	C[a]	Ibuprofen	B[c]
Codeine phosphate and acetaminophen (Tylenol No. 3)	C[a]	Indomethacin	B[d]
		Ketorolac tromethamine	C[c]
Fentanyl	B[a]	Nabumetone	C[c]
Hydrocodone	C[a]	Nalbuphine hydrochloride	B[a]
Hydromorphone hydrochloride	B[a]	Naproxen	B[a]

Narcotic	FDA class	NSAID/analgesic	FDA class
Meperidine hydrochloride	B[a]	Pentazocine hydrochloride	C
Methadone hydrochloride	B[a]	Sulindac	B[c]
Morphine sulfate	B[a]		
Nalbuphine hydrochloride	B[a]		
Oxycodone	B[a]		
Oxycodone hydrochloride and acetaminophen (Tylox)	B[a]		
Propoxyphene	C[a]		

[a]Class D if used for prolonged periods of time or high doses at term.
[b]Class D if full-dose aspirin is used in the third trimester.
[c]Class D if used in the third trimester or near delivery.
[d]Class D if used longer than 48 hours, or after 34 weeks' gestation, or close to delivery.

B. **Antiasthmatics.** Terbutaline sulfate and theophylline are both considered safe medications in pregnancy. Prednisolone and prednisone are mostly inactivated by the placenta and have minimal if any effect on the developing fetus. Due to lessened maternal systemic effects, inhaled steroids are considered preferable to oral steroids.

Antiasthmatic	FDA class	Antiasthmatic	FDA class
Albuterol	C	Ipratropium bromide	B
Aminophylline	C	Metaproterenol sulfate	C
Beclomethasone dipropionate	C	Methylprednisolone	C
Cromolyn sodium	B	Prednisone	B
Epinephrine	C	Terbutaline	B
Fluticasone propionate	C	Theophylline	C
Hydrocortisone	B	Triamcinolone	C

C. **Anticoagulants.** Heparin sodium is the drug of choice for anticoagulation as it does not cross the placenta. Warfarin sodium, which crosses the placenta, causes chondrodysplasia punctata (nasal hypoplasia, ophthalmologic abnormalities, bone stippling, and mental retardation) in 5% of exposed infants.

Anticoagulation	FDA class	Anticoagulation	FDA class
Warfarin sodium (Coumadin)	D/X	Heparin sodium	B
Enoxaparin sodium	B	Nadroparin	B

D. **Anticonvulsants.** There is an increased risk of fetal malformations in epileptic women, whether or not they take anticonvulsant therapy. Use of multiple anticonvulsants (more than three) by the patient, however, is associated with increased risk of congenital anomalies. For those patients on anticonvulsants, 4 mg/day of folic acid should be started 1–3 months before pregnancy and taken up to at least 12 weeks' gestation. Ingestion of 10 mg/day of vitamin K has been recommended during the last month of pregnancy, although this is somewhat controversial. Anticonvulsant plasma levels should be assessed regularly to assure that the lowest effective dose is maintained.

Anticonvulsant	FDA class	Anticonvulsant	FDA class
Carbamazepine	C	Phenytoin	D
Gabapentin	C	Valproic acid	D
Phenobarbital	D		

E. **Antiemetics, antiulcer drugs, antidiarrheals, laxatives.** It is best to initially treat GI symptoms of pregnancy conservatively with change in diet and eating habits. If the patient requires medical management of her symptoms, then any of the following medications are considered nonteratogenic during pregnancy and may be taken.

Antiemetics	FDA class	Antiulcer drugs	FDA class
Dimenhydrinate	B	Calcium carbonate	*
Metoclopramide	B	Cimetidine	B
Ondansetron hydrochloride	B	Famotidine	B
Prochlorperazine	C	Lansoprazole	B
Promethazine hydrochloride	C	Aluminum hydroxide (Maalox)	*
Simethicone	C	Nizatidine	B
Sucralfate	B	Omeprazole	C
		Ranitidine	B

Antidiarrheals	FDA class	Laxatives	FDA class
Diphenoxylate hydrochloride	C	Bisacodyl	B
Kaopectate	*	Docusate sodium	C
Loperamide hydrochloride	B	Docusate sodium plus casanthranol (Peri-Colace)	C
Bismuth subsalicylate	C	Lactulose	B
Psyllium	B	Magnesium sulfate	B
Senna	C	Mineral oil	C

*Generally accepted as safe.

F. **Antimicrobials.** Most antibiotics readily cross the placenta. Common antimicrobials are listed here, including contraindicated medications. Prolonged use of aminoglycosides for more than 2 weeks should be avoided if at all possible due to the potential risk of ototoxicity to the mother and fetus.

Aminoglycoside	FDA class	Antifungals	FDA class
Amikacin sulfate	C/D	Amphotericin B	B
Gentamicin	C	Clotrimazole	B
Kanamycin sulfate	D	Fluconazole	C
Neomycin	C	Griseofulvin	C
Streptomycin	D	Itraconazole	C
Tobramycin	C/D	Ketoconazole	C
Terbinafine hydrochloride	C	Miconazole nitrate	C
		Nystatin	B

Antivirals	FDA class	Antivirals	FDA class
Acyclovir	C	Nevirapine	C
Amantadine hydrochloride	C	Rimantadine hydrochloride	C
Didanosine	B	Stavudine	C
Famciclovir	B	Valacyclovir hydrochloride	B
Foscarnet sodium	C	Vidarabine	C
Ganciclovir	C	Zidovudine	C
Lamivudine	C	Zidovudine with lamivudine (Combivir)	C
Nelfinavir mesylate	B		

G. **Cephalosporins.** All first-, second-, and third-generation cephalosporins are FDA class B medications, except moxalactam, which is a class C drug.
H. **Fluoroquinolones.** All quinolones are FDA class C medications. They are not recommended for use during pregnancy, however, due to the association with cartilage disorders in the joints of young animals, and because safer antibiotics are usually available.
I. **Macrolides**

Macrolide	FDA class	Macrolide	FDA class
Azithromycin	B	Erythromycin	B
Clarithromycin	C		

J. **Penicillins.** All penicillins are FDA class B medications.

K. **Sulfonamides.** All sulfonamides are FDA class B medications throughout pregnancy except near term, when they become class D. Sulfa drugs should not be prescribed for women with glucose-6-phosphate dehydrogenase deficiency due to possible hemolysis in the patient and fetus. Also, they should not be used in the third trimester due to the theoretical possibility of hyperbilirubinemia in the newborn (sulfonamides compete with bilirubin for albumin binding sites).

L. **Tetracyclines.** All tetracyclines are class D medications and are contraindicated in pregnancy.

M. **Other antimicrobials**

Agent	FDA class	Agent	FDA class
Alpha interferon	C	Isoniazid	C
Aztreonam	B	Mefloquine hydrochloride	C
Bacitracin zinc	C	Metronidazole	B
Chloramphenicol	C	Nitrofurantoin	B
Chloroquine (hydrochloride or phosphate)	C	Polymyxin B sulfate	B
Clindamycin	B	Quinine sulfate	D/X
Ethambutol hydrochloride	B	Rifampin	C
Hydroxychloroquine sulfate	C	Spectinomycin hydrochloride	B
Imipenem	C	Trimethoprim	C
		Vancomycin hydrochloride	C

N. **Antipsychotics and antimanics.** Phenothiazines do not appear to have teratogenicity. Due to the possibility of serious side effects, however, their use should be reserved for patients with severe symptoms requiring medical treatment. Lithium use is associated with congenital birth defects (i.e., cardiovascular defects, Ebstein's anomaly), and its use should be avoided if possible during pregnancy, especially during organogenesis. Lithium should be avoided in pregnancy unless the patient is at greater risk of affective instability than of fetal congenital malformations. If a patient must be maintained on lithium, a fetal echocardiography should be performed, as the fetus is at greater risk for cardiac anomalies.

Antipsychotic/antimanic	FDA class	Antipsychotic/antimanic	FDA class
Chlorpromazine	C	Mesoridazine besylate	C
Clozapine	B	Olanzapine	C
Fluphenazine hydrochloride	C	Risperidone	C
Haloperidol	C	Thioridazine hydrochloride	C
Lithium	D	Trifluoperazine hydrochloride	C
Loxapine	C		

O. **Anxiolytics and antidepressants.** Benzodiazepines should be used very cautiously during pregnancy. Diazepam has been associated with respiratory depression, hypotonia, and hypothermia. Amitriptyline hydrochloride appears to be relatively safe during pregnancy with the majority of evidence supporting its safety. Fluoxetine hydrochloride has to date shown no evidence of increased risk of congenital anomalies.

Drug	FDA class	Drug	FDA class
Anticholinergic/antihistaminic		Tricyclic antidepressants	
Diphenhydramine	B	Amitriptyline hydrochloride	D
Hydroxyzine	C	Clomipramine hydrochloride	C
Barbiturates		Desipramine hydrochloride	C
Pentobarbital sodium	D	Doxepin hydrochloride	C
Phenobarbital	D	Imipramine	D
Secobarbital sodium	D	Nortriptyline hydrochloride	D
Benzodiazepines		Other	
Alprazolam	D	Amoxapine	C
Chlordiazepoxide	D	Bupropion hydrochloride	B
Clonazepam	D	Buspirone hydrochloride	B
Diazepam	D	Chloral hydrate	C
Lorazepam	D	Fluphenazine hydrochloride	C
Midazolam hydrochloride	D	Lithium	D
Oxazepam	D	Nefazodone hydrochloride	C
Temazepam	X	Trazodone hydrochloride	C
Triazolam	X	Valproic acid	D
Selective serotonin reuptake inhibitors		Venlafaxine hydrochloride	C
Fluoxetine hydrochloride	B	Zolpidem tartrate	B
Fluvoxamine maleate	C		
Paroxetine hydrochloride	B		
Sertraline hydrochloride	B		

P. **Cardiovascular drugs.** Angiotensin-converting enzyme inhibitors should be avoided in the second and third trimesters of pregnancy as they can cause fetal limb contractures, craniofacial deformities, hypoplastic lung development, oligohydramnios, and fetal death in utero. Digoxin, methyldopa, propranolol hydrochloride, and hydralazine hydrochloride have no apparent teratogenic effects in the fetus. Diuretics should be used with extreme caution as they have the potential to deplete intravascular volume and alter electrolyte balance.

Drug	FDA class	Drug	FDA class
Antiadrenergics		Diuretics	
Clonidine	C	Amiloride hydrochloride	B
Doxazosin mesylate	C	Bumetanide	C
Methyldopa	C	Furosemide	C
Prazosin hydrochloride	C	Hydrochlorothiazide	D
Reserpine	C	Methazolamide	C
Terazosin hydrochloride	C	Spironolactone	D
Antidysrhythmics		Nitrates	
Adenosine	C	Isosorbide (mono- or dinitrate)	C
Amiodarone hydrochloride	C	Nitroglycerin (all forms)	B
Atropine sulfate	C	Pressors/inotropes	
Digitalis	C	Dobutamine hydrochloride	C
Digoxin	C	Dopamine hydrochloride	C
Epinephrine	C	Ephedrine	C
Isoproterenol	C	Epinephrine	C
Lidocaine	C	Norepinephrine bitartrate	D
Procainamide hydrochloride	C		
Antihyperlipidemics			
All of the "statins" are contraindicated in pregnancy.			
Colestipol hydrochloride	B		
Gemfibrozil	C		
Niacin	A[a]		
Antihypertensives			
Amlodipine besylate	C		
Atenolol	D		
Carvedilol	C		
Diazoxide	C		
Diltiazem hydrochloride	C		
Felodipine	C		
Hydralazine hydrochloride	C		
Labetalol hydrochloride	C[b]		
Methyldopa	C		
Metoprolol	C		
Nifedipine	C		
Nitroprusside sodium	C		
Prazosin hydrochloride	C		
Propranolol hydrochloride	C		
Terazosin hydrochloride	C		
Verapamil hydrochloride	C		

[a]Class C if used above the recommended daily allowance.
[b]Class D if used in second or third trimester.

Q. **Drugs for the treatment of diabetes mellitus.** For women with diabetes mellitus, whether type 1 or type 2, maintaining strict glycemic control is the goal. Insulin is the drug of choice during pregnancy. Human insulin is recommended, as animal insulin (bovine or porcine) crosses the placenta as an insulin-antibody complex. Human insulin (semisynthetic) is far less immunogenic and may be better tolerated by those women receiving insulin for the first time. Oral hypoglycemics (i.e., glipizide, glyburide) are FDA class C medications and may have prolonged hypoglycemic effects in the fetus or neonate. Glyburide does not cross the placenta in measurable amounts, however, and is not associated with neonatal hypoglycemia. Glyburide also does not lower blood glucose levels adequately. Insulin is the preferred antidiabetic medication.

Antidiabetic/hypoglycemic	FDA class	Antidiabetic/hypoglycemic	FDA class
Chlorpropamide	C	Insulin (all forms)	B
Glimepiride	C	Metformin hydrochloride	B
Glipizide	C	Tolazamide	C
Glyburide	C	Tolbutamide	C

R. **Other agents.** The list of medications given here is not meant to be an exhaustive compilation of drugs. There are many medications that have been omitted, most of which are less commonly used in pregnancy.

Agent	FDA class	Agent	FDA class
Acarbose	B	Estrogens	X
Alpha interferon	C	Ethanol	D/X
Amphetamines	C	Folic acid	A
Baclofen	C	Guaifenesin	C
Beclomethasone dipropionate	C	Heroin	B
Benztropine mesylate	C	Hydroxyprogesterone	D
Betamethasone	C	Immune globulin	
Bromocriptine mesylate	C	IM/IV IgG	C
Caffeine	B	Hepatitis B	C
Calcitonin	B	Rabies	C
Carbidopa	C	Tetanus	C
Clomiphene citrate	X	Varicella zoster	C
Cocaine hydrochloride	C/X	Indigo carmine	B
Cortisone acetate	D	Iodine	D
Dexamethasone	C	Lamotrigine	C
Epoetin alfa	C	Leucovorin calcium	C
Ergotamine tartrate	D	Leuprolide acetate	X

Agent	FDA class	Agent	FDA class
Levodopa	C	Reserpine	C
Levothyroxine	A	Ribavirin	X
Lidocaine	C	Ritodrine hydrochloride	B
Lindane	B	Saccharin	C
Liothyronine sodium	A	Scopolamine	C
Loratadine	B	Silicone breast implants	C
Lysergic acid diethylamide (LSD)	C	Simethicone	C
Magnesium sulfate	B	Streptokinase	C
Mannitol	C	Sulfasalazine	B
Marijuana	C	Sumatriptan succinate	C
Meclizine hydrochloride	B	Tamoxifen citrate	D
Mesalamine	B	Thioridazine hydrochloride	C
Methadone hydrochloride	B	Thyroglobulin	A
Methamphetamine hydrochloride	C	Urokinase	B
Methimazole	D	Vaccines	
Methylene blue	C	Bacille Calmette-Guérin	C
Mifepristone	X	Cholera	C
Misoprostol	X	*Escherichia coli*	C
Naloxone hydrochloride	B	Group B streptococcus	C
Niacin	A	*Haemophilus* B	C
Nitrofurantoin	B	Hepatitis A and B	C
Octreotide acetate	B	Influenza	C
Opium	B	Measles	X
Oxybutynin chloride	B	Meningococcus	C
Penicillamine	D	Mumps	X
Phenazopyridine hydrochloride	B	Plague	C
Phenytoin	D	Pneumococcus	C
Podophyllum	C	Polio (inactive and live)	C
Prednisolone	B	Rabies (human)	C
Prednisone	B	Rubella	X
Probenecid	B	Smallpox	X
Propofol	B	Tularemia	C
Propylthiouracil	D	Typhoid	C
Protamine sulfate	C	Yellow fever	D
Pseudoephedrine	C	Vasopressin	B
Pyridoxine hydrochloride	A*		

*Class C if used above the recommended daily allowance.

S. **Preeclampsia and tocolytic drugs.** Medications for treatment of preeclampsia and for tocolysis are considered separately in Chaps. 14 and 9, respectively.

Appendix B. PRACTICAL MEDICAL SPANISH FOR GYNECOLOGY AND OBSTETRICS

Brandon J. Bankowski and Jairo Garcia

I. **Introduction**

Hello, I'm Dr. Smith.
Hola, yo soy el (male)/la (female) doctor/doctora Smith.

What's your name?
¿Cómo se llama usted?

Do you speak English?
¿Habla usted inglés?

How old are you?
¿Cuántos años tiene?

II. **History of the present illness**

Do you have **pain**? Where is it?
¿Tiene **dolor**? ¿Dónde siente el dolor?

Did it begin today/yesterday/last week?
¿Empezó hoy/ayer/la semana pasada?

How many times have you had the pain?
¿Cuántas veces ha tenido el dolor?

What is the **pain** like? (Mild? strong? sharp?)
¿Cómo es el **dolor**? (¿Leve? ¿fuerte? ¿agudo?)

Does it come and go?
¿Se va y regresa el dolor?

Like **pressure**? Does it burn?
¿Como presión? ¿Le arde?

Have you had a **fever**? **headaches**?
¿Ha tenido **fiebre**? ¿dolor de cabeza?

. . . Rash? ulcers? itching?
. . . ¿Ronchas? ¿úlceras? ¿picazón?

. . . Cough? wheezing?
. . . ¿Tos? ¿ronquido en el pecho?

. . . Nausea? vomiting? diarrhea?
. . . ¿Nausea? ¿vómitos? ¿diarrea?

Does your vision get blurry?
¿Ve borroso a veces?

Are you short of breath?
¿Le falta el aire?

Does it **burn/hurt** when you urinate?
¿Le **arde/duele** al orinar?

III. **Past medical history**

Do you have any other medical problems?
¿Tiene algun otro problema médico?

. . . Diabetes? asthma? seizures?
. . . ¿Azúcar en la sangre? ¿asma? ¿convulsiones?

. . . Thyroid problems?
. . . ¿Problemas con la tiroides?

Have you had surgery?
¿La han operado alguna vez?

. . . for your appendix?
. . . ¿del apendice?

. . . hysterectomy?
. . . ¿histerectomia (de la matriz)?

. . . ectopic pregnancy?
. . . ¿embarazo ectopico/tubarico?

Do you take any medicine?
¿Toma alguna medicina o medicamento?

Are you using any birth control?
¿Usa algun método anticonceptivo?

. . . Oral contraceptives/pills? condoms?
. . . ¿Pastillas? ¿píldora? ¿condones?

Do you have allergies to drugs?
¿Es alérgica a alguna medicina?

Do you **smoke**?
¿**Fuma** usted?

How many **packs** a day?	¿Cuántas **cajetillas** fuma al día?
Do you drink?	¿Toma bebidas alcohólicas?
Do you use **drugs**?	¿Ha usado **drogas** alguna vez?
How many **pounds** have you gained/lost?	¿Cuántas **libras** ha ganado/perdido?

IV. **Obstetric history**

Have you ever been pregnant?	¿Ha estado embarazada alguna vez?
How many children have you had?	¿**Cuántos** niños ha tenido?
Have you had	¿Ha tenido
. . . any abortions/miscarriages?	. . . algun aborto provocado o espontaneo?
. . . problems with the **pregnancy**?	. . . algun problema durante el **embarazo**?
When is your due date?	¿Cual es la fecha esperada del parto?
Is the baby moving?	¿Se ha movido el bebé hoy?
Have you had contractions?	¿Ha tenido contracciones? dolores de parto?
How much time is there between pains?	¿Cuánto tiempo pasa entre cada dolor/ contracción?
Have you had vaginal **bleeding**?	¿Ha **sangrado** por la vagina?
Have you broken your water?	¿Se le rompió la bolsa de agua?
Push . . . Don't push.	Puje . . . No puje más.
Breathe slowly.	**Respire** lentamente.
We have to do a cesarean section.	Tenemos que hacer una cesarea.

V. **Gynecologic history**

At what age did you begin to menstruate?	¿A qué edad tuvo la primera regla?
How long do your **menses** last?	¿Cuántos días le duran sus **reglas**?
When was your last menstrual period?	¿Cuándo fué su última regla?
Are your periods regular?	¿Son sus reglas regulares?
Have you **bled** between periods?	¿Ha **sangrado** entre las reglas?
Do you have a vaginal **discharge**?	¿Tiene **flujo** vaginal?
. . . with bad odor?	. . . ¿fétido?
As usual or different?	¿Cómo siempre o diferente?
Have you had more than one sexual partner?	¿Ha tenido relaciones sexuales con varias personas?
When was the last time you had **sex**?	¿Cuándo fué la última vez que tuvo **relaciones sexuales**?
. . . two days/**weeks**/months ago?	. . . ¿Hace dos dias/**semanas**/meses?
Have you ever had a sexually transmitted disease?	¿Ha tenido alguna enfermedad venerea?
. . . Chlamydia? gonorrhea?	. . . ¿Clamidia? ¿gonorrea?
. . . Syphilis? AIDS? another?	. . . ¿Sifilis? ¿SIDA? ¿alguna otra?

VI. **Physical examination**

Take off your clothes, please.	Desvístase, por favor.
Put on this **gown**.	Póngase esta **bata**.

Put your feet in the **stirrups,** please.	Ponga los pies en los **estribos,** por favor.
Move toward me. **Relax.**	Muévase hacia mí. **Relájese.**
Separate your **legs,** please.	Separe las **piernas,** por favor.
I'm going to insert the **speculum.**	Voy a introducirle el **espéculo.**
I need to do a **pelvic exam.**	Necesito hacerle un **examen interno/ pélvico.**

VII. Numbers

1	uno	10	diez	30	treinta
2	dos	11	once	40	cuarenta
3	tres	12	doce	50	cincuenta
4	cuatro	13	trece	60	sesenta
5	cinco	14	catorce	70	setenta
6	seis	15	quince	80	ochenta
7	siete	16	dieciséis	90	noventa
8	ocho	20	veinte	100	cien(to)
9	nueve	21	veintiuno	1000	mil

Brandon J. Bankowski and Amy E. Hearne

AC	abdominal circumference
ABOG	American Board of Obstetrics and Gynecology
ACOG	American College of Obstetricians and Gynecologists
AFI	amniotic fluid index
AFP	alpha-fetoprotein
ANC	absolute neutrophil count
AROM	artificial rupture of membranes
BBT	basal body temperature
BMI	body mass index
BOA	birth out of asepsis, born on arrival
BPD	biparietal diameter
BPP	biophysical profile
BPS	bilateral partial salpingectomy
BSE	breast self-examination
BSO	bilateral salpingo-oophorectomy
BTL	bilateral tubal ligation
CEA	carcinoembryonic antigen
CMV	cytomegalovirus
CNM	certified nurse midwife
CP	cerebral palsy
CRL	crown-rump length
C/S	cesarean section
CST	contraction stress test
D & C	dilation and curettage
D & E	dilation and evacuation
DHEAS	dehydroepiandrosterone sulfate
DMPA	depomedroxyprogesterone acetate
DNR	do not resuscitate
DUB	dysfunctional uterine bleeding
E_1	estrone
E_2	estradiol
E_3	estriol
EBV	Epstein-Barr virus
ECC	endocervical curettage
EDC	estimated date of confinement
EDD	estimated date of delivery

EMBx	endometrial biopsy
ER/PR	estrogen receptor/progesterone receptor
Exlap	exploratory laparotomy
FDIU	fetal death in utero
FENa	fractional excretion of sodium
FL	femur length
FM	fetal movement
FSH	follicle-stimulating hormone
FTA	fluorescent treponemal antigen
FTSVD	full-term spontaneous vaginal delivery
5-FU	5-fluorouracil
GBS	group B *Streptococcus*
GC	*Gonococcus*
GCT	glucose challenge test
GDM	gestational diabetes mellitus
GIFT	gamete intrafallopian transfer
GnRH	gonadotropin-releasing hormone
GTT	glucose tolerance test
HBsAg	hepatitis B surface antigen
HC	head circumference
hCG	human chorionic gonadotropin
hPL	human placental lactogen
HPV	human papillomavirus
HSG	hysterosalpingogram
HSV	herpes simplex virus
I & D	incision and drainage
ICSI	intracytoplasmic sperm injection
IUD	intrauterine device
IUFD	intrauterine fetal demise
IUGR	intrauterine growth retardation
IUP	intrauterine pregnancy
IVF	in vitro fertilization
LAVH	laparoscopically assisted vaginal hysterectomy
LBW	low birth weight
LDR	labor, delivery, recovery (room)
LFAVD	low forceps–assisted vaginal delivery
LGA	large for gestational age
LH	luteinizing hormone
LMP	last menstrual period
L-S ratio	lecithin-sphingomyelin ratio
MFM	maternal fetal medicine
$MgSO_4$	magnesium sulfate
MMT	mixed müllerian tumor
MSAFP	maternal serum alpha-fetoprotein

MSO$_4$	morphine sulfate
MTX	methotrexate sodium
NEFG	normal external female genitalia
NOS	night of surgery
NST	nonstress test
OCP	oral contraceptive pills
Para	parity
PID	pelvic inflammatory disease
PIH	pregnancy-induced hypertension
POD	postoperative day
pp	postpartum
PPD	purified protein derivative
PRL	prolactin
PROM	premature rupture of membranes
PRN	as needed
RDS	respiratory distress syndrome
ROM	rupture of membrane
RPR	reactive plasma reagin
RU-486	mifepristone
SAB	spontaneous abortion
SBE	subacute bacterial endocarditis
SBO	small bowel obstruction
SGA	small for gestational age
SROM	spontaneous rupture of membranes
STD	sexually transmitted disease
STS	serum test for syphilis
TAB	therapeutic abortion
TAH	total abdominal hysterectomy
TOA	tubo-ovarian abscess
TPN	total parenteral nutrition
TVH	total vaginal hysterectomy
TZ	transformation zone
U/S, US	ultrasonography
VAIN	vaginal intraepithelial neoplasia
VDRL	Venereal Disease Research Laboratory
VIN	vulvar intraepithelial neoplasia
Vtx	vertex

Appendix D. SELECTED WEB SITES

Brandon J. Bankowski and David Nagey

I. **General obstetrics and gynecology**
   www.obgyn.net—The Obstetrics and Gynecology Network
   www.acog.org—American College of Obstetricians and Gynecologists, district and section sites
   www.arhp.org—Association of Reproductive Health Professionals
   www.plannedparenthood.org—Planned Parenthood Federation of America
   www.EndometriosisAssn.org—Endometriosis Association
II. **Obstetrics**
   www.smfm.org—Society for Maternal Fetal Medicine
   www.thefetus.net—Prenatal Diagnosis
   www.thelaboroflove.com—The Labor of Love—Resource for new parents
   www.parentsplace.com—iVillage/Parents Place—Resource for new parents
   www.aap.org—American Academy of Pediatrics
III. **Reproductive endocrinology and infertility**
   www.asrm.com—American Society for Reproductive Medicine
   www.menopause.org—The North American Menopause Society
   www.resolve.org—Resolve: The National Infertility Association
IV. **Oncology**
   www.sgo.org—Society for Gynecologic Oncologists
   www.medem.com—ACOG medical library
   www.cancer.gov—Thorough guide from National Cancer Institute
   www.sharecancersupport.org—Self-help for women with breast or ovarian cancer
   www.oncolink.com—Free oncology site from the University of Pennsylvania Cancer Center
V. **Research**
   www.geneclinics.org—NIH site on genetic disorders
   www.harrisonsonline.com—Harrison's updated medical text
   www.hivatis.org—HIV/AIDS treatment information
   www.cdc.gov—Centers for Disease Control and Prevention
   www.ncbi.nlm.nih.gov—PubMed (MEDLINE), genetic database (OMIM)
   www.cochrane.org—Free abstracts of clinical trial results
VI. **Johns Hopkins**
   www.hopkins-abxguide.org—Johns Hopkins infectious disease antibiotics guide
   www.hopkinsmedicine.org—Johns Hopkins medical institutions
   www.welch.jhu.edu—Welch Medical Library at Johns Hopkins

INDEX

Page numbers followed by the letter *f* refer to figures; page numbers followed by the letter *t* refer to tables.